Tackling Health Inequities through Public Health Practice

Tackling Health Inequities through Public Health Practice

Theory to Action

SECOND EDITION

A Project of the National Association of County and City Health Officials

Edited by

Richard Hofrichter and Rajiv Bhatia

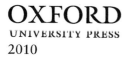

OXFORD
UNIVERSITY PRESS
2010

OXFORD
UNIVERSITY PRESS

Oxford University Press, Inc., publishes works that further
Oxford University's objective of excellence
in research, scholarship, and education.

Oxford New York
Auckland Cape Town Dar es Salaam Hong Kong Karachi
Kuala Lumpur Madrid Melbourne Mexico City Nairobi
New Delhi Shanghai Taipei Toronto

With offices in
Argentina Austria Brazil Chile Czech Republic France Greece
Guatemala Hungary Italy Japan Poland Portugal Singapore
South Korea Switzerland Thailand Turkey Ukraine Vietnam

Published by Oxford University Press, Inc.
198 Madison Avenue, New York, New York 10016
www.oup.com

Oxford is a registered trademark of Oxford University Press

Library of Congress Cataloging-in-Publication Data
Tackling health inequities through public health practice : theory to action : a project of the
National Association of County and City Health Officials / edited by Richard Hofrichter and
Rajiv Bhatia.—2nd ed.
p. cm
Includes bibliographical references.
ISBN 978-0-19-534314-4
1. Health services accessibility—United States.   2. Social medicine—United States.
3. Public health—United States.   I. Hofrichter, Richard.   II. Bhatia, Rajiv.
III. National Association of County & City Health Officials (U.S.)
[DNLM: 1. Healthcare Disparities—United States.   2. Health Services Needs and
Demand—United States.   3. Minority Health—United States.   4. Public Health
Practice—United States.   5. Social Justice—United States. W 84 AA1 T118 2010]
RA418.3.U6T33 2010
362.1—dc22
2009049204

9 8 7 6 5 4 3 2

Printed in United States of America
on acid-free paper

Preface

Health practitioners, particularly in local health departments (LHDs), face many dilemmas in seeking to protect public health. As the front line of the public health in local communities, they must cope with immediate crises as well as chronic issues, limited resources, restrictive statutory mandates, categorical funding, and political pressures. Even more daunting, persistent and severe inequities in health outcomes compromise the health of the nation. Most recently, Hurricane Katrina and the crises in the nation's financial markets have made these inequities and their underlying causes (embedded in racism, class exploitation, and sexism) salient to a wide population.

Addressing the social injustice underlying the distribution of disease and illness should not be viewed as a task outside the role of a public health institution. The day-to-day consequences of health inequities are a direct threat to the health of all as well as to broader social and economic well-being. The public health community must acknowledge and challenge these inequities directly and forcefully. Taking leadership to meet this challenge means being vocal about the problems, causes, and solutions, forging strategic alliances with sister institutions and community-based organizations, organizing public support, and creating supportive work environments for these tasks within public health institutions.

Social justice has always been one of the major values driving public health. Today, much of the etiology of avoidable disease is rooted in inequitable social conditions brought on by disparities in wealth and power and reproduced through ongoing forms of oppression. Social justice has been a motivating force in drawing many people to the field. Elizabeth Fee notes in her introduction to George Rosen's *A History of Public Health*, "When the history of public health is seen as a history of how populations experience health and illness, how social, economic, and political systems structure the possibilities for healthy or unhealthy lives, how societies create the preconditions for the production and transmission of disease, and how people, both as individuals and social groups, attempt to promote their own health or avoid illness, we find that public health history is not limited to the study of bureaucratic structures and institutions but pervades every aspect of social and cultural life." Progress toward the elimination of health inequities will therefore require an expanded and expansive view of the scope of public health practice.

Tackling Health Inequities raises questions and provides a starting point for health practitioners ready to reorient public health practice to address the root causes of health inequities. This reorientation involves restructuring the organization, culture, and daily work of public health. *Tackling Health Inequities* is meant to inspire readers to imagine or envision public health practice and their role in ways that question contemporary thinking and assumptions, as emerging trends, social conditions, and policies generate increasing inequities in health. No predefined set of protocols or tools can eliminate health inequity. It will require reimagining practice, taking risks, and active and strategic engagement of the public health community in the political process. Recent experience in many jurisdictions suggests that many health practitioners are ready and able to act.

This second edition of the book has benefited from recent initiatives and experience of both editors. Many chapters remaining from the previous edition have been updated and expanded, including those by Doak Bloss, Anthony B. Iton, Adewale Troutman, Baker Salsbury et al., and Makani Themba-Nixon. The book has been completely reorganized into four parts. In Part I, "Frameworks, Perspectives, Evidence," new chapters have been added by Sen, Peter, and Kubzansky et al., while Hofrichter's original introductory chapter has been expanded and updated to include the chapter on transforming practice. Part II is completely new with chapters by Kubisch et al. and Wallace et al. on racism; Muntaner et al. and Coburn on class; and Sen and Ostlin on gender inequity. Part III on practice includes new chapters by Thomas and Prentice, Bhatia, Oleru et al., Corburn, and Christopher et al. Finally Part IV, "Shifting Consciousness and Paradigms" includes new chapters by Adelman, Iton, and Muntaner and Chung.

Acknowledgments

Many people provided ideas, insight, and support in the production and review of this book, including both substantive and editorial suggestions. First and foremost, we would like to thank our colleagues at the National Association of County & City Health Officials (NACCHO) and members of the staff Health Equity and Social Justice Team. Members of NACCHO's advisory group and The Health Equity and Social Justice Strategic Direction Team offered significant guidance. This volume builds on the experience of many local health officials across the country committed to health equity in their everyday work.

In addition, we wish to express our gratitude to the W.K. Kellogg Foundation for their continuing support of our work, including the first edition of this publication. Special thanks to Barbara Sabol for her insights and efforts on our behalf, as well as Gail Christopher.

We would also like to thank Ruth Etzel and Bob Prentice for their comments and insights on various parts of the book.

Special thanks to Regan Hofmann and Bill Lamsback at Oxford University Press for their advice and diligence in helping to ensure the publication of this work.

Finally, the editors acknowledge the contemporary and historic social justice struggles of diverse individuals, civil society organizations, and progressive social movements around the world. Their efforts and accomplishments are the inspiration and ultimately the vehicle for a movement for health equity.

Richard Hofrichter and Rajiv Bhatia
Editors

Contents

Contributors xiii

Part I Introduction: Frameworks, Perspectives, Evidence

1 Tackling Health Inequities: A Framework for
  Public Health Practice   3
  Richard Hofrichter

2 Why Health Equity?   57
  Amartya Sen

3 Health Equity and Social Justice   71
  Fabienne Peter

4 United States: Social Inequality and the Burden of Poor Health   86
  *Laura D. Kubzansky, Nancy Krieger, Ichiro Kawachi, Beverly Rockhill,
  Gillian K. Steel, and Lisa F. Berkman*

5 A Framework for Measuring Health Inequity   112
  Yukiko Asada

6 Promoting Social Justice through Public Health Policies, Programs,
  and Services   126
  Alonzo Plough

Part II Racism, Class Exploitation, Sexism, and Health: Exposing the Roots

7 Structural Racism and Community Building   *143*
   Keith Lawrence, Stacey Sutton, Anne Kubisch,
   Gretchen Susi, and Karen Fulbright-Anderson

8 Coronary Heart Disease, Chronic Inflammation, and Pathogenic
   Social Hierarchy: A Biological Limit to Possible Reductions in
   Morbidity and Mortality   *162*
   Rodrick Wallace, Deborah Wallace, and Robert G. Wallace

9 Social Sources of Racial Disparities in Health   *166*
   David R. Williams and Pamela Braboy Jackson

10 Class Exploitation and Psychiatric Disorders   *179*
   Carles Muntaner, Carme Borrell, Haejoo Chung, and Joan Benach

11 Beyond the Income Inequality Hypothesis: Class,
   Neo-Liberalism, and Health Inequalities   *196*
   David Coburn

12 Gender Inequity in Health: Why It Exists
   and How We Can Change It   *225*
   Gita Sen and Piroska Ostlin

Part III Practitioners Take Action: Strategies for Organizational Change and Working with Communities

13 Initiating Social Justice Action through Dialogue in a
   Local Health Department: The Ingham County Experience   *241*
   Doak Bloss

14 The Metro Louisville Center for Health Equity:
   Expanding the Circle of Engagement   *272*
   Adewale Troutman

15 Exploring the Intersection of Public Health and Social Justice:
   The Bay Area Regional Health Inequities Initiative   *283*
   Bob Prentice and Njoke Thomas

16 Using Our Voice: Forging a Public Health Practice
   for Social Justice   *296*
   Rajiv Bhatia, June Weintraub, Lili Farhang, Karen Yu, and Paula Jones

17 Estimation of Health Benefits from a Local Living
   Wage Ordinance   *324*
   Rajiv Bhatia and Mitchell Katz

18 Protecting Health with Environmental Impact Assessment:
A Case Study of San Francisco Land Use Decision Making *336*
Rajiv Bhatia

19 The Community Action Model in a Public Health Department
Setting Case Study: Tobacco Divestment on College Campuses *356*
Mele Lau Smith, Alma Avila-Esparza, Alyonik Hrushow,
Susana Hennessey Lavery, Diane Reed, and Melinda Moore

20 Tackling the Root Causes of Health Disparities through
Community Capacity Building *370*
Anthony B. Iton, Sandra Witt, Alexandra Desautels, Katherine Schaff,
Mia Luluquisen, Liz Maker, Kathryn Horsley, and Matt Beyers

21 Institutionalizing Health Equity and Social Justice in
King County, Washington *404*
Ngozi Oleru, Michael Gedeon, and Matías Valenzuela

22 Street Science: Local Knowledge and Environmental Justice *417*
Jason Corburn

23 Measuring Social Determinants of Health Inequities:
The CADH Health Equity Index *442*
Baker Salsbury, Elaine O'Keefe, and Jennifer Kertanis

24 *Place Matters*: Building Partnerships among Communities
and Local Public Health Departments *458*
Gail C. Christopher, Vincent Lafronza, and Natalie Burke

Part IV Shifting Consciousness and Paradigms

25 *Unnatural Causes*: Using Media to Build a Constituency
for Health Equity *477*
Larry Adelman

26 Talking about Public Health: Developing America's "Second
Language" *495*
Lawrence Wallack and Regina G. Lawrence

27 Helping Public Health Matter: Strategies for Building Public
Awareness *504*
Makani Themba-Nixon

28 The Ethics of the Medical Model in Addressing the Root
Causes of Health Disparities in Local Public Health Practice *509*
Anthony B. Iton

29 Teaching Social Inequalities in Health: Barriers
and Opportunities *517*
Carles Muntaner and Haejoo Chung

Appendices

A. *Selected References*   527
B. *Guidelines for Achieving Health Equity in Public Health Practice*   549
C. *How Social Justice Becomes Embodied in Differential Disease and
   Mortality Rates*   555
D. *Eliminating Health Inequity: The Role of Local Public Health
   and Community Organizing*   557
E. *People's Charter for Health*   559

Index   569

Contributors

Larry Adelman is Executive Producer, California Newsreel, San Francisco, CA.

Yukiko Asada is Assistant Professor, Department of Community Health and Epidemiology, Dalhousie University, Nova Scotia.

Alma Avila-Esparza is Director, Community Health Worker Program, Health Education and Community Health Studies Department, City College of San Francisco, CA.

Joan Benach is Associate Professor, Social Inequalities in Health Research Unit, (GREDS) and EMCONET, Universitat Pompeu Fabra, Barcelona, Spain.

Lisa F. Berkman is Director, Center for Population and Development Studies Thomas D. Cabot Professor of Public Policy and of Epidemiology, Department of Society, Human Development, and Health, Harvard University, Cambridge, MA.

Matt Beyers is Epidemiologist for the Alameda County Health Department, Oakland, CA.

Rajiv Bhatia is the Director of Occupational and Environmental Health, San Francisco Department of Public Health, and an Assistant Clinical Professor of Medicine at the University of California at San Francisco.

Doak Bloss is Health Equity and Social Justice Coordinator, Ingham County Health Department, Lansing, MI.

Carme Borrell is Head of Surveillance, Barcelona Public Health Agency, Barcelona, Spain.

Pamela Braboy Jackson is Professor of sociology at Indiana University in Bloomington, IN.

Natalie Burke is Principal of CommonHealth ACTION, a nonprofit organization in Washington, DC, dedicated to helping people and organizations maximize their potential to improve the health of communities, families, and individuals.

Gail C. Christopher is Vice President for Programs, W. K. Kellogg Foundation, Battle Creek, MI.

Haejoo Chung is CIHR Health Policy Research Fellow, Department of Political Science, University of Toronto, Canada.

David Coburn is Professor Emeritus, Department of Public Health Sciences, Faculty of Medicine, University of Toronto, Canada.

Jason Corburn is Associate Professor, Department of Regional Planning, University of California, Berkeley, CA.

Alexandra Desautels is Policy Analyst for the Alameda County Public Health Department, Oakland, CA.

Lili Farhang is Senior Epidemiologist for the Program on Health Equity and Sustainability at the San Francisco Department of Public Health, San Francisco, CA.

Karen Fulbright-Anderson is Senior Fellow, Roundtable on Community Change, The Aspen Institute, New York.

Michael Gedeon is Senior Policy Analyst, King County Office of Strategic Planning and Performance Management, Seattle, WA.

Susana Hennessey Lavery is Health Educator, Tobacco Free Project, San Francisco Department of Public Health, San Francisco, CA.

Richard Hofrichter is Senior Analyst, Health Equity, National Association of County & City Health Officials, Washington, DC.

Kathryn Horsley is Epidemiologist, Epidemiology Planning and Evaluation Unit, Public Health—Seattle & King County, Seattle, WA.

Alyonik Hrushow is Director, Tobacco Free Project, San Francisco Department of Public Health, San Francisco, CA.

Anthony B. Iton is Senior Vice President for Healthy Communities, The California Endowment, Oakland, CA.

Paula Jones is the Director of Food Systems at the San Francisco Department of Public Health, San Francisco, CA.

Mitchell Katz is Director of the San Francisco Department of Public Health, San Francisco, CA.

Ichiro Kawachi is Chair, Department of Society, Human Development, and Health, and Professor of Social Epidemiology and Department of Society, Human Development, and Health, Harvard University, Cambridge, MA.

Jennifer Kertanis is Executive Director, Connecticut Association of Directors of Health, Hartford, CT.

Nancy Krieger is Professor of Society, Human Development, and Health, Department of Society, Human Development, and Health, Harvard University, Cambridge, MA.

Anne Kubisch is Director of the Aspen Roundtable on Community Change, The Aspen Institute, New York.

Laura D. Kubzansky is Assistant Professor, Department of Health and Social Behavior, Harvard School of Public Health, Cambridge, MA.

Vincent Lafronza is Principal of CommonHealth ACTION, a nonprofit organization in Washington, DC, dedicated to helping people and organizations maximize their potential to improve the health of communities, families, and individuals.

Mele Lau Smith is Health Program Coordinator, Tobacco Free Project, San Francisco Department of Public Health, San Francisco, CA.

Keith Lawrence is Research Associate at the Aspen Institute, Roundtable on Community Change, The Aspen Institute, New York.

Regina G. Lawrence is Chair and Professor of Mass Communication/Political Science, Louisiana State University, Baton Rouge, LA.

Mia Luluquisen is Deputy Director of the Community Assessment, Planning, Education, and Evaluation Unit, Alameda County Health Department, Oakland, CA.

Liz Maker is Evaluation Specialist for the Alameda County Health Department, Oakland, CA.

Melinda Moore is Project Evaluator, M. K. Associates, Marin, CA.

Carles Muntaner is Psychiatric and Addictions Nursing Research Chair, Social Equity and Health, Center for Addictions and Mental Health, and Full Professor, Bloomberg School of Nursing, Dalla Lana School of Public Health & School of Medicine University of Toronto, Canada.

Elaine O'Keefe is Executive Director, Office of Community Health, Yale School of Public Health, and Executive Director of the Yale Center for Interdisciplinary Research on AIDS, Yale University, New Haven, CT.

Ngozi Oleru is Environmental Health Director, Seattle-King County Department of Public Health, Seattle, WA.

Piroska Ostlin is Senior Researcher at the Karolinska Institute in Stockholm, Sweden and a Research Associate at the Harvard Center for Population and Development, Cambridge, MA.

Fabienne Peter is Professor of Philosophy, University of Warwick, Coventry, United Kingdom.

Alonzo Plough is Director of Emergency Preparedness, Los Angeles County Department of Public Health Los Angeles, CA.

Bob Prentice is Director of the Bay Area Regional Health Inequities Initiative (BARHII), Oakland, CA.

Diane Reed is Project Evaluator, Richmond, CA.

Beverly Rockhill is Associate Professor of Public Health Education at University of North Carolina, Greensboro, NC.

Baker Salsbury is Director, Lightbridge Health Department, Groton, CT.

Katherine Schaff is Health Equity Specialist for the Alameda County Health Department, Oakland, CA.

Amartya Sen is Thomas W. Lamont University Professor and Professor of Economics and Philosophy at Harvard University. He is also a Fellow of Trinity College, Cambridge University.

Gita Sen is Professor at the Indian Institute of Management in Bangalore, India, and has been a visiting professor at the Center for Population and Development Studies, Harvard University and a Fellow of the Centre for Development Studies in Trivandrum, India.

Gillian K. Steel is Research Scientist, Department of Health Policy and Management, Harvard University, Cambridge, MA.

Gretchen Susi is Research Associate, Roundtable on Community Change, The Aspen Institute, New York.

Stacey Sutton is Assistant Professor of Urban Planning, Graduate School of Architecture, Planning and Preservation, Columbia University, New York.

Makani Themba-Nixon is Director, The Praxis Project, Washington, DC.

Njoke Thomas is Project Director for the Equality in Health Initiative at the Partnership for Families and Children in Denver, CO.

Adewale Troutman is Director of the Louisville Health Department, Louisville, KY.

Matías Valenzuela is Public Education Coordinator, Public Health—Seattle & King County, WA.

Deborah Wallace is Associate Research Scientist, Department of Sociomedical Sciences Joseph Mailman School of Public Health, Columbia University, New York.

Robert G. Wallace is Post Doctoral Researcher, Department of Ecology and Evolutionary Biology, University of California, Irvine.

Rodrick Wallace is Research Scientist, New York State Psychiatric Institute, New York.

Lawrence Wallack is Dean, College of Urban and Public Affairs, Portland State University, Portland, Oregon, and Emeritus Professor of Public Health at the University of California, Berkeley, CA.

June Weintraub is Supervising Epidemiologist for the Program on Health Equity and Sustainability at the San Francisco Department of Public Health, San Francisco, CA.

David R. Williams is Professor of Sociology, Professor of Epidemiology, and Senior Research Scientist at Harvard University, Cambridge, MA.

Sandra Witt is Deputy Director for Planning, Policy and Health Equity, Alameda County Health Department, Oakland, CA.

Karen Yu is Senior Environmental Health Inspector at the San Francisco Department of Public Health, San Francisco, CA.

PART I

Introduction: Frameworks, Perspectives, Evidence

1

Tackling Health Inequities: A Framework for Public Health Practice

RICHARD HOFRICHTER

Public health practitioners confront growing and unacceptable inequities in the distribution of chronic diseases, illness, and longevity.[1] These health inequities are systematic differences in health status "which are unnecessary and *avoidable*, but in addition are considered *unfair* and *unjust*."[2] They are sustained over time and generations beyond the control of individuals.

Health inequities, we argue in this book, result from an unequal structuring of life chances, based on growing social and economic inequality. That inequality derives from structural features regarding how we organize our social, economic, and political institutions. It is not simply about biased attitudes and discrimination or the distribution of income; rather, it concerns the exercise of political power. Why is that important? Social and economic inequalities injure health, absolutely and relatively, based on long-term reproduced forms of exploitation and social exclusion. In order to take effective action, it is necessary to grasp what drives health inequities. Identifying a way forward toward reforming practice requires theory on a number of levels: sources of conditions in which people live, how social inequalities become embedded in our biology, and theory about social change.

Since the mid-1970s social and economic inequality has increased dramatically in the United States.[3] Globally, gaps in income and wealth between rich and poor within the industrialized countries is widening.[4] Nations with the greatest inequality often show signs of social disintegration, deregulation of labor and financial markets, and weaker social safety nets.[5] Perhaps most strikingly, income inequality in the United States is greater than in any other industrialized country in the world, particularly for African Americans.[6] Furthermore, according to the U.S. Bureau of the Census, almost 18% of all children under the age of 18 in the United States live in poverty.[7] Inequalities in wealth are even wider than those in income and are steadily increasing.[8] Socially, the United States has poor rankings on indicators such as homicide rate, number of prisoners as proportion of the population, mental illness, voting turnout, and public social expenditure.[9]

The presence and growth of social and economic inequalities parallels that for health inequity. Life expectancy and morbidity rates for people with low income are significantly worsening.[10] Jurisdictions with the greatest social and economic inequality typically have the worst life expectancy and mortality rates.[11] The more egalitarian countries experience the best health status, not the richest.[12] Thus, the highly unequal United States ranks 30th in life expectancy for men, 21st for women, and 28th in infant mortality.[13]

What is the significance and implications of these economic and social inequities for public health practice and for social policy? They suggest that public health practitioners must transform the way they approach their work. While a difficult undertaking, nevertheless, public health practitioners in collaboration with others are also in a unique and powerful position to respond. We also suggest, given the evidence, that public health has a moral obligation and duty to act. In the early days of public health, the link between such knowledge and the necessity of social reform was second nature, but today it is not part of most training of the public health workforce. *Tackling Health Inequities through Public Health Practice: Theory to Action* offers guidance that will hopefully spur critical thinking on the relation between theory and practice. A central challenge is to identify feasible alternative methods of organizing public health practice, organization, and culture to eliminate these inequities with the urgency it deserves.

Purpose and Assumptions

Many practitioners, particularly in local public health departments, increasingly recognize the need to address health inequities through action on root causes generated by deep social divisions and oppression. Yet they remain stymied by bureaucratic structures, statutory requirements, limited funding, and constraints on surpassing the seemingly traditional disciplinary boundaries. Many lack confidence in the capacity of public health institutions to challenge the powers and interests responsible for the maintenance and reproduction of inequities.

Tackling Health Inequities in Public Health Practice: Theory to Action suggests approaches for acting effectively on the sources of health inequities, even if in small ways, at the level of practice, in partnership with other institutions that influence health. It offers a framework, based on principles of social justice, and examples for those in the public health system to strengthen their capacity for influencing the root causes through a social justice perspective.

Social justice is a concept, with roots that date at least from the earliest days of the industrial revolution, concerned both with meeting human need and with fundamental aspects of equality—social and economic as well as political, the latter referring to democracy (see section on Developing a Framework, for a more detailed examination of social justice). Such a perspective "explicitly analyzes who benefits from—and who is harmed by—economic exploitation, oppression, discrimination, inequality, and degradation of natural resources."[14]

The purpose of *Tackling Health Inequities in Public Health Practice* is threefold:

1. To provide a conceptual framework, raise questions, and spur thought for exploring the nature and causes of health inequity and what to do about it
2. To explore the social processes that generate and repeatedly reproduce health inequities
3. To offer a knowledge base, resources, case studies, and suggestions for transforming everyday public health practice, bureaucratic structure, and organizational culture in ways that may advance the realization of health equity

Tackling Health Inequities in Public Health Practice presents a rationale for incorporating the elimination of health inequities into public health practice within a social justice framework, as part of public health's core mission. It emphasizes the way practitioners can and do organize the content and structure of their work and relations with their communities, rather than primarily programs and services or remedial interventions. However, no simple correspondence exists between the core social injustices and the forms of practice that will succeed in eliminating the resulting inequity in the distribution of disease. Many routes may get there and they may vary among jurisdictions. A central concern is to identify the essence of public health practice for health equity distinctive from traditional practice.

The seven basic assumptions that guide the work are as follows:

1) Health is more than an end in itself; it is also an asset or resource required for human development and well-functioning communities.
2) Equity in health status benefits everyone because health is a public good necessary to a well-functioning society.
3) Health is a socially and politically defined construct; individual and medical definitions ignore relationships between individual health and healthful social and environmental conditions.
4) Inequities in population health outcomes are primarily the result of social and political injustice, not lifestyles, behavior, or genes.
5) Health is a collective public good, actively produced by institutions and social policies.
6) An accumulation of negative social conditions and lack of fundamental resources contribute to health inequities, and include economic and social insecurity, racial and gender inequality, lack of participation and influence in society, unfavorable conditions during childhood, absence of quality and affordable housing, unhealthy conditions in the workplace and lack of control over the work process, toxic environments, and inequitable distribution of resources from public spending.
7) Tackling health inequities effectively will require an emphasis on root causes and social injustice, the latter concerning inequality and hierarchical divisions within the population.

Consequences of Health Inequity for Society and Action for the Health Professions

For society
- Limits people's ability to have access to the resources and experiences that would provide them good health and well-being, that would enable them to achieve their potential, use their full capabilities—in getting well-paid, productive employment, in being able to participate fully in the social and political life of the community
- Creates psychological stresses that weaken the immune system
- Limits democracy by limiting access to decision-making processes that affect health
- Reduces the quality of life for everyone
- Lowers life expectancy in the jurisdiction in question as the income gap widens

Action for health practitioners

- Recognize that treating the consequences through programs and services will never eliminate health inequity
- Mandate a reexamination of public health priorities, practices, and use of resources
- Communicate facts about the forces that produce or undermine health to their constituencies, responsible public institutions, and political leaders
- Develop a policy agenda for health equity and identify strategic activities with constituencies that supports this agenda
- Engage with communities to develop their capacity and resources to participate fully in social and political processes

Reclaiming History: Equity and Pubic Health

The modern institution of public health resulted from a planned response to the ill effects of an expanding industrial capital and associated urbanization.[15] Historically, major advances in health status occurred from major social reforms such as the abolition of child labor, the introduction of housing and factory codes, the eight-hour work day, reductions in poverty, improvements in living standards, and a guaranteed minimum wage, as well as improvements in sanitation, adequate housing, and a safe food supply. Many of these gains were based on coordinated public health actions in conjunction with social movements.[16] Improvements in living and working conditions led to reductions in death from major infectious diseases, as well as medicine and immunizations.[17] Later, legislative developments such as the Social Security Act, Clean Air Act, and the establishment of the *Occupational Safety and Health Administration* (OSHA), were major steps that improved health for millions of people. Dan Beauchamp reminds us, "Public health stands for collective control over conditions affecting the common health."[18]

The history of public health has also always been closely associated with themes of social justice and social movements designed to achieve social equality and democracy, as well as self-determination and liberation from oppression.[19] Even independent of a social justice perspective, the social origins of disease connected with political and economic systems have long been known.[20] The idea of a basic public responsibility for social health and welfare and the responsibility of those in public health to be advocates for social justice and collective action is integral to public health.[21] Public health practitioners have historically been advocates for social change. They have understood that health is not an individual privilege but a social good belonging to everyone as a *social right*. Demands for better working conditions and good wages, racial and sexual equality, affordable housing, social services, improved sanitation, an end to segregation, and quality education are some examples of the backbone of social movements for change.[22]

However, today the delegitimizing of public action to protect the public interest (deregulation of financial services, decline in health and safety standards for workers, upward redistribution of wealth through the tax system, etc.) has led to de-emphasis on the broad aspects of social and economic life on the deeply rooted social and political determinants of health inequities. Political leaders do not ask public health officials to attend to health inequity nor are either held accountable for it. The direction of public health for decades has been toward a more managerial and technical role within a model to promote individual and population health, which rarely focuses on social injustice and the forces that structure the possibilities for health. Health practitioners work under categorically funded programs within specialized subdisciplines. They are often not held accountable for health inequity. While bureaucratic technical and managerial approaches have been useful in many fields of work, including public health, in providing necessary expertise and advances in knowledge, they also limit the ability to address changes and trends in society that affect health, similar to the way specialists in medical practice sometimes fail to see the whole patient. As Nancy Krieger notes, citing numerous senior epidemiologists, "...modern epidemiology often seems more concerned with intricately modeling complex relationships among risk factors than with understanding their origins and implications for public health."[23] In short, health inequities involve phenomena not easily amenable to scientific measurement and bureaucratic management. But this does not mean that public health has only a minimal role to play or that its practice cannot change to meet new or intensified threats. Global climate change is a relatively new threat. Yet health practitioners know that they must respond and that their response will require new kinds of practice grounded in analyses of social organization and political power. Still, unlike the case for health inequity, political commitment to address climate change has given public health practice the legitimacy to act.

In order for public health to reclaim its historical mission, realize its mandate to protect and improve public health, prevent a decline in health status, and remain accountable, it may be useful to explore methods for reducing the widening and persistent social and economic inequities that affect the entire society. Identifying where exposures come from and why some population groups are more likely to be exposed than others is a central task, which can inevitably lead to acting on the material conditions that create inequities in the distribution of disease and illness. This will likely require rethinking basic tenets in the contemporary theory and practice of public health, some of which has already begun.[24]

Class, Racism, Sexism, and Health: The Research

While life expectancies may have increased dramatically over the past century, so have inequities in health status. What are the origins of health inequity? What social processes generate it? Inequities do not occur randomly. They are not primarily the result of accidents of nature or individual pathology, but result from socially patterned, long-standing historical conditions generated by social and economic inequality.[25] Communities, for example, which suffer significant economic disinvestments, with longer firefighting response times, poor quality of housing, decreased access to nutritious foods, and other multiple stressors, will be more likely to have populations with higher blood pressure and other chronic illnesses. Regardless of specific diseases, those with socioeconomic disadvantage are more susceptible to early death and preventable disease. Since the time of Rudolf Virchow, a public health pathologist, and sanitary reformer Edwin Chadwick in the nineteenth century, health practitioners have known about the importance of the relationship between social class and mortality and morbidity.[26]

A significant body of research, especially since 1990, clearly documents that socioeconomic inequality, including institutional racism and sexism, poor quality of life, and low socioeconomic status are principal causes of morbidity and mortality.[27] Negative socioeconomic and cultural conditions create multiple chronic stressors, from the physical environment to housing, transportation, education, tax policy, and working conditions, which produce inequitable health outcomes. In addition, those that live in poor neighborhoods are likely to experience more health problems, regardless of their own socioeconomic status.[28] As Beaglehole notes, "...a population's health reflects more than the simple summation of the risk-factor profile and health status of its individual members."[29] Moreover, inadequate medical care accounts for only 10 to 15% of premature deaths.[30]

The particular pathways to illness by which health inequities link to exposures are not easy to establish, based on traditional methods in public health science. Yet they remain influenced by the way in which production and investment decisions, labor market policies, activities within financial markets, neighborhood conditions, sexism and racism connect with individual histories to produce health disadvantages.[31] Admittedly, it is difficult to evaluate precisely and scientifically how given social contexts interact with multidimensional biological and psychological exposure pathways to make people susceptible to disease. Systematic disadvantages are cumulative, persistent, intergenerational, and associated with lower capacity for full participation in society.

While class, race, and gender relations interact and overlap, it is useful to separate the threads for purposes of explanation. Debate exists within the research community on how these relations precisely affect population health and also on the conceptualization of the issue more generally. However, class, racism, and gender exploitation remain the fundamental, originating injustices through which power imbalances take hold and influence living conditions. These oppressions vary over time and place, and lack uniform expression. But they remain central to understanding health inequity.

How are inequalities produced and maintained? The sources of inequities in health outcomes remain deeply embedded in the structure of major economic and social institutions. Social determinants of health inequity themselves are not causes of social injustice and inequity. They reflect deeper social divisions that generate multiple social risks, reproduced over time. Public health practitioners need to choose among competing conceptual foundations to explain the dynamics of the social structure that link most determinants of inequities in health to social injustice. Hierarchies of power considered through a perspective of class exploitation, racism, and sexism provides a central base for explaining the seemingly abstract connections between social and economic determinants (poverty, housing, access to transportation), their distribution, and the basis of inequality more adequately. Society's class structure and inequality of property and wealth clearly intertwine with gender and racial hierarchies. However, racism and sexism take root in various forms of material exploitation. Therefore, it may be inappropriate to isolate the social determinants of inequities in health as a list of subjects for "interventions." But if we are to make interventions in the midst of planning broader social changes, it is still necessary to do that within a larger narrative that would link those interventions.

Often practitioners express disinterest in theory; they want to know what to do. But no practice exists without some theory. More than technique, effective practice requires recognition of the social context in which it functions; it must be related to a vision and a way of thinking. Because health is socially produced, related to economic and political forces, conceptual and theoretical issues demand attention. Given recent economic and political conditions, for example, the mortgage crisis, credit crisis, lower living standards, expansion of chronic disease and return of older diseases, global climate change, questions arise about the responsibilities of local public health to engage with such developments. Should public health practice ameliorate the symptoms of such conditions or should public health play a more active role in social change? Recommendations for policy or action plans to tackle the source of health inequity will depend on a clear grasp of what they are and how they function.

Class

Class is about ongoing, historical social divisions over production and distribution and the organization of society. It is important because it creates a persistent, continuous clustering of mortality advantage throughout life for many people and cannot be reduced to proximal individual level causes.[32] In the United States, unlike other parts of the world, analysts often avoid class analysis or relegate inequities to the inevitable result of impersonal and inevitable market forces. Or they define it in relation to either static descriptions of education, occupation, and income levels or in psychological, subjective terms associated with identity regarding social stratification and status.[33] Yet class has a deeper, more objective meaning, connected to property relations and exploitive labor relations.[34] Classes (intimately linked to race and gender relations) involve dynamic relations ordered by ongoing struggle about a way of life in a hierarchy. They represent the organized collective power of a well-resourced group to shape social processes, institutions, economic development, and the built environment, direct society's investments, manipulate policy, and governing rules of the game (laws, regulations, and ideologies that determine the boundaries of permissible political action and visions for change), not the individual characteristics of people. Classes are associated with "structured social processes which position people along social axes. These axes generate status, power, and opportunity for the development of capacities....[they] concern the social division of labor hierarchies of decision-making power...and the arrangement of persons in physical and social space."[35] As Robert Wade Hunter comments, "the rich can translate their income differential into a political oligarchy that sets rules that continuously fortify these differentials."[36] Classes only exist in conflict with other classes in the production and circulation of capital. But class relations change over time because of endless struggle. New forms of subjugation, exploitation, and domination constantly arise, along with new types of resistance to meet them, within an increasingly chaotic economic order and shifting locations of power. For understanding health inequities, the structure of class relations is a more crucial determinant than income categories.[37]

Class relations involve ongoing conflict and are connected to social power, specific interests, and the ability to influence society's decisions beyond simply a greater capacity to consume goods and services. Moreover, class inequality is not the inevitable result of impersonal market forces. Classes have agendas. The outcomes of conflict between classes concern access to society's productive resources, capital, and assets—to the capabilities that enable people to live a full and healthy life.[38]

Class analysis provides an approach for analyzing the regularity of social processes that generate continuing reproduction of health inequities within various forms of exploitation. It enables the development of methods for evaluating strategies to eliminate health inequities through progressive social change. This includes an emphasis on linked policies such as full employment, availability of quality education, public transit, investment in children, access to social assets, and social services.[39]

In addition, class concerns the relationship of organized privilege between social groups. This relationship demands an examination of the implications resulting from variations in the distribution of labor, the conditions of labor, the extraction of labor, labor's market power, the control of production, levels of financial speculation, cultural dispossession, and the structures of political power tied to the state. Class power is expressed, exercised, and manifested in organized political projects such as an end to capital gains taxes, the privatization of schools, campaigns to weaken Medicare and Social Security, and so-called free trade, which enables cheap imports from overseas. An example of the exercise of class power might also include the ability of a real estate developer, with the backing of trade associations, influence over legislative bodies, in collaboration with banking interests, to destroy a neighborhood in order to build condominiums for the wealthy. On the other hand, working people typically seek liberation, autonomy, life, stable social networks, and well-being, including the infrastructure to support it. They want a living wage, safety, and environmental standards and institutions that enable them to act against things like resource depletion, global climate change, unregulated financial activities, and pollution.

A strong connection exists between work and health, particularly given its connection to family life and the well-being of communities, and the documented relation between socioeconomic status and health.[40] With rapidly changing patterns of employment, job requirements, and declining social supports that would guarantee income in new welfare provisions, increasing levels of stress exacerbate inequities among those already made vulnerable, excluding them from full participation in society's major institutions. Unemployment and underemployment have long been associated with serious health risks, including suicide, depression, violence, and alcohol consumption.[41] In addition, the level of control employees have over their work conditions and labor markets matters for health. Those with less control, who tend to be among those with lower socioeconomic status (SES), have worse health outcomes and greater opportunity for injuries and illness. But the notion of exploitation goes beyond workplace conditions. Labor productivity has increased over 75% since the mid-1970s, yet wages for most people have remained stagnant.

An international study examining relationships among political variables and health indicators found a high correlation between working class power and good population health.[42] Since 1973, the power of the working class and labor has been weakening in the United States. The exporting of production, the decline of labor unions, reduction in the social wage (such as welfare and Medicaid), and reduced voter turnout, have influenced this weakening. As employers seek to limit social protections and the economy fails to create necessary levels of employment, populations have thus become more vulnerable to unregulated and chaotic labor markets. Wage cuts, welfare reform, benefit reductions, and threats to privatize social security are examples. They contrast with policies to invest in workers, neighborhoods, or child development.

The incessant drive for endless economic growth generates disruptions to ordinary social life, thus destabilizing communities. Economic growth depends on subjecting people to market forces rather than meeting their needs. Constant and rapid shifting of capital, resources, and jobs to locations of lowest production costs and cheap labor anywhere in the world accelerates the disintegration of communities, creating higher unemployment, dislocation, insecurity, and other stressors associated with illness.

Among many possibilities that influence health inequities, which are related to class: discriminatory practices by banks, economic disinvestment in communities with significant poverty, failure to invest in urban infrastructures (bridges, electrical grids sewer systems), downsizing and restructuring, gentrification, targeting of industrial and toxic waste facilities in many low-income African American communities, profiteering by drug companies seeking to maintain control of patents, and shifting the tax burden to those with limited resources. As neighborhoods decline, the possibilities for healthy lives disappear. Stated another way, the nation's social immune system, the infrastructure of its well-being, declines in an unequal manner.

Within the accelerated patterns of globalization in the social order (outsourcing of jobs, greater extraction of natural resources, more intensive use of chemicals and toxic production processes, expansion of unproductive speculative investment), ever greater pressures accelerate degradation of the environment, life-support systems, and the capacities of the ecosystem more generally, weaken, leading to the return of infectious diseases and new risks to health that affect those with fewer resources. These developments are distributed unevenly in poorer communities as people must manage their own risk.[43] For example, with the elimination of most pension plans, people must manage their own retirements at a time when social obligations are in decline. In addition, poor communities must also bear the burden of structural inequalities designed through corporate or public policy, such as layoffs or the location of toxic waste. In 2008, banks were given protections against loss due to their risky, speculative behavior, while the public paid for their failures.

Moreover, inequitable health outcomes do not function separately from the overall pathology of stressors in an economic system that transforms and organizes time and space in our everyday lives in harmful ways. Examples include speed up in the workplace, accelerating money exchanges and the circulation of capital around the world, moving the locations of production, mechanisms of resource extraction, increasing discriminatory land use policies, and otherwise shifting social and ecological costs onto society thereby creating social disintegration. Capital may be able to move in nanoseconds, but people cannot. These phenomena get written differentially into the body's biology and immune system through physical and social exposure pathways that create stress and can occur over a lifetime.[44]

In recent years, severe cutbacks in social spending across the country, especially for public health and critical infrastructural supports including affordable housing, education, and mass transportation, have exacerbated health problems in already deteriorating communities. Even though new federal resources have been targeted for bioterrorism, funding for addressing the root causes of health inequities and even some traditional public health practices has not increased; rather it has decreased. With lack of investments in areas such as child development, job creation, education, and increasing layoffs, health status for many disadvantaged communities is worsening. Continuing segregation resulting from zoning and policies of gentrification, combined with low income, further contribute to deteriorating health status. Unstable and changing labor markets, tax policies that favor the wealthy, chaos in credit and housing markets, and subsidies to large corporations that redistribute wealth upwards, increases marginalization and has led to greater exposure to health hazards and susceptibility to disease.[45] These conditions occur in one of the most unequal nations in the world with respect to both income and wealth.[46]

Racism

Racism, according to Camara Jones, "is a system of structuring opportunity and assigning value, based on how we look...Through various institutions, laws, and policies, restricting access to knowledge, resources, and representation in the political system, it disadvantages communities and advantages others through unearned white privilege.... It saps the whole society of its strength through a waste of human resources."[47] Nancy Krieger also explains racism as concerning "practices that create and reinforce oppressive systems of race relations whereby people and institutions engaging in discrimination adversely restrict, by judgment and action, the lives of those against whom they discriminate."[48] Racial and gendered structures of power and inequalities profoundly influence health status because hierarchies of all kinds determine life chances.[49] Racial and gender discrimination and oppression become systematically embedded in all social institutions, policies and cultural practices, rules, and conditions in everyday life, although they differ widely across different racial groups. The cultural practices that occur within these identities often obscure their connection to class interests. This sometimes hinders sorting out the primacy of one over the other, although they remain mutually reinforcing. For epidemiology, the issue of race and addressing health inequities is not to confuse racial differences in health outcomes with biological/genetic differences but instead to recognize the effects of racism on health and how racism gets into the body.[50] Racial segregation is an example of structural inequality—supported by the real estate industry, the banks, and federal housing policies. Segregation leads to isolation and economic deprivation resulting from the poor quality of education and lack of good jobs. In poor, segregated communities the lack of investment, along with disinvestments creates stressors leading to health inequities.

A vast amount of data also demonstrates the relation of racism to inequality in health status and the continuing high mortality rates of African Americans and people of color more generally.[51] The racial gap begins early, before life begins, given the stresses of racism on the mother, and continues throughout. In addition, when controlling for socioeconomic status, racial disparities in health remain due to factors such as segregation and discrimination, which adversely affects mental health and leads to cardiovascular disease and hypertension.[52] As David Williams argues, "...black–white differences in [socioeconomic status] SES...are a direct result of the systemic implementation of institutional policies based on the premise of the inferiority of blacks and the need to avoid social contact with them."[53] Racism is manifested in many ways, restricting opportunities and limiting survival rates. The targeting of industrial polluting industries in African American and some Latino communities, as a consequence of segregation and low levels of political power is one example.[54] Segregated housing, unfair banking practices, and poor quality schools have cumulatively created severe stress and unhealthy conditions. In 2008, blacks were three times as likely to have received a subprime loan as whites.[55] More critically, whole communities experience the effects as services decline, the tax base erodes and foreclosures expand. The systematic character of these outcomes expresses their structurally racist character. In addition, racial prejudice itself is a force, collectively, for poorer health outcomes. At every level of income, racial differences in health status persist.

Advances in political power influence conditions that affect health status. Improvements in the living conditions of African Americans during the 1960s and 1970s based on the civil rights movement, resulted in a decline in their mortality rates.[56] But later, beginning in the early 1980s, inequities increased and continue to increase due, among other things, to the effects of subprime mortgage loans and neglect of neighborhoods where many African Americans live, as well as early effects of globalization and cut backs in social services that began during the Reagan administration. Extensive social costs arise from these inequities—threats to economic development, democracy, and the social health of the nation.

Sexism

Gender is also a varied social construct embedded in a series of patterned relations (divided by race and class) often used to justify various traditions, roles, behaviors, laws, and most importantly the constitution of power between and among the sexes. Differentials in health outcomes and well-being between the sexes vary across jurisdictions, age, and ethnic groups, so one cannot speak of an essential concept of gender. However, these differentials are most often attributable to sexism and various cumulative, synergistic gender inequalities than to biological differences.[57] Systematic gender discrimination results from inequities in political representation, the social division of labor, and social stratification, among others, which limit access to resources compared to men and within different groups of women. According to Sen and Ostlin, "Gender relations of power constitute the root causes of gender inequality and…determine whether people's health needs are acknowledged, whether they have voice or a modicum of control over their lives and health, whether they can realize their rights."[58] These inequities themselves place many women in positions leading to violence and exploitation.

The division of labor (occupational segregation), limited patterns of employment according to gender, unequal pay, job discrimination, and changing household structures has often led many women, particularly of low income, to be denied access to resources and advantages available to men and thereby create systemic disadvantages that may limit life chances and negatively influence health.[59] Often limited to service work, domestic labor, and part-time work, limited job benefits, economic insecurity, and the stress of sexual harassment on the job can lead to severe psychosocial stress.[60] Many women are also primary caregivers, doing unpaid work for the family, and single parents, often making them less mobile. All sorts of government policies (welfare) and definitions (the family, mental health), implemented through gendered rules and practices within predefined roles, determine life chances. The socialization girls receive in the institutions of civil society more generally sets women up for restricted roles, constraining options, and potentially generating disadvantage.

Major health inequities are found among women across socioeconomic status and race, particularly among African American women, with respect to life expectancy, morbidity and mortality rates, rates of depression, and chronic conditions such as hypertension and diabetes.[61] These findings suggest that interrelated conditions and experiences, including low social status, limited employment opportunities, and neighborhood safety are important determinants of health inequities that require action. Moreover, women bear the burden of disproportionate levels of domestic unpaid labor through familial relations. As Arline Geronimus notes, "American women in ethnically marginalized or economically disadvantaged populations have not enjoyed improved health or prolonged life in equal measure to those in more advantaged groups...especially among African-American women."[62] Gender inequities in health, overall, result from inequities in political representation, the division of labor, lack of economic autonomy, and gendered hierarchy and social stratification, which limit access to resources compared to men and within different groups of women.[63]

Barriers to Advancing Health Equity in Concepts and Paradigms

The cumulative health impact of racism and class exploitation operates across the life course. Governments mainly offer ameliorative responses or limited regulation when considering health inequity, rather than transformations of institutions that will eliminate the causes. The realization of healthy communities is thus an ongoing process, involving challenges to long-term historical forces and progress will not always be conducive to measurement. It is certainly easier to measure improvements in service delivery than achieving well-being in specific populations. In addition, policy makers and health professionals are usually more comfortable discussing program delivery to so-called "high-risk" populations (rather than high risk conditions) and clinical responses that avoid political conflict or contingent historical and economic dynamics that remain outside the boundaries of scientific analysis.

Why is it difficult to imagine alternatives to the current system and name them? At one level, the historical time line of inequality and its insinuation in all of our institutions obscures the structure of disadvantage. But the limited public debate about health inequities has also become domesticated, preoccupied in the measurement and characterization of the problem, the search for medical and technological solutions, programs to educate those in poverty, and policies to change behavior, avoiding long-term injustices. Yet the language used to explain inequality will determine strategies and highlight the level of plausible social transformation. Effective transformation will involve, as Amartya Sen suggests, equalizing access to capabilities and advantages, leveling the playing field—that is, access to the means of achievement and the freedom to achieve, enabling people to participate effectively in everyday political and social life.[64]

The social sciences and epidemiology

The social sciences, the health professions, and the discipline of epidemiology, tend to avoid the study of macrosocial phenomena. As in most professions, critical reflection on its own historical and political development, presuppositions, and epistemological traditions is often lacking. Until recently, epidemiology as a discipline primarily examined risk factors, the agents of disease, within methodological approaches emphasizing observed phenomena, particularly on the body, not structured social relations. Its theoretical paradigms, driven by the biomedical sciences, leave little room to question the values that shape its perspectives; such paradigms have downplayed the historical conditions and social context that make populations vulnerable, including ecology, sexism, class, and racism.[65] Although "individual risk factors or increased molecular understanding is likely to be extremely limited in understanding variations in disease incidence or prevalence between groups," most of the professional discourse on low-income individuals and high risk populations focuses, as we have noted, on service delivery, access to care, and modification of individual behavior.[66]

These limitations in professional discourse are due partly to the dominance of the biomedical paradigm. Many analysts still consider ill health only in relation to altered biochemical processes, lifestyles, and/or random events in the environment, absent social, economic, and cultural context. Epidemiology, until recently, has been uninterested in developing useful explanations to deal with social forces. The continuing commitment to a biomedical paradigm limits investigations into complex historical issues connected with racism, ecology, social class, and gender discrimination. Public health practice cannot isolate itself from these concerns, but rather must incorporate them within the appropriate scope of public health practice.[67]

Finally, framing injustices as social problems, as if the issue is a puzzle with programmatic, technical solutions limits critical thinking. The effects of social injustice become treatable disorders. Using the term health disparity instead of health inequity makes it appear as if injustice has nothing to do with it; it's just a difference. Focusing on contaminants and hazards similarly obscures the social relations that produce them.

Remedial interventions and reform versus structural systems change

The reduction of inequality requires an exploration of the social processes that generate wealth, poverty, power, and risk. Yet much of the public discussion on inequality, instead of examining root causes and the political strategy that demands, remains almost exclusively focused on access to health care and improving social cohesion, within an underlying assumption that market forces will resolve the issue. Opinion leaders and policy makers give minimal attention to these root causes. Thus, public policy and funding emphasize primarily on diseases and tracking diseases rather than the conditions and social processes that produce disease and chronic illness. The emphasis of programmatic interventions responds to the consequences of inequality instead of inequality itself. Supporters of remedial approaches tend to accept social conditions without exploring how they got that way. Prior to identifying the necessary practices, it seems necessary to integrate political and social analysis into the thinking that might define public health at the level of institutions in order to prevent future inequities.

Developing a Framework: Health and Social Justice

What has social justice to do with health? Health is a basic human need. Social justice and equity have been central to the mission and vision of public health because health is a prerequisite for human development. The idea of a basic public responsibility for social health and welfare and the responsibility of those in public health to be advocates for social justice and collective action have been foundational values of public health.[68] The so-called disparities in health status between different population groups are unjust and inequitable because they resulted from preventable, systemic conditions and policies, as noted earlier. Thus, effective action to eliminate them demands a perspective and conceptual framework grounded in principles of social justice. Otherwise responses will likely remain in a reactive mode, continuing to rely on cures, treatments, or individual interventions, rather than transforming institutions, policies, and practices that cause health inequities. While behavior clearly influences premature mortality and health, behavior always occurs within a socioeconomic context and conditions that continue over time. Although the pathways by which inequality develop are intricate, they are still tied to the way systemic forces such as investment decisions, labor market policies, and neighborhood conditions become linked with individual life histories.

But what is social justice and what is its connection to public health? At least two basic themes constitute its core principles, social and economic equality and democracy—or inclusive participation in social decision making.[69] The first requires an equitable distribution of advantages across society: collective goods, institutional resources (e.g., social wealth), and life opportunities. Excluding income distributional questions, equality means ensuring the development of everyone's capacities to experience life fully. This includes a fair distribution of advantages, as well as greater control of the conditions of social and environmental conditions.[70] But the idea of equality in this conception transcends equal treatment. As Iris Marion Young contends, social justice concerns structural issues related to "deep material differences in social position, division of labour, socialized capacities, normalized standards and ways of living that continue to disadvantage members of historically excluded groups."[71] She reminds us that beyond questions of distribution, social justice is ultimately about liberation from domination and oppression. Many institutions, public and private are involved in reproducing social injustice.

The second theme, democracy (or political equality) concerns the ability to participate effectively, based on principles of inclusion rather than exclusion. It requires access to and sharing productive resources and power. Greater democracy means subjecting more issues and investment decisions to public decision making, collective action, and expanding the political agenda. Achieving social justice requires a type of social change that enables claims for freedom, equality, and democracy to be adequately expressed.[72] For public health, the level of democracy in the political system and the prioritization of public health needs among participants will determine which public health goals make it onto the political agenda.

Social injustice is a negative consequence of unequal privilege, power, and exploitation and reflects deep social divisions in society. The broader context involves not just changes in government policy but the whole range of our commercial and cultural institutions. Thus, the inequalities to eliminate are those of authority, power, influence, material conditions, access to resources, and so on. In practice, social justice requires meeting fundamental human needs and minimizing exploitation and marginalization, and creating a just ecology.[73] Social justice means more than rights because rights can never transcend a society's economic structure and power imbalances; rights are mainly corrective and embedded within the legal system.

A central question from a social justice perspective is "Why is there inequality and how can our organizational structure, policies, and practices change to eliminate health inequities?" The social world is contingent upon an ever-shifting political and social environment, not fixed for all time. The achievement of the end of slavery, women's right to vote, the eight-hour work day, and health and safety laws, were major transformations involving long struggles and conscious strategies. They also depended on a shift in consciousness and values that legitimized new ways of thinking. Support for equality has increased and eroded in different historical moments. Advancing health equity will necessitate rethinking the mission of public health and realize that health inequities are avoidable, not inevitable. At the same time, change will not occur without taking risks and organized action. Nor will it happen without an analysis and questioning of power relations at all levels. How can this or a similar framework advance public health practice? What can be learned from the state of the art now?

Transforming Elements of Public Health Practice: Preliminary Considerations[74]

Developing the capacity of public health practitioners, especially in local health departments (LHDs) to address the root *causes* of health inequities and not merely the consequences may demand changing several major features of public health practice and organizational structure as a whole. Such revaluation involves ways to affect the production of health and illness within specific population groups, to expand the definition of public health practice as a social enterprise,[75] to create systems integrating relevant organizational entities, and to engage in planning and prevention activities, in conjunction with other community organizations and agencies. Unfortunately, no simple one-to-one correspondence exists between principles and practice; no one model can easily describe, for example, how to conduct the ten essential public health services differently or offer a protocol of specific steps. However, it is possible to examine some of the challenges and possible directions and approaches to changing the organization and conduct of public health practice, rather than specific programs or interventions. A guiding principle is a commitment to a public, collective responsibility for establishing the conditions that produce health.[76] A basic assumption is that today's dominant public health paradigm does not incorporate fully the requirements for tackling health inequities because their sources remain outside both the scope of public health institutions and practices. Thus, it is necessary to expand the mandate, voice, and practice of public health to tackle structural inequality.

Public Health Practice at a Crossroads: The Evidence and the Response

The work and value of public health, often unfamiliar to most Americans, is now coming under increasing scrutiny, in the wake of increasing threats to population health, from global climate change, and disasters such as Hurricane Katrina, to West Nile Virus, Avian flu, and E.coli 0157:H7. As more people come into contact with cancer causing agents and pollution, as well as a greater level of chronic illness, the importance of establishing the conditions for health over time, beyond prevention, at the level of social decision making, has become clearer. At the same time, LHDs, and institutions on the front lines of defense, are experiencing greater pressures as their boundaries and scope expand, along with rapid social change, in their efforts to adapt. How can they cope with health inequity?

As noted earlier, the social etiology of disease suggests that patterns of inequity in the distribution of disease and illness correspond to patterns of social and economic inequality. As such, rethinking certain features of public health practice is essential. Yet, public health practice as presently constituted is often unprepared to respond to these inequities. More important, the type of infrastructure, workforce, community capacity building and tracking systems, among other elements needed to tackle health inequities, remains unexamined and underdeveloped. For practitioners, examining the sources of health inequity and its relationship to practice in order to take appropriate action is a necessity. Although public health does not own this issue, its role must be explicit.

Difficulties Faced by Local Health Departments in Addressing Health Equity

Local health departments (LHDs) face many problems in seeking to address health inequity. A necessary relationship is absent between what we know about the degree and character of health inequities and the capacities of the public health system that remain underdeveloped. LHDs often lack both human and financial resources, given already overburdened staff, as well as the capacity for research and policy development. The work takes time, commitment, and consistent participation. A major issue is how to allocate resources, plan, and set priorities for a health-equity-oriented agenda. Agencies whose policies and procedures have serious health consequences may not want public health to interfere. Establishing relationships with those institutions, keeping them informed, and working with them for change is an ongoing challenge.

Legal and bureaucratically defined mandates, institutionalized rules and regulations also limit the range of practice, leading many departments to believe that acting on health inequity is not within their capacity or scope of work. Others avoid the issue because they believe that the success of such work cannot be evaluated sufficiently to demonstrate its value. Political pressure and bureaucratic inertia to stick to traditional activities under the core functions plays a role, and many times internal agency support is absent. Public health always operates in a politicized environment with responsibilities to boards and commissions, and political leaders typically do not hold LHDs accountable for health equity. Rural areas with conservative climates pose special problems. Staff typically lacks training and function under fragmented authority. Orienting a sympathetic county leadership still takes time and effective communication strategies. New responsibilities such as dealing with bioterrorism affect or restrict the possibility for other work.

A dissonance appears to exist in the workforce between expectations and requirements to tackle health inequity. A clinically oriented workforce may not wish to contend with health inequity or may not be prepared to accept a new organizational culture. At a broader level, the public sphere has shrunk. The disease focus, the absence of vision, and fragmentation within the discipline has often led to pessimism in public health, without agents of change for support. Public health practitioners, not used to risk taking and often driven by crises, sometimes find that they are calming people down rather than firing them up for the kind of activism that would lead to change. Different skills are needed for this work.

Limited knowledge of and clarity about the subject and principles of social justice, as well as an inability to frame the issue and communicate it effectively is an important factor hindering LHDs. This includes the absence of research on the specific nature of local inequities or tools to monitor them. Equally important, many practitioners may view their progressive programs on various diseases such as diabetes as based on social justice principles; yet however vital and effective such programs may be, they often remain symptomatic and remedial, rather than focused on targeting the determinants of inequities. It is not always easy or self-evident to distinguish between acting on symptoms and acting on the source or even articulate the types of interventions necessary.

In more general terms, great difficulty exists in articulating an independent role for public health, compared with other sectors already directly linked to the social determinants of inequities in health, such as inadequate housing or poor education. Public health may seek to define its value either independently or in conjunction with many institutions. At the same time, it might be counterproductive or even unfair to frame injustices through a public health perspective in its most traditional role.[77] Governmental public health as presently constituted would benefit from an expanded definition of its role by state and local executives to provide legitimacy for its workforce to transform itself as necessary to act on health inequity.

Standard workforce recruitment and training practices pose difficulties as well. Often existing job classifications and accreditation rules limit the ability to hire people with the necessary background for acting on health inequities. Moreover, the talents and attitudes necessary for success, beyond technical skills, such as creativity and commitment to the issues, may be overlooked in hiring decisions.

Attempts to formalize and standardize public health practice, while necessary in part to evaluate performance, can also create inflexibility in acting on health inequity. This is because the difficulty lies in the need to expand the boundaries of public health practice in ways that connect separate programs and services so as to confront imbalances of power that generate inequity in communities.

Finally, the general public has little knowledge or appreciation of what public health is or does. These difficulties place boundaries on the sustained practices necessary for tackling health inequities. As a result, public health has been forced to retreat from its historical mission, hindered by immediate needs to focus on microbiology and clinical medicine. Yet there is much that public health can do to broaden its capacity to address the social context in which disease and illness occur.

Opportunities

Local public health practitioners function as crucial first responders in their communities and are held in high esteem, as a resource for data, analysis, and expertise. Communities have expectations about the role of public health departments, especially in times of crisis, as new threats such as global climate change, disruption of ecosystems, disasters such as Hurricane Katrina, and the recurrence of old diseases loom. These realities are the foundation upon which to develop a role for LHDs in eliminating health inequity. At the same time, initiatives in the last few years, such as those noted below, suggest a growing momentum for innovative action.

In 2008, the Public Broadcasting Service (PBS) broadcasted *Unnatural Causes: Is Inequality Making Us Sick?*, a 4-hour documentary series on the social determinants of health inequity (see Chapter 25). Over 140 LHDs committed to conducting town-hall events screening the film and engaging in dialogue with community residents and elected officials, thereby raising awareness and offering the potential for constructing compelling messages about the sources of health inequity.

An increasing number of LHDs are offering new models for practice. In 2002, San Francisco County established the first local public health agency health equity initiative—the Program on Health Equity and Sustainability—to effect change through public policy analysis, collaboration, and advocacy. The Louisville Metro Department of Public Health and Wellness, subsequent to establishing their Center for Health Equity in an LHD, commissioned a study to explore "the discrepancies between what public health experts want people to understand, and what the public currently believes about health and health disparities," in order to translate media stories by journalists more effectively, as well as influence those stories. A number of LHDs around the country are testing new strategies, including Multnomah County, OR; Alameda County, CA; New York City, Amherst, MA; Milwaukee, WI; Los Angeles County, CA; Shasta County, CA; Boston, MA; and Chicago, IL among others. The Bay Area Regional Health Inequities Initiative (BARHII), a consortium of ten LHDs in northern California has developed a conceptual framework for exploring and measuring health inequities. They also have devised an organizational assessment tool, which includes a survey for staff to determine general knowledge of health equity (see Chapter 16). Some states (Virginia, Oklahoma, Ohio, and Massachusetts) have established divisions, offices, or staff positions dedicated to eliminating health inequity.

In 2008, *National Association of County and City Health Officials* (NACCHO), with an initial grant from the W. K. Kellogg Foundation, established the LHD National Coalition for Health Equity in an attempt to mobilize LHDs around the country to formulate strategies collectively, build solidarity among them and provide a mechanism for LHDs to inform each other about effective practices and policies.

Transforming Public Health Practice

Given our framework, as well the characterization of LHDs in the 2003 Institute of Medicine report[78] and the analysis of other scholars,[79] what changes to public health practice and its infrastructural components that might advance the elimination of health inequity more effectively and make use of available knowledge? How can LHDs gain traction on this issue to link their commitment to action? How can a social justice framework be incorporated into the overall design of an approach to practice in all parts of the LHD, rather than remain isolated as a special initiative? How do practitioners translate the extensive knowledge on the relation between social and economic inequalities and health inequities in a way that will lead to a transformation in the practice, structure, culture, and knowledge base of public health?

The task does seem daunting. Realizing the changes necessary to eliminate health inequities does not require quick, massive action all at once, but rather taking action on foundations of health, even if in small steps. Social inequalities cannot be reduced primarily through programmatic interventions or services, given research findings about the relation between social hierarchy and chronic stress. In addition, different questions may arise when institutional change rather than individual behavior change is the objective. For example, as Doak Bloss notes in Chapter 13, in addition to asking "Why do people smoke?" the social justice question should be "What social conditions and economic policies, along with systematic practices of tobacco companies, predispose people to the stress that encourages smoking?" In addition to asking "How do we connect isolated individuals to a social network?" we can ask "What institutional policies and practices maintain rather than counteract people's isolation from social supports?" As well as asking, "How do we create more green space, bike paths, and farmers' markets in high-risk neighborhood?" we can ask "What policies and practices by government and commerce discourage or support access to transportation, resources, and nutritious food in neighborhoods where health outcomes are poorest."

Essentially, a major objective is to transition from an improvisational approach to a more comprehensive one, returning to the larger social context that defined the origins of public health. A tension or contradiction that remains unresolved is the extent to which necessary changes can evolve from practice as it exists or instead require an entirely new approach. Whatever road is taken, resolving the dilemma and establishing an effective organizational structure and culture is crucial to success.

We can explore some of the core elements or arenas for change within departments that would enable them to address health inequities. Because social justice practice seeks to change conditions outside of public health institutions, organizational transformation does not necessarily require large financial resources; it concerns instead conducting the work of public health differently, developing a supportive infrastructure within the agency, and creating the space for action. Stated another way, the dimensions through which transformation needs to occur, as discussed below, depend on capacity building within and outside of the public health institution, as a means to legitimize and naturalize a practice based on social justice.

The following discussion briefly outlines specific areas or elements of practice and offers a rationale for change, along with general suggestions and questions about possibilities. For each of the often overlapping elements and components of practice, including organizational structure, I explain their importance and hypothetical options, recognizing that many of these pose challenges for implementation and few have taken action. Appendix B presents "Guidelines for Achieving Health Equity in Public Health Practice," which represents a tentative statement of reflective strategies to build on, based on some of the suggestions in this section.

How do we link the principles of social injustice to people's everyday action? While the analysis may appear overly broad and visionary, a detailed blueprint or protocol would be inappropriate if not impossible. Change in any given health department will emerge in at least two ways: (1) from a separate dialogue process with staff and community members on practice, based on a model similar to that in Chapter 13 that focuses on gaining insight about the relation between social and economic inequality and social injustice; and (2) the naturally occurring reflection from these dialogues that may lead to questioning contemporary procedures and practices.

Internal Organizational Structure: Establishing a Health Equity Team

Working through all levels, an LHD can establish a core, diverse, cross-disciplinary team that would provide leadership to the effort to address the root causes of health inequity. To create real change in the way a department addresses health inequity in its daily practice, it may be necessary to build ownership of and investment in such work from within the organization. Senior management could authorize a group of action-oriented employees to work together to drive the change process forward. The team would be charged with investigating health inequities and the department's responsiveness to root causes, including a survey of employee attitudes and knowledge of the issues (see for example Chapter 15). In that way, they could more effectively identify actions that will change the institutional culture to one that integrates principles of social justice into daily practice. Hypothetically, a department may begin with assumptions about how to proceed, which would include working at the upper end of "the spectrum of prevention," to set the conditions for healthy communities, shifting resources if needed, with a recognition that the root causes involve deep-rooted social divisions and injustices embedded in social processes, not a random accumulation of bad conditions or factors. Working with staff, they would establish a process for envisioning an ideal LHD, anchored in practice, that has reorganized its structure and practice to tackle health inequities in a comprehensive way. As described in Chapter 13, the next step could include an engaging, participatory, democratic dialogue process with selected staff on the root causes of health inequities, including a community

forum, based on the evidence. This would be followed by a subsequent dialogue process, starting with current practice, on how to translate the knowledge of the causes of health inequity into specific public health practices
and standards for them aimed at collective change. Peer networks could be
used to reinforce ideas, tied to technical assistance and mentoring.

Leadership

Advocating for health equity demands leadership and commitment in a
public health institution, along with a willingness to mobilize the necessary
resources. Thus, health officials would first establish health equity as a priority, followed by seeking greater decision-making authority and support
for public policy directed specifically at the elimination of health inequities. On a daily basis, officials would speak publicly and often to reinforce
the messages regarding health equity. Leadership also means ensuring
accountability to institutional commitments. Progress on reducing health
inequities would be measured and reported on a regular basis. Ultimately,
a way must be found to institutionalize and sustain the work.

Even though the LHD is one among many entities that have a role, it
will need to build support among colleagues in other agencies and organizations, as a means to give priority to the health impact of many activities
and decisions at the state and local level. Leadership also means inspiring
others and enabling their voice. Because the causes of population ill health
result primarily from conditions created by long-standing injustices, such
as racism, sexism, and exploitation in the labor process rather than individual behavior, health professionals must advocate for a configuration of
public policies that distinguish those necessary to protect living standards
and correct growing inequities from those that establish the system rules
that will structure the possibilities for health equity linked to broad social
change connected to things like labor markets and land use policy.

Health officials are in a position to demonstrate the links between health
and unemployment, social exclusion (from resources necessary for healthy
lives), poverty, quality education, and central features associated with the
organization of society. Staff would be given latitude to work on health
equity. Finally, agency directors can seek grants related to eliminating
health inequity. That is, they can consider activity related to health equity
as a screen in budget decisions.

The support for health equity as a goal of public health practice and a
basic social right requires explicit expression, along with a rationale and
a method to ensure its implementation. Evidence alone will not result in
change without commitment. This expression would include support for
the enforcement of laws and regulations associated with housing, the
environment, the workplace, and basic sanitation. Doing so would enable

practitioners to review and evaluate priorities, policies, and resources to determine their effect on population health and address health inequities more effectively. It would also generate the momentum to transcend remedial action in favor of more fundamental, coordinated practices directed at root causes.

Establishing a strategic planning process

The challenge for practitioners is to rethink the framework that guides the work of public health. Such a framework would include, at a minimum, meeting basic human needs and equitable distribution of social resources. More than ever, population health depends on the provision of public resources. Supporting equity in action involves establishing goals that target the social determinants of inequalities in health, instead of diseases or mortality rates. An LHD needs to establish its goals and needed capacity for engaging with health inequities.

A health equity team at the LHD may be placed to initiate such a strategic planning process.[80] It may begin with an assessment, relying on surveys and discussions asking questions about what reforms would enable the agency to tackle root causes. For example, BARI III has developed a departmental assessment tool and piloted it in the Berkeley City Health Department, based on a staff survey (Chapter 15).The Alameda County Public Health Department in California has also developed an internal process for evaluating its capacity to address health inequity. It includes a "Public Health 101" interactive training for staff with exercises and modules on racism, community capacity building, and the history of public health. A visioning exercise involving all staff considers organizational changes required, particularly the skills and capabilities necessary, along with a method for implementing new competencies for achieving health equity. Community organizations must be brought into the process at the outset to establish priorities.

Interagency/multidisciplinary coordination

The production of health depends on a variety of conditions, processes, institutions and knowledge, beginning in childhood and overlapping many jurisdictions. Thus, health is never about the work of one agency but requires a system of institutions. In orchestrating action to eliminate health inequities, public health practitioners in an ideal department, would collaborate and coordinate with the many agencies and entities that constitute the system of public health. We might find health practitioners linking their practice with city planning, economic redevelopment, transportation, housing, social welfare, and education, beyond the health professions, along with neighborhood and nonprofit organizations. A major challenge is to determine the unique role and contribution of public health, for example, public health should engage with other institutions, but does not take on the work or role of that institution. The location of public health practice, often perceived as within organizations designated as health departments inhibits the capacity to establish fully the conditions for healthy communities. Intersectoral collaboration efforts would involve, at a minimum, sharing data across agencies, which would link to health outcomes and exposures. For example, data on housing and labor market conditions and investment in community infrastructure could inform public policy.

Workforce development and education

How can the public health workforce respond more systematically and effectively to the source of health inequities? What is the necessary infrastructure? What competencies are necessary? In order to eliminate inequities in health outcomes, the theory, practice, and scope of work within the field of public health would change its focus to the structures that influence the quality of life, addressing the prerequisites for population health. This includes a range of activities from seeking to integrate public health into social policy to redefining through expansion the content of public health practice, recognizing the contribution of many disciplines and skills to success. Practitioners would support the redirection of social and political priorities and resources. They would begin to link activism and science more effectively. Health departments would strive to institutionalize health equity throughout all divisions.

Recruitment (hiring criteria, job descriptions, and qualifications). New staff have multidisciplinary training, (e.g., the social sciences, community organizing, urban planning, public policy, advocacy, negotiation) ability to conduct qualitative research, and an understanding of health inequities, especially the connection between racism, class, and sex discrimination as underlying causes. They are racially and ethnically diverse. Their competencies are appropriate to tackling the root causes of health inequities. Beyond technical and communication skills, the department seeks sensibilities, attitudes, creativity, commitment, and connectedness. Thus, staff must be good listeners, willing to learn, passionate, able to mobilize people, serve as mentors, build trust, promote leadership in the community, and engage in policy advocacy. Job descriptions are rewritten to reflect the changes.

Training and education: Dialogue. Staff members would engage in facilitated dialogue about social justice and its historical link to public health, as well as a revised public health practice. Dialogue occurs over a period of time, with regular updates, within a permanent, ongoing activity. In this process, staff comes to conclusions on their own as a group through a collective building of knowledge. Staff members would participate in regular meetings with neighborhood coalitions and would learn how to interact, as well as the basics of community-based participatory research. Educational materials and mentoring of staff are critical. Some departments, as part of their education, provide workshops on Undoing Racism. A major challenge for many departments is continuity when there is significant turnover and finding methods of educating all staff. Decisions must also be made about how and when to invite all levels of staff into the discussion. Another challenge is the difficulty of educating on systems change and macro policy change. Few come to public health with such a background or in subject areas not traditionally part of public health.

The LHD would collaborate with the local school of public health to ensure inclusion of social justice in the curriculum. Equally important, it would reach out to departments of social sciences in local universities seeking to have public health included in the curriculum outside of public health and the undergraduate curriculum.

Integration of disciplines. Public health practice cannot advance health equity without a more coherent philosophy and theory—one that links economics, ecology, sociology, and geography and avoids disciplinary boundaries. Schools of public health would cross-train on environmental concerns to overcome overspecialization. Workforce recruitment—hiring criteria, job descriptions, and qualifications of new recruits—must consider people with multidisciplinary training, (e.g., the social sciences, community organizing, urban planning) ability to conduct qualitative research, and an understanding of health inequities.

Working and collaborating with communities

The LHD cannot perform its work in isolation from its constituent communities. A necessary step is to identify organizations that engage in social justice struggles and support their alliances, particularly as part of broad social movements—civil rights, human rights, environmental justice, advocates for affordable and safe housing, and so forth. The idea is to establish common ground on related issues, create solidarity, mobilize supporters, and their networks, and develop a coherent agenda. It may be possible to form an association of social justice activists outside the boundaries of the LHD. Consider, for example, the establishment of a community advisory board on health equity. Whatever the specific method, it is important for staff to work with grassroots organizations on a regular basis. The public health agency can thus facilitate or support existing coalitions in communities under stress. In addition, the agency can conduct strategic planning processes with community members with planners, convene and facilitate meetings with other agencies, and provide health data. In supporting alliances, it may be useful to conduct an analysis of power relations among allies for strategic purposes. Thus, depending on the specific objectives, identify who has power to move the agenda or pressure those who do have power. In supporting alliances, it is important to determine whether potential allies have power, what risks they are willing to take, how strongly their interests correlate with those of the LHD, and what the department can offer them. At the same time, the LHD is constrained; it cannot, for example, likely sign on to positions against their local government.

The relationship with community organizations is ongoing, organic, not based on formulas or techniques, but principles and a principled way of interacting and making decisions. Community residents and their organizations must be active partners in any efforts to eliminate health inequities and the LHD must be accountable to the community. The entire staff would work to make common cause with those who are most marginalized and the social movements associated with them. Thus, public health professionals must advocate for social change that transforms the conditions that cause ill health and by strengthening community assets, skills, and capacities. The work begins by building trust and solidarity with community and workers' organizations. In part this may mean breaking with a hierarchical command and control model of operating in the health department to one based on a more participatory, democratic approach to setting priorities and conducting research within neighborhoods. This type of relationship also contrasts with pure service delivery or programs attempting to control diseases. The LHD becomes, in this model, more of a facilitator, while still able to apply its expertise. Most important then is how LHDs work with communities: how they support and assist the community against threats to health. Establishing a long-term relation will require, in most cases, that LHDs change their organizational culture from one with a rigid, predefined set of rules, job classifications, and passive definition of surveillance, to a more flexible, multidisciplined one that can meet new challenges.

Community collaboration is in this model inescapably a method of community organizing for social change. It requires a long-term commitment; it's an alliance. The terms of the relationship are always being negotiated; in part that's because conditions are fluid as is the concept of community. It requires shared decision making, and mutual disclosure of information, particularly at the beginning phases of conducting activities. A clarification of interests and values is always necessary because conflicts are many times not just about misunderstandings or misperceptions. If community residents say that they are being poisoned and their goal is getting assistance, they do wish the health department to argue with them about risk levels, or comparing risks and supposed benefits. A toxic waste site in the neighborhood is a problem of toxic waste, not risk. The community does not wish to debate about probability theory; it wants a remedy. More specifically, responding to health concerns requires working with the community to determine risk, not merely communicating it, and providing an explanation/analysis of findings, not just the findings. The methodology or analysis by the experts may be flawed. Setting priorities and designing research must also be a prerogative of communities. Determining what data to collect depends in part of how the community defines its priorities. These priorities may be different from the LHD.

The field of popular epidemiology emerging in recent years (whereby laypersons take charge of collecting and interpreting data and invite experts to work with them), along with the concept of "street science" (see Chapter 22) supports innovative approaches to improving community health, including consideration of disproportionate risks in exposure experienced by many African Americans and those with low income. Eliciting and using community knowledge through qualitative assessments, dialogue, and insight, popular epidemiology is a philosophy and a method or practice—a type of public participation whereby laypeople detect and act on environmental hazards, and learn to collect data on conditions in the community that create health inequities. According to sociologist Phil Brown, popular epidemiology is "the process whereby laypersons gather scientific and other information, and also direct and marshal the knowledge and resources of experts in order to understand the epidemiology of disease…yet [it is] more…since it emphasizes social structural factors as part of the causal disease chain. Also, it involves social movements, uses political and judicial approaches to remedies, and challenges basic assumptions of traditional epidemiology, risk assessment, and health regulation."[81] It enables people to determine how they know what they know. Community knowledge provides a rich, historical source unavailable from purely technical knowledge or ordinary perception. It may be useful to suggest actions that neighborhood residents can take to bring about change. This will potentially lead to further engagement and create commitment. Similarly, the principles of community-based participatory research represent an important step toward clarifying values, collaborative methods, and relationships in how LHDs will work on research projects with the community.

Given these approaches, perhaps the most important way LHDs can assist communities is to assist in strengthening indigenous leadership capable of mobilizing neighborhood residents to collective action to address health inequities. This means community organizing and involves providing resources that would shift power out of bureaucratic institutions directly into communities. It also means an offer of technical assistance to groups engaged in population health work and the deployment of permanent resources at neighborhood level.

Communications strategy and public education: Shifting consciousness

Gaining support and generating public debate on health inequities will require that health practitioners work with the mass media and develop strategies that would lead to a greater emphasis on root causes of ill health and poor quality of life, particularly the way in which social policy can make a difference. The media must, however, be ready to hear a new message and that message must come from constituents, especially an organized public. The objective is to raise awareness about and explore the sources of health inequities and the collective action necessary to generate dialogue and take action to eliminate those inequities.

What are some possible messages that would resonate with the mass media and the public in trying to shift the focus to the institutional story and trends behind health inequities? Messages might include, "health problems reflect socioeconomic conditions and the standard of living;" "social inequality leads to health inequality;" and "everyone benefits from equality." The goal is to challenge the dominant discourse that emphasizes risk, behavior, and victim blaming. At the same time, basic messages also explain that health is about more than health care, healthy behaviors, and public health programs. The legitimacy of being health experts can get traction for the issue of health inequity, along with a confident, moral message. The basic elements of the social justice message are the following: (1) injustice exists; (2) it is systemic—meaning that there are institutions and policies responsible; and (3) something can be done about it.[82] That something would foster a sense of collective responsibility for health equity.

Find a headline such as "Does poverty cause disease" or "Economic inequality related to health status." The object is to find a way to make the issue compelling by reframing it so that people think about health in ways that link it to actionable social conditions and more fundamental injustices. However, new and more formal relationships with the media may be necessary to tell the story of health differently. The work is not so much about persuasion with facts as providing insights that will shift consciousness. However, critical understanding of health inequity is about more than producing messages; it concerns how people identify themselves and recognize the role that institutions play in establishing health. Health professionals can provide context that gives meaning to seemingly disparate experiences. This involves, at a minimum, posing questions about such things as the sources of toxicity in society and neighborhoods that draws the link between policy, health outcomes, and the capacity to imagine alternative futures. Only in this way will it be possible to reclaim the necessary concept of collective, social responsibility and challenge individualism and the culture of self-help. For LHD success, leadership, internal consensus, and commitment will be a prerequisite, as well as the availability of tools such as the PBS documentary series *Unnatural Causes: Is Inequality Making Us Sick?* (see Chapter 25).

A Good Framing Strategy Should:
   Translate individual problem to social issue. The first step in framing is to make sure that what you say is consistent with your approach. It's hard to justify an environmental approach to an issue if all media interviews frame it from an individual perspective. Further, a social issue is news, an individual problem is not. Translating an issue helps others to see why it is important and newsworthy.
   Assign primary responsibility. Consistency is key. If the issue is tobacco sales to kids, it's hard to justify a new ordinance if spokespeople assign primary responsibility for the problem to parents. Framing for content means framing your message in ways that support your initiative goal and explain to others why the target you chose is the right entity to address the issue.
   Present solution. The message should clearly articulate what the initiative can address. To use youth access to tobacco as an example, the solution offered is to make it harder for merchants to profit from youth smoking.
   Make practical policy appeal. This is where the initiative comes in. It should be communicated as practical, fair, legal, affordable and the right thing to do.
   Develop pictures and images. If a picture is worth a thousand words and the average media bite is seven seconds, developing compelling visuals that illustrate your perspective is critical.
   Tailor to audience. Remember whom you are communicating with in each case. Communities are fragmented with lots of different interests and concerns. Tailor your message to your audience, which is usually your target.
   —Developed by the Berkeley Media Studies Group, Berkeley, CA

Public policy development and analysis

A major goal of public policy to eliminate health inequities is to equalize access to capabilities and advantages, which means, according to Amartya Sen, providing access to the means of achievement and the freedom to achieve, enabling people to engage in the world.[83] Of course many jurisdictions have environmental safety and public health codes that allow public health to intervene to address inadequacies in environmental conditions and housing through structural remediation, for example, replacing mold-damaged material. But practitioners also need to consider how policies relating to taxes, employment, trade, transportation, labor markets, as examples, influence health inequity. Realizing healthy public policy will demand strategizing, not one issue at a time but with a plan for reordering priorities, particularly social investments in the infrastructure to improve the lives of children.

For our purposes, it is important to distinguish the processes of excluding structures (e.g., processes and practices that create inequality) from the excluded groups disadvantaged by those structures. Social inclusion involves a challenge to power rather than an accommodation to it.[84] The achievement of social inclusion includes a broad range of linked policies designed to ensure access to public resources and institutions including quality education, affordable housing, fair distribution of tax expenditures, employment, and social services. It includes both affirmative (resources for training) and protective needs (opposition to redlining by banks and predatory lending in housing, and segregation through land use planning). More important, policies of social inclusion would prohibit vast accumulations of wealth or the purposeful cheapening of the labor force. It would prohibit advantaging the already wealthy and their coordinated capacity to affect everyone else.

Distinguishing among configurations of policy is also important, for example, welfare policies that seek to build solidarity and protect living standards as a corrective to inequity, from those that set the rules of the system and link to broad social changes in areas such as labor markets and land use policy. But no single policy will reduce health inequity significantly without a more comprehensive approach. Moreover, not all policy involves legislation. Administrative rulemaking, moratoria, and mandated research are important areas for potential policy development. Perhaps more important, political conflict includes decision-making arenas beyond government, including within institutions of civil society such as corporations, schools, churches, and workplaces. Young reminds us that these private institutions "often exercise exploitation, domination, and exclusion," just as much as government.

In an article in the *American Journal of Public Health*, James Colgrave asks a critical question associated with the direction of public health:

> Are public health ends better served by narrow interventions focused at the level of the individual or the community, or by broad measures to redistribute the social, political, and economic resources that exert such a profound influence on health status at the population level?...A large and growing body of research [suggests] that broad social conditions must be addressed in order to effect meaningful and long-term improvement in the health of populations.[85]

Broad measures will be necessary that attend to structures and institutions within the social system instead of primarily at-risk individuals. Making major improvements in the health of places and anticipating future increases in health inequities requires policies aimed at structural and institutional change. Such an agenda would focus on the foundations of health and the social roots of suffering, premature death, and disability as they are connected to patterns of disease and illness over time within populations.

What types of strategies aim to remove or lower risk for neighborhoods? Supporting mass transit policies and conducting health impact assessments initiated by affected populations on urban design will be more useful than the traditional emphasis on exercise and diet alone. Public and organizational policies that generally improve the health of populations disadvantaged by social and economic conditions are likely to reduce health inequities. The idea is not only to reverse conditions that lead to inequitable health outcomes, but to produce the conditions that create health before inequities develop.

The supporting evidence for policy must be derived, as Hillary Graham suggests, "beyond the disciplines of social epidemiology and public health to the social science disciplines of sociology, social policy and welfare economics."[86] In each of these areas, it is necessary to explore what we need to know to develop policies that affect public health and health inequity. The intent is to emphasize fundamental, root-based as opposed to ameliorative action aimed at risk "factors." Thus, the focus is necessarily on the social, cultural, and environmental context of patterned negative health outcomes.

Attention to the values that underlie policy and policy menus are critical, given the principle that people have a social right to healthy conditions and that the patterns of illness are not a function of choice or fixed conditions. Healthy public policy must therefore be supported, even though policy effects are difficult to measure over time, particularly when seeking to change institutions, structures, and factors such as air and water quality. Success is also difficult to evaluate because narrowing the gap between socioeconomic groups is a long-term objective, rather than general improvements in health status. However, an objective is to move policy in a different direction, at a macro level, even if measurement is difficult or impossible.

To begin the examination of decision making, LHDs would identify local policies and arenas that affect the social determinants of health and then, in conjunction with their communities, establish policy agendas linked to reducing health inequity. Social policies would be evaluated according to their effect on health equity. But what is the appropriate role for public health?

On one hand, the social injustices that influence health outcomes seem intractable. Involvement in public policy may seem new territory as practitioners are typically not trained or inclined toward policy. However, as noted, the social context has always been critical to determining health and it must engage with these issues through its assessment, assurance, and direct policy development function. Practitioners will find that they have options. The first and most important is assembling, analyzing, and interpretating evidence and the implications for health inequity in the distribution of disease and illness, such as measures of life expectancy, infant mortality, and well-being. The second is mobilizing affected populations and involving them in policy development, as well as exposing the public to the relation between health and policy (see Chapter 18). Third, health practitioners can articulate consistent, informed positions, given the evidence. They can provide documentation and testimony to local city councils and agencies as well as state health departments on the social determinants of health inequities. But such testimony involves more than showing up at hearings. It involves engineering questions and getting invited to testify as a strategy to create interest, with the backing of the public and affected populations. Fourth, as the public voice to the mass media, they can articulate the importance of a public health paradigm, including the representation of public health and the character of communities. The object is essentially to promote a broadened, collective view of health and its relation to major economic and social decisions. In addition, public health departments can publicize the negative processes, decisions, and practices engaged in by corporations. In coalition with each other, LHDs can formulate model policies and principles to establish a national agenda for health equity. Finally, the public health department can contribute to debate and dialogue in the development and implementation of policy that would not exist without their participation. Such a role clarifies the way that health is socially produced through institutions and public decision making. At the same time, risks must be taken to deal with the reality that action will be required in the face of uncertainty. As such, public health can mobilize political will for change and support greater accountability. Public health practitioners have the legitimacy, leverage, and evidence to take action. They have stories to tell that can explain the deep-rooted sources of inequities and thereby influence policy.

Advocacy and organizing

To realize the values of social justice it is necessary for health practitioners to be advocates, which means working with communities to support engagement in political processes that impact health. This objective was clearly stated in the *Institute of Medicine (*IOM) report of 1988 and reinforced in the 2003 IOM report.[87] In seeking to inform opinion makers, shape the debate, support coalitions, and influence decision makers through both the agency's expert role and the community's knowledge, advocacy cannot be mere passive dissemination of information; it demands a strategic plan to deploy information to build social momentum. The basic advocacy role can be described along the following dimensions: (1) inclusion of health equity and social justice in the statutory authority for public health; (2) health equity in performance standards and accreditation; (3) support conferences for and by community members and health workers and invite to conferences; (4) support communities seeking better quality housing or getting landlords to make repairs or increasing the affordability and availability of housing; and (5) offer community organizations technical assistance with things like conducting their own health assessments, planning and evaluation, and guidelines for community development.

Overall, a strategy is necessary for building political will through consolidating political support for addressing the root causes of health inequity at the local, state, and national level. LHDs can attempt to create legitimacy for this work through elected bodies. At the local level, this could take the form of a resolution by the Board of Supervisors directing departments to address the systematic and unjust distribution of illness and disease. At the state and national level, the department might engage with and present information to key elected officials to (1) make them aware of the link between social injustice and health inequity; and (2) encourage formal action to legitimize this work as a responsibility of public health.

Tracking and monitoring

As Chen et al., note, "An important function of public health surveillance and monitoring is the identification of systematic disparities in who experiences the burden of disease and death in the population...[which] reflect underlying social inequalities."[88] Monitoring patterns of socioeconomic inequalities more effectively requires analysis of the measurement of group deprivation over time. As a means to build the capacity of LHDs and their communities to address health inequities, it is necessary to monitor the nature and level of health inequity in a community and the sources of health inequity.

In the past few years, a number of organizations such as the Global Health Equity Alliance,[89] and other researchers,[90] have begun to develop approaches to measuring health inequity that offer innovative tools. Traditional business and economic indicators that receive wide coverage in the news provide a limited and skewed view of the nation's well-being. Thus, an effective, systematic, and official narrative that provides a full picture of social well-being or health equity is lacking. It also requires a coherent system of social reporting that can provide direction and guidance for effective social change. These tools are a way to measure, monitor, and communicate a concept of health equity that can inspire people to action and place health equity on the national agenda. They offer a portrait of conditions to focus public attention on health inequities and make rational assessments to move public policy.

In addition, these tools can facilitate the community's capacity to express its voice on community health concerns related to inequity. What is a health equity index? According to the Equity Gauge Alliance, "An *Equity Gauge* [herein called a health equity index] is an active approach to addressing inequity in health that not only monitors equity, but also incorporates concrete actions to bring about sustained reductions in unfair disparities in health and health care....This active approach requires the involvement of a range of actors in society including researchers, health workers, policy makers, the media, the general public, and nongovernmental organizations (NGOs) concerned with development and justice."[91] More generally, data collection and analysis is a means to inform decision making by building equity into a standard, everyday process that creates consciousness about the issue of health inequity. Since science is not neutral—the choice of scientific questions depends on values about what is important—alliances will need to be developed between scientists, health departments, and social movement activists.

What should we measure? It may be useful to include the forces that generate inequity, such as decisions concerning patterns in the production of toxics, the reduction of occupational and safety standards, changes in living standards and the targeting of toxic waste sites. In addition, we would want to measure the ongoing accumulation of poor conditions and how they influence health. Going further, it is then necessary to demonstrate how political decisions shape those conditions, generating flows of resources favoring some populations over others. Inequities in health outcomes are not random; they reflect patterns of decision making. Often there's an emphasis by researchers on measuring characteristics of people or things (toxicants) rather than the institutions that affect them. Indicators of community health would be useful, beyond medical profiles and demographics of individuals, because well-being depends on a healthy social system, on the prerequisites for self realization. Our social immune system—the infrastructure of social welfare, natural resources, transportation, public education systems—are being dismantled, along with maintenance of the infrastructure such as repairs to bridges and electrical grids.

It is crucial to explore what would constitute indicators of social injustice. Measures of social exclusion that marginalize access to public resources or that document the redistribution of wealth upward are examples. It is important to express the context that perpetuates and enables impoverishment, which in turn influences health. Identifying such indicators requires a macro-level analysis, exploring a broad range of forces, rather than isolated categories. What types of indicators might be used? What could we discover about the etiology of disease and its pathways, which offer clues about causes that could lead to action? Some possibilities are as follows:

- The turbulence of deregulated markets and investment/disinvestment and tax decisions
- Political influence that lead to a pattern of decisions that generates inequity
- Financial speculation, ecosystem destruction, decline in levels of literacy, labor market changes such as the economic division of labor, segmentation, and flows of capital, which have a tremendous impact on health
- Labor market events such as unemployment, changes in the labor supply, changes in earnings, especially the linked indicators of growing economic insecurity that create health risks
- Indicators of corporate decision patterns—such as layoffs, outsourcing, union busting, price fixing, mergers, and so forth, and health outcomes in given communities
- Production and industry processes that expose the population to unhealthy conditions
- Marketing techniques that expose populations to unhealthy products by targeting specific populations[92]

Many people in public health do not think it is possible to measure social structure, which is really about a pattern of social arrangements across a wide variety of institutions that relate to power and public resources. We can do this by asking different kinds of questions, linking the results to mortality rates and measures of life expectancy by race, ethnicity gender, and geography, which is crucial for public health practice. (The National Center for Health Statistics has standards for such measurements.)

Another promising approach to monitoring inequity is Health Impact Assessment (HIA), particularly as initiated by affected populations.[93] It is a method to engage communities and generate attention to public health consequences both of specific projects as well as public policy. The most common elements involve an "attempt to predict the future consequences for health of possible decisions; and that it seeks to inform decision-making."[94] This definition emphasizes a multidisciplinary and qualitative approach, focused primarily on indirect impacts, beyond biomedical perspectives, that can examine social and economic conditions, however difficult. Communities must participate fully in the process if it is to be legitimate and successful.

Overall, research methodologies must incorporate qualitative measures appropriate to the level of analysis for addressing health inequities and population health. Such methodologies would have a more macro-level perspective related to the characteristics of the larger social system and its institutions. Otherwise it will be extremely difficult to transcend individualist, behavioral lifestyle approaches to health policy.

A Brief Note: What Is a Social Justice Practice?

While no bright white line distinguishes a social justice-related intervention from one that is not, it seems useful to offer some general guidelines. Beyond "interventions" a social justice perspective concerns a philosophy, an approach, a way of working, as well as coordinated activity to tackle health inequities. Because health inequities derive from social and economic inequality, a social justice approach stresses imbalances in the distribution of power and targets its efforts to change that imbalance.

Thus, initiatives associated with social justice in relation to root causes of health inequity would be those that primarily emphasize fundamental public resources for healthy communities that address the reduction of social and economic inequality affecting disadvantaged populations. They might include the following:

- A living wage campaign—approximately 70 cities are now engaged in such campaigns and 121 ordinances have been enacted since about 1994. Essentially, these campaigns are about enacting local ordinances requiring private businesses that benefit from public money to pay their workers a living wage, above the minimum wage. The campaigns usually call for some degree of research into work and poverty in the area, research on city contracts, subsidies and related wage data, and often cost of living studies.
- Development of a health equity index, report card, gauge or other analytic tools to measure and promote the level and source of health inequities and indicators such as local resource distribution, housing, education, zoning, and other determinants of health inequity (see Monitoring and Surveillance).
- A comprehensive staff training program or dialogue on health inequity.
- Land use planning initiative to ensure that economic redevelopment produces health places and reduces place-based inequities in living conditions.

- Development of a method or system to ensure access to healthy food, transportation, or high-quality education.
- Addressing institutional racism (segregation, redlining by banks, legacy of slavery, toxic environments) through an educational campaign within the department and in the community that explains how racism affects health status.
- Mobilizing the population to action, forums for discussion, and mechanisms to involve residents in evaluating and monitoring conditions.

This perspective contrasts with treating primarily the consequences or symptoms of the social and economic inequalities that create health inequities, even though such actions would be valuable. Thus, for example, a rat elimination program would not qualify if it fails to address the source of a rat problem related to crowding and lack of affordable housing, which in turn may be related to discrimination. Similarly, seeking to educate the target population to change their behavior, or lifestyles, or other individualistic interventions through traditional health promotion, for example, an asthma program to provide vacuum cleaners to poor people, may be useful in addressing immediate needs, but not the originating injustice. If certain neighborhoods have excessive amounts of certain chemical agents in the water supply, a program to inform citizens to drink bottled water or put filters on their sinks might be useful, but not effective in dealing with the source of the inequity, for example, targeting low-income communities for toxic facilities.

In general, a social justice perspective is activist in its orientation, so that the health department views itself as a change agent, committed to tackling underlying causes, beyond programs and services. With a connection to social movements (civil rights, women's rights, labor, etc.), it requires changing the bureaucratic structures that inhibit moving forward and attending to emerging social trends and political power arrangements that can enhance or constrain an effective approach.

Conclusion

A growing number of LHDs are beginning to experiment with new ways to approach health inequities, many of them improvisational.[95] Success will depend on developing a comprehensive plan of action that will take time. In general, implementing a social justice perspective demands that practitioners ask questions within a broad, developmental conception of social change, such as, what structures and processes cause health inequity? Why is there health inequity?

The transformation of public health practice in the interest of realizing health equity depends on rethinking basic assumptions about what is possible and necessary to break free from limited categorical approaches and a reductive biomedical model focused on genetics and molecular-level analysis. It will mean transcending a crisis mode of functioning to long-range planning for health, recognizing the accumulation of disadvantages over the life course and increased involvement in the design of community development initiatives. Public health is typically on the defensive, expected to prove its case while decisions that make this a less healthy nation seemingly require no evidence about social and health consequences. At a minimum, public health should demand evidence.

A social justice perspective then considers basic causes of health inequity, rather than remediation; the source becomes primary over the effects. It will demand sustained attention to the preservation of natural resources, effects of ecological degradation, and the social disorganization caused by economic decay and other phenomena that create collective, population-related risks. Change will also require reimagining a form of public health practice based on principles of social justice and collective responsibility for the public's health, along with the creation of an infrastructure and network of support to sustain it. Perhaps most importantly, this work cannot be accomplished without full democratic partnerships with affected community constituencies both in deliberative planning processes and providing technical assistance incorporating their knowledge. This is a return to the roots of public health practice.

The Organization of the Book

While *Tackling Health Inequities through Public Health Practice* can be read cover to cover, its design enables readers to select material based on specific needs. Thus, it can be a reference tool in a training exercise or dialogue process, a sourcebook for case studies, or a supplement and background material to other works. Its design is not comprehensive, but instead seeks to inspire practitioners to imagine new possibilities and methodologies for coordinated action to address the root causes of health inequities.

The book is organized into 4 parts and 29 chapters. In Part I, Chapters 1–6 present introductory material as follows:

Part I: Introduction: Frameworks, Perspectives, Evidence presents a series of views on different aspects of health equity, including the underlying philosophical and social justification for it, the evidence, ways to measure it, public policy to eliminate it, and a historical view explaining the current condition of public health and how it can regain its former focus on root causes.

In Chapter 2, Amartya Sen examines the nature of health equity and its relevance for the ability to achieve good health and the connection of health equity to social justice. Fabienne Peter in Chapter 3 explores issues related to making judgments about unfairness and injustice in our institutions generally to those specifically connected to health inequality. Such an examination, in her estimation, may enable us to determine how a society can be made more just. Chapter 4, by Laura D. Kubzansky et al., describes the burden of health inequity and its causes in the United States by applying a population perspective on premature mortality and functional disability. They argue that reducing health inequity will require acting on the entire gradient in health related to family income and devising public policy linked to public health approaches. Yukiko Asada in Chapter 5 proposes a framework for measuring the moral or ethical dimension of health inequity, based on emphasizing logical consistency from conception to measurement. She argues that a link must be made between moral concerns and their quantitative implications. Alonzo Plough in Chapter 6 examines the role of government agencies at all levels, but especially locally, in contributing to the integration of principles of social justice into public health practice, including an agenda and examples.

Part II, Racism, Class Exploitation, Gender Discrimination, and Health: Exposing the Roots, offers a detailed look at the root causes of health inequity, based on class exploitation, racism, and sexism. In Chapter 7, Keith Lawrence and colleagues explore the character of linked policies, across many of our institutions, which sustain racism. Specifically, they consider "how race shapes political, economic, and cultural life in the United States, and offer insights for integrating a racial equity perspective into the work of community building and socioeconomic justice." Chapter 8, by Rodrick Wallace et al., considers how hierarchy, in this case racism, becomes part of human biology, negatively affecting many biological systems over the life course. David Williams and Pamela Braboy Jackson, in Chapter 9, outline how various social factors can "initiate and sustain racial disparities in health." They then evaluate policy implications related to segregation and reducing income differentials. Chapter 10 by Carles Muntaner et al. examines the evidence on the relation between social class and psychiatric disorders in order to clarify the importance and role of class exploitation in the production of illness. Chapter 11 by David Coburn, critiques the income inequality approach to health inequalities, emphasizing a class-based approach emphasizing causes over consequences. He contends that neoliberal policies associated with the power of business have increased inequalities with negative affects on health. In Chapter 12, Gita Sen and Piroska Ostlin analyze how gender relations of power in daily life generate gender inequalities that negatively influence women's health. Beyond issues of economic distribution, they explore connections to race, class, caste, and sexual orientation.

Part III, Practitioners Take Action: Strategies for Organizational Change and Working with Communities presents examples and experiences from selected LHDs in the midst of identifying promising strategies to tackle health inequities and engaging in partnerships with their community constituents. These practitioners' stories, experiments, emerging efforts, and descriptive accounts reflect an attempt to respond to theory but in no way match the perspectives in Part II. Practitioners are offering their own conceptual frameworks and interpretations in the context of how they took action. The variety demonstrates many ideas of translating theory to practice. Most of their initiatives have not yet been evaluated. We are at the beginning of a movement in public health where recognition exists of connections to larger movements. However, these examples are challenges and express the difficulty of making changes and gaining support within existing structures. Moreover, these practitioners are not typically theoreticians with well worked out frameworks. But their aim and objective suggest opportunities and options.

Chapter 13 by Doak Bloss outlines a methodology for engaging employees in an LHD and neighborhood residents in a long-term dialogue process to address the root causes of health inequities based in class, racism, and gender exploitation. Adewale Troutman, in Chapter 14 outlines the development and potential of the Center for Health Equity in the Louisville Public Health Department, one of the first in the country. Bob Prentice and Njoke Thomas in Chapter 15 describe the workings and objectives of the BARHII, an effort to establish a regional organization that would explore ways to transform public health practice to achieve health equity. In Chapter 16, Rajiv Bhatia and colleagues offer "practice stories," principles, and actions from San Francisco, to guide LHDs to engage effectively in health equity work. In Chapter 17 Rajiv Bhatia and Mitchell Katz explore the health benefits of a living wage and the role a health department can play in documenting and supporting its implementation. They estimate the magnitude of health improvements due to a proposed living wage ordinance. In Chapter 18, Rajiv Bhatia analyzes the role of the health impact assessment in accounting for social determinants of health not often considered in land use decisions. Mele Lau Smith and colleagues in Chapter 19 analyze their efforts to implement the Community Action Model (CAM) as part of the San Francisco Tobacco Free Project, a social justice approach based on the theory of

Paulo Freire. Anthony B. Iton, et al., in Chapter 20, explore a community-led, multicomponent public health intervention to build neighborhood level community capacity in the Alameda County Public Health Department in California. Ngozi Oleru and colleagues in Chapter 21 offer a description of perhaps the first effort in the United States explicitly to incorporate principles of equity and social justice in all major county-wide decision making in Seattle-King County, WA. Chapter 22 by Jason Corburn explores the centrality of community-generated knowledge as a means to improve environmental decision making, particularly as it relates to issues of environmental justice. He argues for a comprehensive fusing of professional and lay knowledge in order to democratize inquiry in ways that meet community needs. Baker Salsbury and colleagues in Chapter 23, also examine an initiative begun in Connecticut, the Health Equity Index, designed to document the root causes of health inequity by engaging fully with community residents. Finally, Gail Christopher and colleagues in Chapter 24 describe the objectives of a foundation-funded initiative *Place Matters*, which established partnerships among health departments, community organizations, and county governments in 22 jurisdictions to design collaborative strategies for addressing health inequity.

Part IV, Shifting Consciousness and Paradigms examines efforts to shift the paradigm of how practitioners and the public think about health equity and suggests ways to break out of traditional understandings of why some populations get sick and others do not.

Larry Adelman, in Chapter 25, detail how the PBS documentary series *Unnatural Causes: Is Inequality Making Us Sick?* can be used effectively as a consciousness raising and organizing tool. He highlights how the series was part of a larger, broad-based public campaign, working collaboratively with many constituencies. Chapter 26 by Lawrence Wallack and Regina Lawrence examine the importance of identifying a "language of human interconnection" in order to advance egalitarian values in public policy that would support efforts to achieve health equity. Makani Themba-Nixon in Chapter 27 outlines the elements of an effective communications plan and describes how to develop compelling stories in reaching out to the mass media. Anthony Iton critiques the biomedical paradigm in Chapter 28 and its limits for addressing health inequities. Finally, Carles Muntaner and Haejoo Chung in Chapter 29 examine the barriers and opportunities to teaching social inequalities in health, including effective teaching methods to overcome them. He explores both epistemologies that constrain critical thinking as well as labor practices that exploit those who teach about inequity and funding sources that dictate research questions.

Notes

1. See for example, Joannes Siegrist and Michael Marmot eds., *Social Inequalities in Health: New Evidence and Policy Implications* (Oxford: Oxford University Press, 2006); T.A. LaVeist, "Segregation, Poverty, and Empowerment: Health Consequences of African Americans, in *Race, Ethnicity, and Health: A Reader*, ed. T.A. LaVeist (San Francisco, CA: Jossey-Bass, 2002).

2. Margaret Whitehead, "The Concepts and Principles of Equity and Health," 22(3) *International Journal of Health Services* (1992): 430; See Margaret Whitehead, *The Health Divide: Inequalities in Health in the 1980s* (London: Health Education Council, 1987); G. Dahlgren and M. Whitehead, *Policies and Strategies to Promote Social Equality in Health* (Stockholm: Institute of Future Studies, 1991); M. Whitehead and F. Diderichsen, "International Evidence on Social Inequalities in Health," in *Health Inequalities—Decennial Supplement*, ed. F. Drever and M. Whitehead, DS Series No. 15, Office for National Statistics (London: The Stationery Office, 1997): 45–69. NACCHO uses the term health inequities rather than disparities because the latter does not convey the injustice underlying the differences in health status. That is, the needed response is not to any difference but to those that are actionable, avoidable, and unjust. At the same time, we seek to highlight the way in which social and organizational policy as well as institutional discrimination and oppression affect population health.

3. See, for example, Steven H. Woolf, Robert E. Johnson, and Jack Geiger, "The Rising Prevalence of Severe Poverty in America: A Growing Threat to Public Health," 31(4) *American Journal of Preventive Medicine* (2006): 332–341; Edward N. Wolff, "Racial Wealth Disparities: Is the Gap Closing?" Policy Brief No. 66. (New York: Levy Institute, 2001); Edward N. Wolff, "Recent Trends in Living Standards in the United States," (New York: The Jerome Levy Economics Institute, May, 2001); John Schmitt, "Labor Markets and Economic Inequality in the United States Since the End of the 1970s," in *Neoliberalism, Globalization, and Inequalities: Consequences for Health and Quality of Life*, ed. Vicente Navarro (Amityville, NY: Baywood, 2007); Richard Wilkinson, *The Impact of Inequality: How to Make Sick Societies Healthier* (New York: The New Press, 2005), 6. See also Thomas LaVeist ed., *Race, Ethnicity, and Health: A Public Health Reader* (San Francisco, CA: Jossey-Bass, 2002); Hilary Graham ed., *Understanding Health Inequalities* (Buckingham: Open University Press, 2000), 4; G. Pappas, S. Queen, W. Hadden, and G. Fisher, "The Increasing Disparity Between Socioeconomic Groups in the United States." 329 *New England Journal of Medicine* (1993): 103–109. For an analysis of more recent data see Jared Berenstein, "Updated U.S. Congressional Budget Office Data Reveal Unprecented Increase in Inequality" 38(3) *International Journal of Health Services* (2008): 431–437.

4. Gary Teeple, *Globalization and the Decline of Social Reform: Into the Twenty-First Century* (Aurora, ON: Garamond Press, 2000); Robert Beaglehole and Ruth Bonita, *Public Health at the Crossroads: Achievements and Prospects* (Auckland, Cambridge: Cambridge University Press, 1997); Ronald Labonte, "International Governance and World Trade Organization (WTO) Reform" 12(1) *Critical Public Health* (1998): 93–104; R.Wilkinson and M. Marmot, eds., The Social Determinants of Health (Oxford: Oxford University Press,

1998); Peter Arno and Janis Barry Figueroa, "The Social Determinants of Health," in *Unconventional Wisdom: Alternative Perspectives on the New Economy*, ed. Jeff Madrick (New York: New Century Foundation Press, 2000) 93–104; Alex Callinicos, *Equality* (Cambridge: Polity Press, 2000); P.H. Lindert, "When Did Inequality Rise in Britain and America?" 9(1) *Journal of Income Distribution* (2000): 11–25.

5. John Schmitt, "Labor Markets and Economic Inequality in the United States Since the End of the 1970s," in ed. V. Navarro, Note 1; Bruce Kennedy and Ichiro Kawachi, *Is Inequality Bad for Our Health?* (Boston, MA: Beacon Press, 2000).

6. See Lawrence Mishel, Jared Bernstein, and Sylvia Allegreto, *The State of Working America 2006–2007* (Ithaca, NY: Cornell University Press, 2007); "The Wealth Divide: The Growing Gap in the United States Between the Rich and the Rest," an Interview with Edward Wolff, Multinational Monitor (May, 2003), available at http://www.multinationalmonitor.org/mm2003/03may/may03interviewswolff.html; Edward N. Wolff, "Recent Trends in Household Wealth in the United States: Rising Debt and the Middle-Class Squeeze," The Levy Economics Institute Working Paper No. 502 (New York: Levy Economics Institute, June 2007).

7. U.S. Bureau of the Census, *U.S. Census Bureau News* (Washington, DC, August 26, 2004). See also Nancy Krieger, "Why Epidemiologists Cannot Afford to Ignore Poverty," 18(6) *Epidemiology* (November, 2007): 658–663.

8. Sarah Burd-Sharps, Kristen Lewis, and Eduardo Borges Martins, *The Measure of America: American Human Development Report, 2008–2009* (New York: Columbia University Press, 2008); Sheldon Danziger, Sandra Danziger, and Jonathan Stern, "The American Paradox: High Income and High Child Poverty," in *The Political Economy of Inequality*, ed. Frank Ackerman,. Neva Goodwin, Laurie Dougherty, and Kevin Gallagher, (Washington, DC: Island Press, 2000): 351–354; George A. Kaplan, Susan A. Everson, and John Lynch, "The Contribution of Social and Behavioral Research to an Understanding of the Distribution of Disease: A Multilevel Approach," in *Promoting Health: Intervention Strategies from Social and Behavioral Research*, ed. Brian D. Smedley and S. Leonard Syme (Washington, DC: Institute of Medicine, National Academy of Sciences, 2000): 37–81; Edward N. Wolff, *Top Heavy: A Study of the Increasing Inequality of Wealth in America* (New York: The Twentieth Century Fund, 1995); Robert Reich, "The Missing Options" 35 *The American Prospect* (1997): 6–13.

9. See Dennis Raphael, "A Society in Decline: The Political, Economic and Social Determinants of Health Inequalities in the United States," in *Health and Social Justice: Politics, Ideology, and Inequity in the Distribution of Disease*, ed. Richard Hofrichter (San Francisco. CA: Jossey-Bass, 2003); RWJ Commission.

10. See Commission to Build A Healthier America, "Overcoming Obstacles to Health," Report from The Robert Wood Johnson Commission to the Commission to Build A Healthier America, New Jersey, 2008; Robert Pear, "Gap in Life Expectancy Widens for the Nation," *New York Times* (March 23, 2008); David R. Williams and A.M. Chung "Racism and Health," in *Health in Black America*, ed. R. Gibson and J.S. Jackson (Thousand Oaks, CA: Sage, 2001).

11. G. A. Kaplan, E. Pamuk, J.W. Lynch, J.W. Cohen, and J.L. Balfour, "Income Inequality and Mortality in the United States: Analysis of Mortality and

Potential Pathways" 312 *British Medical Journal* (1996): 999–1003; John W. Lynch, George Davey Smith, George A. Kaplan, and James S. House, "Income Inequality and Mortality: Importance to Health of Individual Income, Psychosocial Environment, or Material Conditions" 320 *British Medical Journal* (April 29, 2000): 1200–1204; Howard Waitzkin, "Political Economic Systems and the Health of Populations: Historical Thought and Current Directions," in *Macro Determinants of Population Health*, ed. Sandro Galea, (Secaucus, NJ: Springer, 2007), Chapter 5; Robert Hunter, "Should We Worry about Income Inequality," in ed. V. Navarro, 2007, Note 3.

12. Stephen Bezruchka, "Improving Economic Equality and Health: The Case of Postwar Japan," 98(4) *American Journal of Public Health* (April, 2008): 1–6; Richard Wilkinson, *Unhealthy Societies: The Afflictions of Inequality* (New York: Routledge, 1996). See also Stephen Bezruchka, "Societal Hierarchy and the Health Olympics," 164(12) *Canadian Medical Association Journal* (June 12, 2001): 1701–1703.

13. World Health Organization, "WHO Issues New Healthy Life Expectancy Rankings," Press Release WHO, Washington, DC and Geneva, Switzerland (June 4, 2000). In 2005, the United State has dropped to 29th; see also Bezruchka, 2001, Note 12.

14. Nancy Krieger, "A Glossary for Social Epidemiology," 55 *Journal of Epidemiology and Community Health* (2001): 693–700.

15. See George Rosen, *A History of Public Health* (London: Johns Hopkins University Press, 1993 [1958]); Christopher Hamlin, *Public Health and Social Justice in the Age of Chadwick: Britain 1800–1854* (London: Cambridge University Press, 1998); Vincente Navarro, "Health and Inequalities Research," 34 *International Journal of Health Services* (2004): 87–99; Dorothy Porter, *Health Civilization and the State: A History of Public Health from Ancient to Modern Times* (London: Routledge, 1999).

16. Burd-Sharps et al., Note 8: 163.

17. See Note 15.

18. Dan E. Beauchamp, *Health of the Republic: Epidemics, Medicine and Moralism as Challenges to Democracy* (Philadelphia, PA: Temple University Press, 1988) 17.

19. Porter, Note 15; Rosen, Note 15; Nancy Krieger and Anne-Emannuelle Birn, "A Vision of Social Justice as the Foundation of Public Health: Commemorating 150 Years of the Spirit of 1848," 88(11) *American Journal of Public Health* (November, 1998): 1603–1606.

20. See for example Frederick Engels, *The Condition of the Working Class in England* (London: Allen and Unwin, 1952); George Rosen, Note 1; Rudolph L. Virchow, *Disease, Life and Man: Selected Essays* (Stanford, CA: Stanford University Press, 1958); Christopher Hamlin, Note 15.

21. Beauchamp, Note 18; Note 19.

22. Christopher Hamlin, Note 15; I. Sram and J. Ashton, Millennium Report to Sir Edwin Chadwick, 317 *British Medical Journal* (1998): 592–596.

23. Nancy Krieger, "Epidemiology and the Web of Causation: Has Anyone Seen the Spider?," 39(7) *Social Science & Medicine* (1994): 887–903.

24. Nancy Krieger, "Researching Critical Questions on Social Justice and Public Health: An Ecosocial Perspective," in *Social Injustice and Public Health*, ed. Barry Levy and Victor Sidel (New York: Oxford University Press, 2006): 460–479.

25. See for example, Donald Acheson, *Independent Inquiry into Inequalities in Health* (London: The Stationery Office, 1998); Benjamin Amick, C. S. Levine, A.R. Tarlov, and D.C. Walsh eds., *Society and Health* (New York: Oxford University Press, 1995); George Davey Smith, Daniel Dorling, and Mary Shaw, eds., *Poverty, Inequality and Health in Britain: 1800–2000, A Reader* (Bristol: Policy Press, 2001); F. Diderichsen, T. Evans, and M. Whitehead, "The Social Basis of Disparities in Health," in *Challenging Inequities in Health: From Ethics to Action*, ed. Timothy Evans, Margaret Whitehead, Finn Diderichsen, Abbas Bhuia, and Meg Wirth (New York: Oxford University Press, 2001): 13–23; Paul Farmer, *Infections and Inequalities: The Modern Plagues* (Berkeley, CA: University of California Press, 1999); Arline T. Geronimus and J. Phillip Thompson, "To Denigrate, Ignore, or Disrupt: Racial Inequality in Health and the Impact of a Policy-Induced Breakdown of African American Communities" 1 *Du Bois Review* (2004): 247–79; G. A. Kaplan, E. Pamuk, J.W. Lynch, J.W. Cohen, and J.L. Balfour, "Income Inequality and Mortality in the United States: Analysis of Mortality and Potential Pathways" 312 *British Medical Journal* (1996): 999–1003; Diana Kuh, Rebecca Hardy, Claudia Langenberg, Marcus Richards, and Michael E.J. Wordsworth, "Mortality in Adults Aged 26–54 Years Related to Socioeconomic Conditions in Childhood and Adulthood: Post War Birth Cohort Study," 325 *British Medical Journal* (November 9, 2002): 1076–1080.
26. Hamlin, Note 15.
27. Dennis Raphael, *Social Justice is Good for Our Hearts: Why Societal Factors—Not Lifestyles—are Major Causes of Heart Disease in Canada and Elsewhere* (Toronto: CSJ Foundation for Research and Education, 2002); David Coburn, "Beyond the Income Inequality Hypothesis: Class, Neo-liberalism, and Health Inequalities." 58 *Social Science & Medicine* (2004): 41–56; C. R. Ronzio, E. Pamuk, and G.D. Squires, "The Politics of Preventable Deaths: Local Spending, Income Inequality, and Premature Mortality in U.S. Cities" 58 *Journal of Epidemiology and Community Health* (2004): 175–179; Peter S. Arno and Janis Barry Figueroa. "The Social and Economic Determinants of Health," in *Unconventional Wisdom: Alternative Perspectives on the New Economy*, ed. Jeff Madrick (New York: The Century Foundation Press, 2000) 93–104; Nancy E. Adler, Michael Marmot, Bruce S. McEwen, and Judith Stewart eds., *Socioeconomic Status and Health in Industrial Nations: Social, Psychological, and Biological Pathways* (New York: New York Academy of Sciences, 1999).
28. Mindy Fullilove, *Root Shock: How Tearing Up City Neighborhoods Hurts America and What We Can Do About It* (New York: One World, 2004); Ichiro Kawachi and Lisa F. Berkman, *Neighborhoods and Health* (New York: Oxford University Press, 2003).
29. Robert Beaglehole, *Global Public Health: A New Era* (Oxford: Oxford University Press, 2003): 3.
30. J. M. McGinnis and William H. Foege, "Actual Causes of Death in the United States" 270 *Journal of the American Medical Association* (1993): 2207–2212.
31. Robert Chernomas, *The Social and Economic Causes of Disease*, (Manitoba: Canadian Centre for Policy Alternatives, March, 1999).
32. Nancy Krieger, "Proximal, Distal, and the Politics of Causation: What's Level Got To Do With It," 98(2) *American Journal of Public Health* (February, 2008): 221–230.

33. See Eric Olin Wright, *Class Counts* (Cambridge: Cambridge University Press, 2000); Graham Scambler, *Health and Social Change: A Critical Theory* (Buckingham: Open University Press, 2002).
34. See Muntaner, Chapter 10, this volume; Stanley Aronowitz, *How Class Works* (New Haven, CT: Yale University Press, 2003).
35. Iris Marion Young, "Structural Injustice and the Politics of Difference," in *Social Justice and Public Policy: Seeking Fairness in Diverse Societies*, ed. Gary Craig, Tania Burchardt, and David Gordon (Bristol: The Policy Press, 2008): 80.
36. Hunter, Note 11: 114.
37. See M. Norman Oliver and Carles Muntaner, "Researching Health Inequities Among African Americans: The Imperative to Understand Social Class," 35(3) *International Journal of Health Services* (2005): 485–498.
38. Amartya Sen, *Inequality Reexamined* (Cambridge, MA: Harvard University Press, 1992); Stanley Aronowitz, Note 29.
39. Graham Scambler and Paul Higgs, "Stratification, Class and Health: Class Relations and Health Inequalities in High Modernity," 33(2) *Sociology* (1999): 275–296;
40. See Ruth Brousseau and Irene Yen, "On the Connections between Work and Health," in *Reflections* 1(3) (Woodland Hills, CA: The California Wellness Foundation, June, 2000); Ben Amick and J. Lavis, "Labor Markets and Health: A Framework and Set of Applications," in *Society and Population Health*, ed. Alvin Tarlov (New York: The New Press, 2000).
41. D. Dooley, J. Fielding, and L. Levi, "Health and Unemployment" 17 *Annual Review of Public Health* (1996): 449–465.
42. Vicente Navarro and Leiyu Shi, "The Political Context of Social Inequalities and Health" 31(1) *International Journal of Health Services* (2001): 1–21.
43. Vicente Navarro, "Health and Equity in the World in the Era of 'Globalization' " 29(2) *International Journal of Health Services* (1999): 215–226.
44. Nancy Krieger ed., *Embodying Inequality: Epidemiologic Perspectives* (Amityville, NY: Baywood Publishing, 2004). See also Rodrick Wallace et al., Chapter 8 of this volume.
45. Graham Scambler and Paul Higgs, Note 29; Graham Scambler, *Health and Social Change: A Critical Theory* (Buckingham: Open University Press, 2002).
46. See, for example, Edward N. Wolff, Note 1; Edward N. Wolff, *Top Heavy: A Study of the Increasing Inequality of Wealth in America* (New York: The Twentieth Century Fund, 1995); www.inequality.org
47. Personal conversation and presentation by Camara P. Jones at The Consumer Health Foundation Annual Meeting, Washington, DC, 2007.
48. Nancy Krieger, "Does Racism Harm Health? Did Child Abuse Exist Before 1962? On Explicit Questions, Critical Science, and Current Controversies: An Ecosocial Perspective," 93(2) *American Journal of Public Health* (2003): 194–199.
49. Rodrick Wallace, Deborah Wallace, and Robert Wallace, "Coronary Heart Disease, Chronic Inflammation, and Pathogenic Social Hierarchy: A Biological Limit to Possible Reductions in Morbidity and Mortality," 96(5) *Journal of the National Medical Association* (2004): 609–619. See also Amy Schultz and Leith Mullings eds., *Gender, Race, Class, and Health: Intersectional Approaches* (San Francisco, CA: Jossey-Bass, 2005): Chapter 1.

50. Ibid.
51. See Arline T. Geronimus and J. Phillip Thompson, "To Denigrate, Ignore or Disrupt: Racial Inequality and the Impact of a Policy-Induced Breakdown of African American Communities," 1(2) *Du Bois Review* (2004): 247–279; V. Cain, "Investigating the Role of Racial/ethnic Bias in Health Outcomes," 93(2) *American Journal of Public Health* (2003), 191–192; N.J. Waitzman and K.R. Smith, "Separate But Lethal: The Effects of Economic Segregation on Mortality in Metropolitan Areas," 76(3) *Milbank Quarterly* (1999): 341–373.
52. Waitzman, Ibid. See also Rodrick Wallace, Note 41.
53. David R. Williams, "African-American Health: The Role of the Social Environment," 75(2) *Journal of Urban Health: Bulletin of the New York Academy of Medicine* (June, 1998): 308.
54. Mary E. Northridge and Peggy Shepard, "Environmental Racism and Public Health," 87 *American Journal of Public Health* (1997): 730–732. Robert D. Bullard, *Unequal Protection: Environmental Justice and Communities of Color* (San Francisco, CA: Sierra Club Books, 1994); United Church of Christ, *Commission for Racial Justice, Toxic Waste and Race in the United States: A National Report on the Socioeconomic Characteristics of Communities with Hazardous Waste Sites* (New York: United Church of Christ, 1987); Center for Policy Alternatives, *Toxic Waste and Race Revisited* (Washington, DC, 1995). See also Delores Acevedo-Garcia, "Zip Code Level Risk Factors for Tuberculosis: Neighborhood Environment and Residential Segregation in New Jersey, 1985–1992," 91 *American Journal of Public Health* (2001): 734–741.
55. Amad Rivera, Brenda Cotto-Escalera, Anisha Desai, Jeanette Huezo, and Dedrick Muhammad, *Foreclosed: State of the Dream 2008* (Boston: United for A Fair Economy, 2008).
56. Douglas Almond, Kenneth Chay, and Michael Greenstone, "Civil Rights, the War on Poverty, and Black–White Convergence in Infant Mortality in the Rural South and in Mississippi," Paper No. 07–04, 2006; L. Mullings, "Inequality and African-American Health Status: Policies and Prospects," in *Twentieth Century Dilemmas—Twentieth Century Prognoses*, ed. W.A. VanHome and T.V. Tonnesen (Madison, WI: University of Wisconsin Institute on Race and Ethnicity, 1989): 154–182; David R. Williams, "Race and Health: Trends and Policy Implications," in *Income, Socioeconomic Status, and Health: Exploring the Relationships*, ed. James A. Auerbach and Barbara K. Krimgold (Washington, DC: National Policy Association, 2001): 71–72.
57. Arline T. Geronimus, "Understanding and Eliminating Inequalities in Women's Health in the United States: The Role of the Weathering Conceptual Framework," 56 *Journal of the American Medical Women's Association* (2001): 133–136. See Gita Sen and Piroska Ostlin, Chapter 12, this volume; Lesley Doyal, *What Makes Women Sick?: Gender and the Political Economy of Health* (Basingstoke: Macmillan, 1995).
58. Sen and Ostlin, this volume.
59. See Mel Bartley, Amanda Sacker, David Firth, and Ray Fitzpatrick, "Dimensions of Inequality and the Health of Women," in Understanding Health Inequalities, ed. Hilary Graham (ed.), (Philadelphia, PA: Open University Press, 2000): 58–78.

60. Ichiro Kawachi, B. Kennedy, V. Gupta, and D. Prothrow-Stith, "Women's Status and the Health of Men and Women: A View From the States," 48 *Social Science & Medicine* (1999): 21–32; Amy Schulz, Edith Parker, Barbara Isreal, and Tomiko Fisher, "Social Context, Stressors and Disparities in Women's Health," 56 *Journal of the Medical Women's Association* (2001): 143–149.

61. Denise Spitzer, "Engendering Health Disparities," 96 (Suppl. 2) *Canadian Journal of Public Health* (March–April, 2005): 578–596.

62. Geronimus, Note 51: 133.

63. Kawachi, et al 1998, Note 60.

64. Amartya Sen, Note 38; see also Amartya Sen, "Economic Progress and Health," in *Poverty, Inequality, and Health: An International Perspective,* ed. David Leon and Gill Walt (Oxford: Oxford University Press, 2001): 333–345.

65. See Nancy Krieger, Note 24; Lynn Weber, "Reconstructing the Landscape of Health Disparities Research: Promoting Dialogue and Collaboration between Feminist Intersectional and Biomedical Paradigms," in *Gender, Race, Class, and Health: Intersectional Approaches,* ed. Amy J. Schulz and Leith Mullings (San Francisco, CA: Jossey-Bass, 2006): 21–59.

66. John B. McKinlay, "Paradigmatic Obstacles to Improving the Health of Populations: Implications for Health Policy," 40(4) Salud Publica Mex (July–August, 1998).

67. Ibid.

68. Nancy Krieger and Anne-Emannuelle Birn, "A Vision of Social Justice as the Foundation of Public Health: Commemorating 150 Years of the Spirit of 1848," 88(11) *American Journal of Public Health* (November, 1998): 1603–1606; Bernard Turnock, *Public Health: What It Is and How It Works,* 4th ed. (Sudbury, MA: Jones and Bartlett, 2008).

69. Autonomy and liberation are two other central features of social justice.

70. For a discussion of the philosophical relation between social justice and health equity see Sudhir Anand, Fabienne Peter, and Amartya Sen eds., *Public Health, Ethics, and Equity* (New York: Oxford University Press, 2004): Introduction and Chapters 1, 2, 3, and 5.

71. Young, Note 35: 78.

72. See Phillip Green, *Equality and Democracy* (New York: New Press, 1998).

73. See David Harvey, *Justice, Nature and the Geography of Difference* (Cambridge, MA: Blackwell, 1996).

74. "Public health, suggests the Institute of Medicine (IOM), is what we do collectively to assure the conditions for people to be healthy. This conception of public health extends to societal activities well beyond those performed by governmental public health authorities....Even when confined to government, public health practice is broad in scope....[Citing the Model State Public Health Act] public health...means 'assuring the conditions in which the population can be healthy. This includes population-based or individual efforts primarily aimed at the prevention of injury, disease, or premature mortality, or the promotion of health in the community such as assessing the health needs and status of the community through public health surveillance and epidemiological research, developing public health policy, and responding to public health needs and emergencies." –James G. Hodge and Lawrence O.

Gostin, *Public Health Practice vs. Research: A Report for Public Practitioners Including Cases and Guidance for Making Decisions* (Atlanta, GA: May 24, 2004); Bernard Turnock defines public health practice as "The development and application of preventive strategies and interventions to promote and protect the health of populations," Note 68: 517.

75. Turnock, Note 68.

76. Dan E. Beauchamp, *Health of the Republic: Epidemics, Medicine and Moralism as Challenges to Democracy* (Philadelphia, PA: Temple University Press, 1988); Brian Barry, *Why Social Justice Matters* (New York: Routledge, 2005): Chapter 6.

77. I wish to thank Adam Karpati for these points.

78. National Academy of Sciences, Institute of Medicine, *The Future of the Public's Health in the 21st Century* (Washington, DC, 2003).

79. Turnock, Note 68.

80. The Genesee County Health Department has initiated such a process, as well as the Office of Minority Health and Public Policy in the Virginia Department of Public Health.

81. Phil Brown, "Popular Epidemiology and Toxic Waste Contamination: Lay and Professional Ways of Knowing," in *Illness and the Environment: A Reader in Contested Medicine*, ed. Steve Kroll-Smith, Phil Brown, and Valerie J. Gunter (New York: New York University Press, 2000): 366.

82. Berkeley Media Studies Group and The Praxis Project, *Meta Messaging: Framing Your Case and Reinforcing Your Allies* (Berkeley, CA, 2005); Hunter Cutting and Makani Themba-Nixon, *Talking the Walk: A Communications Guide to Racial Justice* (Oakland, CA: AK Press, 2005).

83. Sen, Note 38.

84. Ronald Labonte, "Social Inclusion/Exclusion and Health: Dancing the Dialectic," in *The Social Determinants of Health: Canadian Perspectives*, ed. Dennis Raphael (Toronto: Canadian Scholars Press, 2004): 253–266.

85. James Colgrave, "The McKeown Thesis: A Historical Controversy and Its Enduring Influence," 92(5) *American Journal of Public Health* (2002): 725–729.

86. Note 65: 295

87. Smedley and Syme, Note 8.

88. Jarvis T. Chen, David H. Rehkopf, Pamela D. Waterman, et al., "Mapping and Measuring Social Disparities in Premature Mortality: The Impact of Census Tract Poverty Within and Across Boston Neighborhoods, 1999–2001" 83(6) *Journal of Urban Health: Bulletin of the New York Academy of Medicine* (2006): 1063–1084.

89. see http://www.gega.org.za/index.php

90. See for example, Marianne M. Hillemeier, John Lynch, Sam Harper, and Michele Casper, "Measurement Issues in Social Determinants: Measuring Contextual Characteristics for Community Health," 38(6) Part II: *Health Services Research* (December, 2003): 1645–1718.

91. Note 89.

92. Nicholas Freudenberg and Sandro Galea, "Corporate Practices," in ed. Galea, Note 11.

93. Alex Scott-Samuel and Eileen O'Keefe, "Health Impact Assessment for Healthy Public Policy: The Way Ahead," Contributing Papers, the 3rd HIA

International Workshop on Global and Regional Challenges for Healthy Society, Nakhon Pathom, Thailand (July 19–21, 2006).

94. John Kemm, "Perspectives on Health Impact Assessment," 81(6) *Bulletin of WHO* (2003): 387.

95. Some of the most promising practices include: Louisville, KY; Alameda County, CA; Shasta County, CA, and San Francisco, CA.

2

Why Health Equity?

AMARTYA SEN

'The world...is not an inn, but a hospital,' said Sir Thomas Browne more than three and half centuries ago, in 1643. That is a discouraging, if not entirely surprising, interpretation of the world from the distinguished author of *Religio Medici and Pseudodoxia Epidemica*. But Browne may not be entirely wrong: even today (not just in Browne's 17th century England), illness of one kind or another is an important presence in the lives of a great many people. Indeed, Browne may have been somewhat optimistic in his invoking of a hospital: many of the people who are most ill in the world today get no treatment for their ailments, nor the use of effective means of prevention.

In any discussion of social equity and justice, illness and health must figure as a major concern. I take that as my point of departure – the ubiquity of health as social consideration – and begin by noting that health equity cannot but be a central feature of the justice of social arrangements in general. The reach of health equity is immense. But there is a converse feature of this connection to which we must also pay attention. Health equity cannot be concerned only with health, seen in isolation. Rather it

This chapter is reprinted with permission from *Health Economics*, 11(8)(2002): 659–666.

must come to grips with the larger issue of fairness and justice in social arrangements, including economic allocations, paying appropriate attention to the role of health in human life and freedom. Health equity is most certainly not just about the distribution of health, not to mention the even narrower focus on the distribution of health care. Indeed, health equity as a consideration has an enormously wide reach and relevance.

I shall consider three sets of issues. First, I shall begin by discussing the nature and relevance of health equity. Second, I shall go on to identify and scrutinize the distinct grounds on which it has been claimed that health equity is the wrong policy issue on which to concentrate. I hope to be able to argue that these grounds of skepticism do not survive close scrutiny. Finally, in the section dealing with general considerations and particular proposals, I shall consider some difficult issues that have to be faced for an adequate understanding of the demands of health equity. It is particularly important in this context to see health equity as a very broad discipline which has to accommodate quite diverse and disparate considerations.

Health Equity and Social Justice

I have tried to argue in an earlier work, *Inequality Reexamined*, that a theory of justice in the contemporary world could not have any serious plausibility if it did not value equality in some space – a space that would be seen as important in that theory.[1] An income egalitarian, a champion of democracy, a libertarian, and a property-right conservative may have different priorities, but each wants equality of something that is seen as valuable – indeed central – in there respective political philosophy. The income egalitarian will Prize an equal distribution of incomes; the committed democrat must insist on equal political rights of all; the resolute libertarian has to demand equal liberty; and the property-right conservative must insist on the same right of all to use whatever property each has. They all treasure – and not just by accident – equality in terms of some variable which is given a central position in their respective theories of justice. Indeed, even an aggregative focus, as Benthamite utilitarianism has, involves a connection with equality in so far as everyone would have to be treated in the same way in arriving at simple aggregates (such as the utility total). In fact, equality, as an abstract idea, does not have much cutting power, and the real work begins with the specification of what is it that is to be equalized. The central step, then, is the specification of the space in which equality is to be sought, and the equitable accounting rules that may be followed in arriving at aggregative concerns as well as distributive ones. The content of the respective theories turns on the answers to such questions as 'equality of what?' and 'equity in what form?'[2]

This is where health becomes a critical concern, making health equity central to the understanding of social justice. It is, however, important to appreciate that health enters the arena of social justice in several distinct ways, and they do not all yield exactly the same reading of particular social arrangements. As a result, health equity is inescapably multidimensional as a concern. If we insist on looking for a congruence of the different aspects of health equity before we make unequivocal judgments, then often enough health equity will yield an incomplete partitioning or a partial ordering. This does not do away with the discipline of rational assessment, or even of maximization (which can cope within completeness through reticent articulation), but it militates against the expectation, which some entertain, that in every comparison of social states there must be a full ranking that places all the alternative states in a simple ordering.[3] Indeed, even when two alternative states are ultimately ranked in a clear and decisive way, that ranking may be based on the relative weighing – and even perhaps a compromise – between divergent considerations, which retain their separate and disparate relevance even after their comparative weights have been assessed.

So what, then, are the diverse considerations? First, health is among the most important conditions of human life and a critically significant constituent of human capabilities which we have reason to value. Any conception of social justice that accepts the need for a fair distribution as well as efficient formation of human capabilities cannot ignore the role of health in human life and the opportunities that persons, respectively, have to achieve good health – free from escapable illness, avoidable afflictions and premature mortality. Equity in the achievement and distribution of health gets, thus, incorporated and embedded in a larger understanding of justice.

What is particularly serious as an injustice is the lack of opportunity that some may have to achieve good health because of inadequate social arrangements, as opposed to, say, a personal decision not to worry about health in particular. In this sense, an illness that is unprevented and untreated for social reasons (because of, say, poverty or the overwhelming force of a community-based epidemic), rather than out of personal choice (such as smoking or other risky behaviour by adults), has a particularly negative relevance to social justice. This calls for the further distinction between health achievement and the capability to achieve good health (which may or may not be exercised).This is, in some cases, an important distinction, but in most situations, health achievement tends to be a good guide to the underlying capabilities, since we tend to give priority to good

health when we have the real opportunity to choose (indeed even smoking and other addictive behaviour can also be seen in terms of a generated
'unfreedom' to conquer the habit, raising issues of psychological influences
on capability – a subject I shall not address here).

It is important to distinguish between the achievement and capability, on
the one side, and the facilities socially offered for that achievement (such
as health care), on the other. To argue for health equity cannot be just a
demand about how health care, in particular, should be distributed (contrary to what is sometimes presumed). The factors that can contribute to
health achievements and failures go well beyond health care, and include
many influences of very different kinds, varying from genetical propensi-
ties, individual incomes, food habits and lifestyles, on the one hand, to the
epidemiological environment and work condition, on the other.[4] Recently,
Sir Michael Marmot and others have also brought out the far-reaching
effects of social inequality on health and survival.[5] We have to go well
beyond the delivery and distribution of health care to get an adequate
understanding of health achievement and capability. Health equity cannot
be understood in terms of the distribution of health care.

Second, in so far as processes and procedural fairness have an inescapable relevance to social justice, we have to go beyond health achievement
and the capability to achieve health. As someone who has spent quite a bit
of effort in trying to establish the relevance of the capability perspective
(including health capabilities) in the theory of justice, I must also stress
that the informational basis of justice cannot consist only of capability
information, since processes too are important, in addition to outcomes
(seen in isolation) and the capability to achieve valued outcomes.[6] For this
reason, inequalities even in health care (and not just in health achievement) can also have relevance to social justice and to health equity, since
the process aspect of justice and equity demand some attention, without
necessarily occupying the centre of the stage.

Let me illustrate the concern with an example. There is evidence that
largely for biological reasons, women tend to have better survival chances
and lower incidence of some illnesses throughout their lives (indeed even
female fetuses have a lower probability of spontaneous miscarriage). This
is indeed the main reason why women predominate in societies with
little or no gender bias in health care (such as West Europe and North
America), despite the fact that more boys are born than girls, everywhere
in the world (and an even higher proportion of male fetuses are conceived).
Judged purely in terms of the achievement of health and longevity, this is a
gender-related inequality, which is absent only in those societies in which
anti-female bias in health care (and sometimes in nutrition as well) makes
the female life expectancy no higher than male. But it would be morally

unacceptable to suggest that women should receive worse health care than men so that the inequality in the achievement of health and longevity disappears.[7] The claim to process fairness requires that no group – in this case women – be discriminated in this way, but in order to argue for that conclusion we have to move, in one way or another, away from an exclusive reliance on health achievement.

Third, health equity cannot only be concerned with inequality of either health or health care, and must take into account how resource allocation and social arrangements link health with other features of states of affairs. Again, let me illustrate the concern with a concrete example. Suppose persons A and B have exactly similar health predispositions, including a shared proneness to a particularly painful illness. But A is very rich and gets his ailment cured or completely suppressed by some expensive medical treatment, whereas poor B cannot afford such treatment and suffers badly from the disease. There is clearly a health inequality here. Also, if we do not accept the moral standing of the rich to have privileged treatment, it is plausible to argue that there is also some violation of health equity as well. In particular, the resources used to cure rich A could have been used instead to give some relief to both, or in the case of an indivisibility, to give both persons an equal chance to have a cure through some probabilistic mechanism. This is not hard to argue.

Now, consider a policy change brought about by some health egalitarians, which gives priority to reducing health inequality. This prevents rich A from buying a cure that poor B cannot buy. Poor B's life is unaffected, but now rich A too lives with that painful ailment, spending his money instead on, say, having consoling trips on an expensive yacht on esoteric seas. The policy change does, in fact, reduce the inequality of health, but can it be said that it has advanced health equity? To see clearly the question that is being asked, note that it is not being asked whether this is a better situation overall (it would be hard to argue that it is so), nor am I asking whether it is, everything considered, a just arrangement (which, again, it is not – it would seem to be a Pareto worsening change, given A's desire to use his money to buy health, rather than a yacht). I am asking, specifically, is there more health equity here than in the former case?

I would argue that health equity has not been enhanced by making rich A go around exotic seas on his costly yacht, even though inequality in the space of health as such is reduced. The resources that are now used by rich A to go around the high seas on his yacht could have been used instead to cure poor B or rich A, or to give them each some relief from their respective painful ailments. The reduction of health inequality has not advanced health equity, since the latter requires us to consider further the possibility of making different arrangements for resource allocation, or social institutions or policies. To concentrate on health inequality only in assessing health equity is exactly similar to approaching the problem of world hunger (which is not unknown) by eating less food, overlooking the fact that any general resource can be used to feed the hungry better.

The violation of health equity cannot be judged merely by looking at inequality in health. Indeed, it can be argued that some of the most important policy issues in the promotion of health care are deeply dependent on the overall allocation of resources to health, rather than only on distributive arrangements within health care (for example, the 'rationing' of health care and other determinants of health), on which a good deal of the literature on health equity seems, at this time, to concentrate. Resources are fungible, and social arrangements can facilitate health of the deprived, not just at the cost of other people's health care or health achievement, but also through a different social arrangement or an altered allocation of resources. The extent of inequality in health cannot give us adequate information to assess health equity.

This does not, of course, imply that health inequality is not a matter of interest. It does have interest of its own, and it certainly is a very important part of our understanding of health equity, which is a broader notion. If, for example, there are gross inequalities in health achievement, which arise not from irremediable health preconditions, but from a lack of economic policy or social reform or political engagement, then the fact of health inequality would be materially relevant. Health inequalities cannot be identified with health inequity, but the former is certainly relevant to the latter. There is no contradiction here once we see health equity as a multidimensional concept.

Contrary Arguments

The claim that health equity is important can be resisted on various different grounds, involving empirical as well as conceptual arguments. In various forms these contrary arguments have been presented in professional as well as popular discussions. It is useful to examine the claims of these different arguments and to assess the relevance of health equity in the light of these critical concerns. I do this through posing some skeptical questions as a dialogic device.

Are Distributive Demands, in General, Really Relevant?

It could be argued that distributive requirements in general, including equity (not just health equity), lack ethical significance as a general principle.

Utilitarians, for example, are not particularly bothered by inequality in utilities, and concentrate instead on maximizing the distribution-independent sum-total of utilities. A fundamental rejection of inequality as a concern would inter alia reduce the relevance of health equity.

There are several different counter arguments that have to be considered in response. First, as John Rawls has argued in disputing the claims of utilitarianism, distribution in difference does not take the distinction between persons adequately seriously.[8] If a person remains miserable or painfully ill, her deprivation is not obliterated or remedied or overpowered simply by making someone else happier or healthier. Each person deserves consideration as a person, and this militates against a distribution-indifferent view. The Rawlsian counterargument is as relevant to health inequalities as it is to the inequality of well-being or utility.

Second, specifically in the field of health, there are some upper bounds to the extent to which a person can be made more and more healthy. As a result, even the engineering aspect of the strategy of compensating the ill-health of some by better and better health of another has some strict limits.

Third, even if we were somehow convinced by the distribution-indifferent view, there would still be some form of equity consideration in treating all persons in the same way in arriving at aggregate achievements (as utilitarianism does). Distribution-independent maximization of sum-total is not so much a denial of equity, but a special – and rather limited – way of accommodating equity within the demands of social justice.

Are Distributional Demands Really Relevant for Health Achievement in Particular?

It could be argued that equity may be important in some fields, but when it comes to ill-health, any reduction of illness of anyone must be seen to be important and should have the same priority no matter what a person's overall level of health, or of general opulence, is. Minimization of a distribution-independent disability-adjusted life years (DALY), which is now used quite widely, is a good example of this approach.[9]

In responding to this query, it is useful to begin by explicitly acknowledging that any improvement in anyone's health, given other things, is a good ground for recognizing that there is some social betterment. But this need to be responsive to everyone's health does not require that exactly the same importance be attached to improving everyone's health – no matter how ill they presently are. Indeed, as Sudhir Anand and Kara Hansen have argued, distribution indifference is a serious limitation of the approach of DALY.[10] The use of distribution indifference in the case of DALY works, in fact, with some perversity, since a disabled person, or one who is chronically ill, and thus disadvantaged in general, also receives less medical attention for other ailments, in the exercise of DALY minimization, and this has the effect of adding to the relative disadvantage of a person who is already disadvantaged. Rawls's criticism of the distribution indifference of utilitarianism (in not taking the difference between persons sufficiently seriously) would apply herewith redoubled force.

It is interesting to note in that context that the founders (such as Alan Williams and Tony Culyer) of the quality-adjusted life years (QALY) approach, which has some generic similarity with the DALY approach, have been keen on adjusting the QALY figures by distributional considerations.[11] Indeed, Alan Williams notes, in the context of expounding his views on what he calls the 'fair innings' argument (on which, more presently), he had 'for a long time' taken 'the view that the best way to integrate efficiency and equity considerations in the provision of health care would be to attach equity weights to QALYs.'[12] There is no particular reason to be blind to health equity while being sensitive to equity in general.

Given the Broad Ideas of Equity and Social Justice in General, Why Do We Need the More Restricted Notion of Health Equity?

It can be argued that equity-related considerations connected with health are conceptually subsumed by some broader notion of equity (related to, say, utilities or rights). Health considerations may figure inter alia in the overall analysis of social equity, but health equity, in this view, does not have a status of its own. This criticism would have considerable cogency if the idea of health equity were intended to be detached from that of equity and justice in general.

But as has been already argued in this essay, the discipline of health equity is not confined to concentrating only on inequalities in health. Health equity may well be embedded in a broader framework of overall equity, but there are some special considerations related to health that need to come forcefully into the assessment of overall justice. In doing this exercise, the idea of health equity motivates certain questions and some specific perspectives, which enrich the more abstract notion of equity in general. The fact that health is central to our well-being needs emphasis, as does the equally basic recognition that the freedoms and capabilities that we are able to exercise are dependent on our health achievements. For one thing, we are not able to do much if we are disabled or ceaselessly bothered by illness, and we can do very little indeed if we are not alive. As Andrew Marvel had noted in his 1681 poem 'To His Coy Mistress': 'The grave's fine and private place, / But none, I think, do there embrace.'

The penalty of illness may not be confined to the loss of well-being only, but also include one's lack of freedom to do what one sees as one's agency responsibilities and commitments.[13] Health and survival are central to the understanding not only of the quality of one's life, but also for one's ability to do what one has reason to want to do. The relevance of health equity for social justice in general is hard to overstress.

Is It Not the Case That Health Equity Is Subsumed by Considerations of Equity in the Distribution of Resources (Such as Incomes or What Rawls Calls 'Primary Goods')?

In this line of reasoning, it is argued that health equity may have, in principle, some importance, but it so happens that this consideration is empirically subsumed by the attention we have to pay to equity in the distribution of resources or 'primary goods', since these economic and social resources ultimately determine the state of people's health. In response, we can begin by noting that the state of health that a person enjoys is influenced by a number of different considerations which take us well beyond the role of social and economic factors. An adequate policy approach to health has to take note not only of the influences that come from general social and economic factors, but also from a variety of other parameters, such as personal disabilities, individual proneness to illness, epidemiological hazards of particular regions, the influence of climatic variations, and so on. A proper theory of health equity has to give these factors their due within the discipline of health equity. In general, in the making of health policy, there is a need to distinguish between equality in health achievements (or corresponding capabilities and freedoms) and equality in the distribution of what can be generally called health resources. While the latter has relevance, I have argued, through process considerations, it is the former that occupies a central territory of equity in general and health equity in particular.

General Considerations and Particular Proposals

I turn finally to questions and debates on substantive claims about the content of health equity. Since health equity has to be seen, as I have tried to argue, as a broad discipline, rather than as a narrow and formulaic criterion, there is room for many distinct approaches within the basic idea of health equity. But the breadth of the idea of health equity is itself in some need of defence. The problems and difficulties in taking a particularly confined interpretation of health equity do not typically lie in the relevance of what that interpretation asserts (this is, often enough, not in doubt), but rather in what it denies. It is possible to accept the significance of a perspective, without taking that perspective to be ground enough for rejecting other ways of looking at health equity, which too can be important.

Consider Alan Williams's powerful idea of a 'fair innings'[14] which relates to – but substantially extends – the approach to health equity as developed by Culyer and Wagstaff.[15] Williams develops the case for fair innings with great care, pointing to the ethics underlying the approach: 'the notion of a 'fair innings' is based on the view that we are each entitled to a certain level of achievement in the game of life, and that anyone failing to reach this level has been hard done by, whilst anyone exceeding it has no reason to complain when their time runs out'.[16] Developing this insight, Williams arrives at the position that 'if we think (as I do) that a fair innings should be defined in terms of quality adjusted life expectancy at birth, and that we should be prepared to make some sacrifice to reduce that inequality, it is quite feasible to calculate a set of weights representing the differential social value of improvements in quality-adjusted life years delivered to different sorts of people in our current situation'.

Through this procedure, Williams neatly captures the important equity issue related to the fact that the differences in prospects of a fair innings can be very large between different social classes.

There is no doubt that this approach has much to commend, and in particular it seems to deal with inter-class inequality in a fulsome way. And yet the question can be asked whether this is all that needs to be captured in applying the idea of health equity. Just to raise an elementary question, let me return to the issue of less health hazards and greater survival chances that women have compared with men. Williams notes this fact, and notes that 'the difference in life expectancy at birth between men and women in the UK is even greater than that between social classes!' He goes on to point out that the gender difference in quality-adjusted life years is comparatively less than in unadjusted life expectancy (women seem to have a tougher time than men while alive), but also notes that 'whereas nearly 80% of women will survive long enough to enjoy a fair innings (which in this case I have taken to be 60 QALYs), less than 60% of men will do so'.

Williams point out, using this line of reasoning, 'We males are not getting a fair innings!'[17] The difficult issues arise after this has been acknowledged. What should we then do? If, as the fair innings approach presumes, this understanding should guide the allocation of health care, then there has to be inequality in health care, in favour of men, to redress the balance. Do we really want such inequality in care? Is there nothing in the perspective of process equality to resist that conclusion, which would militate against providing care on the basis of the gender of the person for an identical ailment suffered by a woman and a man?

The issue of gender difference illustrates a more general problem, namely that differences in quality-adjusted life expectancy need not give us ground enough to ignore the demands of non-discrimination in certain vital fields of life, including the need for medical care for treatable ailments. Sometimes the differences are very systematic, as with gender contrasts, or for that matter with differences in age: indeed as Williams notes, 'whatever social group we belong to, the survivors will slowly improve their chances of achieving a fair innings, and as their prospects improve, the equity weights attached to them should decline.'[18] Fair innings is a persuasive argument, but not the only persuasive one. We do not, for example, refuse to take King Lear to be a tragedy on the ground that Lear had, before Shakespeare starts his story, along and good life, with many excellent 'quality-adjusted life years', adding up to more than a 'fair innings'.

This problem is not special only to Williams's proposal, but applies generally to all approaches that insist on taking a single-dimensional view of health equity in terms of achievement of health (or, for that matter, the capability to achieve health). For example, it applies just as much to the policy conclusion arrived at by Culyer and Wagstaff in their justly celebrated paper on 'equity and equality in health and health care'[19] that 'equity in health care should… entail distributing care in such a way as to get as close as is feasible to an equal distribution of health'. But should we really? A gender-check, followed by giving preference to male patients, and other such explicit discriminations 'to get as close as is feasible to an equal distribution of health' cannot but lack some quality that we would tend to associate with the process of health equity.

I should make it clear that I am not arguing for giving priority to process equity over all other considerations, including equity in health and the capability to achieve good health. Culyer and Wagstaff are right to resist that, and they would not have done better if instead they were to give absolute priority, in general, to equity in health delivery, irrespective of consequences. They take us not from the frying pan to fire, but rather from fire to the frying pan. But I want to be neither in the fire, nor in the frying pan. Health equity is a broad and inclusive discipline, and any unifocal criterion like 'fair innings' or 'equal distribution of health' cannot but leave out many relevant concerns.[20] The assertive features of what Williams, Culyer, Wagstaff and others recommend deserve recognition and support, but that should not be taken to imply the denial of the relevance of other claims (as they seem to want, through giving unconditional priority to their unifocal criterion).

To conclude, health equity has many aspects, and is best seen as a multidimensional concept. It includes concerns about achievement of health and the capability to achieve good health, not just the distribution of health care. But it also includes the fairness of processes and thus must attach importance to non-discrimination in the delivery of health care. Furthermore, an adequate engagement with health equity also requires that the considerations of health be integrated with broader issues of social justice and overall equity, paying adequate attention to the versatility of resources and the diverse reach and impact of different social arrangements.

Within this broad field of health equity, it is, of course, possible to propose particular criteria that put more focus on some concerns and less on others. I am not trying to propose here some unique and preeminent formula that would be exactly right and superior to all the other formulae that may be proposed (though it would have been, I suppose, rather magnificent to be able to ordain one canonical answer to this complex inquiry). My object, rather, has been to identify some disparately relevant considerations for health equity, and to argue against any arbitrary narrowing of the domain of that immensely rich concept. Health equity is a broad discipline, and this basic recognition has to precede the qualified acceptance of some narrow criterion or other for specific – and contingently functional – purposes. The special formulae have their uses, but the general and inclusive framework is not dispensable for that reason. We need both.

Acknowledgements

For helpful discussions, I am most grateful to Sudhir Anand, Lincoln Chen, Anthony Culyer and Angus Deaton. I would also like to acknowledge support from the Rockefeller Foundation funded project on Health Equity at the Harvard Center for Population and Development Studies.

Notes

1. A. Sen, *Inequality Reexamined* (Cambridge, MA: Harvard University Press; Oxford: Clarendon Press, 1992).
2. A. Sen, 'Equality of What?', in *Tanner Lectures on Human Values*, ed. S. McMurrin (Cambridge: Cambridge University Press, Salt Lake City: University of Utah, 1980) and see Note 1.
3. I have discussed the need for incomplete orderings and reticent articulations in A. Sen, *Collective Choice and Social Welfare* (San Francisco: Holden-Day, 1970; republished, A msterdam: North-Holland, 1979); and A. Sen, 'Maxim   is at ion and the Act of Choice', 65 *Econometrica* (1997): 745–779. Guest Editorial 665.

4. The importance of the distinction between health and health care for the determination of public policy has been well discussed, among other issues, by Jennifer Prah Ruger, *Aristotelian Justice and Health Policy: Capability and Incompletely Theorized Agreements*, (PhD diss., Harvard University, 1998).
5. See M.G. Marmot, M. Shipley, and G. Rose, 'Inequalities in Death—Specific Explanations of a General Pattern', 323 *The Lancet* (1984): 1003–1006; M.G. Marmot, G.D. Smith, S.A. Stansfeld, et al., 'Health Inequalities among British Civil Servants: The Whitehall II Study,' *Lancet* 337 (1991):1387–1393; and M.G. Marmot, M. Bobak, and G. Davey Smith, 'Explorations for Social Inequalities in Health', in *Society and Health*, ed. B.C. Amick, S. Levine, A.R. Tarlov, and D. Chapman (London: Oxford University Press, 1995), 172–210. See also R.G. Wilkinson, *The Unhealthy Societies: The Afflictions of Inequality* (New York: Routledge, 1996).
6. A. Sen, 'Well-being, Agency and Freedom: The Dewey Lectures 1984', 82 *Journal of Philosophy* (1985): 169–221; A. Sen, 'Consequential Evaluation and Practical Reason', 97 *Journal of Philosophy* (2000): 477–502.
7. Sen, 1992, Note 1.
8. J. Rawls, *A Theory of Justice* (Cambridge, MA: Harvard University Press, 1971).
9. See C.J.L. Murray, 'Quantifying the Burden of Disease: The Technical Basis for Disability Adjusted Life Years', 72 *Bulletin of World Health Organization* (1994), 429–445; C.J.L. Murray and A.D. Lopez, 'The Global Burden of Disease: A Comprehensive Assessment of Mortality and Disability From Disease, Injuries, and Risk Factors, in 1990 and Projected to 2020' (Geneva: World Health Organization, 1996); WHO, *World Health Report 2000* (Geneva: World Health Organization, 2000).
10. S. Anand and K. Hansen, 'Disability Adjusted Life Years: a Critical Review', 16(6) *Journal of Health Economics* (1997): 685–702; S. Anand and K. Hansen, 'DALYs: Efficiency versus Equity', 26(2) *World Development* (1998): 307–310.
11. The exponents of the QALY and DALY strategies have discussed their differences rather prominently in recent debates between New York and Geneva. I shall not, however, go into those differences in this Chapter.
12. A.I. Williams, 'Few are Going to Get Fair Innings, Someone Needs to Keep the Score,' in *Health, Health Care and Health Economics,* ed. M.L. Barer, T.E. Getzen, and G.L. Stoddart (New York: John Wiley and Sons, 1998), 319–330. See also A.J. Culyer and A. Wagstaff, 'Equity and Equality in Health and Health Care', 12 *Journal of Health Economics* (1993), 431–437; A.J. Culyer, 'Equality of What in Health Policy? Conflicts between Contenders', Discussion Paper No. 142, (New York: Centre for Health Economics, University of York, 1995).
13. On this see Sen, 1992, Note 1. See Gavin Mooney, 'Economics, Communitarianism, and Health Care', in *Health, Health Care, and Economics*, ed. M.L. Barer et al.(New York: John Wiley and Sons, 1998): 397–414. In the same volume see Claude Schneider-Bunner, 'Equity in Managed Competition'; Han Bleichrodt, 'Health Utility Indices and Equity Considerations'; Jeremiah Hurley, 'Welfarism, Extra-Welfarism and Evaluative Economic Analysis in the Health Sector'; and Thomas Rice, 'The Desirability of Market-Based Health Reforms: A Reconsideration of Economic Theory.'

14. A.I. Williams, 'Intergenerational Equity: An Exploration of the 'Fair Innings' Argument', 6 *Health Economics* (1997): 117–132; A.I. Williams, 'Few are Going to Get Fair Innings, Someone Needs to Keep the Score,' in *Health, Health Care and Health Economics,* ed. M.L. Barer, T.E. Getzen, and G.L. Stoddart (New York: John Wiley and Sons, 1998): 319, 330.
15. A.J. Culyer and A. Wagstaff, 1993, Note 12; and Culyer, Note 12.
16. Williams, 1998, Note 14: 319.
17. Ibid., 327.
18. Ibid., 326–327.
19. Culyer and Wagstaff, 1993, Note 12.
20. P. Anand and A. Walloo, 'Utilities versus Right to Publically Provided Goods: Arguments and Evidence from Health Care Rationing', 67 *Economica* (2000): 543–577.

3

Health Equity and Social Justice

FABIENNE PETER

I. Introduction

There is consistent and strong empirical evidence for social inequalities in health, as a vast and fast-growing literature shows. Social inequalities in health are significant variations in health outcomes (as measured by life-expectancy at birth, infant mortality, morbidity, etc.) across different social groups. Typically, the lower a group's social position, the worse the average health status of its members.[1] Gender, race, social class, occupational status, and socio-geographic location are examples of social categories that define social groups. More recently, a new set of studies has emerged that focuses on the relationship between income inequality and population health. Though still contested, the findings suggest that the more unequal a society, the worse its achievements in (aggregate) health.[2] Explanations for the occurrence of social inequalities in health are manifold and often difficult to establish.[3] The principal upshot of these studies is that one explanation that seems at first plausible, namely differences in access to

This chapter is reprinted from *Journal of Applied Philosophy*, 18(2)(2001): 159–70. Copyright 2001 John Wiley and Sons. Reproduced with permission of Blackwell Publishing Ltd.

health care, does not get us very far. Access to health care is only one social factor among others that influences people's health. The goal of empirical studies of social inequalities in health is to understand *social determinants* of health, and, increasingly, to explain the *mechanisms* or *pathways* that lead to the observed social differences in health outcomes. The latter is accompanied by a renewed interest in the social sciences and a move towards more interdisciplinary analysis of the social processes underlying inequalities in health.[4]

This development is often labelled a 'new public health', but, as for example Ann Robertson stresses, "[m]any would argue that this is not so much a new public health as a return to the historical commitments of public health to social justice."[5] In the public health field, the concern with health equity and social justice is recognized as having a normative dimension, i.e. as involving value judgements in an explicit way. According to the frequently quoted definition by Margaret Whitehead, health inequities are "differences [in health] which are unnecessary and avoidable but, in addition, are also considered unfair and unjust."[6] While it points in the right direction, this definition leaves open how we should go about making judgments of unfairness and injustice. The problem a theory of health equity faces is, therefore, how to go from the *empirical* identification of *social inequalities* in health to a *normative* judgment about *health inequities*. What is needed is a framework within which the ethical issues raised by the empirical literature can be addressed and which helps in determining which inequalities in health outcomes are unjust.

Until recently, there has been little work in ethics and political philosophy that deals with these issues. Many general theories of justice, such as John Rawls theory of justice as fairness, do not address health specifically.[7] In bioethics, efforts have tended to concentrate on access to *health care*.[8] There are, of course, good reasons for focusing on health care. The premise for any theory of justice is that there is some good that can be (re) distributed, that something can be changed about the situation that is considered unjust. If, in the context of health, the allocation of health care is perceived to be the instrument that is best suited to correct health outcomes, then conceptions of equity will concentrate on health care—not health. Furthermore, we may regard people's access to health care as being important in and of itself, independently of its contribution to an equitable distribution of health outcomes.[9] If, however, we are concerned not just with health care but also with health outcomes, and if there are serious social inequalities in health outcomes that cannot be traced back to differential access to health care, then conceptions of health equity have to go beyond health care.

The situation has started to change and a literature on public health ethics is emerging.[10] This chapter seeks to contribute to this literature by putting forward a theoretical framework for making health equity judgments.

The chapter defends what I call an *indirect* approach. I call an approach *direct* if it isolates health from other social spheres and is defined with respect to particular distributions of health outcomes—most existing approaches to health equity, as I shall explain later, are direct. An indirect approach, in contrast, is based on the premise that social inequalities in health are wrong not simply because actual health outcomes deviate from some pattern of health outcomes that is considered ideal, but rather because, and insofar as, they are the expression and product of unjust economic, social, and political institutions. It thus embeds the pursuit of health equity in the pursuit of social justice in general. In addition, the approach I shall present also stresses the reverse relationship between inequalities in health and social justice: an understanding of social inequalities in health and the mechanisms by which they are produced, may reveal something important about how the institutions of society work and may hence inform our assessment of the justice of these institutions. The emphasis placed on the larger social processes that bring about social inequalities in health is in line with the development in public health research to focus more on the 'upstream' influences on people's health.[11]

The approach I shall present is based on John Rawls theory of justice as fairness, in particular as it is presented in his later book *Political Liberalism*.[12] Although Rawls has not himself addressed the topic of health, I shall argue that the conception of justice as fairness provides a useful framework for evaluating social inequalities in health.

I shall elaborate on the distinction between direct and indirect approaches to health equity in section III and will highlight some important concepts of Rawls theory of justice as fairness in section IV. Section V synthesizes the previous two sections in a framework for health equity analysis. Before pursuing further the question of how to make judgments of health equity, it will be important to discuss the notion of health itself—this is the subject of the next section.

II. Health

What makes thinking about health equity difficult from the outset is that the concept of health itself is not easy to grasp and varies considerably across places and times. Although general observations can be made with respect to the meaningfulness of different definitions of health, it is likely that their adequacy will vary with the context in which we refer to it.

As, for example, the authors of the Black Report stress, a relationship between health and society is present not only at the level of social
inequalities in health but already at the level of health itself.[13] They argue
that the medical professions approach to health is only one among others,
and its partiality may impede finding solutions to pressing health problems. Instead of the "medical model," they advocate a "social model" of
health—grounded in the social sciences. They suggest that the role of social
studies of health problems should be "in part, to increase understanding of
the social and socio-economic factors which play a part in the promotion
of health and the causation of disease and in part to take the natural next
step and relate these factors themselves to the broader social structure."[14]

A general criticism of the medical model is that it directs too much
attention to diseases and their remedy. There is thus a danger of losing
sight of such issues as why good health is important for people, what good
health means to them, and what the broader social context is in which
the pursuit of health and the response to disease are shaped.[15] In some
sense, the WHO definition, according to which "health is a state of complete physical, mental and social well-being and not merely the absence
of disease or infirmity,"[16] and quality-of-life approaches to health can be
read as a reaction against this paradigm.[17] A definition of health as extensive as the one by WHO runs into problems of its own, however. It is
not clear in what ways health is distinct from other components of well-
being. The definition thus does not allow for the possibility that (some)
well-being might be achieved while health is bad, or that health might be
good yet well-being low. Nor is it clear how well-being can be defined in
a way that is consistent with a plurality of conceptions of the good life—a
characteristic of modern democratic societies. A further objection to the
WHO definition is that such a broad conception of health bears the danger of overly medicalizing social problems.[18] As Vincanne Adams writes in
a related context, it may treat the social pursuit of health "as a technical
problem with technical solutions, rather than a political problem with a
political solution."[19]

Amartya Sen's capability approach offers a fruitful alternative for
assessing health problems in society.[20] The idea underlying the capability
approach is that in policy evaluation, the appropriate information is
not individual utility or well-being, nor the resources people have access
to (e.g., medical care), but something in between. Sen argues that what
matters is what people can *do* with the resources they have access to—a
notion of freedom. A person's capability tries to capture that. Capability
is the set of 'functionings'—the various doings and beings'—that a person
can achieve (but may decide not to). Examples of functionings are being
adequately nourished, being able to read, or, more complex, achieving

self-respect. Sen often cites good health as an example of a functioning.[21] It may, however, be more promising to see health as a capability of its own, or, more precisely, as a sub-set of a person's capability. The idea is that health itself is composed of several functionings—such as, for example, being able to move around, not being tired, etc.

Sen leaves it largely open, which functionings should be included when assessing a particular social situation. What is more, he stresses that in each case, this will require a process of selecting the relevant functionings and weighing the relative importance.[22] Seeing health as a capability (sub-set) in this way thus accommodates the insight that defining a concept of health is a process that involves value judgments and which is potentially subject to political contestation—an issue that has just recently been stressed by Robertson in her paper on the "politics of need" and its implications for public health.[23] It recognizes that defining health and determining what counts as a health problem and what as another type of social problem is not a task that can be resolved by health specialists alone, but depends on other aspects of social institutions, and may change over time. Medicine and public health can contribute to the resolution of certain social problems, but they cannot, by themselves, determine goals and priorities for individuals and for society as a whole.

III. Direct and Indirect Approaches to Health Equity

Returning to the main subject of this paper, namely to the question of how to assess the justice or injustice of social inequalities in health, let me start by discussing the distinction between direct and indirect approaches to health equity. A direct approach sees health equity as an end in itself.[24] This is to say that the goal is to achieve justice with respect to the distribution of health outcomes, independently of, but in parallel with, justice in other spheres, such as, for example, income or education.

To give an example for a direct approach, it is sometimes assumed that what is disturbing about social inequalities in health is that the health of the population *overall* is lower than it could be. The Black Report, for example, uses this language.[25] Such an approach is informed by the utilitarian principle of maximizing overall well-being—in our case the health of the population. Utilitarianism is, however, often criticized for being blind to distributive considerations.[26] In the case of population health, a maximizing approach implies that we are indifferent between health benefits to, say, the poor and to the rich, as long as these benefits have the same impact on overall population health.

More explicitly concerned with equity are principles of *specific egalitarianism*—another family of direct approaches to health equity.[27] Egalitarian principles recognize that equality of health outcomes is hardly obtainable, but postulate it as a goal that we should strive for insofar as possible. For the bioethicist Robert Veatch,[28] for example, egalitarianism in the context of health encompasses any number of closely related positions that among other things include the moral rule that justice requires that persons be given an opportunity to have equal net welfare insofar as possible and that, applied to health care, *justice requires that persons be given an opportunity to have equal health status insofar as possible* (emphasis added).

Whitehead seems to be defending an approach of that kind when she writes that health equity is "concerned with creating equal opportunities for health and with bringing health differentials down to the lowest level possible."[29] Davidson Gwatkin, finally, articulates a third possible approach to health equity by suggesting that we should focus primarily on the health of the poor.[30] This view is akin to what is known as the "priority view" in moral philosophy. It is articulated by Derek Parfit and put forward as an alternative to egalitarianism.[31] Parfit argues that our moral concern should not be with differences in and of themselves, but rather with absolute deprivation. Improving the lot of those who suffer most will yield the greatest gain in social utility or well-being. The priority view is thus a variant of utilitarianism. Adapted to health equity—and given the premise that there is a link between health and poverty—this approach would imply giving priority to improving the health of the poor.[32]

In spite of the many differences, what characterizes such direct approaches is that a situation is judged inequitable if the health status of the population differs from what is perceived to be the ideal—whether judged by a measure of aggregate population health or by a measure that is sensitive to the distribution of health outcomes (or a combined measure).

An indirect approach, in contrast, treats the pursuit of health equity as embedded in and interlinked with the pursuit of social justice. Let me explain the idea in more detail.

There are two forms of potential interlinkage between social inequalities in health and justice. First, an indirect approach sees differences in health outcomes as inequitable if they are the result of unjust social arrangements. The emphasis thus lies not on the pattern of distribution of health outcomes, but to on the broader social processes underlying health inequalities. An indirect approach can thus make sense of the intuition that there is more reason to be concerned if we find that whites have significantly higher life-expectancy than blacks in similar socio-economic positions, than if we find that women have higher life-expectancy than men.

The second form of interlinkage pulls in the opposite direction. It is based on the premise that a society's achievements and failures in health may contain important information about the injustice of particular social arrangements and thus supplement our assessment of these arrangements in general. A couple of recent publications have explored this line of reasoning.[33] At this level, even in an indirect approach, there is a role for examining distributive patterns of health outcomes. They can provide a starting-point for an in-depth analysis of how social institutions work and the injustices they may embody.

One advantage of the indirect approach is that it provides a basis for selecting relevant social groups in the assessment and explanation of social inequalities in health. What the above example underlines is that even if a direct approach is adopted prima facie, the choice of relevant social groups is based on an implicit judgment about unjust social arrangements that disadvantage certain groups. An indirect approach makes such judgments explicit.

Moreover, by stressing interlinkages between the health sphere and other social spheres, the indirect approach avoids elevating health to an organizing principle of society, nor does it strictly privilege another social sector over health. It was argued above that health is not a static concept and that an approach to health equity should be able to accommodate this. A conception of health equity that builds exclusively on the medical model of health tends to downplay the inevitable biases and value judgments inherent in the disciplines of medicine and public health. An indirect approach to health equity is more compatible with a social model of health, which takes into account the influence of a variety of social factors on health.

It should be noted, however, that the direct and indirect approaches to health equity overlap. For it is clear that an indirect approach will need some justification for why health is considered a relevant indicator and such a justification will draw upon the nature of the good of health.[34] In other words, both need some account of why health is an important good. But they differ with respect to the context in which such an account is given and to the type of account given. While there is a tendency implicit in direct approaches to take health as an unambiguous, objective social goal, the indirect approach can better deal with the inherent complexity of health, which makes it difficult to confine health to a sphere of its own, independent of all other social spheres.

IV. A Theoretical Framework for Social Justice

Rawls' theory of justice as fairness has been the most influential theory of social justice put forward in this century.[35] As already mentioned, however, it does not specifically address the issue of health. What is more, Rawls explicitly rules out situations such as those we are interested in here. He assumes the healthy and able-bodied person as the norm and that accidents and illness are randomly distributed in society—precisely what the empirical literature on social inequalities in health shows is not the case. Rawls concedes that because accidents and illness have the potential to induce great suffering, and to hinder a person from pursuing his or her goals in life, they may require social action. But in Rawls view, social action takes the form of restoring people to good health—of providing health care.[36]

In spite of this I shall argue that the conceptions of justice as fairness and of political liberalism that Rawls has developed can provide guidelines for how to assess social inequalities in health. This section provides some necessary background. What a theory of justice must do, according to Rawls, is provide principles for the regulation of "the inequalities in life prospects between citizens that arise from social starting positions, natural advantages, and historical contingencies."[37] A key premise of Rawls theory of justice as fairness is that of society as a *fair system of co-operation*—to be understood in contrast with society as a loose association of individuals.[38] The idea of co-operation stresses a functional relation between the social division of labour in the production and distribution of social goods and the social roles and positions into which individuals are slotted. According to this view, the social conditions into which somebody is born have a profound impact on what she or he can achieve and aspires to achieve. From the point of view of justice, there is thus a limit on the claims people who do well have on their achievements. By the same token, people who do not do well may have a claim on social goods.

The principles of justice aim at regulating the terms of social co-operation. However, their scope is limited to what Rawls calls the *basic structure* of society—society's main political, social, and economic institutions. There are several reasons why Rawls focuses on the basic structure.[39] In *A Theory of Justice* Rawls explains it as follows[40]:

> The basic structure is the primary subject of justice because its effects are so profound and present from the start. The intuitive notion here is that this structure contains various social positions and that men [*sic!*] born into different positions have different expectations of life determined, in part, by the political system as well as by economic and social circumstances. In this way the institutions of society favor certain starting places over others. These are especially deep inequalities. Not only are they pervasive, but they affect men's initial chances in life; yet they cannot possibly be justified by an appeal to the notions of merit or desert. It is these inequalities, presumably inevitable in the basic structure of any society, to which the principles of social justice must in the first instance apply.[41]

The basic structure of society affects not only the distribution of material resources and through this peoples chances to carry out different life plans, but also, as Rawls emphasizes, the talents and abilities people have.[42] Moreover, what Rawls does not mention but what the literature on social inequalities in health suggests, is how social arrangements affect peoples life-expectancy and general prospects of health. I shall come back to this issue in the next section.

The main idea expressed in the principles of justice as fairness is that social and economic inequalities are tolerated in the basic structure of society insofar as they do not jeopardize the fundamental equality of all members of society. More precisely, justice is seen as undermined if society's main economic, social and political institutions require sacrifices from the worse-off groups purely to the benefit of the better-off groups. Such a social division of labour would not be compatible with the idea of society as a "fair system of cooperation."

V. Health Equity and the Justice of Society's Basic Institutions

What does this interpretation of justice imply for an approach to health equity? I will argue that it would be incompatible with what I called a direct approach to health equity. The principal reason is related to taking as a starting-point for a theory of justice the premise that societies are characterized by a pluralism of religious, philosophical, and moral doctrines.[43] This implies that justice cannot be based on some notion of the common good, nor on some shared notion of individual well-being. Rawls explicitly rejects assessing justice on the grounds of some account of well-being.[44] In consequence, an interpretation of health that stresses well-being, such as the WHO definition, would not be compatible with Rawlsian justice. Similarly, a notion of health that claims to be objective and value-free, but that in fact is not, would not be appropriate.

Moreover—and again in respect of pluralism—justice as fairness refrains from specifying a particular distributive pattern for certain goods:

> [T]he two principles of justice do not insist that the actual distribution conform at any given time...to any observable pattern, say equality, or that the degree of inequality computed from the distribution fall within a certain range, say of values of the Gini coefficient.[45]

For this reason, a Rawlsian approach to health equity is necessarily an indirect approach.[46] In the passage just quoted, Rawls continues: "What is enjoined is that (permissible) inequalities should make a certain functional contribution to the expectations of the least favored, where this functional contribution results form the working of the system of entitlements set up in public institutions." The idea here is that how basic social institutions work is more important than the resulting outcomes—as characterized by distributive patterns—that are observed. In Rawlsian justice, the focus is thus shifted from health outcomes to the mechanisms implicit in basic social institutions that produce social inequalities in health.

Above, I introduced two forms of interlinkage between social inequalities in health and justice. How do they relate to Rawlsian justice? On the one hand, justice as fairness offers a framework for evaluating social inequalities in health—for making health equity judgments. It points to the particular weight of inequalities that can be traced back to society's principal social and economic institutions. And it identifies as unjust those class, race, gender or socio-geographical inequalities in health that originate in the basic structure of society and are the result of a social division of labour that benefits the better-off groups at the expense of the worse off. Again, the goal is not to achieve a specific pattern of health outcomes, but a just basic structure of society. If the basic structure is just, then all outcomes these institutions produce can be considered just.[47]

On the other hand, research on social inequalities in health and their causes may tell us something about whether basic social arrangements have the effect of undermining the fundamental equality of all members of society— whether these arrangements do or do not constitute a "fair system of social cooperation." Because of the links the empirical literature on social inequalities in health demonstrates between cultural, social, and economic parameters and health outcomes, such information can supplement economic and sociological information about the achievements of different social arrangements in the basic structure of society and their changes over time.

At this stage, it will be important to discuss a possible objection to this approach. It may be argued that the correct way to apply Rawlsian justice is to say that since health does not enjoy special status in justice as fairness, all social inequalities in health must be regarded as just, provided that the basic structure of society is just. In other words, this argument perceives only a one way relationship between justice as fairness and social inequalities in health and fails to recognize how information about social inequalities in health may help one in assessing the justice of the basic structure. This particular link between justice as fairness and social inequalities in health requires further justification, therefore. In principle, justice as fairness suggests that the basic structure of society should be evaluated on the basis of 'primary goods.'[48] The list of primary goods includes basic rights and liberties, and income and wealth, among other things, but not health. The most important primary good, according to Rawls, is the social basis for self-respect.[49]

This stems again from the idea of society as a fair system of co-operation, which requires that nobody is excluded a priori. If inequalities in the basic social arrangements which shape individual lives express a disvaluation of certain social positions and occupations in such a way that people cannot gain a sense of self-respect, then these structures are unjust.

The notion of social bases of self-respect is of course very ambiguous and needs specification. In general, it can be said that the *implementation* of Rawlsian justice cannot avoid taking into account information that reaches beyond the primary goods framework that Rawls has laid out. Health information—in particular, research that attempts to uncover the more "upstream" causes of social inequalities in health—may play an important role in gaining understanding about how the organization of the basic structure of society affects people and groups of people. For instance, discrimination and lack of social respect seem to show in health outcomes (among other variables), as recent studies on inequalities between blacks and whites in the US demonstrate.[50]

VI. Concluding Remarks

This paper has outlined an approach to health equity that proceeds indirectly and embeds health equity within the general pursuit of social justice. Building on Rawls theory of justice as fairness, it was argued that social inequalities in health are unjust or inequitable if they result from an unjust basic structure of society—i.e. a basic structure that imposes sacrifices to the worse-off only to benefit the already better-off groups. This entails that to be able to form a judgment on social inequalities in health, we need an understanding of the underlying causes. At the same time, information about the health status of people may give us important information to assess the justice of social arrangements. Understanding the effects the basic structure has on people's prospects of health may help us decide whether or not these institutions ensure the social bases for self-respect for everybody. While justice as fairness cannot offer a complete blueprint of what a just society would look like, it certainly provides a framework for thinking about issues related to social justice.

Acknowledgements

I have benefited from so many people, that it is impossible to acknowledge everybody. But I would like to thank those in the Global Health Equity Initiative who made me start thinking about these issues; I am particularly grateful to Ben Amick, Sudhir Anand, and Tim Evans. I would also like to thank Sissela Bok, Norman Daniels, and Dan Wikler for very helpful comments.

Notes

1. See Michael Marmot, G. Rose, M. Shipley, and P. Hamilton, 'Employment Grade and Coronary Heart Disease in British Civil Servants,' 32 *Journal of Epidemiology and Community Health* (1978):244–249; Sir Douglas Black, J.N. Morris, Cyril Smith, and Peter Townsend *Inequalities in Health: The Black Report*, ed. Peter Townsend and Nick Davidson (London: Penguin, 1990); Nancy Krieger, D. L. Rowley, A.A. Herman, B. Avery, and M.T. Phillips, 'Racism, Sexism, and Social Class: Implications for Studies of Health, Disease and Well Being,' 9(Supplement) *American Journal of Preventive Medicine* (1993): 82–122; Davidson R. Gwatkin and Michel Guillot, *The Burden of Disease among the Global Poor: Current Situation, Future Trends, and Implications for Strategy* (Washington D.C.: International Bank for Development and Reconstruction and World Bank, 2000).
2. See R. Wilkinson, *Unhealthy Societies: The Afflictions of Iinequality* (London and NewYork: Routledge, 1996); Ichiro Kawachi, Bruce Kennedy, and Richard G. Wilkinson, *Income Inequality and Health* (New York: New Press, 1999).
3. For a good review, see Michael Marmot, Martin Bobak, and George Davey Smith, 'Explanations for Social Inequalities in Health,' in *Society and Health*, ed. Benjamin C. Amick, S. Levine, A.R. Tarlov, and D. Chapman Walsh (New York and Oxford: Oxford University Press, 1995):172–210.
4. C.F. Lisa, F. Berkman, Thomas Glass, Ian Brissette, and Teresa E. Seeman, 'From Social Integration to Health: Durkheim in the New Millenium,' 51 *Social Science and Medicine* (2000): 843–857.
5. Ann Robertson, 'Critical Reflections on the Politics of Need: Implications for Public Health,' 47(10) *Social Science and Medicine* (1998): 1419–1430. On this, see also N. Krieger and A.-E. Birn, 'A Vision of Social Justice as the Foundation of Public Health: Commemorating 150 Years of the Spirit of 1848,' 88(11) *American Journal of Public Health* (1998): 1603–1606.
6. Margaret Whitehead, *The Concepts and Principles of Equity and Health* (Copenhagen: World Health Organization, 1990): 5.
7. John Rawls, *A Theory of Justice* (Cambridge, MA: Harvard University Press, 1971).
8. See Norman Daniels, *Just Health Care* (Cambridge: Cambridge University Press, 1985).
9. As Poland et al. have stressed, the population health perspective should not be read as implying that health care is not important. See B. Poland, D. Coburn, A. Robertson, and J. Eakin, 'Wealth, Equity and Health Care: a Critique of a Population Health Perspective on the Determinants of Health,' 46(7) *Social Science and Medicine* (1998): 785–798.
10. Joao Pereira, 'What Does Equity in Health Mean?' 22(1) *Journal of Social Policy* (1993): 19–48; Sarah Marchand, Daniel Wikler, and Bruce Landesman, 'Class, Health, and Justice,' 76(3) *The Milbank Quaterly* (1998): 449–468;

Dan Beauchamp and Bonnie Steinbock, *New Ethics for the Publics Health* (New York: Oxford University Press, 1999); Norman Daniels, Bruce Kennedy, and Ichiro Kawachi, 'Health and Inequality, or Why Justice is Good for Our Health,' in *Public Health, Ethics, and Equity,* ed. Sudhir Anand, Fabienne Peter, and Amartya Sen (Oxford: Oxford University Press, 2004): 63–92.

11. See for example the contributions in Amick, et al., Note 2.

12. John R. Rawls, *Political Liberalism* (New York: Columbia University Press, 1993).

13. Black et al., Note 1.

14. Ibid., 36.

15. Rene Leriche wrote: 'in disease, when all is said and done, the least important thing is man' (quoted in G. Canguilhem) *The Normal and the Pathological* (New York: Zone Books, 1991): 92. Critical medical anthropology in particular examines the meaning of illness for people. See, for example, A. Kleinman, *The Illness Narratives: Suffering, Healing, and the Human Condition* (New York: Basic Books, 1988); E. Corin, 'The Cultural Frame: Context and Meaning in the Construction of Health,' in *Society and Health,* ed. B. Amick III, S. Levine, A. Tarlov, and D.C. Walsh (New York and Oxford: Oxford University Press, 1995): 272–304; A.W. Frank, *The Wounded Storyteller: Body, Illness, and Ethics* (Chicago: University of Chicago Press, 1995). See also M. Foucault, *The Birth of the Clinic* (New York: Pantheon Books, 1973) for an account of the development of the biomedical model and its political context.

16. World Health Organization, *World Health Organization: Basic Documents,* 26th ed., (Geneva: World Health Organization, 1976): 1.

17. Brock discusses the switch that has taken place in the public policy context from the biomedical model to a quality-of-life approach for evaluating health and the implications thereof for social evaluation ingeneral. See D. Brock, 'Quality of Life Measures in Health Care and Medical Ethics' in *Quality of Life,* ed. M. Nussbaum and A. Sen (Oxford: Clarendon Press, 1993): 95–132.

18. H.T.J. Englehardt writes: 'Medicine medicalizes reality. It translates sets of problems into its own terms. Medicine molds the ways in which the world of experience takes shape; it conditions reality for us,' in *The Foundations of Bioethics* (Oxford and New York: Oxford University Press, 1986): 157. A few pages below (ibid, 163) he adds, 'Seeing an element of life as a medical problem raises more than issues of scientific medicine. The medicalization of reality raises issues of public policy and of ethics.'

19. V. Adams, *Doctors for Democracy: Health Professionals in the Nepal Revolution* (Cambridge: Cambridge University Press, 1998): 6. See also V. Das, *What Do We Mean by Health?* (Baltimore: Johns Hopkins University, n.d., *mimeo*).

20. Sen provides a good overview of the capability approach, see M. Nussbaum and A. Sen eds., Note 17.

21. For example, Sen, ibid.: 31.

22. Nussbaum, in some contrast to Sen, argues for a specific set of capabilities. See M.C. Nussbaum, 'Morality, Politics, and Human Beings: II. Human Functioning and Social Justice: In Defense of Aristotelian Essentialism' 20(2) *Political Theory* (1992): 202–246.

23. Robertson, Note 5.

24. For a good review of such approaches, see Marchand, Wikler, and Landesman, Note 10.
25. Black et al., Note 1. I owe this point to Marchand, Wikler, and Landesman, Note 10.
26. A critique of utilitarianism can be found in Rawls, Note 7: 22–33; Rawls formulated his theory of justice as fairness as an alternative to utilitarianism. See also B. Williams, 'A Critique of Utilitarianism,' in *Utilitarianism: For and Against*, ed. J.J.C. Smart and B. Williams (Cambridge: Cambridge University Press, 1973): 77–150.
27. I borrowed the term 'specific egalitarianism' from Marchand, Wikler, and Landesman, Note 10. On various forms of specific egalitarianism in health, see, for example, B. Williams, 'The Idea of Equality,' in *Problems of the Self* (Cambridge: Cambridge University Press, 1973); M. Waltzer, *Spheres of Justice* (Oxford: Blackwell, 1983); R.M. Veatch, 'Justice and the Right to Health Care: An Egalitarian Account,' in *Rights to Health Care,*, ed. T.J. Bole and W.B. Bondeson (Dordrecht: Kluwer, 1991): 83–102; Nussbaum, Note 22; R. Dworkin, 'Justice in the Distribution of Health Care,' 38(4) *McGill Law Journal* (1992): 883–898, in contrast, argues against what he calls the insulation thesis—the tendency to single out health as a special good.
28. Veatch, ibid.: 83.
29. Whitehead, Note 6: 9.
30. D.R. Gwatkin, 'Health Inequalities and the Health of the Poor: What Do We Know? What Can We Do?' 78(1) *Bulletin of the World Health Organization* (2000): 75–85.
31. D. Parfit, 'Equality or Priority,' 10 *Ratio* (1997): 202–221.
32. If there is no such empirical link, the priority view would require focusing on the sickest, independently of their social situation, and one would have to distinguish from that view one that focuses on the health of the poor. On this, see Marchand, Wikler, and Landesman, Note 10.
33. A. Sen, 'Mortality as an Indicator of Economic Success and Failure,' 108 *The Economic Journal* (1998): 1–25; J.Y. Kim, J.V. Millen, A. Irwin, and J. Gershman, *Dying for Growth* (Monroe, ME: Common Courage Press, 2000).
34. What I am concerned with here is not so much the *empirical* correlation between health outcomes and some indicator of general performance. The issue is, rather, the *theoretical* question whether performance in the health space might tell us something important about social arrangements. I thank Sudhir Anand for pointing this difference out to me.
35. See in particular Rawls (1971), Note 7 and (1993), Note 12.
36. [W]e assume that persons as citizens have all the capacities that enable them to be cooperating members of society.... [W]e do not mean to say, or course, that no one ever suffers from illness and accident; such misfortunes are to be expected in the ordinary course of life, and provision for these contingencies must be made. Rawls (1993), Note 12: 20.
37. Ibid. (1993): 271.
38. See, for example, Rawls (1993): 15.
39. I cannot discuss this issue in full here, but see in particular Rawls (1993), Note 12: 257–288.
40. Rawls (1971), Note 7: 7.

41. Just to avoid confusion: when Rawls speaks of expectations of life, he is not alluding to mortality, but to the chances people have of carrying out different life plans.

42. [W]e cannot view the talents and abilities of individuals as fixed natural gifts. To be sure, even as realized there is presumably a significant genetic component. However, these abilities and talents cannot come to fruition apart form social conditions, and as realized they always take but one of many possible forms....So not only our final ends and hopes for ourselves but also our realized abilities and talents reflect, to a large degree, our personal history, opportunities, and social position Rawls (1993), Note 12: 270.

43. Ibid.: 3f.

44. Rawls, 'Social Unity and Primary Goals,' in *Utilitarianism and Beyond,* ed. A. Sen and B. Williams (Cambridge: Cambridge University Press, 1982): 159–186.

45. Rawls, Note 12: 283.

46. Justice as fairness is often called a *procedural* conception of justice—in contrast to consequentialist theories. Consequentialism requires us to assess different social arrangements with respect to the goodness of the consequences in which they result. Given that the approach to health equity sketched here builds on Rawls theory of justice, one may call it a procedural approach to health equity, I decided against using this term, and called my approach 'indirect' instead, to underline the need to include considerations of goodness in assessing health equity.

47. It may be added that justice as fairness does not translate into a right to health. In general, it can be said that the interpretation of justice as fairness presented here is less threatened by the bottomless pit' problem that is sometimes discussed in relation to the maxim in principle—a reductionist version of Rawls' difference principle.

48. For a list of primary goods, see Rawls (1993), Note 12: 181.

49. See Rawls, Ibid: 440.

50. N. Krieger and S. Sidney, 'Racial Discrimination and Blood Pressure: The CARDIA Study of Young Black and White Women and Men,' 86 *American Journal of Public Health* (1996): 1370–1378; B.P. Kennedy, I. Kwachi, K. Lockner, C. Jones, and D. Prothrow-Smith, '(Dis)respect and Black Mortality,' 7(3) *Ethnicity and Disease* (1997): 207–214.

4

United States: Social Inequality and the Burden of Poor Health

LAURA D. KUBZANSKY, NANCY KRIEGER, ICHIRO KAWACHI, BEVERLY
ROCKHILL, GILLIAN K. STEEL, AND LISA F. BERKMAN

If life was a thing that money could buy, the rich would live
and the poor might die
—1830s English folk song, cited by Hobsbawm[1] (1996: 208)

The United States has the dubious distinction of ranking first among industrialized nations in inequalities in both income and wealth.[2,3] Between 1974 and 1994, the top 5% of the U.S. households increased their share of the nation's aggregate household income from 16% to 21%. The top 20% of U.S. households' share of aggregate income rose from 44% to 49%, while the share among the bottom 20% shrank from 4.3% to 3.6%.[4] Such a concentration of and disparity in wealth in the United States has not been seen since the 1920s,[2] and these trends have continued through the late 1990s.[5,6]

Growing national inequalities in income and wealth portend growing socioeconomic inequalities in health. Studies have compared data from the 1960s, the late 1970s, and 1980s and have found that even as mortality rates overall are declining in the United States, there are widening disparities in mortality by educational level[7,8] and by income level.[9] Concomitantly, the U.S. population attributable death rate due to poverty increased between the early 1970s and early 1990s, especially among black men and women.[10] Additional research suggests that these socioeconomic disparities in health may underlie many observed racial/ethnic and some gender inequalities in health.[9,10]

United States

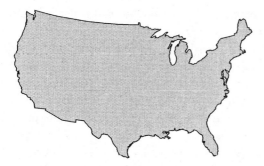

Total population (millions), 1997	271.8
Human development index, 1999	0.927
Human development index rank, 1999	3
Infant mortality rate (per 1,000 live births), 1997	7
Real GDP per capita (PPP$), 1997	29,010
Public spending on health	
as percentage of GDP, 1995	6.5

FIGURE 4.1 United States.
SOURCE: UNDP 1999. (Human Development Report)

Despite its greater wealth and proportion of national income spent on health care, the United States manifests poorer health than many other developed nations (see Figure 4.1). The United States is ranked first in the world in the percent gross national product (GNP) spent on health care. In 1995, national health care expenditures totaled $989 billion and comprised 13.6% of the gross domestic product (GDP). Average life expectancy from birth in the United States in 1990 was, however, 75.4 years (for men and women combined), below that of 15 other World Health Organization (WHO)-participating countries. Because inequalities in health are inextricably intertwined with social inequalities, the health of the U.S. population is painfully unequal.[11,12,13,14,15]

To date, much public health research on social inequalities has focused on who is at greatest risk for poor health outcomes. The goal has been to quantify the magnitude of the effect of deprivation on health. Understanding and acting to reduce the population's burden of disease, however, requires more than estimates of risk. Also important, as suggested by what has been called a "population perspective," is distribution of risk across a population.[16] This approach takes into account both magnitude of and proportion exposed to a given risk. Those with the highest levels of risk fall in the tail of the population distribution and therefore are small in number. Those with moderate levels of risk comprise the bulk of the distribution. Rose[16] argued that small shifts in average individual risk can lead to large population effects. Focusing solely on the ill health burden of the poor (tail of the income/wealth distribution) may underestimate the true impact of the social gradient in health, because each step up in the socioeconomic hierarchy is associated with better health than the level below. While Rose[16] suggested improvements might come about by shifting the population to lower risks, a population perspective in which the distribution is altered by shifts toward the mean (e.g., reducing disparity) is also compatible with his arguments. In either case, a population perspective would consider the burden of poor health over the entire socioeconomic distribution of the population.

The importance of analyzing social inequalities in health in relation to both magnitude and distribution of risk is underscored by an increasing concern with health equity, the idea that everyone should have an opportunity to attain their full potential for health.[17] The necessity of research on social inequalities and health is also heightened by the current focus on health as a human right.[18] Adding urgency is the trend of growing economic inequalities in the United States. These economic inequalities have widened considerably over the past two decades at the same time that the social safety net of welfare and related programs has been partially dismantled.[2,12,19]

In this context, a population perspective directs attention to the importance of recognizing that different interventions may be required for a small number of people at highest risk and for the large number of people at moderate risk for poor health outcomes. At issue is consideration of both the effect and impact of socioeconomic position on health. Measures of effect compare specific socioeconomic groups (such as people with a household income less than $10,000 versus those with a household income greater than $50,000) to see how a fixed change in socioeconomic status influences some health outcome (e.g., mortality rates). Measures of impact compare specific socioeconomic groups in terms of their absolute differences in inequalities, taking into account the size of the groups being compared.[20] Examination of effects of social factors can tell us who is at highest risk for adverse health outcomes (e.g., magnitude of inequality in outcome), whereas consideration of the distribution of social conditions across the population can tell us where the greatest population burden of poor health may be carried (impact). Both matter, and the simultaneous consideration of effect and impact may inform our thinking about social inequalities and health outcomes.

Conducting research on socioeconomic position and health in the United States, however, is not easy. Research on socioeconomic position has been difficult historically because of the virtual absence of adequate information on socioeconomic position in health data.[21] Socioeconomic data typically have not been a component of published U.S. vital statistics (for a comprehensive review, see Krieger et al.[21]). Instead, data have been stratified solely by age, sex, and what is referred to as "race."[22] There are a number of national surveys containing data on both socioeconomic position and health (for a detailed discussion, see Krieger et al.[19]). These vary in the measures of socioeconomic position and health outcomes that are included, as well as in how representative they are of the U.S. population. Thus, merging across data sets is difficult, limiting the ability of any study to be inclusive of multiple measures of both exposures and outcomes.

Conceptual Framework

Although a great deal of research has identified the effect of socioeconomic position and other social conditions on health outcomes, little attempt has been made to estimate the population burden of social inequality on poor health outcomes. Link and Phelan[23] and others[24,25] have suggested that some social factors are "fundamental causes" of disease and, as such, are critically related to health inequalities. A cause may be considered fundamental when it involves access to resources that can be used to avoid risks or to minimize the consequences of disease once it occurs. These resources, frequently distributed unevenly across society, include money, power, prestige, and various kinds of interpersonal relationships. Given the importance of these resources in structuring daily lives, the effects of fundamental causes will endure, although the intervening risk factors and, in fact, specific diseases may change over time. Investigators have suggested that social conditions as defined by socioeconomic position, race/ethnicity, and gender strongly influence individuals' access to resources and may therefore be considered social determinants of health.[26,27]

In previous work, health effects of individual social factors have often been examined. Because social circumstances are interrelated in basic and important ways, however, their relationship to health outcomes may be understood most comprehensively by considering the joint effects of membership in two or more social categories. By social category we mean the various ways of classifying the different combinations of age, gender, race/ethnicity, and income groups, for example, black women with income less than $10,000.[28,29] With regard to conceptualizing social determinants of health, we have opted to examine the effect and the impact of socioeconomic position on health in relation to age, gender, and race/ethnicity. Given our desire to utilize data representative of the U.S. population and based in part on the availability of data, we have chosen annual household income as a basic indicator of socioeconomic position. For the purposes of this research, we consider income to be a marker of socioeconomic position rather than a mediator of the effect of socioeconomic position on health.

Despite the numerous expressions of poor health, one of the most commonly used outcomes in work on social inequality and health is age-adjusted and sometimes age-specific mortality rates. [7,30,31] Although these mortality rates are the "common denominator" of health statistics because of their universal assessment across diverse populations, they are insufficient to describe the consequence of inequalities for health and well-being. Of greater relevance in a context of increasing life expectancy is premature mortality. We all eventually die, but the relevant question is "at what age?" In addition, as "rectangularization" of the survival curve appears in the growing elderly U.S. population (and in other countries), it becomes important to consider other critical health outcomes beyond mortality.[32] These include functional limitations and disability related to both aging and work exposures, health among infants and young children related to developmental abilities, selected chronic conditions among adults, and mental health. Thus, to draw attention to ways that inequality both shortens and impairs people's lives, we focused on two outcomes, premature mortality and functional disability, as experienced in representative samples of the U.S. population. In this study, the measure of health inequity is the disparity in these health outcomes across race/ethnicity (restricted to blacks and whites), gender, and income group.

Methods

We present analyses framed by a population perspective to look at the effect and impact of socioeconomic inequality on two outcomes, premature mortality and functional limitations (disability). Analyses are stratified by age, gender, and race/ethnicity (restricted to blacks and whites due to sample size limitations). These analyses were conducted using data from two large-scale studies based on nationally representative samples of U.S. blacks and whites (see Box 4.1 for details on methods). The National Longitudinal Mortality Study (NLMS) was used for analyses of premature mortality, and the National Health Interview Survey was used for cross-sectional analyses of disability. The 1980 population estimates were obtained from the U.S. Census Bureau. These estimates were used to represent the population distribution across the adjusted 1980 income levels derived from the NLMS.

Box 4.1 Methods

Study Populations

The National Longitudinal Mortality Study (NLMS) is a long-term prospective study of mortality in the United States.[33] The study population for the NLMS consists of samples drawn from the Current Population Surveys (CPS) between 1979 and 1985. Follow-up times range from 4 to 11 years for any individual. NLMS data were obtained from the National Heart, Lung and Blood Institute. Further details on the NLMS have been provided elsewhere.[31,33]

The National Health Interview Survey (NHIS) is a continuous nationwide multistage probability design sample survey in which data about health and other characteristics of each member of the household are collected through personal household interviews of the civilian noninstitutionalized population residing in the United States. Weighted data were used for our analyses. The combined sample for 1988–1990 comprised 139,672 households containing 358,870 persons living at the time of the interview. Further description of the survey design, the methods used in estimation, and general qualifications of the data obtained from the survey are available elsewhere.[34, 35]

Determinants

Socioeconomic position was indicated by family income, as categorized by either the NLMS or the NHIS. The income categories are different in these two sources. In the NLMS, family income was adjusted to reflect 1980 dollars and was assigned to one of seven categories: $0 to $4999, $5000 to $9999, $10,000 to $14,999, $15,000 to $19,999, $20,000 to $24,999, $25,000 to $49,999, or over $50,000. In the NHIS, family income was assigned to one of four categories: under $10,000, $10,000 to $19,999, $20,000 to $34,999, or $35,000 or more (1988–1990).

Age was categorized into 5-year age groups in the NLMS. Two age groups were included in the NHIS, 45 to 65 years and 65 years and over.

Race/ethnicity included categories white and black, as reported by respondents. Neither category is exclusive of Hispanics. Other race/ethnicity categories were not included in the analyses due to unavailable data and small sample sizes.

Gender was categorized as male or female in both surveys.

Outcomes

Average YPLL[75] per person was calculated using data from the NLMS. Following methods used by the National Center for Health Statistics,[35] $YPLL_{75}$ was derived using ten 5-year age groups and was not age

(Continued)

standardized. Deaths in age groups under 25 years were not included due to instability of the data obtainable for these groups. To compute the total YPLL for each group, the number of deaths in each 5-year age stratum in race/ethnicity–gender–income group was multiplied by the years of life lost, calculated as the difference between age 75 years and the midpoint of the age stratum. For example, the death of a person 45 to 49 years of age counted as 27.5 years lost. To derive a per person YPLL in each race/ethnicity–gender–income group, this number was then divided by the number of persons in the race/ethnicity–gender–income group. $YPLL_{75}$ is an average per person per year measure. For example, 0.20 means that the average person loses approximately 2.5 months every year before the age of 75 years.

Prevalence of disability was calculated using data from NHIS and was measured as the proportion of each group that reported limitations in activities of daily living at the time of the survey. Questions were asked in reference to the last year. People were classified in terms of the major activity usually associated with their particular age group. The major activities were paid working or keeping house for those aged 18 to 69 years old and the capacity for independent living (e.g., the ability to bathe, shop, dress, or eat without needing the help of another person) for those 70 years of age and over. Each person was classified into one of two categories with regard to their performance of age-related activities: (1) unable to perform the major activity; or able to perform the major activity, but limited in the kind or amount of this activity; or not limited in the major activity, but limited in the kind or amount of other activities; and (2) not limited in any way.

Slope Index of Inequality (SII) is a measure that uses the slope of a weighted regression line to indicate the average relationship between income and individual health across the distribution of income.[36] Because the size of each socioeconomic group is considered, the SII represents the absolute effect on health of moving from the lowest socioeconomic position through to the highest.[37]

Years of potential life lost ($YPLL_{75}$) per person is a measure of premature mortality and serves as an indicator of effect in our study. The utility of a measure of YPLL has been recognized by the U.S. General Accounting Office as the best single indicator for reflecting differences in the health status of states' populations. This office recommended that it be used to assist the distribution of federal funding for core public health functions.[38] Methods that take account of the longer life expectancy of women or whites, for example, make it more difficult to demonstrate how far short any group falls of a benchmark that we believe should be attainable by everyone. Thus, our method of calculating $YPLL_{75}$ does not consider known differences between groups in life expectancy, but takes an upper age limit that should be attainable (such as age 75 years) as a benchmark for everyone and shows how much we are falling short of the benchmark.

Functional disability is our second health outcome and is also an indicator of effect. Activity limitation was used to ascertain disability, which is a long-term reduction in a person's capacity to perform the average kind or amount of activities associated with his or her age group.

The slope index of inequality (SII) is a measure that takes into account both the effect and the impact of the income distribution on health. We use the SII in our analysis because it allows us to capture explicitly and clearly the gradient in health, as opposed to other measures of effect (e.g., the population attributable risk for mortality).

Estimates of YPLL$_{75}$ per person and disability prevalence for each age–racial/ethnic–gender–income stratum (effect measures) were calculated. To demonstrate who is at highest risk and how many people bear the risk burden, we contrasted YPLL$_{75}$ per person and disability estimates with the population distribution across income categories. Slope indices of inequality for both premature mortality and disability were calculated and presented to exemplify a measure that takes account of both effect and impact.

Results

Effect of Social Inequality on Premature Mortality

Figure 4.2 indicates the income distribution across race/ethnicity and gender categories. In general, there is an inverse and concave relationship between income and YPLL$_{75}$ per person that is similar in all racial/ethnic–gender groups; as family income decreases, YPLL$_{75}$ increases at an increasing rate (see Table 4.1 and Figure 4.2). At least twice as many YPLL$_{75}$ were lost per person at the lowest income levels (less than \$5,000) versus the highest levels (greater than or equal to \$50,000), and this ratio steadily decreases as income increases. For example, on average, black men with less than \$5,000 income who are aged 50 years can expect to lose 7.75 (0.31 x 25) potential years of life, whereas black men with an income greater than \$50,000 at age 50 can expect to lose 1.75 (0.07 x 25) potential years of life.

Considering both the effect of income on premature mortality and the income distribution (impact), the slope index of inequality suggests that as individuals advance from the lowest to the highest income groups, at each level of income (as defined above), on average, there is a gain of 5 days of life per person per year (b = –0.0137, p < 0.01).

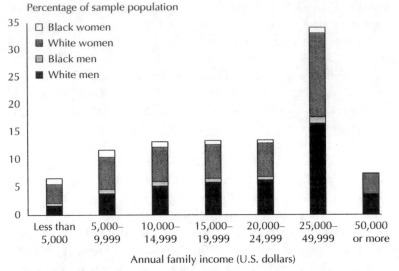

Figure **4.2** Distribution of Sample Population across Income Levels, by Race/
Ethnicity and Gender, in the United States, 1980.
Source: Based on data from the U.S. Census Bureau.

Analysis of Joint Effects

Additional analyses examined the joint effects of race/ethnicity, gender, and
income on $YPLL_{75}$ (see Table 4.1). With regard to the effect of socioeconomic position on premature mortality (estimate of $YPLL_{75}$ per person), the
overall pattern described above was largely similar in each racial/ethnic–
gender group (see Figures 4.3 and 4.4). Figure 4.3 is designed to juxtapose
visually both the income distribution and the risk of premature mortality
in each race/ethnicity and gender category. Risks were highest in the low-
income group. Although the pattern was similar across subgroups, there are
several differences worth noting. For instance, the population distribution
of income among whites and blacks differs strikingly (see Figure 4.2). For
both black women and black men, the population is concentrated largely
in the lower income strata, and this is particularly true for black women;
15% of blacks (19% of black women) had a family income under $5,000
compared with 6% of the white population. Because of the greater concentration of the black population at lower income levels, in terms of premature mortality, more blacks than whites experience adverse effects of low
income. In addition, among the lower four income strata for both men and
women, blacks are generally one and a half times more likely to lose years
of life prematurely than whites. Because the proportion of the population

TABLE 4.1. Premature Mortality by Race/Ethnicity, Gender, and Income Level in the United States, 1979–1989

FAMILY INCOME LEVEL AND SOCIAL CATEGORY	POPULATION (THOUSANDS)	SHARE OF SAMPLE POPULATION (PERCENT)	AVERAGE YEARS OF POTENTIAL LIFE LOST (YPLL$_{75}$) PER PERSON PER YEAR
Less than $5,000	7,985	6.61	0.15
Black women	1,308	1.08	0.16
White women	4,058	3.36	0.10
Black men	616	0.51	0.31
White men	2,003	1.66	0.19
$5,000–$9,999	14,155	11.71	0.12
Black women	1,572	1.30	0.11
White women	6,960	5.76	0.07
Black men	975	0.81	0.21
White men	4,648	3.85	0.17
$10,000–$14,999	15,947	13.20	0.10
Black women	1,146	0.95	0.10
White women	7,565	6.26	0.06
Black men	922	0.76	0.19
White men	6,314	5.22	0.12
$15,000–$19,999	16,192	13.40	0.08
Black women	877	0.73	0.08
White women	7,383	6.11	0.05
Black men	832	0.69	0.14
White men	7,100	5.88	0.10
$20,000–$24,999	16,300	13.49	0.07
Black women	672	0.56	0.06
White women	7,352	6.08	0.05
Black men	692	0.57	0.13
White men	7,584	6.28	0.09
$25,000–$49,999	41,231	34.12	0.07
Black women	1,270	1.05	0.07
White women	18,651	15.43	0.05
Black men	1,384	1.15	0.14
White men	19,926	16.49	0.09
$50,000 or more	9,034	7.48	0.06
Black women	112	0.09	0.06
White women	4,185	3.46	0.05
Black men	153	0.13	0.07
White men	4,584	3.79	0.08

Note: Family income levels are in 1980 U.S. dollars

Source: Based on data from the National Longitudinal Mortality Study.

represented by blacks is small, however, they account for a smaller percentage of the total years of life lost than whites.

With regard to gender, men lose more years of life than women in virtually all but the highest income stratum; this is true for both blacks

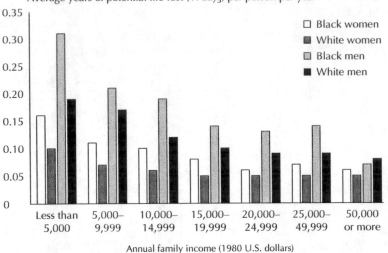

Average years of potential life lost (YPLL$_{75}$) per person per year

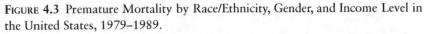

Annual family income (1980 U.S. dollars)

FIGURE 4.3 Premature Mortality by Race/Ethnicity, Gender, and Income Level in the United States, 1979–1989.
SOURCE: Based on data from the National Longitudinal Mortality Study.

and whites. Although the SII suggests on average a gain of 5 days of life per person per year as individuals advance from the lowest to the highest income groups, this varies across gender and race/ethnicity from as much as 11.42 days of life for black men per year to 6.21 days of life for white man per year to 6.61 days of life per black women per year to a low of 2.41 days of life for white woman per year. Thus, while patterns are similar across racial/ethnic–gender–income groups, because of distributional differences in income in the population and differences in the magnitude of effects, further insight may be gained by examining the socioeconomic gradient in premature mortality separately by gender and race/ethnicity.

Effect of Social Inequality on Disability

Similar to the patterns identified with premature mortality, there is a monotonic inverse relationship between income and disability in both age groups (see Tables 4.2 and 4.3, and Figure 4.5). Among individuals age 45 to 64 years, approximately 26% had an income of less than $20,000, 26% had an income between $20,000 and $34,999, and 48% had an income greater than $35,000. In contrast, among individuals aged 65 years and over, approximately 60% had an income less than $20,000, 24% had an

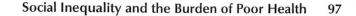

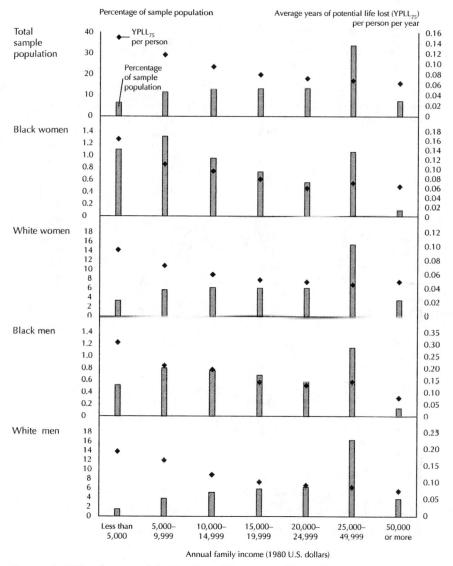

FIGURE 4.4 Distribution of the Burden of Premature Mortality across Income Groups, by Race/Ethnicity and Gender, in the United States, 1979–1989. SOURCE: Based on data from the National Longitudinal Mortality Study.

income between $20,000 and $34,999, and 17% had an income greater than $35,000. Among all subgroups aged 45 to 64 years, disability was approximately four times more prevalent in the lowest income level (less than $10,000) compared with the highest levels ($35,000 or more). Although this difference remained among individuals aged 65 years and

TABLE 4.2. Prevalence of Disability among Adults Age 45–64 by Race/Ethnicity, Gender, and Income Level in the United States, 1988–1990

FAMILY INCOME LEVEL AND SOCIAL CATEGORY	POPULATION (THOUSANDS)	SHARE OF SAMPLE POPULATION (PERCENT)	PREVALENCE OF DISABILITY (PERCENT)
Less than $10,000	3,206	8.79	56.72
Black women	533	1.46	56.70
White women	1,511	4.14	53.90
Black men	293	0.80	60.10
White men	869	2.38	60.50
$10,000–$19,999	6,262	17.18	33.36
Black women	559	1.53	31.50
White women	3,149	8.64	30.40
Black men	417	1.14	32.40
White men	2,137	5.86	38.40
$20,000–$34,999	9,628	26.41	21.27
Black women	478	1.31	18.00
White women	4,580	12.56	20.90
Black men	453	1.24	21.90
White men	4,117	11.29	22.00
$35,000 or more	17,361	47.62	13.27
Black women	449	1.23	15.10
White women	7,580	20.79	13.50
Black men	500	1.37	11.00
White men	8,832	24.23	13.10

Source: Based on data from the National Health Interview Survey.

older, the magnitude was reduced; disability was 1.7 times more prevalent among those with the lowest versus the highest incomes. Of note, the income distribution shifted for individuals aged 65 years or more so that 60% of the aged 65 years and over population had an income under $20,000 versus 26% of the aged 45 to 64 years population (see Table 4.3).

Among those aged 45 to 64 years, considering both the effect of income on disability and the income distribution, the SII was significant. This result suggests that as individuals advance from the lowest to the highest income groups, there is, on average, a 12% decrease in prevalence of disability (b 0.12, p 0.05). Among individuals aged 65 years or older the SII was significant and suggested that as individuals advance from the lowest to the highest income groups at each level of income, on average there is a 7% decrease in prevalence of disability (b = −0.07, p < 0.05).

TABLE 4.3. Prevalence of Disability among Adults Age 65 and over by Race/
Ethnicity, Gender, and Income Level in the United States, 1988–1990

FAMILY INCOME LEVEL AND SOCIAL CATEGORY	POPULATION (THOUSANDS)	SHARE OF SAMPLE POPULATION (PERCENT)	PREVALENCE OF DISABILITY (PERCENT)
Less than $10,000	5,532	25.06	48.83
Black women	599	2.71	55.90
White women	3,380	15.31	46.60
Black men	296	1.34	53.40
White men	1,257	5.69	50.40
$10,000–$19,999	7,642	34.62	38.88
Black women	316	1.43	45.30
White women	3,948	17.88	37.50
Black men	293	1.33	43.00
White men	3,085	13.97	39.60
$20,000–$34,999	5,195	23.53	33.01
Black women	112	0.51	36.60
White women	2,582	11.70	31.60
Black men	103	0.47	32.00
White men	2,398	10.86	34.40
$35,000 or more	3,708	16.80	28.52
Black women	77	0.35	36.40
White women	1,737	7.87	29.60
Black men	70	0.32	32.90
White men	1,824	8.26	27.00

Source: Based on data from the National Health Interview Survey.

Analysis of Joint Effects

Similar patterns are observed in each racial/ethnic–gender group, with
black women again the most likely to be in the lower income strata.
Although broadly comparable, these patterns nonetheless hid important
distinctions among the different racial/ethnic and gender groups. In both
age groups, women (black and white combined) comprised a higher percentage of the total population with an income under $10,000, than did
blacks (women and men combined). Given this income distribution and the
effect of income on disability, women and blacks were more likely to experience disability. For example, Table 4.2 indicates that approximately 57%
of black women aged 45 to 64 years with an income less than $10,000
are disabled. Also, although the prevalence of disability among blacks and
whites was similar across men and women of similar incomes in the age
group 45 to 64 years, disability was more prevalent among blacks (men
and women) versus whites in the 65 years and over age group (see Tables

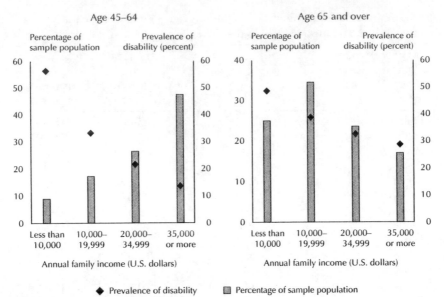

FIGURE 4.5 Distribution of the Burden of Disability across Income Groups, by Age Group, in the United States, 1988–1990.
SOURCE: Based on data from the National Health Interview Survey.

4.2 and 4.3). In the age 65 years and over group, black women reported the highest levels of disability across all income strata, while in the lowest income stratum white women reported the lowest levels of disability, although white women comprise a large proportion of the population with an income less than $10,000. Among individuals aged 45 to 64 years, however, disability was more prevalent among men (both black and white) than among women at each income level except the highest. This finding would suggest that a large part of the disability prevalence among women may be more strongly related to income than to gender in this age group.

Discussion

Key Findings: Effect and Impact of Socioeconomic Position on Health

In this study, we consider the health effects of socioeconomic position using a population perspective.[16] A robust effect of income on health is evident in all age, racial/ethnic, gender, and income groups and across two different markers of health status—premature mortality and disability. Those with less income consistently live more disabled and less healthy lives, and die at younger ages, than their wealthier counterparts. Similar to other studies, our findings indicate that adverse health effects appear to be potentiated with increasing levels of deprivation. Our findings are also in line with other research on socioeconomic position and race/ethnicity. For example, a recent study reported that life expectancy for whites exceeded that of blacks at every income level. Furthermore, at age 45 years, black women with an income of $25,000 or more could expect to live 3.8 years longer than those with an income of less than $10,000.[39]

As reported in other studies examining racial/ethnic and gender differences in health within socioeconomic strata,[11,12] effects of income on premature mortality and disability varied by both race/ethnicity and gender. For example, within socioeconomic strata, blacks generally lost more years of life than whites, and men lost more years of life than women. In terms of premature mortality, black men in the lowest income stratum fared worse than any other group. In contrast, blacks and whites did not differ significantly in levels of disability within each income stratum among those aged 45 to 64 years. Among individuals aged 65 years or more, however, within each income stratum black women generally reported the highest levels of disability while white women reported the lowest levels. The pattern of findings with regard to gender also depends on which health outcome was considered. Differences between men and women across income strata were less consistent when disability rather than premature mortality was the health indicator.

An understanding of the overall influence of socioeconomic position on health is obtained by taking into account both the magnitude of the effects and the size of the group in which they occur. The slope index of inequality can be interpreted as the absolute effect of moving from the lowest to the highest income group while taking into account the actual distribution of income. This study, based on a nationally representative sample of the U.S. population, demonstrates that low income significantly increased risk of premature mortality and disability despite the fact that the lowest income groups were often composed of the fewest people.

Although the effect of socioeconomic position on health may be relatively stable, the impact will be significantly influenced by the distribution of income (or whatever marker of socioeconomic position is being considered) in the population. Given that income inequality in the United States is increasing, taking into account and tracking changes in the income distribution is particularly crucial in order to develop effective policies that address the health effects of socioeconomic position. For example, in our examination of disability in the 1988–1990 U.S. population, we find a marked difference in income distribution between those aged 45 to 64 years and those aged 65 years or older. A similar income distribution shift between younger and older individuals occurs in the 1980 U.S. population. More individuals aged 65 years and older were likely to have low incomes, and this is particularly true for women. Because those with low incomes are disproportionately burdened with poor health outcomes, older blacks and women, who are likely to have little income, are particularly disadvantaged. Despite the wealth of the U.S. population and the proportion of U.S. GNP spent on health care, good health eludes an unacceptably high proportion of the population, and the distribution of this disadvantage is socially determined.

Attention to both the effect and the impact of socioeconomic position on health leads to some unexpected findings. For example, previous work has suggested that women experience higher levels of disability than men in older populations.[14] Our study indicates that men aged 45 to 64 years (both black and white) generally have higher prevalence rates of disability than women in all but the highest income stratum. Data on income distribution, however, suggest that those with low incomes are disproportionately women and that those with low incomes are more likely to be disabled. Thus, the impact of disability on 45- to 64-year-old women in low-income groups is greater than for men even though male prevalence rates of disability are greater. Differences in income distribution may not be completely controlled even when socioeconomic position is included as a covariate in analyses of gender and disability. In this study, a greater understanding of the distribution of income across relevant social conditions was gained by stratifying simultaneously across race/ethnicity, gender, and age groups. Thus, studies on gender variations in disability that fail to take into account the potential confounding effect of income for men and women may be biased. Alternatively, income may be considered a mediating factor in the relationship between gender and health. Further research, however, is needed to confirm this finding while controlling more carefully for the effects of age.

Possible Biases and Limitations

The unavailability of relevant data severely constrains investigation of both the effect and the impact of socioeconomic position on health (for review, see Krieger et al.[18]). For example, in this analysis, although we would have preferred to use more recent data, the data available for YPLL calculations were collected between 1975 and 1985. Given that income inequality has been increasing over the last decade, however, we feel some confidence that the direction of the effects we found are valid, although the magnitude may be somewhat underestimated.

Although research has suggested that family income does provide important information about social and health inequalities,[40,41] there are nevertheless some concerns about the use of family income as an indicator of socioeconomic position. The family income variable does not adjust for family size or account for different family structures (single parenthood, extended family, and so forth), may fluctuate widely over time,[42] and may be a poor proxy for purchasing power or income available to family members.[43] For example, goods and services available to whites and residents of higher income neighborhoods in the United States tend to be higher quality and lower priced than those available to blacks and residents of lower income neighborhoods.[44,45]

Additional limitations may arise from the potential for racial/ethnic misclassification. Some investigators have raised concerns about the quality of race/ethnicity data.[46,47] For example, because the distribution of a study population into different race/ethnicity categories varies depending on the assessment technique, respondent self-report of his or her race/ethnicity identification may differ substantially from an observer's assessment. Moreover, few data are available on racial/ethnic groups other than blacks and whites. It is also important to note that socioeconomic position should not be used as a proxy for race/ethnicity. Although race/ethnicity and socioeconomic position may be correlated, a number of studies have demonstrated that the effects of one cannot fully be explained by the other.[48] As the data reported here suggest, even within each income stratum, blacks often have a worse health status than whites.

In addition, our analyses were limited because the data with regard to disability are cross-sectional. As a result, some component of the association with income may be a function of reverse causation because it is likely that some people were ill or disabled and unable to work. Certainly, ill health may significantly affect income. Similarly, some of the variation in YPLL may be due to differences in access to care. Longitudinal and prospective studies of other populations, however, show that neither reverse causation nor access to care is likely to explain fully our results.[14,16,48] Our findings may also be limited because our analyses of premature mortality did not take into account the age structure of the population. Many of the age-relevant differences occur at younger ages, however, which were not included in our analyses due to data limitations. In addition, we cumulated the number of years of life lost up to age 75 for each group and found the number to be consistent with other findings of differences in life expectancy between groups. Thus, we are confident that our results accurately represent the direction of the effects found.

Finally, effects of social inequality may not be uniform across all types of health outcomes. Our analyses were limited by the focus on only two health outcomes, premature mortality and disability. Social factors may affect health through multifaceted and dynamic processes, and examination of only one health outcome may result in an incomplete understanding and underestimation of their effects. Because fundamental social causes of disease involve resources that are important determinants of multiple risk factors, fundamental social causes are linked to multiple health outcomes.[23] A greater understanding of social inequality in health would be gained by considering an array of health outcomes beyond premature mortality, such as mental health, healthy aging, positive well-being, and incidence of specific diseases. Further gains may be made by examining trends in the effect and impact of the socioeconomic gradient in health over time, although at present such analyses are limited by available data.

Pathways

The manner in which socioeconomic position operates to influence health outcomes has not yet been fully elucidated,[3,25] although it is known that it shapes a wide array of physical, occupational, environmental, behavioral, social, and psychological factors.[11,23,46,50] Through efforts to understand how social inequalities influence health, we may begin to address some of these health inequalities. It is theoretically possible that the empirical link between socioeconomic position and health reflects merely a spurious association whereby underlying, genetically based factors give rise to both socioeconomic position and health outcomes. Alternatively, the "drift" hypothesis suggests that the effects of socioeconomic position on health may be due to downward mobility among persons in poor health. A variety of research has suggested, however, that these explanations are not satisfactory.[51,52] Here, we briefly review some of the mechanisms (or pathways), in addition to material deprivation, by which various aspects of socioeconomic position (measured with a variety of markers) may influence health outcomes.

Based on the assumption that education is a critical component of socioeconomic position, the cumulative advantage perspective argues that educational attainment increases resources that accumulate through life, ultimately producing a larger socioeconomic gap in health among older individuals than younger.[53,54] Ross and Wu[55] suggest that educational attainment influences more proximate determinants of health. For example, well-educated people are more likely to have more economic resources (full-time jobs, fulfilling work, high incomes) and more social psychological resources (high sense of personal control and social support) and to engage in better health behaviors (more likely to exercise, drink moderately, and receive preventive medical care; less likely to smoke).[50] By accumulating health-promoting resources over time, those with more education are likely to have better health outcomes.[50,55]

Others have argued that income inequality is itself deleterious for population health.[5,56,57] In more affluent countries, what seems to predict life expectancy reliably is the extent of relative deprivation, as measured by the size of the income gap between the rich and the poor.[57,58] One's relative socioeconomic position, rather than simply the absolute level, may also be importantly associated with health.[58,59] A number of mechanisms by which income inequality influences health have been proposed, such as underinvestment in human capital,[60] erosion of social cohesion and social capital,[56,61] and the potentially harmful consequences of frustration brought about by relative deprivation.[59]

If different social groups (e.g., black men vs. white women) systematically experience differential health outcomes, it is because their options for living healthy lives are constrained by the fact of—and social processes involved in—perpetuating social inequality. These restricted options are manifested through experiences of discrimination, living and working in adverse conditions, stress, and access to medical care, as well as mediated through a range of social, psychological, cultural, and religious resources that are influenced by membership in these groups.[47]

Group membership as summarized by the various social categories is associated with a social identity, a set of obligations, and accessibility of resources, which individually or jointly may influence health outcomes. To clarify how membership in specific social categories influences health outcomes, we will need to unpack the psychological and social ramifications of category membership and examine their effects on health. For example, psychosocial factors such as feelings of control, hostility, sense of confidence, loneliness, and isolation have shown consistent relationships with both socioeconomic position and health.[24,52] Certain groups (e.g., blacks) are also more likely to experience discrimination (and its attendant stresses), which is known to adversely affect physiological and psychological functioning.[43,62,63] Moreover, individuals with fewer resources may be exposed to greater levels of stress or are more vulnerable to stressors and are therefore more likely to experience adverse health outcomes.[64]

Recommendations

We have sought to integrate inequality in the social structure with inequality in health outcomes to give a sense of both the relative unfairness and the burden of poor health in the United States. According to the population perspective, the occurrence of common diseases and exposures reflects the behavior and circumstances of a whole society, and "moderate and achievable change by the population as a whole might greatly reduce the number of people with conspicuous problems...as many people exposed to a small risk generate more disease than a few exposed to a conspicuous risk."[16] To implement programs that might change the distribution of risk in a population, one must understand the specifics of the population distribution across social conditions and health outcomes.[16] Our findings suggest that the burden of disease is much larger than the effect of disproportionate ill health on the very poor. Some strategies aimed at moving the entire distribution or reducing disparities may in the end be more effective than those that are focused solely on the tail of the distribution (e.g., those living in poverty). Policies that deal with the growing inequalities in income distribution, for example, may have a considerable impact on health inequalities.[65,66] More informed decisions may be made when information on both effect and impact is available.

One key to documenting and evaluating systematically how socioeconomic position, race/ethnicity, gender, and age combine to produce social inequalities in health will be to improve the data available for answering these critical questions. This information will allow us to incorporate into policies an understanding that some gender and racial/ethnic differences are due to socioeconomic position differences, as well as to consider both direct and indirect effects of socioeconomic position. In a recent review, Krieger and colleagues[19] make a number of recommendations regarding the measurement of social class and other aspects of socioeconomic position for public health research and surveillance. Among them are recommendations to include consistent measures of socioeconomic position in all public health databases, to use theoretically grounded measures of socioeconomic position with careful consideration of measurement level, to consider contextual effects and multilevel analyses, and to consider pathways by which socioeconomic position and other social factors may influence health. Given the many pathways of influence, it is also vital that policies carefully consider early life versus adult exposures, because early childhood exposures can affect adult life dynamics in terms of achieved social status. Thus, monitoring health status in relation to socioeconomic status is key in the United States as in many other nations.

Policies may also be more effective in improving population health when they take into consideration the entire gradient in health related to family income instead of just the tail. For example, if we use estimates for a family of three in a midsized city in Massachusetts, such a family on welfare and food stamps earns $10,272 a year. The federal poverty level is $13,330. Current policies provide strong incentives to work. If the head of this household succeeds in working and earns minimum wage, then working full time and obtaining income tax credit, she or he will earn

$14,017.[67] Although these earnings put the family about $700 above the poverty line, working is also likely to incur additional offsetting expenses related to transportation, health insurance, and child care. Given that the family remains so near the poverty line, members of a working class family with earnings around minimum wage are still at considerable health risk. This example illustrates how focusing only on the extreme tail of the income distribution, while important, hardly solves the problem related to the observed gradient in mortality, especially among lower-middle-class families. The United States lacks policy strategies enabling families to move substantially closer to the median income or even to modest standards of self-sufficiency. Public and private sector policies related to work and family issues may further enable adults to take care of dependents while maintaining long-term work commitments. Other policies related to housing, income tax, and neighborhood revitalization also hold the potential to reduce inequalities in health stemming from social inequalities. A critical next step will be to integrate policy-related disciplines with epidemiological and public health approaches.

In a time of growing income inequality in the United States and other countries, it is all the more important to document contingent inequalities in health so as to spur action to reduce these inequalities and improve health equity. A population perspective may inform research on health equity and social inequalities. Armed with this knowledge, and with a sense of who bears the burden of poor health, we may address the issue of health inequity in a targeted and comprehensive way.

References

1. Hobsbawm, E., *The Age of Revolution, 1789–1848* (New York: Vintage Books, 1996).
2. Wolff, E.N., *Top Heavy: A Study of the Increasing Inequality of Wealth in America* (New York: The Twentieth Century Fund Press, 1995).
3. Smeeding, T. and P. Gottschalk, "The International Evidence on Income Distribution in Modern Economies: Where Do We Stand?" in *Poverty and Inequality: The Political Economy of Redistribution*, ed. J. Neil (Kalamazoo, MI: W.E. Upjohn Institute for Employment Research, 1997): 79–103.
4. DeVita, C.J., "The United States at Mid-Decade," 50 *Population Bulletin* (1996): 2–48.
5. Kawachi, I., B.P. Kennedy, and R.G. Wilkinson, eds., *Income Inequality and Health. The Society and Health Population Reader* (New York: The New Press, 1999).
6. Bernstein, J., E.C. McNichol, L. Mishel, and R. Zahradnik, *Pulling Apart: A State-by-State Analysis of Income Trends* (Washington DC: Center on Budget and Policy Priorities and Economic Policy Institute, 2000).

7. Pappas, G., S. Queen, W. Hadden, and G. Fisher, "The Increasing Disparity in Mortality between Socioeconomic Groups in the United States, 1960 and 1986," 329 *New England Journal of Medicine* (1993): 103–109.
8. Duleep, H.O., "Mortality and Income Inequality," 58 *Social Security Bulletin* (1995): 34–50.
9. Schalick, L.M., W.C. Hadden, E. Pamuk, V. Navarro, and G. Pappas, "The Widening Gap in Death Rates among Income Groups in the United States from 1967 to 1986," 30 *International Journal of Health Services* (2000): 13–26.
10. Hahn, R.A., E.D. Eaker, N.D. Barker, S.M. Teutsch, W.A. Sosniak, and N. Krieger, "Poverty and Death in the United States," 26(4) *International Journal of Health Services* (1996): 673–690.
11. Krieger, N., D.L. Rowley, A.A. Herman, B. Avery, and M.T. Phillips, "Racism, Sexism, and Social Class: Implications for Studies of Health, Disease, and Well-Being," 9(Suppl. 6) *American Journal of Preventive Medicine* (1993): 82–122.
12. Williams, D.R. and C. Collins, "U.S. Socioeconomic and Racial Differences in Health: Patterns and Explanations," 21 *Annual Review of Sociology* (1995): 349–386.
13. Haan, M.N., G.A. Kaplan, and T. Camacho, "Poverty and Health: Prospective Evidence from the Alameda County Study," 125 *American Journal of Epidemiology* (1987): 989–998.
14. Guralnik, J.M., L.P. Fried, and M.E. Salive, "Disability as a Public Health Outcome in the Aging Population," 17 *Annual Review of Public Health* (1996): 25–46.
15. United Nations Development Programme (UNDP), *Human Development Report 1999* (New York: UNDP, 1999).
16. Rose, G., *The Strategy of Preventive Medicine* (Oxford: Oxford University Press, 1992).
17. Calman, K.C., "Equity, Poverty and Health for All," 314 *British Medical Journal* (1997): 1187–1191.
18. Mann, J.M., S. Gruskin, M.A. Grodin, and G.J. Annas, eds., *Health and Human Rights: A Reader* (New York: Routledge, 1999).
19. Krieger, N., D.R. Williams, and N.E. Moss, "Measuring Social Class in Public Health Research," 18 *Annual Review of Public Health* (1997): 341–378.
20. Kunst, A., *Cross-National Comparisons of Socio-economic Differences in Mortality* (Rotterdam: Erasmus University, 1997).
21. Krieger, N. and E. Fee, "Social Class: the Missing Link in U.S. Health Data," 24(1) *International Journal of Health Services* (1994): 25–44.
22. Krieger, N., J.T. Chen, and G. Ebel, "Can We Monitor Socioeconomic Inequalities in Health? a Survey of U.S. Health Departments' Data Collection and Reporting Practices," 112 *Public Health Reports* (1997): 481–494.
23. Link, B.G. and J. Phelan, "Social Conditions as Fundamental Causes of Disease," *Journal of Health and Social Behavior* (1995): 80–94.
24. Anderson, N.B. and C.A. Armstead, "Toward Understanding the Association of Socioeconomic Status and Health: a New Challenge for the Biopsychosocial Approach," 57 *Psychosomatic Medicine* (1995): 213–225.

25. Kaplan, G.A., "Where Do Shared Pathways Lead? Some Reflections on a Research Agenda," 57 *Psychosomatic Medicine* (1995): 208–212.
26. Standing, H., "Gender and equity in health sector reform programmes: A review," 12(1) *Health Policy and Planning* (1997): 1–18.
27. Williams, D.R., "Race and Health: Basic Questions, Emerging Directions," 7 *Annals of Epidemiology* (1997): 322–333.
28. Krieger, N., "Epidemiology and the Web of Causation: Has Anyone Seen the Spider?" 39(7) *Social Science and Medicine* (1994): 887–903.
29. Susser, M. and E. Susser, "Choosing a Future for Epidemiology: Ii. from Black Box to Chinese Boxes and Eco-Epidemiology," 86(5) *American Journal of Public Health* (1996): 674–677.
30. Marmot, M.G., M.J. Shipley, and G. Rose, "Inequalities in Death: Specific Explanations of a General Pattern?" 1 *Lancet* (1984): 1003–1006.
31. Backlund, E., P.D. Sorlie, and N.J. Johnson, "The shape of the relationship between income and mortality in the United States," 6 *Annals of Epidemiology* (1996): 12–20.
32. Berkman, L.F., "The Changing and Heterogeneous Nature of Aging and Longevity: a Social and Biomedical Perspective," 8 *Annual Review of Gerontology and Geriatrics* (1988): 37–68.
33. Rogot, E., P.D. Sorlie, N.J. Johnson, and C. Schmitt, *A Mortality Study of 1.3 Million Persons by Demographic, Social, and Economic Factors: 1979–1985 Follow-Up* (Bethesda, MD: National Institutes of Health, 1992).
34. Collins, J.G. and F.B. LeClere, *Health and Selected Socioeconomic Characteristics of the Family: United States, 1988–90* (Hyattsville, MD: National Center for Health Statistics, 1996).
35. National Center for Health Statistics, *Health, United States, 1996–1997 and Injury Chartbook* (Hyattsville, MD: U.S. Government Printing Office, 1996).
36. Wagstaff, A., P. Paci P., and E. van Doorslaer, "On the Measurement of Inequalities in Health," 33(5) *Social Science and Medicine* (1991): 545–557.
37. Preston, S.H., M.R. Haines, and E. Pamuk, *Effects of Industrialization and Urbanization on Mortality in Developed Countries,* 19th International Population Conference (Manila, Liege: IUSSP, 1981).
38. Selik, R.M. and S.Y. Chu, "Years of Potential Life Lost Due to Hiv Infection in the United States," 11 *Aids* (1997): 1635–1639.
39. National Center for Health Statistics, *Health, United States, 1998* (Hyattsville, MD: U.S. Government Printing Office, 1998).
40. Coulter, E.J. and L. Guralnick, "Analyses of Vital Statistics by Census Tract," 54 *Journal of the American Statistical Association* (1959): 730–740.
41. Nagi, M.H. and E.G. Stockwell, "Socioeconomic Differentials in Mortality by Cause of Death," 88 *Health Services Reports* (1973): 449–456.
42. Duncan, G., "Income Dynamics and Health," 26 *International Journal of Health Services* (1996): 419–444.
43. Williams, D.R., Y. Yu, J.S. Jackson, and N.B. Anderson, "Racial Differences in Physical and Mental Health: Socioeconomic Status, Stress, and Discrimination," 2 *Journal of Health Psychology* (1997): 335–351.
44. Macintyre, S., S. Maciver, and A. Sooman, "Area, Class, and Health: Should We Be Focusing on Places or People?" 22(2) *Journal of Social Policy* (1993): 213–234.

45. Kaplan, G., "People and Places: Contrasting Perspectives on the Association between Social Class and Health," 26 *International Journal of Health Services* (1996): 507–519.
46. Hahn, R.A., "The State of Federal Health Statistics on Racial and Ethnic Groups," 267 *Journal of the American Medical Association* (1992): 268–271.
47. Williams, D.R., R. Lavizzo-Mourey, and R.C. Warren, "The Concept of Race and Health Status in America," 109 *Public Health Reports* (1994): 26–41.
48. Seeman, T.E., P.A. Charpentier, M.E. Tinetti, et al., "Predicting Changes in Physical Performance in a High-Functioning Elderly Cohort: Macarthur Studies of Successful Aging," 49(3) *Journal of Gerontology: Medical Sciences* (1994): M97–M108.
49. Kaplan, G.A., "You Can't Get There from Here: Understanding the Association between Socioeconomic Status and Health Requires Going Upstream," 11 *Advances: The Journal of Mind–Body Health* (1995): 15–16.
50. Ross, C.E. and C.-L. Wu, "The Links between Education and Health," 60 *American Sociological Review* (1995): 719–745.
51. Wilkinson, R.G., *Class and Health: Research and Longitudinal Data* (London: Tavistock, 1986).
52. Adler, N.E., T. Boyce, M.A. Chesney, et al., "Socioeconomic Status and Health: the Challenge of the Gradient," 49 *American Psychologist* (1994): 15–24.
53. Merton, R.K., "The Matthew Effect in Science," 159 *Science* (1968): 56–63.
54. Ross, C.E. and C.-L. Wu, "Education, Age, and the Cumulative Advantage in Health," 37 *Journal of Health and Social Behavior* (1996): 104–120.
55. Blane, D., "Editorial: Social Determinants of Health—Socioeconomic Status, Social Class, and Ethnicity," 85(7) *American Journal of Public Health* (1995): 903–904.
56. Wilkinson, R.G., *Unhealthy Societies: The Afflictions of Inequality* (New York: Routledge, 1996).
57. Kawachi, I. and B.P. Kennedy, "The Relationship of Income Inequality to Mortality: Does the Choice of Indicator Matter?" 45(7) *Social Science and Medicine* (1997): 1121–1127.
58. Wilkinson, R.G., "Income Distribution and Life Expectancy," 304 *British Medical Journal* (1992): 165–168.
59. Kawachi, I., S. Levine, S.M. Miller, K. Lasch, and B. Amick, *Income Inequality and Life Expectancy—Theory, Research and Policy*, No. 94–92 (Boston: Harvard School of Public Health, 1994).
60. Kaplan, G.A., E.R. Pamuk, J.W. Lynch, R.D. Cohen, and J.L. Balfour, "Inequality in Income and Mortality in the United States: Analysis of Mortality and Potential Pathways," 312 *British Medical Journal* (1996): 999–1003.
61. Kawachi, I., B.P. Kennedy, K. Lochner, and D. Prothrow-Stith, "Social Capital, Income Inequality, and Mortality," 87 *American Journal of Public Health* (1997): 1491–1498.
62. Anderson, N.B., H.F. Myers, T. Pickering, J.S. Jackson, "Hypertension in Blacks: Psychosocial and Biological Perspectives," 7 *Journal of Hypertension* (1989): 161–172.
63. Krieger, N. and S. Sidney, "Racial Discrimination and Blood Pressure: the Cardia Study of Young Black and White Adults," 86 *American Journal of Public Health* (1996): 1370–1378.

64. Thoits, P.A., "Life Stress, Social Support, and Psychological Vulnerability: Epidemiological Considerations," 10 *Journal of Community Psychology* (1982): 341–362.
65. Kennedy, B.P., I. Kawachi, and D. Prothrow-Stith, "Income Distribution and Mortality: Cross Sectional Ecological Study of the Robin Hood Index in the United States," 312(7037) *British Medical Journal* (1996): 1004–1007.
66. Kawachi, I. and B.P. Kennedy, "Health and Social Cohesion: Why Care about Income Inequality?" 314(7086) *British Medical Journal* (1997): 1037–1040.
67. Gerwin, C., "How Much Is Enough?" Fall *CommonWealth* (1998): 13–14.

5

A Framework for Measuring Health Inequity

YUKIKO ASADA

Researchers and policymakers worldwide have demonstrated longstanding interest in health inequality. Why are they interested in health inequality? Just as in any other scientific pursuit, some of them may simply be interested in describing how health is distributed. Others may be interested in understanding the mechanism of health inequality so they can improve population health.

The interest in health inequality, however, is not always limited to describing and understanding it. Some health inequalities are of moral concern because of the value we place on health.[1-3] This moral concern distinguishes health inequality as a topic of both policy and ethical inquiry. The moral or ethical dimension of health inequality is generally termed health inequity, although no consensus on a precise definition of health inequity exists.[4]

Given the importance of moral concern in health inequality, it is surprising that a comprehensive conceptual framework for measuring health inequality capturing moral concern has yet to be developed. Although philosophers have long discussed equality and justice, until recently they have rarely addressed health in their discussion.[2,5] This is primarily because of

This chapter is reprinted with permission from *Journal of Epidemiology and Community Health* 59(2005): 700–705. Copyright 2005 BMJ Publishing Group Ltd.

the assumption that health distribution is beyond human control. Bioethics has concentrated on individual patient–physician issues and, until recently, has failed to address ethical issues at the population level.[2,6–8]

In the multi-disciplinary health sciences field, measuring differences in health by group, for example, income, education, or race/ethnicity, has become the standard method for health inequality analysis. The World Health Organisation recently challenged this standard method by proposing individuals, instead of groups, as the unit of analysis.[9,10] The WHO researchers asked: why should you not measure health inequality across individuals, irrespective of individuals' group affiliations, in much the same way as income inequality? The WHO approach has caused much controversy [9,11–16] but evidently stimulated discussion on why and how we measure health inequality.

This chapter responds to the current growing interest in and need for developing a framework for measuring health inequality sensitive to relevant moral and quantitative concern. The proposed framework suggests various ways to think morally about health inequality and emphasises the logical consistency from conception to measurement.

Terminology

Health sciences researchers have increasingly distinguished health inequity from health inequality.[3,4,17] However, confusion over the terminology still persists, especially when researchers with different disciplinary training assemble to collaborate. In addition, words that seem to suggest similar meanings, for example, difference, disparity, heterogeneity, and injustice, aggravate the confusion.

The framework in this chapter refines the terminology common among health sciences researchers. The most frequently cited clarification of terminology in the health sciences literature is that of Whitehead and Dahlgren: health inequalities that are avoidable and unfair are health inequities.[18] Since they proposed this classification in 1991, a consensus has emerged among health sciences researchers as schematically explained in Figure 5.1. Suppose we select a population of interest, for example, a country or province, and the unit of analysis, either the individual or group. Health distribution is a way in which health is spread among the unit of analysis in the population. Health equality is the health distribution in which health is spread equally to every unit of analysis in the population, and health inequality is all health distributions that are otherwise. Reducing health inequality is the same as increasing health equality. Despite the different

Within a population of concern (for example, country, county),
among the unit of analysis (individual or group)

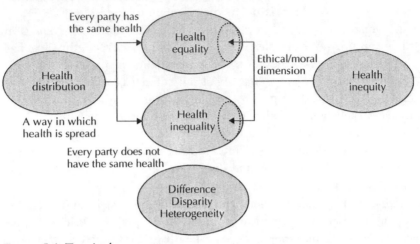

FIGURE 5.1 Terminology.

connotation of each word, terms such as difference, disparity, and heterogeneity have the same meaning here as inequality. Some health distributions are of moral concern, and the moral dimension of health distribution
is health inequity.

A Framework for Measuring Health Inequity

I propose to consider that measuring health inequity entails three steps: (1)
defining when a health distribution becomes inequitable, (2) deciding on
measurement strategies to operationalise a chosen concept of equity, and
(3) quantifying health inequity information. Steps 1 and 2 extract the information concerning health inequity from the health distribution and allow
us to draw such figures as those in Figure 5.2. Quantifying the extent of
health inequity by means of a single number (step 3) is a strategy to facilitate examination, comparison, and understanding of the health inequity in
question. All three steps ask distinct questions, and a decision made at one
step does not always guide a decision at another step.

Step 1: Defining Health Inequity

A variety of perspectives on health equity exist. They can be loosely cat-
egorised as: health equity as equality in health, and health inequality as

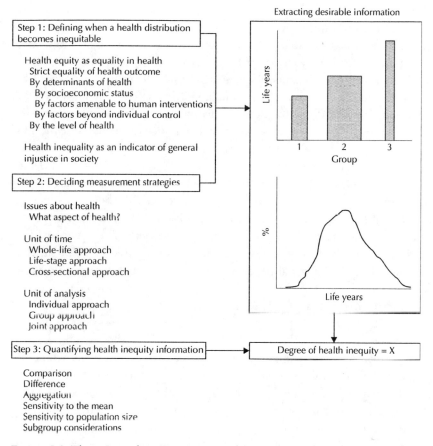

Extracting desirable information

Step 1: Defining when a health distribution becomes inequitable

Health equity as equality in health
  Strict equality of health outcome
  By determinants of health
    By socioeconomic status
    By factors amenable to human interventions
    By factors beyond individual control
    By the level of health

Health inequality as an indicator of general injustice in society

Step 2: Deciding measurement strategies

Issues about health
  What aspect of health?

Unit of time
  Whole-life approach
  Life-stage approach
  Cross-sectional approach

Unit of analysis
  Individual approach
  Group approach
  Joint approach

Step 3: Quantifying health inequity information   ⟶   Degree of health inequity = X

Comparison
Difference
Aggregation
Sensitivity to the mean
Sensitivity to population size
Subgroup considerations

FIGURE 5.2 Three Steps for Measuring Health Inequity.

an indicator of general injustice in society. No perspective is free from conceptual challenges. Yet, identifying a perspective on health equity that motivates measurement is an inevitable task.

Health equity as equality in health

Perspectives in the first group derive the moral significance of health distributions from the value of health. The simplest view in the first group is the perspective on health equity as strict equality of health outcome for all persons. If we believed that health is to some degree special, equality of health outcome among everyone, just as equality of political liberty among everyone, might seem to be the most straightforward criterion for health equity. Strict equality for all, however, is not an attractive view for various reasons. For example, it denies personal choice. It would be unrealistically expensive. Moreover, it would be unachievable because some determinants of health are beyond human control. Unlike political liberty, strict equality in health-for-all would not be a feasible nor agreeable goal. Accordingly, popular accounts of health equity relax the strictness in one way or another.

The most common way to depart from strict equality in health outcome is to look at health determinants. We can define health inequalities caused by certain determinants as inequitable.[2,3] Inequalities in health associated with socioeconomic status (SES), for example, to many people present an intuitive moral concern.[17,19] The WHO researchers consider determinants more broadly than SES [9,20] and propose to view health inequality caused by factors amenable to human interventions as inequitable.[12] Le Grand and Whitehead define health inequity as health inequality by factors beyond individual control.[3,21]

Measurement strategy would differ depending on the choice of determinants of health as well as the reason for the choice. There are, for example, various reasons why health inequality associated with SES is inequitable. We might extend the theory of justice as fairness proposed by John Rawls[22] and include health as a social primary good along with income and wealth, offices, and the bases of self respect. Should we measure health inequity based on the extended Rawlsian framework, we would look at the average health of the worst off group, for example, life expectancy of the lowest quintile income group. If, on the other hand, we adopted a view that systematic, pervasive, or structural inequalities are inequitable,[17,19,23,24] the focus would be on the correlations between health and such other factors as SES and sex.

Another way to define health equity as equality in health is to focus on the level of health. This approach is based on the idea of the minimally adequate level of health, a multi-purpose resource that is useful for any life plan. Society would be concerned about whether each person satisfies the minimally adequate level of health regardless of how each person realises her health. Society would not be concerned about health above this level as it accepts that people may trade off health with other goods depending on their preferences and conceptions of good life. In other words, adopting this view we would not measure health inequalities above this level.

Norman Daniels's normal species functioning[5] and the capability approach[25,26] are examples of the idea of the minimally adequate level of health. The right to health perspective, popular in international health circles,[27] is also compatible with this view.

Health inequality as an indicator of general injustice in society

Perspectives in the second group emphasise relations between health and other important goods. Multiple factors directly or in complex combination determine health. The exact mechanism of health production is beyond our understanding. But health is an ultimate outcome of how society distributes multiple determinants of health. We can regard health inequality as an indicator of general injustice in society.[2] Amartya Sen, for example, suggests mortality as a supplement to the conventional economic indicators.[28] Daniels et al. are intrigued by a coincidence that the social primary goods that Rawls suggests in his theory of justice[22] happen to be important determinants of health. "Social justice is good for our health"[7] they therefore claim. In this view, the primary concern is just distribution of social primary goods. Extended, we may use the distribution of health as an indicator of a just society.

Step 2: Deciding on Measurement Strategies

To operationalise an equity perspective as a measurement strategy, we need to consider further issues, namely, issues about health, the unit of time, and the unit of analysis. Empirically, these are measurement questions based on data availability. When measuring health inequity, moral considerations should also guide measurement strategy.

Issues about health

We cannot measure health equity without measuring health. In deciding the measurement of health in health equity analysis, we must consider a fundamental question: why does health distribution cause moral concern? Two widely shared views exist. Firstly, health in itself is one component of welfare. Secondly, health is a multi-purpose good that is useful for any life plan. These characteristics of health form the fundamental basis for moral interests in health distribution.

These fundamental values of health support functionality as the aspect of health to consider, thereby, the use of health-related quality of life measures. In the understanding of health as one component of welfare and a multi-purpose resource, what is relevant is what a person can or cannot do or whether a person exhibits general symptoms such as pain or anxiety. A different disease category in itself does not affect the level of health-related welfare or the potential use of health as a multi-purpose resource.

Unit of time

To decide the unit of time in health inequity analysis, you must ask: within what time period should health equity be sought? Three approaches exist.[29,30] The whole life approach looks at the entire health experiences of people from birth to death. The life stage approach compares health experiences of people within the same age group. The cross sectional approach takes a snapshot of health experiences of people at a certain time all together, irrespective of their life stages.

Which of these three approaches is the most appropriate time unit in health equity analysis? To examine this question, it is once again useful to recall why we seek health equity. In the understanding of health as a resource, it is reasonable to think that we appreciate opportunities that health brings differently at different stages of life. The same good health, for example, may bring more opportunities in youth than in senescence. Furthermore, empirical studies show that good health in earlier life stages is in itself an opportunity for good health in later life stages.[4,31]

The understanding of health as a multi-purpose resource endorses the life stage approach and rejects the whole life and cross sectional approaches. By focusing on the overall health experience, the whole life approach loses important information on when and in what way a person is healthy in life. The cross sectional approach, although perhaps most commonly used in health inequity analysis, is too crude as it neglects the age distribution of a population. "Age weight" is necessary properly to combine different life stages as the whole life experience or as the snapshot of health experiences of a population. The issue of relative value of each life stage is controversial.[32-34] Until we resolve the question of age weight, the life stage approach best reflects our fundamental value of health while leaving the unsettled issues open.

Unit of analysis

Three key issues distinguish the individual and group approach. The first and the most fundamental question is among whom—individuals or groups—you wish to seek health equity. The second issue relates to comparability of health inequity analysis. The individual is the ultimate unit of analysis, while an unlimited number of group choices are possible, and group definitions vary.[9,35] The third issue concerns the use of the average in

---

Box 5.1 What This Chapter Adds

- This chapter refines classification of such words as health inequality, health inequity, difference, disparity, and heterogeneity.
- This chapter proposes a framework for measuring the moral dimension of health inequality where important moral and quantitative questions are identified and other significant questions can be further built upon, rather than defending one particular measurement based on a certain normative position.
- The framework suggests various ways to think morally about health inequality and emphasises the logical consistency from conception to measurement.

the group approach. What does the average of a group represent? Should we be worried about the information neglected by the use of the average?

Researchers often consider the choice of the unit of analysis as dichotomous. Should both individual and group data be available, however, researchers could examine health equity across individuals as well as groups.[16] By simultaneously measuring health equity across individuals and groups, researchers can identify what proportion of the overall health inequity is attributable to a particular group characteristic and, among many group characteristics, which one contributes most to the overall health inequity. Recent studies have increasingly used this approach.[36–38]

While this approach is promising, it does not resolve all the three issues mentioned above. Researchers still need to examine the philosophical question of among whom they wish to seek health equity and the issue of comparability.

Step 3: Quantifying Health Inequity Information

To quantify the degree of health inequity, various measures are available, for example, the range measures,[39] the concentration index,[40,41] and the Gini coefficient.[35,42] How can researchers choose among them? Convenience, rather than principle, often drives this decision. But different measures can conclude different degrees of health inequity even when used for the same health distribution.[41] Among the issues discussed in the so-called axiomatic approach in the income inequality literature,[39,43] philosophical work by Larry Temkin,[30] and small but pioneering work in the health sciences field,[20,41,44–47] the following six questions deserve significant thought when quantifying health inequity information.

Comparison

How many units are to be compared, and what is the basis of comparison? Figure 5.3 illustrates four different ways to make comparisons. In Figure 5.3 a small circle represents a person or a group, placing it horizontally from the sickest to the healthiest or the worst off to the best off, and arcs between them represent the comparisons we make. Concept A considers the range between the highest and the lowest, the extremes of the distribution. Concept B compares everyone to an established norm and considers differences as shortfalls in achievement. Concept C compares every unit against the mean. In concept D, every individual or group is compared with each other. Obviously, these four choices are not exhaustive and are intended only to illustrate the discussion points.

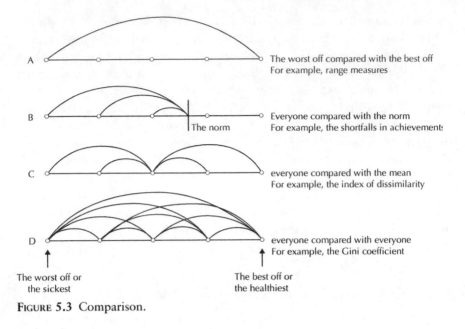

FIGURE 5.3 Comparison.

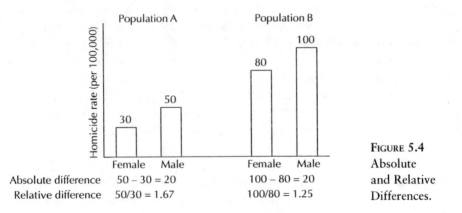

FIGURE 5.4 Absolute and Relative Differences.

Absolute or relative differences

Do we look at differences absolutely or relatively? In Figure 5.4, absolute sex differences in homicide are the same in these two populations, but population A has greater relative difference than population B. While nothing is wrong in expressing differences absolutely or relatively, it is not clear which provides a better expression of health inequity.

Aggregation

How do we aggregate differences at the population level? Imagine that small circles in each of A, B, C, and D in Figure 5.3 represent income

Box 5.2 Policy Implications

- Without clearly defining health inequity and logically consistently applying the chosen concept to measurement, no one can move onto effective policymaking for health equity.
- This chapter helps researchers and policymakers to define health inequity and points to key questions that they need to address when applying the chosen concept to measurement of health inequity.

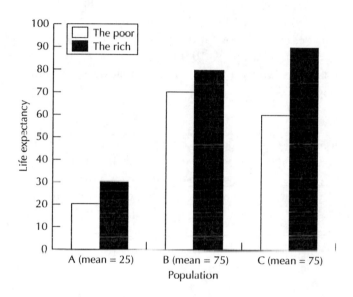

FIGURE 5.5
Sensitivity to
the Mean.

quintile group and their life expectancies are 55, 60, 65, 70, and 75 years old from the lowest to the highest group. Should all five year differences between the successive income groups be considered the same? Or might we wish to "value health differently along the distribution,"[44] for example, providing a greater weight to the five year difference at the lower tail?

Sensitivity to the mean

Should the assessment of health inequity be sensitive to the population's mean health? In other words, is health inequity worse in a sicker population?[30] Figure 5.5 illustrates three populations, each of which presents life expectancies of the poor and the rich. Population B and C have the same mean. Both the poor and the rich in population B have 50 years more than the poor and the rich in population A. Life expectancies of both the poor and the rich in population C are three times those of the poor and the rich in population A. Is health inequity worse in population A than population B and C? So-called mean independent measures, such as the concentration index and the Gini coefficient, judge that health inequity in population A and C is the same while health inequity is worse in population A than B. Whether this is the right judgment for health inequity is a moot point requiring philosophical investigation.

Sensitivity to population size

Should the assessment of health inequity be sensitive to the population size? Most inequity comparisons do not take this into account. But the same shortfall of 10% of the total population below a certain norm, for example, makes up a different number of people in populations with different sizes: 10 persons below the norm in the population of 100 people, and 1000 persons in the population of 10,000. If you were concerned about suffering from health inequity, you might judge that health inequity is worse in a larger population.[30]

Subgroup considerations

How should overall inequity of a population correspond to inequities between and within subgroups? Suppose overall health distributions are identical in population A and B. However, these same overall distributions are made up from very different subgroup contributions. In population A the rich are healthy and the poor sick, while health is not correlated with income in population B. Are population A and B the same in terms of health inequity?

Conclusions

Researchers and policymakers in various fields have increasingly recognised health equity as an important issue. Despite the growing recognition, what health inequity means is still often unclear, and how best the moral consideration can be brought into the measurement needs further investigation. Aiming to fill this gap, this paper proposed a framework for measuring health inequity consisting of three steps. Health inequity implies social responsibility and calls for policy action. Without clearly defining health inequity and logically consistently applying the chosen concept to measurement, no one can move onto effective policymaking for health equity.

This chapter admittedly raised more questions than it answered. Given the excitingly multi-disciplinary nature of the topic of measuring health inequity, future work examining the questions left open will be only possible through a dynamic, collaborative effort by researchers from different disciplines.

Acknowledgements

I am indebted to Professors David Kindig, John Mullahy, Patrick Remington, Alberto Palloni, Daniel Hausman, and Daniel Wikler for their general assistance for my dissertation, from which this study was derived. I am also grateful to Professor Nuala Kenny for comments on an earlier version of the manuscript.

Funding: this project was supported by grant number 1 R03 HS 13116 from the US Agency for Healthcare Research and Quality, and the Canadian Institute of Health Research Training Program for Ethics and Health Policy and Research.

References

1. Marchand, S., D. Wikler, and B. Landesman, "Class, Health, and Justice," 76 *The Milbank Quarterly* (1998): 449–467.
2. Peter, F. and T. Evans, "Ethical Dimensions of Health Equity," in *Challenging Inequalities in Health: From Ethics to Action*, ed. T. Evans, M. Whitehead, F. Diderichsen, Abbas Bhuiya, and Meg Wirth (New York: Oxford University Press, 2001): 25–33.
3. M. Whitehead, "The concepts and principles of equity and health," 22 *International Journal of Health Services* (1992): 429–445.
4. I. Kawachi, S.V. Subramanian, and N Almeida-Filho, "A Glossary for Health Inequalities," 56 *Journal of Epidemiol Community Health* (2002): 647–652.
5. N. Daniels, *Just Health Care* (Cambridge: Cambridge University Press, 1985): 56.
6. D.W. Brock, "Broadening the Bioethics Agenda," 10 *Kennedy Institute of Ethics Journal* (2000): 21–38.
7. N. Daniels, B. Kennedy, and I. Kawachi, *Is Inequality Bad for Our Health?* (Boston, MA: Beacon Press, 2000): 3–33.
8. D. Wikler, Bioethics, Human Rights, and the Renewal of Health for All: An Overview," in *Ethics, Equity and the Renewal of WHO's health-for-all strategy*," ed. Z. Bankowski, J.H. Bryant, and J. Gallagher (Geneva: CIOMS, 1997): 21–30.
9. C.J.L. Murray, E.E. Gakidou, and J. Frenk, "Health Inequalities and Social Group Differences: What Should We Measure?" 77 *Bulletin of the World Health Organization* (1999): 537–543.
10. World Health Organisation, *The World Health Report 2000: Health Systems: Improving Performance* (Geneva: World Health Organisation, 2000): 215.
11. C. Almeida, P. Braveman, M.R. Gold, et al., "Methodological Concerns and Recommendations on Policy Consequences of the World Health Report 2000," 357 *Lancet* (2001): 1692–1697.
12. Y. Asada and T. Hedemann, "A Problem with the Individual Approach in the Who Health Inequality Measurement," 1 *International Journal for Equity in Health* (2002): 1–5. http://wwwequityhealthjcom/content/1/1/2 (accessed 22 Oct 2004).

13. P. Braveman, N. Krieger, and J. Lynch, "Health Inequalities and Social Inequalities in Health," 78 *Bulletin of the World Health Organization* (2000): 232–233.

14. P. Braveman, B. Starfield, and H.J. Geiger, "World Health Report 2000: How It Removes Equity from the Agenda for Public Health Monitoring and Policy," 323 *British Medical Journal* (2001): 678–681.

15. D. Hausman, Y. Asada, and T. Hedemann, "Health Inequalities and Why They Matter," 10 *Health Care Analysis* (2002): 177–191.

16. M. Wolfson and G. Rowe, "On Measuring Inequalities in Health," 79 *Bulletin of the World Health Organization* (2001): 553–560.

17. P. Braveman and S. Gruskin, "Defining Equity in Health," 57 *Journal of Epidemiology and Community Health* (2003): 254–258.

18. G. Dahlgren and M. Whitehead, *Policies and Strategies to Promote Social Equality in Health* (Stockholm: Institute of Future Studies, 1991).

19. B. Starfield, "Basic Concepts in Population Health and Health Care," 55 *Journal of Epidemiology and Community Health* (2001): 452–454.

20. E.E. Gakidou, C.J.L. Murray, and J. Frenk, "Defining and Measuring Health Inequality: an Approach Based on the Distribution of Health Expectancy," 78 *Bulletin of the World Health Organization* (2000): 42–54.

21. J. Le Grand, *Equity and Choice: An Essay in Economics and Applied Philosophy* (London: Harpercollins Academic, 1991): 62–126.

22. J. Rawls, *A Theory of Justice* (Cambridge, MA: Harvard University Press, 1971): 194.

23. M. Walzer, *Spheres of Justice* (New York: Basic Books, 1983): 3–30.

24. International Society for Equity in Health (ISEqH), *Working Definitions*, http://www.iseqh.org/en/workdef.htm (accessed 4 Feb 2005).

25. M.C. Nussbaum, *Women and Human Development: The Capabilities Approach* (Cambridge: Cambridge University Press, 2000): 110.

26. A. Sen, *Inequality Reexamined,* (Cambridge, MA: Harvard University Press, 1992): 207.

27. J.M. Mann, "Medicine and Public Health, Ethics and Human Rights," 27 *The Hastings Center Report* (1997): 6–13.

28. A. Sen, "Mortality as an Indicator of Economic Success and Failure," 108 *Economic Journal* (1998): 1–25.

29. D. McKerlie, "Equality and Time," 99 *Ethics* (1989): 475–491.

30. L.S. Temkin, *Inequality* (Oxford: Oxford University Press, 1993): 308.

31. C. Power, S. Matthews, and O. Manor, "Inequalities in Self-Rated Health: Explanations from Different Stages of Life," 351 *Lancet* (1998): 1009–1014.

32. A. Tsuchiya, "QALYs and Ageism: Philosophical Theories and Age Weighting," 9 *Health Economics* (2000): 57–68.

33. A. Williams, "Intergenerational Equity: An Exploration of the 'Fair Innings' Argument," 6 *Health Economics* (1997): 117–132.

34. N. Daniels, *Am I My Parents' Keeper?* (Oxford: Oxford University Press, 1988): 176.

35. R. Illsley and J. Le Grand, "Measurement of Inequality in Health," in *Health Economics,* ed. A. Williams (London: Macmillan, 1987): 12–36.

36. E. van Doorslaer and X. Koolman, "Explaining the Differences in Income-Related Health Inequalities across European Countries," 13 *Health Economics* (2004): 609–628.

37. A. Wagstaff and E. van Doorslaer, "Overall Versus Socioeconomic Health Inequality: a Measurement Framework and Two Empirical Illustrations," 13 *Health Economics* (2004): 297–301.
38. P.M. Clarke, U.-G. Gerdtham, and L.B. Connelly, "A Note on the Decomposition of the Health Concentration Index," 12 *Health Economics* (2003): 511–516.
39. A. Sen, *On Economic Inequality* (Oxford: Oxford University Press, 1997): 46.
40. X. Koolman and E. Van Doorslaer, "On the Interpretation of a Concentration Index of Inequality," 13 *Health Economics* (2004): 649–656.
41. A. Wagstaff, P. Paci, and E. van Doorslaer, "On the Measurement of Inequalities in Health," 33 *Social Science & Medicine* (1991): 545–557.
42. J. Le Grand, "Inequality in Health: Some International Comparison" 31 *European Economic Review* (1987): 182–191.
43. F.A. Cowell, "Measurement of Inequality," in *Handbook of Income Distribution*, ed. A.B. Atkinson and F. Burguignon, Vol. 1 (Amsterdam: Elsevier, 2000): 89–166.
44. S. Anand, F. Diderichsen, and T. Evans, et al., "Measuring Disparities in Health: Methods and Indicators," in *Challenging Inequalities in Health: From Ethics to Action,* ed. T. Evans, M. Whitehead, F. Diderichsen, et al. (New York: Oxford University Press, 2001): 49–67.
45. C.A. Mustard and J. Etches, "Gender Differences in Socioeconomic Inequality in Mortality," 57 *Journal of Epidemiology and Community Health* (2003): 974–980.
46. J.P. Mackenbach and A.E. Kunst, "Measuring the magnitude of socio-economic inequalities in health: an overview of available measures illustrated with two examples from Europe," *Social Science & Medicine* (1997): 757–771.
47. O. Manor, S. Matthews, and C. Power, "Comparing measures of health inequality," 45 *Social Science & Medicine* (1997): 761–771.

6

Promoting Social Justice through Public Health Policies, Programs, and Services

ALONZO PLOUGH

Introduction

Public health policies, programs, and services—collectively termed public health practice—in the United States have been the subject of a series of reports by the Institute of Medicine (IOM)[1,2] and considerable commentary by the federal government, professional associations, and academic institutions.[3-5] However, social injustice as a focus of practice is rarely discussed.

Most assessments of the state of public health practice have dealt with such issues as organizational structure, funding shortfalls, and capacity limitation. They have typically focused on defining functional capacity (to provide the 10 essential public health services*) and the growing gaps between population health challenges and resources invested in the public health system.[6]

This chapter is reprinted with permission from *Social Injustice and Public Health*, Barry S. Levy and Victor W. Sidel eds., Oxford University Press, 2006: 418–432.
*The ten essential public health services are: (1) monitor health status to identify community problems; (2) diagnose and investigate health problems and health hazards in the community; (3) inform, educate, and empower people about health issues; (4) mobilize community partnerships and action to identify and solve health problems; (5) develop policies and plans that support individual and community health efforts; (6) enforce laws and regulations that

Broad assessments of a system in "disarray," particularly at the local level, abound. Federal- and state-level attempts to bring coherence to public health practice through standards and performance measures are presented as remedies for the diagnosis of systemic dysfunction. Current strategic planning at the Centers for Disease Control and Prevention (CDC) looks to the private sector and individual health care providers as an underused component of public health practice.[7]

These analyses also mention, one way or another, the imperative of public health to improve the social conditions in specific communities that largely determine health and well-being. Social determinants of health, community-based public health, community-based participatory research, and the social/ecological model** all appear as descriptors of a component of public health practice. However, this domain of practice is not considered essential. No national standards or performance measures explicitly deal with the promotion of social justice as a public health practice core capacity.

To understand better how social justice can and does become an object of public health practice, there must be (a) a recognition that public health practice is overwhelmingly a government activity—in organizational delivery and in financing, and (b) a debunking of much of the conventional judgment that public health practice is in disarray. Because the performance of activities and interventions to promote social justice challenges the broader political economy and explicitly identifies social injustice as a causal element in the poor health status of a particular community, government public health practice is placed in a difficult context. How health departments approach this problem will depend on (a) the level of government—federal, state, or local—in which the agency is located, (b) the political ideology of elected officials who oversee the agency, (c) the capacity and commitment of public health officials, (d) the ability of agency staff members to meaningfully engage community residents in collaborative endeavors, and (e) the competing demands of public health challenges, such as *severe acute respiratory syndrome* (SARS), bioterrorism preparedness, routine outbreaks of disease, inspections of various facilities, and service delivery mandates. An operational focus on root causes of poor health, such as

---

protect health and ensure safety; (7) link people to needed personal health services and assure the provision of health care when otherwise unavailable; (8) assure a competent public health and personal health care workforce; (9) evaluate effectiveness, accessibility, and quality of personal and population-based health services; and (10) research for new insights and innovative solutions to health problems.

**The social/ecological model describes how social, physical, and genetic factors influence health status. This includes contextual and relational influences on health, such as social and community networks, living and working conditions, institutional influences, and political and economic policies, all of which interact to shape population and individual health.

poverty, income and wealth inequality, and racism—all factors related to social injustice—requires a public health capacity not often discussed. This is the capacity to effectively manage the urgent demands of public health practice while simultaneously and explicitly understanding the social context and root causes of the poor health of populations. Importantly, this understanding of social context and root causes must inform both current practice and future strategic planning.

Public Health Agencies and Social Justice

Federal Agencies

The capacity to address social injustice in public health practice, or the ability to develop it, varies with the level of government in which a health agency operates. Federal agencies such as CDC and the Health Resources and Services Administration (HRSA) have a national scope, extensive grants and contracts, and multiple delivery and research programs that could focus on social injustice as a core problem in public health practice. Although there are some isolated examples of social justice as a key component of federal agency policy, these do not represent a central tendency. Too often, such promising policy directions like HRSA's 100 Percent Access and Zero Disparities initiative during the Clinton administration or the environmental justice focus of CDC's National Center for Environmental Health during the same period have had marginal funding and program development. The administration of each U.S. president has a different capacity to envision social injustice as an operational policy and program direction. As a result, there has been little sustained effort to address this fundamental problem at the federal level.

State Health Departments

State-level public health practice faces similar challenges, with frequent changes in governors, high turnover of public health officials, and widespread inability to gain sustained political support for explicit public heath activities to address social injustice. As is the case with federal-level public health practice, state health departments are often not directly connected with community-based public health practice. The default mode of public health practice at the state level is the pass-through of federal funds to local agencies, very general and aggregated statewide policy development, and regulatory activities. Advocacy and activism of health officials—which are essential ingredients for successful policy interventions to reduce social injustice—are very constrained at this level.

The average tenure of state public health directors is only 2.9 years.[8] As a result, directors are usually just starting or about to leave positions, making it quite difficult to provide the sustained and visible leadership needed to address social injustice as an essential function of public health practice. A review of the websites of the 50 state health departments found only one department with an extensive and explicit incorporation of social justice as a standard of practice.[9] The Association of State and Territorial Heath Officials (ASTHO) website contains no reports on or any references to addressing social justice as a core public health practice strategy.

Clearly, federal- and state-level public health agencies could influence critical policy areas that are shaped at the state level of government, such as education, taxation, housing, and economic development. The scale of federal- and state-level bureaucracy and the siloed nature of agency behavior make such direct action and collaboration difficult, especially on politically charged topics.

Federal and state public health agencies, however, can facilitate social justice interventions at the local level through funding that is sufficiently flexible to allow for community-driven approaches to prevention that can address social determinants of health. Funding approaches, such as the Racial and Ethnic Approaches to Community Health (REACH) program that has funded local coalitions to address health disparities in AIDS/HIV, diabetes, and infant mortality, have resulted in effective community-level interventions that address root causes of ill health and represent a social justice framework. The Steps to a Healthier United States (STEPS) grants program holds similar promise, although this program has been implemented too recently to evaluate its impact.

Local Health Departments

The local level of government public health practice is best situated to explicitly address social injustice. Local health departments represent the backbone of the government public health system, but they have been poorly represented in studies and reports on the current and projected status of public health practice.[10] Both of the influential IOM reports indicate that the public health system—from the perspective of conventional standards and technical capacity—is in disarray. Local health departments in particular are cited as having limited public health capacity.

There are a number of flaws, however, in the conventional analysis of local public health capacity.[11] In the United States, 70 percent of the population and almost all highly populous urban areas—where health disparities based on race, ethnicity, and poverty abound—are served by metropolitan health departments that are highly functional and have developed many effective policies, programs, and services. These health departments are also the most community-embedded components of the government public health structure and are beginning to develop public health practice models that explicitly consider addressing social injustice as a core organizational competency.

The best examples of a commitment to social justice as a part of public practice are associated with the policy commitment of the National Association of County and City Health Officials (NACCHO) to social justice. There are numerous references to social justice on the NACCHO website, which operates as a technical resource to local public health practitioners.[12] Its board has adopted a resolution that has, in part, urged "support for ideas, activities, social movements, and policies that advance action to build health equity through social justice."[13] In 2002, NACCHO revised its strategic plan to define as a core strategic action of local public health practice the capacity "to address issues of health equity and social justice, oppose racism, and support diversity and cultural competence."

In the world of public health practice, this dramatic difference in a professional association's explicit support for incorporating social justice as a core competency and providing tools, training, workshops, and other technical assistance to local practitioners to implement strategies and specific actions is profound. This support has provided grants and other resources that build strategic action in many local communities across the nation. Importantly, such a professional practice framework provides a much-needed legitimacy for advocacy work at the local level. When a local board of health member or city official questions why a health department is involved in land use or environmental justice as a policy and program area, the ability to point to a national organization's strategic plans and practice guidelines often provides the evidence for these actions being seen as "standard" public health practice.

Local public health practice is grounded in specific communities and is part of a local network of community-based organizations and public and private institutions with a shared local governmental context. The broad range of social conditions that adversely influence health outcomes—such as unemployment rates, poverty, disinvestments in public education, unsafe neighborhoods, and suburban sprawl (as a deterrent to community cohesion)—have a daily immediacy at this level of public health practice. The definition of public health as a "social enterprise" with a mandate to align the technical tools of epidemiology and assessment with effective community partnerships and advocacy can become operational in local health departments with the leadership and commitment to engage with their communities in challenging social injustice. The much longer tenure of local public health officials, compared with their state counterparts, increases the possibilities for catalytic leadership and sustained practice efforts grounded in a social justice framework. Staff members of local health departments are also members of the community, helping to increase linkages between communities that experience health problems related to social injustice and local public health programs and services that should be accountable to these communities.

Clearly, all government public health agencies—including local health departments—are challenged in creating authentic community partnerships. To be effective in a community-linked approach to addressing social injustice requires public health agencies to incorporate new approaches to collaboration that go far beyond the traditional expert-driven approach to professional public health practice.[14] Roz Lasker and Elisa Weiss[15] present a very thoughtful approach to the essential principles of collaboration required to facilitate activities that address the root causes of health disparities and other social and economic conditions that decrease the well-being of communities. The key components of their community health governance model suggest that effective collaboration requires empowerment, community building (the bridging of social ties), and community engagement. All of these are essential activities of public health practice, without which public health agencies would probably revert to the rhetoric of community engagement without the impact from true power sharing with community members. Too often, public health agencies use the language of the social determinants of health and the need to reduce health disparities but do not internally transform in ways that would allow for the nontraditional actions required to address social injustice as a risk to the public's health. Using the language of social justice while applying the traditional top-down tools of public health practice has a limited impact.

The major challenge of public health practice is to move theoretical knowledge about the relationship of social injustice to increased health risks and poor health outcomes into broad and sustainable changes in agency policies and practices. These changes include (a) providing support and training to staff members in partnership development, and (b) creating the capacity to extend public health practice beyond the agency walls to dynamic partnerships with other disciplines, such as economic development, land use planning, housing, transportation, and education.

Local public health practitioners are particularly effective when local data are generated and communicated through accessible reports that highlight the impact of specific social and economic factors on health outcomes. Effective use of local media is an essential tool of public health practice in broadening the public's awareness of the impacts of social injustice on community health. Careful, data-driven presentations to local elected officials and health board members are essential components of public health practices that address social injustice. However, this type of political advocacy is not always the most significant form of community and political mobilization activities.

Effective local public health practice depends largely on capabilities to (a) build on a general base of community-driven partnerships (some of which are not explicitly health focused), (b) identify root causes and leverage points for change, and (c) select the most effective set of tools and strategies that match specific manifestations of social injustice. Root causes of social injustice are often best addressed by focusing on policies concerning labor and employment, taxation, environmental conditions, housing, land use, and child development and support. The critical responsibility of public health practice that is oriented to social justice is to recognize the broader context of causation and to not constrict programs and interventions to those that are based on individual behaviors or a specific disease.

Public Health Practice Oriented to Social Justice

Two Case Studies

This section examines two examples of how public health policies, programs, and practices can highlight the relationship between social injustice and the public's health. Each example provides some practical insights into how community partnerships can be used to deepen knowledge of root causes of poor health, mobilize and activate political and community leadership, and make initial efforts sustainable. The case studies are drawn from local public health agencies in San Francisco and Seattle. Each case study focuses on a health-related problem with significant social determinants, with each public health agency and its community partners deploying different strategies to link the broader social justice problem with a specific approach to health improvement at the community level. The scale of impact and the possible sustainability of the efforts in each of these case studies are different. They highlight the complexities of addressing social injustice through public health practices and policies that are primarily governmental.

Case Study 1

The San Francisco Department of Public Health is a city and county health department serving a diverse metropolitan population. Its practice framework is linked to the strategies to promote social justice in local public health practice at a national level. For example, its environmental health section supports the Program on Health, Equity, and Sustainability, the goal of which is "to make San Francisco a livable city for all residents and to foster environmental, community, and economic conditions that allow residents to achieve their human potential."[16]

In 2002, the department facilitated a process to address environmental health disparities in asthma, particularly in relation to indoor-air exposure to poor children. Recognizing that some neighborhoods have a high concentration of substandard housing and drawing on published studies relating poor indoor-air quality to the presence of mites, cockroaches, and mold, the department raised the level of community awareness through data presentation and community mobilization. Setting the context with an estimate of 54,000 residents diagnosed with asthma, the department pointed out the disproportionately more severe outcomes among communities of color and placed this risk in a broader community context by stating, "The health and well-being of San Francisco's residents, families, and community are at stake."[17]

An important community-mobilizing strategy was the development of the San Francisco Asthma Task Force. Chaired by a local nongovernment social-service provider, the composition of the group reflected the diversity of the community, including representatives of nonprofit organizations and community-advocacy organizations and community members, many of whom had experienced asthma in their own families. The task force developed focused working groups that had a diversity of members. These working groups gained information from tenants with asthma, property owners, managers, builders, and contractors to develop a community-based definition of the problem. Then teams from the Department of Public Health and the task force applied the interdisciplinary tools of environmental health, environmental epidemiology, building and housing code enforcement, and tenant organizing to further define intervention and policy approaches. Through an open community process, including retreats, the task force developed recommendations that focused on improving indoor-air quality for lower-income tenants. The final report of the task force highlighted the structural deficiencies of buildings that exacerbate asthma by exposure to molds, fumes, and other hazards. These factors, which represent significant forms of housing injustice, were presented by the group as root causes of asthma. There was explicit recognition, based on the findings of the work groups, that low-income people have few housing options and are disproportionately exposed to these factors.[18]

Recommendations resulting from this locally driven public health partnership reflect insights gained and action strategies developed when public health workers and community partners create dynamic collaborations to address social injustice. The major action strategies that it developed to address environmental determinants of asthma included the following:

1. Establishing a cross-agency group to inspect public-housing properties and to create accountability mechanisms that rapidly brought conditions into compliance with the housing code. This strategy involved creating interagency collaborations among the health department, the housing agency, and agencies involved with code enforcement, the police, and the legal and judicial systems, all of which focused on improving the underlying social conditions that account for income-based disparities in asthma.
2. Establishing standards and guidelines for comprehensive healthy housing, including roles for property owners—requiring government entities to strengthen the relationship between building codes and landlords' legal obligation to tenants to reduce housing-related health risks.
3. Instituting a legal housing-advocacy program for poor patients identified with asthma. This intervention implemented a monitoring and engagement strategy that raised awareness about environmental determinants of asthma and linked poor asthma patients using hospital emergency departments with information and housing advocates.

This case study demonstrates how many of the elements of a social justice-oriented public health practice are developed and implemented. While the overall project recognized the clinical and disease control issues, its thrust addressed the root causes of asthma in housing and economic policies. The health department was a key participant, but the project was broadly based in the community and led by community organizations. Finally, recommendations addressed the social context of risk and incorporated nontraditional approaches for providing public health programs and services.

Case Study 2

Public Health–Seattle and King County is a large metropolitan local health department serving nearly 2 million people. The department has long recognized the critical importance of social justice in public health practice, as reflected in its mission and value statements and its organizational structure. A specific interdisciplinary unit—Community-Based Public Health Practice (CBPHP)—was established in 1998 to develop community-driven activities grounded in a deep understanding of the social determinants of health.[19] A major focus of CBPHP was eliminating disproportionately poor health status in communities of color.

To develop an approach to this problem that was oriented to social justice, the department initiated a series of surveys and studies that documented growing disparities among economically marginalized King County racial and ethnic groups. Specific examination of disparities in infant mortality, teen pregnancy, diabetes, and other poor health outcomes set the stage for a more contextual examination of root causes of these problems.[20] The results of these studies were published in an easily accessible form and were made widely available on the Internet and through other communication channels. Health department staff members worked closely with advocates to increase community awareness of these problems and to engage community members in strategies to improve the underlying social and economic bases of the poor health outcomes. This work involved specific community-driven assessment of health and examination of the critical social contexts in specific communities, including American Indians and Alaska Natives, African-Americans, members of specific Asian and Pacific Island groups, and Hispanics.

The King County Ethnicity and Health Survey revealed that discrimination influenced all health disparities. For example, 32 percent of African-Americans thought that they had been discriminated against when receiving health care services at some time.[21] Lower percentages of members of ethnic groups also reported experiencing discrimination. Because discrimination is a potent cause of social injustice, a broader strategy was required for effective advocacy and change. Community partners and health department staff members recognized that racism was the root cause and that how racism influenced health status and health-seeking behavior of specific ethnic populations had to be addressed. In the health care setting, perceptions of discrimination can powerfully impact health-seeking behavior and, potentially, health status.

Giving voice to individuals who had experienced racism in health care settings provided a more grounded presentation of the problem. By presenting the issues in human terms, the report presented a dramatic and compelling sense of the problem—much more than could have been achieved with a presentation of statistical data. As a result, the information was more likely to improve staff behavior in institutions where discrimination had occurred.

The health department contracted with a community-based organization to develop and conduct the Racial Discrimination in Health Care Interview Project.[22] The results were reported in a community report and a public health report that was broadly distributed among health care practitioners and their institutions, as well as political and community leaders.[23] The reports highlighted the extensive range and frequency of perceived discrimination among those interviewed. The discrimination events, which had taken place at nearly 30 different public and private health care facilities throughout King County, included racial slurs and blatant examples of rude behaviors and differential treatment. As the report stated, most interviewees reported changing their behaviors as a result of discrimination they had experienced. Some reported delaying treatment due to their negative experiences and not knowing where else to seek care.

These descriptive and experience-based examples from the survey were presented in numerous public settings, including press conferences with the county executive, community meetings, conferences of health professional associations, and board of health meetings. They generated much media attention. The results of the series of studies on race, ethnicity, and health were presented to the chief executives of the major hospitals and health plans in the region. A call to action was delivered in all of those settings, seeking a broad community consensus to adopt the recommendations of the reports, including training health care providers, establishing uniform institutional policies to enforce nondiscrimination, and collecting data and performing monitoring by including questions regarding discrimination on patient satisfaction surveys. Many of the recommendations were implemented by local institutions. The work to eliminate discrimination continues.

Additional Examples of Public Health Practice That Address Social Injustice

These two case studies provide good examples of how public health practice can incorporate a social justice framework that influences policy and service. There are many other ways that government public health, especially at the local level, can address injustice. One example is using public health surveillance data to identify the adverse health effects of social injustice. Public health agencies can closely monitor a set of social indicators—such as measures of poverty, income inequality, housing costs, parents who read to young children, and unemployment—that are highly related to health and human development. It is increasingly important to link these types of social indicators to the more traditional vital statistics and health status measures and to use census tracts and ZIP codes as units of analysis. By this approach, public health departments can develop, with their community partners, neighborhood-focused assessments that can assist communities in advocating to improve social and economic conditions that underlie health disparities. Sometimes the advocacy might be focused on ensuring access to preventive services, such as prenatal care for poor women through community and public health clinics. Increasingly, such assessments find that addressing factors such as inadequate housing, lack of jobs with a livable wage, unsafe workplaces, and community exposures to environmental hazards are even more important than providing traditional, client-focused public health services. Given recent budget cuts for public health services in most jurisdictions, it is unlikely that public health agencies can directly ensure that all appropriate services are available and accessible. However, public health practice can align funded services to populations with the greatest needs and aggressively present the political and social context for the critical gaps in access to preventive services.

An Action Agenda for a Social Justice Core Competency in Public Health Practice

For public health practice to better address social injustice, there will need to be a fundamental shift in what is currently viewed as core or essential public health activities. Evolving local, state, and federal standards for public health in the United States clearly prioritize the traditional role of disease prevention and health promotion, although this is greatly complicated by the even higher prioritization of bioterrorism preparedness. Although community involvement, even community engagement, is seen as a core public health activity, its goals are articulated and its outcomes are measured primarily as changes in individual behavior that reduce conventional disease risk factors. For example, it may be stated that more people eat a healthy diet or perform physical exercise or that more young people understand the risk factors associated with drug use due to community assessment and partnership activities.

A public health practice competency addressing the impact of social injustice on health goes beyond affecting individual behavior change and improving the effectiveness of practices within the traditional boundaries of health services. It focuses on enabling more accountable public and private decisions concerning the basic needs of groups of people who have poor health because of discrimination based on race, income, language, ethnicity, or sexual orientation. Its outcomes can be measured by sustainable reductions in the social determinants of this discrimination.

What Are Some of the Barriers to Wider Acceptance of a Core Public Health Competency Demonstrating Ability to Reduce Social Injustice?

First, as reflected in curricular and other requirements of schools of public health and public health programs, academic public health faculty members are just beginning to develop courses that train students in methods and skills relevant to reducing the impact of social injustice on health. Research and courses on health disparities, minority health, and social determinants of health are more prevalent than ever before in this country, but these courses focus on description of problems and policy issues—generally not on methods of engaging communities to develop sustainable actions to address the root causes of health disparities. Courses on community-based public health practice should go beyond community-based assessment of conventional health risk factors and should focus on community-organizing and empowered collaborative practices that can address root causes of social injustice. These courses could link to public health practice settings, where people who have suffered poor health due to social injustice could serve as adjunct faculty members.

A second and closely related barrier to wider acceptance of this core public health competency is the lack of federal funding to support the development of public health practice approaches to address social injustice. This inadequacy includes limited funding for campus/practice/community partnerships to develop and disseminate best practices. More extensive federal funding to local health departments is required to enable their staff members to understand how to develop effective community partnerships and to develop expertise in nontraditional areas of practice. Clear but flexible mandates for authentic community partnerships in policy and program development are needed.

State health departments need to recognize that the community-driven nature of the social determinants of health requires a decentralized focus on local leadership and community development. This requires a shift in focus away from aggregated state plans for reducing disparities to legislative and regulatory policy approaches to reduce the impact of social injustice on the public's health. It requires legislators and policymakers at all levels of government to understand, for example, that housing and land-use/zoning decisions have a major influence on the public's health.

The third and final barrier to wider acceptance of this core public health competency involves raising money to support its promotion during a period of budgetary constraints. Public health practitioners at all levels will need to creatively use data on the social determinants of health to inform and influence the decisions of elected officials. The greatest challenge may be the perception that social injustice is rarely eliminated by public health services alone—although services can reduce the impact of social injustice on individuals who receive these services. A public health practice commitment to incorporating social justice as a core capacity means going far beyond providing services—it means being a catalyst for sustainable structural change to reduce social injustice.

References

1. Institute of Medicine. *The Future of Public Health* (Washington, DC: Academy Press, 1988).
2. Institute of Medicine, *The Future of the Public's Health in the 21ˢᵗ Century* (Washington, DC: National Academy Press, 2003).
3. M. Fraser, "State and Local Health Department Structures: Implications for Systems Change and Transformations for Public Health," *Turning Point Newsletter* (Washington, DC, 1998): 1(4).
4. National Association of County and City Health Officials, *Local Public Health Agency Infrastructure: A Chartbook* (October, 2004), http://www.naccho.org/pubs/detail (accessed January 28, 2005).
5. C.G. Freund and Z. Liu, "Local Health Department Capacity and Performance in New Jersey," 6 *Journal of Public Health Management & Practice* (2000): 42–50.
6. G.P. Mays, C.A. Miller, and P.K. Halverson eds., *Local Public Health Practice: Trends and Models* (Washington, DC: American Public Health Association, 2000).
7. Centers for Disease Control and Prevention, *The Futures Initiative: Creating the Future of CDC for the 21ˢᵗ Century*, http://www.cdc.gov/futures/update.htm (accessed January 28, 2005).
8. M.B. Meit, "I'm OK, But I'm Not Too Sure About You: Public Health at the State and Local Levels," 7 *Journal of Public Health Management & Practice* (2001): vii–viii.
9. Minnesota Department of Health, *Benefits of Community Engagement* http://www.health.state.mn.us/communityeng/index.html (accessed January 28, 2005).
10. M.A. Barry, L. Centra, E. Pratt, C.K. Brown, and L.Giordano, *Where Do the Dollars Go? Measuring Local Public Health Expenditures* (Washington, DC, 1998). Submitted to the Office of Disease Prevention and Health Promotion, Department of Health and Human Services, by National Association of City and County Health Officials, National Association of Local Boards of Health, and the Public Health Foundation, http://www.phf.org (accessed January 28, 2005).
11. A.L. Plough, "Understanding the Financing and Functions of Metropolitan Health Departments: A Key to Improved Public Health Response," 10 *Journal of Public Health Management & Practice* (2004): 421–427.
12. www.naccho.org
13. National Association of County and City Health Officials. *Resolution to Promote Health Equity* (July 2002), http://www.naccho.org/resolution94.cfm (accessed January 28, 2005).

14. A.L. Plough, "Common discourse but divergent actions–bridging the promise of community health governance and public health practice," 80 *Journal of Urban Health* (2003): 53–7.
15. R.D. Lasker and E.S. Weiss, "Broadening Participation in Community Problem-solving: a Multidisciplinary Model to Support Collaborative Practice and Research," 80 *Journal of Urban Health* (2003): 14–47.
16. San Francisco Department of Public Health. Program on Health, Equity and Sustainability 2004, http://www.dph.sf.ca.us/ehs (accessed January 28, 2005).
17. Ibid.
18. The San Francisco Asthma Task Force. *Strategic Plan on Asthma for the City and County of San Francisco* (San Francisco, CA: San Francisco Board of Supervisors, June, 2003): 3.
19. Public Health–Seattle and King County, *Strategic Direction: a Guide to Public Health Programs over the Next 5 Years* (September 1999).
20. Public Health–Seattle and King County, *Data watch: Racial Disparities in Infant Mortality 1990–1998* (August 2000).
21. Public Health–Seattle and King County, *The King County Ethnicity and Health Survey for King County* (October 1998), http://www.metrokc.gov/health/reports/ethnicity/index.htm (accessed January 28, 2005).
22. Public Health–Seattle and King County, *Racial Discrimination in Health Care Interview Project* (January 2001).
23. Public Health–Seattle and King County, *Public Health Special Report: Racial and Ethnic Discrimination in Health Care Settings* (January 2001).

PART II

Racism, Class Exploitation, Sexism, and Health: Exposing the Roots

7

Structural Racism and Community Building

KEITH LAWRENCE, STACEY SUTTON, ANNE KUBISCH, GRETCHEN SUSI, AND KAREN FULBRIGHT-ANDERSON

Race and poverty are still strongly linked in America. Data from the 2000 U.S. Census show that a person of color is nearly three times more likely to be poor than a white person. Similarly, a neighborhood that is largely made up of people of color is more likely to be poor than a predominantly white neighborhood, and racial minorities are overrepresented in the poorest and most disadvantaged neighborhoods.

These facts alone make clear that our national effort to promote a just society and vibrant democracy is not likely to succeed without an honest

*This chapter is reprinted with permission from The Aspen Institute Roundtable on Community Change.

*This publication is the result of collective learning by staff of the Aspen Institute Roundtable on Community Change and advisors to the Project on Structural Racism and Community Revitalization. The authors are Keith Lawrence, Stacey Sutton, Anne Kubisch, Gretchen Susi, and Karen Fulbright-Anderson. But the messages have been developed with the invaluable input of Lisette Lopez, Manning Marable, Khatib Waheed, Andrea Anderson, and J. Phillip Thompson. The authors wish to thank them as well as the many members of the Roundtable and colleagues too numerous to mention for their feedback along the way as these concepts have been developed. The staff and cochairs of the Roundtable thank the Annie E. Casey Foundation for its financial and intellectual support of this work. We also thank the Mott Foundation, the Kellogg Foundation, the Rockefeller Foundation, the Ford Foundation, and the Robert Wood Johnson Foundation, which have also supported this work.

and unflinching appraisal of the role that race plays in all of our lives. At this historical moment, it is both appropriate and important to ask the following questions:

- How is it that a nation legally committed to equal opportunity for all—regardless of race, creed, national origin, or gender—continually reproduces patterns of racial inequality?
- Why, in the world's wealthiest country, is there such enduring poverty among people of color?
- How is it that in our open, participatory democracy, racial minorities are still underrepresented in positions of power and decision making?

Focusing on these questions might seem to be a distraction, or worse, overwhelming, for those working to reduce poverty and build strong communities. To some, they may even seem unnecessary, since there are African Americans, Latinos, Native Americans, and Asians who are highly successful, and many whites who are desperately poor. Yet the successes of a few individuals of color cannot obscure the overall pattern of opportunity and benefit that is defined by race: white Americans remain significantly more likely than racial minorities to have access to what it takes to fulfill their inborn potential to succeed in life, and to be rewarded fairly for their efforts.

Without fully accounting for the historical and ongoing ways in which racial dynamics produce inequities between whites and people of color, those working for social justice risk pursuing misguided, incomplete, or inappropriate strategies to the challenge. This chapter explores how race shapes political, economic, and cultural life in the United States, and offers insights for integrating a racial equity perspective into the work of community building and socioeconomic justice.

The Significance of Race to Poverty and Disadvantage

The Racial Disparity Picture

The statistical portrait of the American population broken out by race reveals persistent disparities between people of color and white Americans in almost every quality of life arena, the most basic being income, education, and health. In some arenas, racial disparities have shrunk over time, but the correlation between race and well-being in America remains powerful.

The Meaning of Race

Scientific studies conclude that race has no biological meaning. The gene for skin color is linked with no other human trait. The genes that account for intelligence, athletic ability, personality type, and even hair and eye color are independent of the gene for skin color. In fact, humans are far more alike than they are different, and share 99.9 percent of their genetic material. Race does, however, have social and political significance. Social scientists call the term *Race* a "social construct," that is, it was invented and given meaning by human beings. Why? Answering that question requires examining the creation of racial categories in history, and what those categories have produced.

In the case of the United States, two primary racial categories—white Europeans and all nonwhite "others"—emerged early in our nation's history. Beginning with the expropriation of Native American lands, a racialized system of power and privilege developed and white dominance became the national common sense, opening the door to the enslavement of Africans, the taking of Mexican lands, and the limits set on Asian immigrants.

Over time, beliefs and practices about power and privilege were woven into national legal and political doctrine. While committing to principles of freedom, opportunity, and democracy, the U.S. found ways to justify slavery, for example, by defining Africans as nonhuman. This made it possible to deny Africans rights and freedoms granted to "all men" who were "created equal." Only when white Southerners wanted to increase their political power in the legislature did they advocate to upgrade Africans' legal status to three-fifths of a human being. Thus, from the earliest moments in our history, racial group identities granted access to resources and power to those who were "white" while excluding those who were "other" legally, politically, and socially.

Expressions of racism have evolved markedly over the course of American history, from slavery through Jim Crow through the civil rights era to today. Racism in twenty-first century America is harder to see than its previous incarnations because the most overt and legally sanctioned forms of racial discrimination have been eliminated. Nonetheless, subtler racialized patterns in policies and practices permeate the political, economic, and sociocultural structures of America in ways that generate differences in well-being between people of color and whites. These dynamics work to maintain the existing racial hierarchy, even as they adapt with the times or accommodate new racial and ethnic groups. This contemporary manifestation of racism in America can be called "structural racism."

Structural Racism

Many of the contours of opportunity for individuals and groups in the United States are defined—or "structured"—by race and racism. The term *structural racism* refers to a system in which linked public policies, institutional practices, cultural representations, and other norms often reinforce the perpetuation of racial group inequity. It identifies dimensions of our history and culture that have allowed privileges associated with "whiteness" and disadvantages associated with "color" to endure and adapt over time.

The concept of structural racism may not immediately resonate with everyone in our diverse society. Most Americans are proud of how far our nation has come on civil rights. Moreover, when most of us think of racism in the United States, two images generally come to mind. First, we see racism as a historical phenomenon, something that was part of America's past, especially slavery and Jim Crow segregation. Second, racism is often understood as a dynamic between whites and African Americans. Few readily filter the histories of Native Americans, Chinese, Latino, and ethnic European immigrants through a structural racism prism. Structural racism, however, touches and implicates everyone in our society—whites, blacks, Latinos, Asians, and Native Americans—because it is a system for allocating social privilege. The lower end of the privilege scale, characterized by socioeconomic disadvantage and political isolation, has historically been associated with "blackness" or "color." Meanwhile, the upper end of the scale that gives access to opportunity, benefits, and power has been associated with "whiteness." Between the fixed extremes of whiteness and blackness, different groups of color at various times have occupied a fluid hierarchy of social and political spaces.

Racial group status can change, but not easily. A group that is subordinated in one era can move closer to power and privilege in another era. In the past century, groups such as the Irish, Italians, and Jews in America started low on the socioeconomic and political ladder and "became white" over time. More recently, "model minority" status has been given to some Asian groups, allowing group members to gain access to some of the privileges associated with whiteness.

Position and mobility within the racial hierarchy, which in some ways resembles a caste system, cannot be determined by the nonwhite or subordinated groups. How those at the lower end of the privilege scale perceive themselves, or how they behave, is less significant to their racial privilege status than broadly held perceptions about them. European immigrants to nineteenth-century America could not "become white" by simply adopting the mainstream habits and declaring themselves its members. They had to be allowed access into occupational, educational, residential, and other settings that had previously excluded them. In other words, racial and ethnic group position reflects the dominant group's exclusionary or inclusionary exercise of political, economic, and cultural power.

The structural racism lens allows us to see more clearly how our nation's core values—and the public policies and institutional practices built on them—perpetuate social stratifications and outcomes that all too often reflect racial group sorting rather than individual merit and effort. The structural racism lens allows us to see and explore:

- the racial legacy of the past;
- how racism persists in national policies, institutional practices, and cultural representations;
- how racism is transmitted and either amplified or mitigated through public, private, and community institutions;
- how individuals internalize and respond to racialized structures.

The structural racism lens allows us to see that, as a society, we often take for granted a context of white leadership, dominance, and privilege. This dominant consensus on race is the frame that shapes our attitudes and judgments about social issues. It has resulted from the way historically accumulated white privilege, national values, and contemporary culture has interacted so as to preserve the gaps between white Americans and Americans of color.

White Privilege: The Legacy and Enduring of Our Racial History

White Privilege refers to whites' historical and contemporary advantage in all of the principal opportunity domains, including education, employment, housing, health care, political representation, media influence, and so on. Whites' have a major advantage in each one of those areas, but the accumulated benefit across all domains results in a pattern that has concentrated and sustained racial differences in wealth, power, and other dimensions of well-being.

An example of the way in which historical privilege has a legacy that carries through to today can be found in comparing average levels of wealth accumulation among groups. Blacks and whites who earn the same salaries today have significantly different wealth levels (capital assets, investments, savings, and so on). Whites, for example, earning between $50,001 and $75,000 have a wealth level that is two-and-one-half times as high as their black counterparts. What explains this difference? Many members of the current generation of adult white Americans, along with their parents, grandparents, and other forebears:

- benefited from access to good educational institutions;
- had access to decent jobs and fair wages;
- accumulated retirement benefits through company programs, union membership, and social security;
- benefited from homeownership policies and programs that allowed them to buy property in rising neighborhoods.

By contrast, significant numbers in the current generation of adults of color, along with their parents, grandparents, and other forbears:

- came from a background of slavery or labor exploitation;
- were limited by de jure or de facto segregation;
- were generally confined to jobs in areas such as agricultural, manual, or domestic labor, and excluded from jobs that allowed them to accumulate savings and retirement benefits;
- were discriminated against by lending institutions and were excluded from owning homes in economically desirable locations through redlining and other policies.

In other words, at pivotal points in U.S. history when socioeconomic factors produced abundant opportunities for wealth and property accumulation—such as the G.I. Bill and home mortgage subsidies—white Americans were positioned to take advantage of them, whereas Americans of color were systematically prohibited from obtaining benefits from them.

These inequalities are likely to continue for some time by examining data about one of the major avenues for wealth accumulation—homeownership—and about access to credit, which is a necessity on the path to homeownership. Lack of homeownership has social effects beyond wealth accumulation. Adults who do not own homes do not have access to home equity that might be tapped for important investments, such as education for their children. Parents who have not had a chance to pay off a mortgage may become dependent on their children in their retirement years and lack a valuable material resource to pass on to their children. In addition, research has shown that regardless of socioeconomic status children of homeowners are less likely to drop out of school, get arrested, or become teen parents than are children of families who are renters.[1]

Race has been and continues to be a valuable social, political, and economic resource for white Americans. It grants them easier access to power and resources and provides them better insulation from negative pre-judgments based on physical features, language, and other cultural factors than their nonwhite counterparts. For whites, whiteness, the "default setting" for race in America, is the assumed color of America. But because the U.S. is deeply invested with strong beliefs about opportunity, the built-in advantages that whites have in most competitive areas are overlooked.

Processes That Maintain Racial Hierarchies

Our history, national values, and culture are the backdrop for under-standing structural racism. But the racial status quo is maintained in part because it adapts and changes over time. Racism in America has its own particular dynamics that sometimes lead to greater racial equity, some-times move us backward, and sometimes change the nature of the problem itself. The two most important of these dynamics are "racial sorting" and "progress and retrenchment."

Racial Sorting

Racial sorting refers to both the physical segregation of racial and eth-nic groups and the psychological sorting that occurs through social and cultural processes and stereotyping. Although federal legislation barring racial discrimination in key domains such as housing, employment, and public accommodation was enacted in 1964, racial and ethnic groups are still largely isolated from one another in contemporary America. Analyses of the 2000 census show that despite increasing racial and ethnic diver-sity in national-level statistics, the country remains as segregated as ever. Most visible is the consistent relationship between race and residence: white Americans live in neighborhoods that are, on average, more than 80 percent white and no more than 7 percent black, while the average black or Hispanic person lives in a neighborhood that is about two-thirds non-white.[2] Because a person's place of residence is strongly linked to access to schools, business districts, jobs, and so on, this residential "hyperseg-regation" translates directly into racial sorting in education, commerce, employment, and other public venues.

Physical proximity to other racial groups may not necessarily create social equity, but hypersegregation is clearly problematic. When groups do not interact, their knowledge of one another is less likely to be based on personal experience and more likely to be informed by hearsay, media portrayals, and cultural stereotypes. Lack of genuine interpersonal contact contributes to a psychological distancing from those who are perceived as "other," which, in turn, undermines opportunities for trust, empathy, and common purpose to develop. This psychological sorting reinforces and compounds the physical and geographic sorting process. Face-to-face interaction among diverse groups, on the other hand, helps to reduce prejudice.[3]

In theory, physical and psychological racial segregation does not need to equate with advantage and disadvantage. But in the United States, historically and today, racial homogeneity of neighborhoods has been highly correlated with income and overall well-being. For the most part, predominantly white neighborhoods enjoy better schools, lower crime rates, better transportation access, better environmental conditions, and so on. Moreover, this racialized "neighborhood gap" in equality actually grew in the past decade as whites who earned more moved to neighborhoods that matched their own economic status while blacks and Hispanics continued to be less mobile and less able to move to better neighborhoods.[4]

As a nation, we have not found a way to make "separate but equal" work. In 1954, the Supreme Court concluded that racially segregated schools were "inherently unequal," and the Court has gone on to reconfirm this opinion with a number of decisions since then. Nonetheless, in our political economy, groups of color are continually "sorted" and experience marginalization, isolation, exclusion, exploitation, and subordination relative to those who are white. The link between whiteness and privilege and between color and disadvantage is maintained, even today, through these sorting processes.

Progress and Retrenchment

Perhaps the most discouraging characteristic of structural racism is its adaptability and resilience. The forces that permit structural racism to endure are dynamic and shift with the times. So as progress is made toward racial equity on a particular policy front, a backlash may develop on another front that could undo or undermine any gains. Or powerful interests may move to preserve the racial order in other ways. The net effect tends to be a repositioning of the color line rather than its erasure.

The clearest examples of this retrenchment have been in the consistent challenges to affirmative action, but there are many more subtle and less direct ways in which equity gains can be counteracted. For example, the Fair Housing Act of 1968 guaranteed equal access to housing for all, but people of color continued to be quietly excluded from high-quality suburban housing by discriminatory lending practices, zoning regulations that dictated the size of a house or restricted multifamily dwellings, and public underinvestment in mass transportation between cities and suburbs. Or while the historic 1954 *Brown vs. Board of Education* U.S. Supreme Court decision prohibited racial segregation in public schools, subsequent judicial, legal, and administrative actions undermined it.[5] As a result of these and continued residential segregation, black and Latino students are more isolated from whites in their schools today than just twenty years ago.[6]

Race is a social construct. Racial hierarchy preserves a social order in which power, privilege, and resources are unequally distributed, and no individual, institution, or policy needs to be activated to preserve the system of privilege: it is built in. Structural racism identifies the ways in which that system is maintained, even as it is contested, protected, and contested again.

Racialized Public Policies and Institutional Practices

The backdrop of white privilege, national values, and contemporary culture is the context within which our major institutions, or opportunity areas—such as health care, education, the labor market, the criminal justice system, or the media—operate today. While we expect the policies and practices of public and private institutions to be race neutral, they are inevitably influenced by this racialized context and, therefore, contribute to the production of racially disparate outcomes. If background forces go unrecognized and unexamined, racial disparities such as those typically seen in the labor market and criminal justice systems are understood simply as unintended consequences of "neutral" or, by and large, "fair" industry policies and practices. Sorting and stereotyping reinforce this, as they work to legitimize, or at least explain, the inequitable outcomes in employment, housing, health care, education, and other opportunity areas. Following are examples of how structural racism operates within the key areas of education and the labor market.

Education

Public education is probably the national system that holds the greatest potential for reducing racial inequities over time. It is universally available and invests in children at an early age when, in theory, environmental influences are less deterministic and thus children can achieve according to individual talents. However, examination of educational systems across the nation reveals that black and Latino students are more segregated now than two decades ago, that the schools they attend are comparatively under-resourced, and that within the schools they are provided fewer academic opportunities and are treated more punitively than their white counterparts. The link between these features and educational outcomes is strong.

Labor Market

Theoretically, the labor market should be race neutral: supply and demand are not racialized concepts. Yet there are myriad examples of how workers of color are excluded, exploited, and marginalized relative to white workers.

Although illegal, active discrimination against workers of color still occurs. Social science studies and newspapers regularly report on experiments where similarly qualified applicants, or testers, of color and testers who are white apply for the same jobs with unequal results. (These experiments are also conducted in the rental, purchase, and mortgage markets and produce similar findings.) Discrimination also comes in more passive forms. Examples include:

- Zip-code or name-based discrimination: Job seekers perceived to live in undesirable locations or perceived as people of color based on their names may be excluded from consideration for job opportunities by employers.
- Occupational segregation based on race, ethnicity, or gender: Racial minorities and women are overrepresented in the lowest paid and least desirable jobs. Researchers have found that occupational segregation has been most pronounced for black male youths.[7]
- Hiring through informal mechanisms such as social networks: These employer practices often disadvantage people without insider connections. Since inside connections for high-quality jobs have been and continue to be racially disproportionate, this is one mechanism that perpetuates labor market differentials.[8]

Finally, many seemingly race-neutral actions taken by employers produce racially inequitable outcomes. Often, these are explained as legitimate industry procedures or norms that are difficult to challenge because they are time honored. But the outcome data are revealing.

A large study regarding racial disparities in corporate firing practices, conducted during the recession of the early 1990s, included nearly five hundred firms. It found that the net job loss for black workers was disproportionately high compared to that for white workers. This case is instructive because the rationales for the job cuts—standard downsizing, last hired-first fired, subcontracting of noncore tasks, globalization—are commonly seen as race neutral, although their effects clearly are not.

Ten years later, the same patterns are still in evidence. In the recession of the early 2000s, blacks lost jobs at twice the rate of whites and Hispanics. Nearly 90 percent of the jobs that were lost were decent-paying jobs in manufacturing that are unlikely to return.[9]

What Does a Structural Racism Perspective Imply for Community Building and Related Social Justice Work?

The structural racism framework describes the many mechanisms that perpetuate the link between race and well-being in the U.S. It evaluates critically the socioeconomic, political, cultural, geographic, and historical contexts in which people of color are located, and demonstrates how and why those contexts affect individual and family outcomes.

For those involved in community building and social justice, the structural racism framework specifically highlights the ways in which racialized institutional, political, and cultural forces can counteract or undermine efforts to improve distressed communities, reduce poverty, and promote equity. The implication for action is that social change leaders must adopt an explicitly race-conscious approach to their work: they must factor race into their analysis of the causes of the problems they are addressing, and they must factor race into their strategies to promote change and equity.

But what exactly does *race-consciousness* mean, and how should practitioners working at the community level—as well as those who support and partner with them—actually begin to apply the insights that are revealed by using a structural racism perspective? It is often difficult to see how individual or organizational actors with limited reach and resources might make any major difference. Structural racism can seem overwhelming and abstract, and racial equity, idealistic. Without question, these formidable issues will not be resolved overnight. Change will not come without deliberate effort, however. The work ahead can be thought of in four parts.

1. Racial Equity Must Be a Central Goal of the Work

Racial equity can only be achieved if whites and Americans of color are equally likely to have positive or negative experiences in employment, education, homeownership, criminal justice, and all the other arenas that determine life outcomes in the United States. The structural racism analysis demonstrates that people of color are so disproportionately harmed by

racialized public policies, institutional practices, and cultural representations that racial equity itself needs to be a priority objective for anyone
committed to promoting social, economic, and political justice. This means
that racial equity should not be just one of many elements of the analysis
and one of many goals of the work but, rather, should be located at the
core, forming part of the mission statement and programmatic goals of all
who are active in antiracism struggles.

It is counterintuitive to consider that individuals, organizations, and initiatives dedicated to improving outcomes for disadvantaged groups need to
be encouraged to make racial equity an explicit part of their work. After
all, their target populations are often people and communities of color. But
analyses of the work of large segments of community building and allied
fields reveal under-attention to racial factors.[10] Moreover, the race-related
issues that do surface tend to focus more on interpersonal dynamics,
emphasizing strategies and actions that address diversity, proportionality,
and cultural competence. They rarely address the structural dimensions of
racism. Some of the hypotheses explaining the relative absence of focus on
structural racism include:

- Race and racism are uncomfortable topics to put on any agenda at any
  time, and the social welfare field, despite deep commitment to justice
  and equity, is no exception.
- Because antipoverty work often focuses on individuals and communities of color, race is assumed to be well integrated into strategies and
  programs; this, in turn, works to relieve pressure to address race deliberately and explicitly.
- Strategies and solutions in the social services, economic development,
  and community building fields tend to be oriented to enhancing individual, family, and community capacities to do better. A structural racism
  analysis suggests that these strategies are necessary but not sufficient,
  and that system-level change needs to be accorded higher priority.
- Community-building approaches are built on principles of cooperative
  problem solving, collaboration, and common enterprise, whereas the
  structural framework raises issues that imply challenging power and
  privilege.
- Many of the key leadership institutions in the social and economic
  development field (such as foundations, banks, corporations, research
  institutes) are themselves products of historically racialized inequities in
  this country, and their ability to take leadership on racial equity issues
  may not come naturally.[11]

A first step is for organizations to ensure that they have their own house in order. It is important for organizations to model racial equity internally if they are to take responsibility for achieving such ends in the wider community. Resources exist to guide organizations aiming to improve their ability to address racial issues and offer strategies for leadership development, staff training, workforce diversification, developing knowledge about constituents, and so on. For those engaged in social change, numerous, relevant training and technical assistance programs are available.[12] Few guides exist, however, for those in community-building who wish to address racial equity,[13] and tools for addressing the structural dimensions of racism are only in the earliest phases of development.

Adopting racial equity as a central tenet of the work suggests that, in addition to attention to internal organizational factors, social change advocates need to focus on racially equitable outcomes produced at all stages of effort. This means that all of the work must consider how a program, initiative, investment, or strategy will contribute to reducing racial inequity. Identifying racially disaggregated data are a critical first step. Since the notion of equity is a comparative one, clearly the basic commitment is to closing outcome gaps between people of color and whites in key opportunity areas, with goals, interim outcomes, and benchmarks specified. Because some of the arenas assumed to provide opportunity and justice in the United States actually work to produce greater racial disparity, no area should remain unexamined.

Recognizing the importance of race may or may not imply racially explicit interventions. Disadvantages experienced by people of color are often also associated with class, nativity, gender, language, and other factors. While race is inextricably linked to all these, it may sometimes make strategic sense to craft interventions or build alliances that do not lead with race explicitly. What ought not be negotiable, however, is the priority placed on racial equity outcomes.

2. Emphasize Capacity Building among Change Agents

The experience of the most recent generation of community-building efforts has demonstrated that community and other social change agents do not have the capacity to promote neighborhood change at a scale that promises to make a serious dent in socioeconomic or racial inequity. The structural analysis explains why this occurs by highlighting how historic and contemporary macro forces overwhelm local efforts, however meritorious they might be, that are designed to intervene at the individual, family, and community levels. One scholar has described community-based work as "swimming against the tide" of major systemic and institutional trends that undermine progress in distressed inner-city neighborhoods.[14]

One immediate strategy is to invest in building the capacity of local organizations to maximize their ability to produce whatever kinds of change that are within their reach and control. For the most part, local-level community development, social service, and other community-building organizations are strapped for resources and, as a result, can barely attain modest programmatic results in fairly narrowly defined arenas. Yet these thousands of organizations, staffed by millions of workers, is a potentially powerful network for achieving significant change. Viewed in this light, investment in their capacity is a critical step toward promoting true democracy, social justice, and racial equity.

Racial equity goals also nudge all strands of the community-building field toward a paradigm that assumes that civic capacities deserve equal priority to functional ones. Broadly, this means accessing and participating in the policymaking and governance processes that allocate public resources. To do this, organizations and individuals first must identify their actual and potential civic engagement capacities: their abilities to gauge the impacts of new policies, to frame their concerns effectively and effectively communicate their messages, to get the attention of policymakers and powerbrokers, and to mobilize support among peers and across other levels.

Many organizations engage in efforts to document and address structural factors that contribute to racial inequities. And there is a need to raise up their work and push the boundaries of current agendas as far as possible given financial and human resources. At the same time, more of those involved in community-change could help lay the groundwork for the type of social change needed. Institutions with high national profiles and resources for research and analysis might, for example, be more effective at defining and promoting policy or regulatory alternatives to the status quo. Individuals or smaller organizations with fewer resources, on the other hand, might exercise responsibility by pressuring peers, and others within their reach who are powerful, to act responsibly.

3. Identify Key Public Policies and Institutional Practices That Need Reform and Develop Alliances That Have the Power to Change Them

A central insight of the structural racism analysis is that racial disadvantage is driven by interrelated policies and systems operating at multiple levels. This makes it unlikely that any single organization would posses all the capacities and resources required to achieve most equity outcomes. Reducing racially biased outcomes when child welfare workers make decisions about removing children from their homes might, for example, call for the development of tools that introduce a greater degree of objectivity into the decision-making process. Getting child welfare systems to use these tools may require legal intervention.[15]

Therefore, we must take into account all that is required to reach our objectives, recognize what we can do effectively, and identify others with capacities we lack who might be potential allies. Addressing the policy, institutional, and cultural barriers associated with racial inequities may almost invariably require networking, communicative, legislative, research, civic, legal, and other kinds of expertise, unlikely to be found in any single organization.

Existing tools and strategies can assist in this work. One is to locate the source of institutional policy and administrative decisions, examine how and when they are made, and how the key actors and processes can be reached and influenced. Another is to strengthen the power and the voice of grassroots constituents to hold key decision makers on that power map accountable for outcomes. Grassroots organizing and advocacy are strategies that have often been left to community organizers and single-issue organizations; the broader community-building field would benefit from developing a comfort level and expertise with that approach to the work. Participation in the electoral process will also be critical.

Operationally, convergence of community building and related practitioners around racial equity would not necessarily compel everyone to meld their agendas and operations into one. Rather, what it might mean is:

- a shared recognition of the systemic sources of disadvantages and disparities among the populations that all are trying to reach;
- identification of the multiple and interrelated levels—cultural, governmental, regional, local, institutional, individual, and so on—at which racist norms, assumptions, policies, and practices pertinent to people of color need to be tackled;
- commitment among the field's principal actors to work deliberately to dismantle or counter structures, policies, and practices that contribute to racial inequities;
- forging alliances with other fields that are concerned about these issues, such as civil rights, social justice, and environmental justice.

Convergence around these ideas would suggest that the community-building is committed as a whole to making our democracy work for all people, even as it pursues its traditional objectives. In concert with others in allied fields, the community-building field seems well positioned to harness an array of civic resources that could be used to influence policies in education, employment, criminal justice, health, the environment, and other public and private institutions that directly shape the life chances of poor people.

4. Counter Popular Assumptions That Work to Reproduce the Status Quo

While few Americans alive today openly sanction racism or consciously engage in practices that maintain structural racism, many benefit from its existence and help to maintain it as they follow society's conventions and participate in its routines. In hundreds of ways—by acquiescing to negative cultural stereotypes, by moving to segregated suburbs, by taking advantage of exclusive job networks, by accepting regressive tax reforms, by neglecting to participate in democratic citizenship, and so on—Americans, in their everyday lives and roles, end up sustaining racial hierarchy. Difficult though this may be to accept, we are responsible in differing degrees for racial inequities simply because we generally participate uncritically in the systems and processes that sustain them.

Taking personal, organizational, and political responsibility for racial equity is not the same as acceptance of blame for racial disadvantage.[16] Rather, taking responsibility for racial equity is the willingness to acknowledge that the nation's enduring racial disparity patterns are inconsistent with its ideals, and thus are unacceptable. It is also a willingness to challenge publicly and privately what may seem to be "normal" and "race-neutral" norms and values in our culture and political economy. Who gets to define what we mean by *equal opportunity, meritocracy,* and *individualism,* and who is responsible for how they play out?

Exploring precisely where and how we fit into a structural racism system requires careful reflection. Demystifying the complex structures and arrangements that are a part of our lives by locating ourselves in them is a critical first step in assessing our capabilities. We might start out by asking ourselves simple questions that focus on different levels of intervention, such as the following:

- In what ways do we—as individuals—accept the notion of the inherent "fairness of the system," that is, that American ideals of equal opportunity and meritocracy work in much the same way for everyone? What mechanisms work to encourage the notion that poor outcomes are the fault of unmotivated individuals, family break up, or the culture of poverty, without connecting that information to broader structural factors? Do we find ourselves making racial or cultural group generalizations, or allowing such generalizations to go unchallenged?

- Where do we fit into, and help sustain, for instance, a media industry that continually underrepresents or produces negative images of Americans of color?
- What role does social service, community development, or philanthropic organizations play in the maintenance of racial inequality? Do programmatic and funding priorities that focus only on remediating racial inequities distract us from the need to address the sources of such inequities? What role do we expect employment initiatives to play in a private sector that keeps African Americans and Latinos at the vulnerable end of the workforce? What role do we expect schools to play in a public education system that underinvests in our poorest children and our children of color?

Conclusion

The structural racism framework offers community builders and social justice workers not only a powerful and promising intellectual tool, but valuable insights for individual, organizational, community, and collective action toward racial equity. The framework can be thought of as a lens that brings into focus new ways of analyzing the causes of the problems that community builders are addressing and new approaches to finding solutions to those problems. Specifically, the structural racism perspective highlights:

- chronic racial disparities, not just race relations;
- specific power arrangements that perpetuate chronic disparities, especially as they exist in public policies and institutional practices;
- general cultural assumptions, values, ideologies, and stereotypes that allow disparities to go unchallenged;
- the dynamics of progress and retrenchment, which highlight how gains on some issues can be undermined by forces operating in other spheres or by oppositional actors;
- political, macroeconomic, regional, and other contextual factors that have enormous influences on outcomes for children, families, and communities.

The promise of this framework lies in its understanding of the embeddedness of modern racism in the normal routines of our private and public lives. Racial hierarchy is interwoven with the laissez-faire processes and mechanisms of twenty-first century America's commerce, politics, and popular culture. Virtually all Americans, in some way, accommodate to the realities of white privilege and operate within socioeconomic templates that guarantee its continuation. Regardless of whose ancestors bear principal liability for our inequitable social evolution to this point, we are now all so invested in the norms and procedures of the status quo that it will not change without the dedicated efforts of everyone—both its beneficiaries and victims. To community builders, already hard-pressed by many funding and operational challenges, this call to responsibility for racial equity should not be perceived as the proposal of a heavier workload. Rather, it is a call to reexamine current goals and methods from a racial equity vantage point, which would bring public policies, institutional practices, and cultural assumptions into the foreground. Thus, for example, those who now seek to expand provision of human services, or low-income housing, might come to see policy analysis, and collective action on various levels to shape policy, as higher priorities. They may also see more value in building strategic alliances beyond the field's imagined boundaries to address other related policies and issues—such as tax and regulatory practices, trade policies, social "safety net" provisions, or federal transportation investment priorities—that tend to be off their screens. Or they might choose to work more directly with the media to counteract negative racialized beliefs and images about welfare or other public support programs and, more generally, to reframe dominant images of poverty and disadvantage in America.

Inattention to racial equity has limited the success of community builders. Continued under-attention to race risks undermining future work. The structural racism framework posits that raising the profile and centrality of racial equity will increase the likelihood that community builders will succeed in improving the well-being of children, families, and communities.

Notes

1. Richard K. Green and Michelle White, *Measuring the Benefits of Homeowning's Effect on Children* (Chicago: University of Chicago, Center for the Study of Economy and State, 1994).
2. John Logan, *Separate and Unequal: The Neighborhood Gap for Blacks and Hispanics in Metropolitan America* (Albany, NY: Lewis Mumford Center for Comparative Urban and Regional Research, October 13, 2003): 3.
3. Nathalie F. P. Gilfoyle, Lindsey Childress-Beatty, Paul R. Friedman, and William F. Sheehan, *Brief Amicus Curiae of the American Psychological Association in Support of Respondents*. In the Supreme Court of the United States, Barbara Grutter, Petitioner v. Lee Bollinger et al., Respondents, and Jennifer Gratz and Patrick Hamacher, Petitioners v. Lee Bollinger et al., Respondents (2003): 14.
4. Logan, Note 2.
5. For a short summary of leading court decisions on desegregation between 1895 and 1995, see Applied Research Center, *46 Years after Brown v. Board of Ed: Still Separate, Still Unequal* (Oakland, CA.: Applied Research Center, 2000, research brief): 10–11.

6. Erica Frankenberg and Chungmei Lee, "Race in American Public Schools: Rapidly Resegregating School Districts" (Cambridge, MA: Civil Rights Project, Harvard University, August 2002): 5.
7. Paul E. Gabriel, Donald R. Williams, and Suzanne Schmitz, "The Relative Occupational Attainment of Young Blacks, Whites, and Hispanics," 57(1) *Southern Economic Journal* (July 1990): 35–46.
8. Katherine O'Regan and John Quigley, "The Effect of Social Networks and Concentrated Poverty on Black and Hispanic Youth Unemployment," 27(4) *Annals of Regional Science* (December 1993): 327–342.
9. Louis Uchitelle, "Blacks Lose Better Jobs Faster as Middle-Class Work Drops," *New York Times*, (July 2003).
10. Rebecca Stone and Benjamin Butler, *Core Issues in Comprehensive Community Building Initiatives: Exploring Power and Race* (Chicago: Chapin Hall Center for Children at the University of Chicago, 2000).
11. Ibid.
12. Ilana Shapiro, *Training for Racial Equity and Inclusion: A Guide to Selected Programs* (Washington, DC: Aspen Institute, 2002).
13. Institute for Democratic Renewal and Project Change Anti-Racism Initiative, *A Community Builder's Tool Kit* (Claremont, CA: Institute for Democratic Renewal, Claremont Graduate Center, n.d.). See also Hedy Nai-Lin Chang, *Community Building and Diversity: Principles for Action* (Oakland, CA: California Tomorrow, 1997).
14. Alice O'Connor, "Swimming against the Tide," in *Urban Problems and Community Development*, ed. Ronald F. Ferguson and William T. Dickens (Washington, DC: Brookings Institute, 1999).
15. This example is drawn from the experiences of the National Council on Crime and Delinquency and the Children's Rights Institute.
16. Iris Young, "From Guilt to Solidarity: Sweatshops and Political Responsibility," *Dissent* (Spring 2003).

8

Coronary Heart Disease, Chronic Inflammation, and Pathogenic Social Hierarchy: A Biological Limit to Possible Reductions in Morbidity and Mortality

RODRICK WALLACE, DEBORAH WALLACE, AND ROBERT G. WALLACE

The origin of "racial," "class," and "ethnic" disparities in health has recently become the center of some debate in the United States, with remedies proposed by mainstream authorities characteristically and predictably focused on individual-oriented "prevention" by altered lifestyle or related medical "magic bullet" interventions. A recent paper finds close correlation of CHD mortality with patterns of racial segregation in New York City, one of the world's most segregated urban centers. More generally, similar works shows that all-cause black-white mortality differences are highest in metropolitan areas with the greatest racial segregation. "[T]he clinical hypothesis that an enhanced immune response results in increased plaque vulnerability begs the question as to why a population distribution of inflammation exists in the first place and what the underlying determinants of this distribution might be."* This question is, precisely, the principal focus of our analysis.

...Social conditions—in this case, a particular form of hierarchy—in fact represent "social exposures" which can be synergistic with other

This chapter of selected excerpts is reprinted with permission from the *Journal of the National Medical Association* (2004), 609–619.
*P. Ridker, "On Evolutionary Biology, Inflammation, Infection, and the Causes of Atherosclerosis," 105 *Circulation* (2002): 2.

physiologically active agents—for example, classic toxic substances. The analysis is, however, complicated by the essential role of culture in human life, which, to reiterate the metaphor used by the evolutionary anthropologist Robert Boyd, "is as much a part of human biology as the enamel on our teeth." CHD seems, then, to be very much a life-history disease associated with a particular kind of sociocultural environment—what we call pathogenic hierarchy. We shall be interested in a model of how such an environment might write itself onto the immune function.

...[T]he special role of culture in human biology, particularly as associated with social hierarchy, becomes directly and organically manifest in the basic biology and dynamics of plaque formation. That is, for human populations, "cultural factors" like racism, wage slavery, and exaggerated social disparity—what we will call pathogenic social hierarchy—are as much a part of the "basic biology" of coronary heart disease as are the molecular or biochemical mechanisms of plaque deposition and development....[I]mmune cognition and cognitive socioculture can become fused into a composite entity—and that...composite, in turn, can be profoundly influenced by embedding systems of highly structured psychosocial and socioeconomic stressors. In particular, we argue that the internal structure of the external stress—its "grammar" and "syntax"—is important in defining the coupling with the Immunocultural Condensation. We suppose that the tripartite mutual information representing the interpenetrative coagulation of immune, CNS, and locally "social" cognition, is itself subjected to a "selection pressure", i.e., influenced by a larger embedding but highly structured process representing the power relations between groups. Most typically, these would constitute pathogenic hierarchical systems of imposed economic inequality and deprivation, the historic social construct of racism, patterns of wage-slavery or, very likely, a coherent amalgam of them all.

We thus propose that chronic vascular inflammation resulting in coronary heart disease is not merely the passive result of changes in human diet and activity in historical times but represents the image of literally inhuman "racial" and socioeconomic policies, practices, history, and related mechanisms of pathogenic social hierarchy imposed upon the immune system, beginning in utero and continuing throughout the life course. Our interpretation is consistent with, but extends slightly, already huge and rapidly growing animal model and "health disparities" literatures. Pathogenic social hierarchy is a protean and determinedly plieotropic force, having many possible pathways for its biological expression: if not heart disease, then high blood pressure; if not high blood pressure, then cancer; if not cancer, then diabetes; if not diabetes, then behavioral pathologies leading to raised rates of violence or substance abuse; and so on. We have explored a particular mechanism by which pathogenic social hierarchy imposes an image of itself on the human immune system through vascular inflammation. [Recent research]... implies, however, the existence of multiple, competing, pathways along which deprivation, inequality, and injustice operate. These not only write themselves onto molecular mechanisms of "basic" human biology, but become, as a result of the particular role of culture among humans, literally a part of that basic biology. The nature of human life in community and the special role of culture in that life ensure that individual psychoneuroimmunology cannot be disentangled from social process, its cultural determinants, and their historic trajectory. Psychosocial stress is not some undifferentiated quantity like the pressure under water but has a complex and coherent cultural grammar and syntax which write themselves as a particular distorted image of pathogenic social hierarchy within the human immune system: chronic vascular inflammation. For marginalized populations, this is not a simple process amenable to magic bullet interventions. Substance abuse and overeating become mechanisms for self-medication and the leavening of distorted leptin/cortisol cycles. Activity and exercise patterns may be constrained by social pathologies representing larger-scale written images of racism. The writing of pathogenic social hierarchy onto human immune function over the life course seems to be a fundamental, and likely very plastic, biological mechanism equally unlikely to respond in the long run to magic bullet interventions. Rather, an extension of the comprehensive reforms which largely ended the scourge of infectious disease in the late 19th and early 20th centuries seems prerequisite to significant intervention against coronary heart disease and related disorders for marginalized populations within modern industrialized societies. This analysis has obvious implications for the continued decline of CHD within the U.S. majority population. Our own studies show clearly that the public health impacts of recent massive deindustrialization and deurbanization in the United States have not been confined to urbanized minority or working-class communities where they have been focused, but have become "regionalized" in a very precise sense so as to entrain surrounding suburban counties into both national patterns of hierarchical and metropolitan regional patterns of spatially contagious, diffusion of emerging infection, and behavioral pathology. In essence, social disintegration has diffused outward from decaying urban centers, carrying with it both disease and disorder.

In precisely the same sense, it seems virtually inevitable that American Apartheid, as expressed in patterns of pathogenic hierarchy entraining all subpopulations, will similarly constitute a very real biological limit, in Robert Boyd's sense, to possible declines in CHD among both white and black subpopulations.... Nobody is more enmeshed in, and hence susceptible to, the pathologies of hierarchy than those of a majority whose fundamental cultural assumptions include the social reality of divisions by class and race.

While the overall structure of diabetes mortality was poverty-driven, the New York metropolitan region, one of the most virulently segregated in the United States, showed a startling decline in the strength of the relation between diabetes mortality rate and poverty rate over the two time periods,....[T]he marked weakening of the relation for the New York metro region is not a sign of improvement in the lot of the poor—rather, it means that high incidence is spilling over into areas with low-to-moderate poverty rates, i.e., high incidence is crossing class lines. The explanation, they infer, may lie in either or both of two hypotheses: the level of stress once associated with poverty is affecting those above the poverty line in this metro region, or the response to stress once concentrated in the population below the poverty line has been adopted by those not living in poverty.

We find that American Apartheid and similar systems of pathogenic social hierarchy are classic double-edged swords which wound both dominant and subordinate communities, placing a very real biological limit to the possible decline of coronary heart disease across the entire social spectrum. Programs of social and cultural reform affecting marginalized populations will inevitably entrain the powerful as well, to the benefit of all.

9

Social Sources of Racial Disparities in Health

DAVID R. WILLIAMS AND PAMELA BRABOY JACKSON

Racial disparities in health in the United States are substantial. The overall death rate for blacks today is comparable to the rate for whites thirty years ago, with about 100,000 blacks dying each year who would not die if the death rates were equivalent.[1]

This chapter outlines factors in the social environment that can initiate and sustain racial disparities in health. Race is a marker for differential exposure to multiple disease-producing social factors. Thus, racial disparities in health should be understood not only in terms of individual characteristics but also in light of patterned racial inequalities in exposure to societal risks and resources.

We illustrate some of these social processes by examining racial differences in mortality from 1950 to 2000 for five causes of death that reveal divergent pathways to current health disparities. Three of these causes of death—homicide, heart disease, and cancer—show wide disparities between black and white populations; two of these causes—pneumonia and flu, and suicide—show virtually no disparities. Data are available for blacks and whites for the 1950–2002 time period only. We present both absolute (black–white differences) and relative (black–white ratios) indicators of disparity.

This chapter is reprinted with permission from *Health Affairs*, 24(2)(March/April 2005): 325–334.

TABLE 9.1. Age-Adjusted Death Rates for Blacks and Whites for Three Causes of Death, and Racial Disparities. 1950–2000

CAUSE	1950	1960	1970	1980	1990	2000
Homicide						
White	2.6	2.7	4.7	6.7	5.5	3.6
Black	28.3	26.0	44.0	39.0	36.3	20.5
Difference	25.7	23.3	39.3	32.3	30.8	16.9
Ratio	10.9	9.6	9.4	5.8	6.6	5.7
Heart Disease						
White	584.8	559.0	492.2	409.4	317.0	253.4
Black	586.7	548.3	512.0	455.3	391.5	324.8
Difference	1.9	–10.7	19.8	45.9	74.5	71.4
Ratio	1.0	1.0	1.0	1.1	1.2	1.3
Cancer						
White	194.6	193.1	196.7	204.2	211.6	197.2
Black	176.4	199.1	225.3	256.4	279.5	248.5
Difference	–18.2	6.0	28.6	52.2	67.9	51.3
Ratio	0.9	1.0	1.2	1.3	1.3	1.3

Source: National Center for Health Statistics, Health, United States, 2003.

Notes: Deaths per 100,000 population. "Difference" is calculated as black death rates minus white death rates for each cause of death. "Ratio" refers to the ratio of black deaths to white deaths.

Persistent Racial Disparities in Health

Homicide

Table 9.1 presents national trend data for black–white disparities in homicide, heart disease, and cancer. The homicide rate in 2000 was almost six times greater for African Americans than it was for whites. However, homicide deaths for blacks were almost 30 percent lower in 2000 than in 1950, and the racial gap in homicide death rates, both absolutely and relatively, was smaller in 2000 than in 1950.

Homicide makes a small contribution to racial differences in mortality. It is the fifteenth leading U.S. cause of death and is responsible for about 17,000 deaths each year. In contrast, the annual death toll for the three leading causes of death—heart disease (700,000), cancer (550,000), and stroke (160,000)—are markedly larger. These illnesses and related chronic conditions, such as hypertension, diabetes, and obesity, are the key contributors to excess levels of ill health, premature mortality, and disability among blacks. Heart disease, for example, is the leading U.S. cause of disability and years of life lost for both men and women.

Heart Disease

Death rates from coronary heart disease were comparable for blacks and whites in 1950, but by 2000, blacks had a death rate that was 30 percent higher than that for whites (Table 9.1). Death rates from heart disease declined markedly from 1950 to 2000 for both racial groups, but because the decline for whites (57 percent) was more rapid than for blacks (45 percent), both the relative and absolute racial differences were larger in 2000 than in 1950.

Cancer

Blacks moved from having a lower cancer death rate than whites in 1950 to having a rate that was 30 percent higher in 2000. Cancer death rates for whites have been relatively stable over time, with the mortality rate in 2000 being almost identical to the rate in 1950. In contrast, cancer mortality for blacks has been increasing, with the rate in 2000 being 40 percent higher than in 1950. Over time, lung and ovarian cancer death rates increased for both racial groups, while mortality from colorectal, breast, and prostate cancer markedly increased for blacks but was stable or declined for whites.[2]

Understanding Racial Differences in Health

Racial differences in socioeconomic status, neighborhood residential conditions, and medical care are important contributors to racial differences in disease.

Socioeconomic Status

Whether measured by income, education, or occupation, socioeconomic status (SES) is a strong predictor of variations in health.[3] Americans with low SES have levels of illness in their thirties and forties that are not seen in groups with higher SES until three decades of age later.[4] All of the indicators of SES are strongly patterned by race, such that racial differences in SES contribute to racial differences in health. Moreover, the differences in health by SES within each racial group are often larger than the overall racial differences in health.

Education. Among adults ages 25–44, homicide rates are strongly patterned by education.[5] The homicide rate for black males who have not completed high school is more than five times that of black males with some college education or more. Similarly, there is a ninefold difference in homicide rates by education for white males, a fourfold difference for black females, and a sixfold difference for white females. At the same time, large racial differences in homicide persist when blacks and whites are compared at similar levels of education. For example, the homicide death rate for African American men with at least some college education is eleven times that of their similarly educated white peers. Strikingly, the homicide rate of black males in the highest education category exceeds that of white males in the lowest education group.

Income. Income also plays a role in understanding racial differences in coronary heart disease and cancer mortality. For example, death rates from heart disease are two to three times higher among low-income blacks and whites than among their middle-income peers.[6] In addition, for both males and females at every level of income, blacks have higher coronary heart disease death rates than whites. Mortality from heart disease among low- and middle-income black women is 65 percent and 50 percent higher, respectively, than for comparable white women.

Health practices. Another pathway underlying the association between race and chronic diseases is the patterning of health practices by race and socioeconomic status.[7] Dietary behavior, physical activity, tobacco use, and alcohol abuse are important risk factors for chronic diseases such as coronary heart disease and cancer. Moreover, changes in these health practices over time are patterned by social status. Disadvantaged racial groups and those with low SES are less likely to reduce high risk behavior or to initiate new health-enhancing practices. For example, people with high SES have been markedly more likely to quit cigarette smoking over the past several decades compared with their lower-SES counterparts. They also have greater health knowledge, are more receptive to new health information, and have greater resources to take advantage of health-enhancing opportunities than their low-SES peers.[8]

Stress. Exposure to psychosocial stressors may be another pathway linking SES and race to health. Chronic exposure to stress is associated with altered physiological functioning, which may increase risks for a broad range of health conditions.[9] People of disadvantaged social status tend to report elevated levels of stress and may be more vulnerable to the negative effects of stressors. In addition, the subjective experience of discrimination is a neglected stressor that can adversely affect the health of African Americans.[10] Reports of discrimination are positively related to SES among blacks and may contribute to the elevated risk of disease that is sometimes observed among middle-class blacks.

Residential Segregation

The persistence of racial differences in health after individual differences in SES are accounted for may reflect the role that residential segregation and neighborhood quality can play in racial disparities in health.[11] Because of segregation, middle-class blacks live in poorer areas than whites of similar economic status, and poor whites live in much better neighborhoods than poor blacks. Other U.S. racial/ethnic minority groups are less segregated than blacks, and although residential segregation is inversely related to income for Latinos and Asians, the segregation of African Americans is high at all levels of income.[12] The most affluent African Americans (annual incomes over $50,000) experience higher levels of residential segregation than the poorest Latinos and Asians (incomes under $15,000). Segregation is a neglected but enduring legacy of racism in the United States. Instructively, blacks manifest a higher preference for residing in integrated areas than any other group.[13]

Impact on income. Residential segregation is a central mechanism by which racial economic inequality has been created and reinforced in the United States.[14] It is a key determinant of the observed racial differences in SES because it determines access to education and employment opportunities. For example, an empirical study of the effects of segregation on young African Americans making the transition from school to work found that the elimination of residential segregation would completely erase black–white differences in earnings, high school graduation rates, and employment and would reduce racial differences in single motherhood by two-thirds.[15]

Violence. In addition, segregation creates health-damaging conditions in both the physical and social environments. Research has identified specific pathways by which neighborhood conditions can encourage violence and create racial differences in homicide.[16] Because of its restriction of educational and employment opportunities, residential segregation creates areas with high rates of concentrated poverty and small pools of employable and stably employed males. In turn, high male unemployment and low wage rates for males are associated with high rates of out-of-wedlock births and female-headed households.[17] Single-parent households are associated with lower levels of social control and supervision of young males, which, in turn, lead to elevated rates of violent behavior.[18]

The association between family and neighborhood factors and the risk of violent crime is identical for blacks and whites.[19] However, because of residential segregation, blacks are more exposed to these conditions than whites. In the 171 largest U.S. cities, there is not even one in which whites live in socioeconomic conditions that are comparable to those of blacks.

As Robert Sampson and William J. Wilson concluded, "The worst urban context in which whites reside is considerably better than the average context of black communities."[20]

Links to disease. Independent of individual SES, factors linked to poor residential environments make an incremental contribution to the risk of a broad range of health outcomes, including heart disease and cancer.[21] Multiple characteristics of neighborhoods are conducive to healthy or unhealthy behavioral practices. The perception of neighborhood safety is positively associated with physical exercise, and this association is larger for minority group members than for whites.[22] Neighborhoods also differ in the existence and quality of recreational facilities and open, green spaces. The availability and cost of healthy products in grocery stores also vary across residential areas, and the availability of nutritious foods is positively associated with their consumption.[23] Also, both the tobacco and alcohol industries heavily market their products to poor minority communities.[24]

Medical Care

Racial differences in SES contribute to reduced levels of health insurance coverage for African Americans, and limited access to medical care plays a role in racial differences in disease. Moreover, the black–white gap in access to and use of health services did not narrow between 1977 and 1996.[25] Also, the racial gap in unemployment, median income, and poverty remained large and fairly stable throughout this period.[26]

Links to homicide. Medical care is a contributor to homicide and the racial disparities in homicide. Rates of violent crime have increased over time, but homicide rates have been fairly stable. The lethality of violent assaults has declined as advances in emergency medicine and trauma care have reduced the likelihood that a violent assault will end as a homicide.[27] However, black assault victims are less likely than their white peers to receive timely emergency transportation and subsequent high-quality medical care.[28] The Institute of Medicine (IOM) report *Unequal Treatment* also found that blacks receive poorer-quality emergency room care than whites.[29] It revealed systematic and pervasive racial differences in the quality of care provided across a broad range of medical conditions, including heart disease and cancer. Racial differences in the quality and intensity of treatment persist after SES, insurance status, patient preference, severity of disease, and coexisting medical conditions are taken into account.

Links to cancer mortality. African Americans are less likely than whites to receive preventive, screening, diagnostic, treatment, and rehabilitation services for cancer, and this probably contributes to racial differences in cancer mortality.[30] Although blacks have higher cancer mortality than whites, the annual incidence (new cases) of cancer is lower for black than for white women. However, when compared at the same stage of cancer diagnosis, black women have poorer survival rates than their white counterparts. Blacks also are more likely than whites to experience delays in the receipt of care after a positive screening test, delays in the initiation of treatment after a biopsy, the receipt of care from inadequately trained providers, and limited access to appropriate follow-up and rehabilitation services.

Impact of segregation. Black Medicare patients are more likely than white ones to reside in areas where medical procedure rates and the quality of care are low.[31] In addition, a small group of physicians, who are more likely to practice in low-income areas, provide most of the care to black patients. These providers are less likely than other physicians to be board certified and less able to provide high-quality care and referrals to specialty care.[32] Also, pharmacies in segregated neighborhoods are less likely to have adequate medication supplies, and hospitals in these neighborhoods are more likely to close.[33]

Disentangling the relative importance of the complex causal processes that lead to disparities in disease is challenging, but renewed efforts are needed to identify key points of intervention.

Where There Are No Disparities

Flu and Pneumonia

Examining racial disparities over time reveals that success stories do exist. Flu and pneumonia is one such story. It is the seventh leading cause of death and is responsible for more than 65,000 deaths annually. However, both the absolute and the relative racial differences for deaths from flu and pneumonia were minimal in 2000 (Table 9.2). In contrast, large racial differences existed in 1950, with black mortality being 70 percent higher than that of whites. Over time, striking declines are evident for both races, with larger declines for blacks than for whites. Flu and pneumonia is an acute respiratory illness that can be prevented by vaccination and treated by antiviral medicines. It differs from the major chronic illnesses that typically have a large behavioral component, are long term in development, and have symptoms that are not always readily evident. The virtual elimination of this disparity suggests that the application of a widely diffused technology (facilitated by Medicare and Medicaid), in which social variations in motivation, knowledge, and resources play a small role, can eliminate a large disparity in health.

TABLE 9.2. Age-Adjusted Death Rates for Blacks and Whites for Flu and Pneumonia and for Suicide. and Racial Disparities. 1950–2000

CAUSE	1950	1960	1970	1980	1990	2000
Flu and Pneumonia						
White	44.8	50.4	39.8	30.9	36.4	23.5
Black	76.7	81.1	57.2	34.4	39.4	25.6
Difference	31.9	30.7	17.4	3.5	3.0	2.1
Ratio	1.7	1.6	1.4	1.1	1.1	1.1
Suicide						
White	13.9	13.1	13.8	13.0	13.4	11.3
Black	4.5	5.0	6.2	6.5	7.1	5.5
Difference	−9.4	−8.1	−7.6	−6.5	−6.3	−5.8
Ratio	0.3	0.4	0.5	0.5	0.5	0.5

Source: National Center for Health Statistics, Health, United States, 2003.

Notes: Deaths per 100,000 population. "Difference" is calculated as Black Death rates minus white death rates for each cause of death. "Ratio" refers to the ratio of black deaths to white deaths.

Suicide

Suicide is a success story of another sort. Suicide is the eleventh leading U.S. cause of death (30,000 deaths annually). Suicide rates for both racial groups have been fairly stable over time, with a slight decline for whites and a slight increase for blacks in recent years. However, black suicide death rates have been consistently lower than those of whites. The suicide data are consistent with national data, which indicate that the prevalence of major psychiatric disorders are lower for blacks than for whites.[34] Suicide is an example of a health condition for which the socially disadvantaged group does not have elevated rates. This pattern highlights the importance of attending to protective resources that may improve health and protect vulnerable populations from at least some of the negative effects of environmental exposures. For example, high levels of self-esteem and religious involvement are potential contributors to blacks' better suicide and mental health profile.

Policy Implications

Persisting disparities in health violate widely shared U.S. norms of equality of opportunity and the dignity of each person. Eliminating health disparities is also important for the overall well-being of the entire U.S. society. First, diseases that are initially more prevalent in disadvantaged geographic areas eventually diffuse and spread into adjacent affluent communities.[35] Second, the illnesses and disabilities associated with racial disparities limit the productive capacities and output of adults in their prime working years. This can negatively affect productivity at the local and national levels and can lead to declines in tax revenues and increased costs of social services.[36] Thus, effectively addressing racial disparities in health likely requires addressing distal social policies and arrangements that create the disparities in the first place.[37]

Addressing Segregation

Racial residential segregation is one of the primary causes of U.S. racial inequality, and although discrimination in the sale and rental of housing was made illegal in 1968, considerable evidence suggests that housing discrimination persists.[38] Current public preferences and opportunities for the enforcement of equal opportunity statutes suggest that U.S. residential patterns are unlikely to change in the foreseeable future. Thus, the elimination of the negative effects of segregation on SES and health may require a major infusion of economic capital to improve the social, physical, and economic infrastructure of disadvantaged communities.[39] Such investment could improve the economic circumstances and productivity of African American families and communities and have spillover benefits for health.

Narrowing the Income Gap

Over the past fifty years, changes in the black–white gap in income have been associated with parallel changes in the black–white gap in health. Between 1968 and 1978, in tandem with the narrowing of racial inequality attributable to the economic gains of the civil rights movement, black men and women experienced a larger decline in mortality than their white counterparts on both a percentage and absolute basis.[40] However, as blacks' median household income fell relative to that of whites from its 1978 level throughout the 1980s, the black–white gap in adult and infant mortality widened between 1980 and 1991.[41]

At the same time, although it is generally recognized that policies that disproportionately assist the disadvantaged are desirable, it is unclear whether those policies are best implemented at the federal, state, or local level and what optimal forms such policies should take.[42] Greater attention needs to be given to rigorously evaluating the extent to which policies in multiple sectors of society have consequences for health and health disparities, so that we can have an improved understanding of the conditions under which specific policy initiatives are more or less likely to achieve desirable results.

Improving Medical Care

Improving access to medical care for vulnerable populations, especially for preventive services, can play a role in reducing racial disparities in health. According to a 2000 study, only half of physicians or fewer routinely counsel patients who smoke about smoking cessation, treat patients with elevated blood lipids for this condition, treat hypertensive patients for their high blood pressure, and routinely screen patients for diabetes.[43] One way to improve medical care might be to provide physicians with incentives to ensure that they use evidence-based guidelines for treatment and follow national standards of care. Also, given that underrepresented minority providers are more likely than others to practice in underserved areas, increasing the numbers of blacks in the health professions is likely to be an effective strategy in improving access to care.[44]

Rethinking Health Policy

There is a need to rethink what constitutes health policy. Given the broad social determinants of health, policies in societal domains far removed from traditional health policy can have decisive consequences for individual and population health. A recent federal report outlines an ambitious agenda to eliminate disparities in cancer.[45] Recognizing that the determinants of cancer disparities transcend its scope, the U.S. Department of Health and Human Services (HHS) called for the creation of a Federal Leadership Council, led by HHS, that would leverage government-wide resources to address disparities. This proposed council would include all federal departments that have policies that can affect health and health disparities, including the Departments of Labor, Education, Defense, Justice, Energy, and Transportation. Similar coordination is necessary at the regional and local levels. There are political, professional, and organizational barriers to such intersectoral collaboration, but multiple strategies to address them have been identified, including the need to establish a permanent locus for intersectoral activity regarding health.[46] Although much is yet to be learned about the specific pathways by which the social environment creates disease, much progress can be made toward eliminating disparities by acting on current knowledge.

Editor's Notes

Research for this chapter was supported by the John D. and Catherine T. MacArthur Foundation Research Network on Socioeconomic Status and

Health and the Robert Wood Johnson Foundation. The authors thank Car Nosel, Trisha Matelski, and Natalie Moran for assistance with preparation of the manuscript.

Notes

1. R.S. Levine, J.E. Foster, R.E. Fullilove, et al., "Black–White Inequalities in Mortality and Life Expectancy, 1933–1999: Implications for Healthy People 2010," 116(5) *Public Health Reports* (2001): 474–483; and National Center for Health Statistics, *Health, United States, 2003* (Hyattsville, MD: U.S. Government Printing Office, 2003).
2. T.A. Piffath, M.K. Whiteman, J.A. Flaws, A.D. Fix, and T.L. Bush, "Ethnic Differences in Cancer Mortality Trends in the U.S., 1950–1992," 6(2) *Ethnicity and Health* (2001): 105–119.
3. M. Marmot, "The Influence of Income on Health: Views of an Epidemiologist," 21(2) *Health Affairs* (2002): 31–46; and N.E. Adler and K. Newman, "Socioeconomic Disparities in Health: Pathways and Policies," 21(2) *Health Affairs* (2002): 60–76.
4. J.S. House, J.M. Lepkowski, A.M. Kinney, R.P. Mero, R.C. Kessler, and A.R. Herzog, "The Social Stratification of Aging and Health," 35(3) *Journal of Health and Social Behavior* (1994): 213–234.
5. E. Pamuk, D. Makuc, K. Heck, and C. Renben, *Health, United States, 1998, with Socioeconomic Status and Health Chartbook* (Hyattsville, MD: NCHS, 1998).
6. Ibid.
7. R. Cooper, J. Cutler, P. Desvigne-Nickens, et al., "Trends and Disparities in Coronary Heart Disease, Stroke, and Other Cardiovascular Diseases in the United States: Findings of the National Conference on Cardiovascular Disease Prevention," 102(25) *Circulation* (2000): 3137–3147.
8. B.G. Link and J. Phelan, "Social Conditions as Fundamental Causes of Disease," (extra issue) *Journal of Health and Social Behavior* (1995): 80–94.
9. B.S. McEwen, "Protective and Damaging Effects of Stress Mediators," 338(3) *New England Journal of Medicine* (1998): 171–179.
10. D.R. Williams, H. Neighbors, and J.S. Jackson, "Racial/Ethnic Discrimination and Health: Findings from Community Studies," 93(2) *American Journal of Public Health* (2003): 200–208.
11. D.R. Williams and C. Collins, "Racial Residential Segregation: A Fundamental Cause of Racial Disparities in Health," 116(5) *Public Health Reports* (2001): 404–416.
12. D.S. Massey, "Segregation and Stratification: A Biosocial Perspective," 1(1) *Du Bois Review* (2004): 7–25.
13. Ibid.
14. D.S. Massey and N. Denton, *American Apartheid: Segregation and the Making of the Underclass* (Cambridge, MA: Harvard University Press, 1993).
15. D.M. Cutler, E.L. Glaeser, and J.L. Vigdor, "Are Ghettos Good or Bad?" 112(3) *Quarterly Journal of Economics* (1997): 827–872.

16. R.J. Sampson and W. Wilson, "Toward a Theory of Race, Crime, and Urban Inequality," in *Crime and Inequality*, ed. J. Hagan and R.D. Peterson (Stanford, CA: Stanford University Press, 1995): 37–54.

17. M. Testa, N.M. Astone, M. Krogh, and K. Nekerman, "Employment and Marriage among Inner-City Fathers," in *The Ghetto Underclass*, ed. W.J. Wilson (Newbury Park, CA: Sage, 1993): 96–108.

18. R.J. Sampson, "Urban Black Violence: The Effect of Male Joblessness and Family Disruption," 93(2) *American Journal of Sociology* (1987): 348–382.

19. Ibid.

20. See Note 16.

21. K.E. Pickett and M. Pearl, "Multilevel Analyses of Neighborhood Socioeconomic Context and Health Outcomes: A Critical Review," 55(2) *Journal of Epidemiology and Community Health* (2001): 111–122.

22. Centers for Disease Control and Prevention (CDC), "Neighborhood Safety and the Prevalence of Physical Inactivity—Selected States, 1996," 48(7) *Morbidity and Mortality Weekly Report* (1999): 143–146.

23. A. Cheadle, B.M. Psaty, S. Curry, et al., "Community-Level Comparisons between the Grocery Store Environment and Individual Dietary Practices," 20(2) *Preventive Medicine* (1991): 250–261.

24. D.J. Moore, J.D. Williams, and W.J. Qualls, "Target Marketing of Tobacco and Alcohol-related Products to Ethnic Minority Groups in the United States," 6(1–2) *Ethnicity and Disease* (1996): 83–98.

25. R.M. Weinick, S.H. Zuvekas, and J.W. Cohen, "Racial and Ethnic Differences in Access to and Use of Health Care Services, 1977 to 1996," 57(Suppl. 1) *Medical Care Research and Review* (2000): 36–54.

26. Office of the President, *The Annual Report of the Council of Economic Advisers* (Washington, DC: Office of the President, 1998).

27. A.R. Harris, S.H. Thomas, G.A. Fisher, and D.J. Hirsch, "Murder and Medicine: The Lethality of Criminal Assault, 1960–1999," 6(2) *Homicide Studies* (2002): 128–166.

28. P.J. Hanke and J.H. Gundlach, "Damned on Arrival: A Preliminary Study of the Relationship between Homicide, Emergency Medical Care, and Race," 23(4) *Journal of Criminal Justice* (1995): 313–323.

29. B.D. Smedley, A.Y. Stith, and A.R Nelson, eds., *Unequal Treatment: Confronting Racial and Ethnic Disparities in Health Care* (Washington, DC: National Academies Press, 2002).

30. Department of Health and Human Services, Trans-HHS Cancer Health Disparities Progress Review Group, *Making Cancer Health Disparities History* (Washington, DC: DHHS, 2004).

31. K. Baicker, A. Chandra, J.S. Skinner, and J.E. Wennberg, "Who You Are and Where You Live: How Race and Geography Affect the Treatment of Medicare Beneficiaries," *Health Affairs*, October 7, 2004, content.healthaffairs.org/cgi/content/abstract/hlthaff.var.33 (accessed December 15, 2004).

32. P.B. Bach., H.H. Pham, D. Schrag, R.C. Tate, and J.L. Hargraves, "Primary Care Physicians Who Treat Blacks and Whites," 351(6) *New England Journal of Medicine* (2004): 575–584.

33. Williams and Collins, Note 11; T.C. Buchmueller, M. Jacobson, and C. Wold, "How Far to the Hospital? The Effect of Hospital Closures on Access to

Care," NBER Working Paper no. w10700 (Cambridge, MA: National Bureau of Economic Research, 2004).

34. R.C. Kessler, K.A. McGonagle, S. Zhao, et al., "Lifetime and Twelve-Month Prevalence of DSM-III-R Psychiatric Disorders in the United States: Results from the National Comorbidity Survey," 51(1) *Archives of General Psychiatry* (1994): 8–19.

35. R. Wallace, D. Wallace, and R.G. Wallace, "Coronary Heart Disease, Chronic Inflammation, and Pathogenic Social Hierarchy: A Biological Limit to Possible Reductions in Morbidity and Mortality," 96(5) *Journal of the National Medical Association* (2004): 609–619.

36. J. Bound T. Waidmann, M. Schoenbaum, and J.B. Bingenheimer, "The Labor Market Consequences of Race Differences in Health," 81(3) *Milbank Quarterly* (2003): 441–473.

37. See Note 8.

38. M. Fix and R.J. Struyk, *Clear and Convincing Evidence: Measurement of Discrimination in America* (Washington, DC: Urban Institute Press, 1993).

39. D.R. Williams and C. Collins, "Reparations: A Viable Strategy to Address the Enigma of African American Health," 47(7) *American Behavioral Scientist* (2004): 977–1000.

40. R.S. Cooper, M. Steinhauer, A. Schatzkin, and W. Miller, "Improved Mortality among U.S. Blacks, 1968–1978: The Role of Antiracist Struggle," 11(4) *International Journal of Health Services* (1981): 511–522.

41. See Note 26 and Note 11.

42. A. Deaton, "Policy Implications of the Gradient of Health and Wealth," 21(2) *Health Affairs* (2002): 13–30; and D. Mechanic, "Disadvantage, Inequality, and Social Policy," 21(2) *Health Affairs* (2002): 48–59.

43. See Note 7.

44. M. Komaromy, K. Grumbach, M. Drake, et al., "The Role of Black and Hispanic Physicians in Providing Health Care for Underserved Populations," 334(20) *New England Journal of Medicine* (1996): 1305–1310.

45. See Note 30.

46. S.L. Syme, B. Lefkowitz, and B.K. Krimgold, "Incorporating Socioeconomic Factors into U.S. Health Policy: Addressing the Barriers," 21(2) *Health Affairs* (2002): 113–118.

10

Class Exploitation and Psychiatric Disorders

CARLES MUNTANER, CARME BORRELL, HAEJOO CHUNG,
AND JOAN BENACH

Psychiatric epidemiologists were among the first scientists to document that the poor suffer from a higher rate of psychiatric disorders than the affluent. Psychiatric disorders and, more precisely, psychiatric research have propelled many studies on social class and psychiatric disorders which reflect the humanistic concerns of psychiatrists. These studies were motivated by a desire to improve the living conditions of workers, immigrants, and racial or ethnic Minorities.[1] The absence or poor quality of psychiatric care for poor working class, immigrant, or racial and ethnic minority populations[2] raised a related set of concerns about the implications of economic inequality for the treatment of psychiatric disorders.

The psychiatric and public health perspective on social class has been characteristically 'pragmatic.'[3] Following the ethos of public health and medical care, the goal has been to 'act upon the world' to reduce suffering and increase well-being.[4] Psychiatric disorders, which have a major worldwide impact on disability, are the leading cause of disability among women and, by 2020, are expected to become the main cause of years lost to disability.[5]

This chapter is reprinted from *Liberatory Psychiatry* (2008), 131–146. Reprinted with the permission of Cambridge University Press.

Overall, the relevance of social class to psychiatry stems from the strength of the association between social class and psychiatric disorders and the severe consequences that working-class life has for the quality of life of psychiatric patients.[6] Most psychiatric research is thus grounded in the medical world with its associated materialism and realism. It is within this context of professional pragmatism and technology that several findings on the relation between social class and psychiatric disorders have emerged within the last century.

This literature can inform social scientists interested in psychiatry because of the clinical relevance of categories which correspond to the most severe forms of disorders seen by psychiatrists. In spite of its narrow conceptualization of stratification (e.g., as in the popular 'status syndrome'[7]), this relatively simple literature on the relations between social class stratification and psychiatric disorders provides important findings that have proved quite robust across time and place. However, we need to inform research on the social inequality and psychiatric disorders by looking beyond education or prestige ranks, such as the urgent need of patients that cannot afford medical care or new drugs in neo-liberal states like the U.S.[8] and, crucially, to consider the explanations for social inequalities.[9]

In this chapter we review the recent evidence on the relation between social stratification, social class, and psychiatric disorders, arguing for the need to distinguish between the concepts of social stratification and social class proper in social psychiatry. Next, we venture into uncharted territories in social class and psychiatric disorders by introducing the concept of exploitation. We note a paradox of this area of knowledge: at least in the U.S., social scientists often adopt the role of social psychologists while epidemiologists and psychiatrists take on the role of social scientists. We end by emphasizing the need for greater cross-fertilization between Neo-Marxian and Neo-Weberian class analyses and psychiatry in the study of social inequalities in psychiatric disorders.

The Status Syndrome: The Empirical Association between Social Strata and Psychiatric Disorders

There is a strong inverse association between economic inequality – based on conventional rank indicators – and psychiatric disorders.[10] The evidence is particularly strong to support the association between economic inequality, measured in terms of income, educational credentials, or occupational social class, (often referred to as indicators of 'socioeconomic status') and the most frequent forms of psychiatric illnesses, such as depression, anxiety disorders, and substance use disorders.[11] For example, a comprehensive meta-analysis of prevalence and incidence studies on socioeconomic position and depression indicated that persons with low educational attainment or low income are at higher risk of depression.[12] In the United States, individuals with annual household incomes of less than $20,000 per year were found to have a prevalence of major depression in the past month that was twice as high as that for individuals with annual household incomes of $70,000 or more.[13] Studies of U.S. metropolitan areas have found even larger differences (with odds ratios of 11 to 16) between high- and low-income respondents' risks of depression.[14]

In a 13-year follow-up study that used psychiatric interviews as a method of assessment, poverty was found to increase the risk of depression by 2.5 times.[15] In the same study in east Baltimore, respondents who did not receive income from property were 10 times more likely to have an anxiety disorder than were those who obtained some income from property.[16]

With regard to occupational social class, the prevalence of depression in the past 6 months among those employed in household services was 7 percent, almost three times that of executive professionals (2.4 percent).[17] More recent studies show that blue-collar workers are between 1.5 and 2 times as likely to be depressed as white-collar workers.[18] Similar risk increases have been reported with a 1-year follow-up period.[19] Being born to parents employed in manual labour occupations confers almost twice the risk of depression for women and almost four times the risk of depression for men compared with those born to at least one parent not in the working class.[20] In addition to depression, similar two- to three-fold differences in prevalence between high and low occupational strata have been reported in the United States for substance use disorders, alcohol abuse or dependence, antisocial personality disorder, anxiety disorders, and all psychiatric disorders combined.[21] Internationally, even larger differences have been found – up to a four-fold higher current prevalence of common psychiatric disorders among 'working-class' respondents compared with their middle-class counterparts.[22]

Poverty is also a consistent risk factor for multiple psychiatric disorders, including depression, anxiety disorders, antisocial personality, and substance-use disorders.[23] Cross-sectional and longitudinal studies have found consistent associations between area poverty and psychiatric disorders. In addition, most income inequality studies have shown an association between income inequality and high rates of psychiatric disorders.[24]

The Proximal Determinants of Psychiatric Disorders: The Contribution of Psychiatric Epidemiology to Social Psychiatry

The challenge for psychiatrists and social scientists alike is to use concepts from stratification research to explain these patterns. There is currently a heated controversy on the relative importance of 'neo-material' determinants (contemporary physical or biological risk or protective factors) and 'psychosocial' determinants, such as perceptions of relative standing in the income distribution, for explaining socioeconomic gradients in health in wealthy countries.[25] In brief 'neo-material' scholars claim that most social inequalities in health are determined by 'material' (socially determined physical and chemical) risk and protective factors linked to poverty and inequality, such as poor housing, poor diet, drugs, environmental and workplace hazards, injuries, poor transportation, lack of access to quality health care, or physical violence.[26] Psychosocial scholars, on the other hand, stress the role of perceptions of inequality, social capital, perceptions of job stress, or social isolation.[27] Research supports both types of explanations.

Neo-material indicators of economic inequality, such as owning a car or a house, and indices of deprivation have recently been incorporated into research on the social epidemiology of psychiatric disorders.[28] For example, in a national survey of United Kingdom households, an independent association was found between housing tenure and access to a car, on the one hand, and neurotic disorder (including some anxiety disorders) and depression, on the other.[29] Also, an analysis of the British Household Panel Survey found that low material standard of living was associated with risk for depression and anxiety disorders.[30] A geographic area deprivation index, including housing tenure and car ownership, has been associated with the prevalence and persistence of risk for depression. Although deprivation indicators suggest that absence of material goods increases the risk of psychiatric disorders, research has yet to uncover the specific mechanisms linking material factors to depression or anxiety (e.g., food insecurity, bad diet; poor housing, fear of being evicted, homelessness; noise, pollution, dirt, physical violence, extreme temperatures at work or in the community; unsafe working conditions, physical overwork, exhaustion, lack of sleep; poor transportation; poor health, chronic diseases; unmet health care needs).

Studies have also provided cross-sectional and prospective evidence of an association between psychosocial factors, such as perceived job demands and perceived financial hardship, on the one hand, and depression, symptoms of depression, or anxiety disorders, on the other.[31] Since the mid-seventies' Whitehall studies, there have been a large number of studies showing that the effects of social stratification on psychiatric disorders are partially mediated by psychosocial factors such as 'job autonomy' or 'lack of control.'[32] A substantial amount of this evidence in social epidemiology comes from the Whitehall studies themselves and constitutes the foundation of the 'status syndrome.'[33] In addition, in social science, a large number of studies have shown compatible results although 'material' risk factors and biomedical indicators are less likely to be included in those studies.[34] Therefore, social scientists might be overstating the importance of psychosocial factors because they do not usually include measures of material resources.

A common limitation of most 'psychosocial' studies is an over-reliance on self-report measures of both psychosocial risk factors and psychiatric disorders outcomes (including questionnaires and lay administered diagnostic interviews), coupled with an infrequent use of clinical diagnostic interviews (e.g., due to lack of psychiatric training), to assess psychiatric disorders. Such methods produce vulnerability to self-report bias (persons might have a tendency to report both 'stress' and 'psychiatric disorder' without having either). Even in prospective studies that take into account reverse causation it is difficult to rule out the possibility that features of the material environment (physical and biological exposures) are confounded with a respondent's perceptions.[35]

Nevertheless, the reported associations of job insecurity or remaining in a downsized organization with symptoms of anxiety and depression suggest that psychosocial exposures can have independent effects on psychiatric disorders.[36] Thus, epidemiology's emphasis on the material and objective as well as on the psychosocial and subjective can help refine both methods and explanations in social psychiatry. The implications of this ongoing debate are important for social psychiatry models and methods: (1) the potential neglect of material resources in the determination of psychiatric disorders would force a reappraisal of sociological 'stress' models; and (2) evidence of self-report bias or confounding as noted above would imply more emphasis on objective assessment of exposures, and less emphasis on self-reports.

Class Structure and Psychiatric Disorders

Although there have been relatively few empirical studies on social class, the need to study social class proper has been noted by epidemiologists and social scientists alike.[37] Thus, while social stratification refers to the ranking of individuals in some economic (e.g., income), political (e.g., power within organizations) or cultural (education) continuum, social class deals with the social relations (owner, worker, self-employed; manager, supervisor, worker; professional, technician, unskilled worker) that generate economic, political and cultural inequalities in a social system.[38] Most research on social inequalities in psychiatric disorders relies on indicators of social stratification (e.g., the 'status syndrome') and does not include any analysis of social class relations.[39] Nevertheless, social class positions based on employment relations (e.g., workers, managers, employers) can be powerful determinants of population health via processes such as the exposure to risk or protective factors such as social and health services or income.[40] In a series of studies,[41] we have examined the relationship between social class and psychiatric disorders within a Neo-Marxian framework which emphasizes class employment relations.[42] To illustrate the conceptual and empirical importance of this approach to class analysis, we underscore the conceptual differences between social stratification and class approaches and provide empirical support for the unique relation between class and psychiatric disorders.

Social stratification usually refers to the ranking of individuals along a continuum of economic attributes such as income or years of education. These rankings are known as 'gradient' indicators in epidemiology.[43] Most researchers use several measures of social stratification simultaneously because single measures have been insufficient to explain social inequalities in the health of populations. There is little doubt that measures of social stratification are important predictors of patterns of morbidity from psychiatric disorders.[44] However, despite their usefulness in predicting psychiatric disorders outcomes, these measures do not reveal the social mechanisms that explain how individuals come to accumulate different levels of economic (and political or cultural) resources.[45]

Class inequality, which includes relations of property and control over the labour process, is also associated with psychiatric illness. Social class, understood as social relations linked to the production of goods and services[46] is conceptually and empirically distinct from social stratification/ socioeconomic status (SES). Moreover, social class is associated with psychiatric disorders over and above SES indicators.[47] One study found a small overlap between SES and social class measures, although the association between social class and depression could not be accounted for by SES.[48] Other studies have found initial evidence of a non-linear relationship between social class and psychiatric disorders, as would be predicted by social class models but not by SES models.[49] Low-level supervisors (who do not have policy-making power but can hire and fire workers) have higher rates of depression and anxiety than both upper-level managers (who have organizational control over policy and personnel) and front-line employees (who have neither). Control over organizational assets is determined by the possibility of influencing company policy (making decisions over number of people employed, products or services delivered, amount of work performed, and size and distribution of budgets) and by sanctioning authority over others in the organization (granting or preventing pay raises or promotions, hiring, and firing or temporally suspending subordinates). The repeated experience of organizational control at work would protect most upper-level managers against mood and anxiety disorders. Low-level supervisors, on the other hand, are subjected to 'double exposure': the demands of upper management to discipline the workforce and the antagonism of subordinate workers, while exerting little influence over company policy. This 'contradictory class location'[50] may place supervisors at greater risk of depression and anxiety disorders than either upper management or non-supervisory workers. The bottom line is that this finding was predicted by the 'contradictory class location' hypothesis but was not predicted or explained by indicators of years of education or income gradients. The gradient ('SES') hypothesis would have led to the expectation that supervisors, because of their higher incomes, would present lower rates of anxiety and depression than workers.

According to the example above, the theoretical and explanatory power of social class stems from social relations of ownership or control over productive resources (i.e., physical, financial, and organizational). Social class relations have important consequences for the lives of individuals. The extent of an individual's legal right and power to control productive assets determines an individual's abilities to acquire income. And income determines in large part the individual's standard of living. Thus, the class position of 'business owner' compels its members to hire 'workers' and extract labour from them, while the 'worker' class position compels its members to find employment and perform labour. Social class provides an explicit relational mechanism (property, management) that explains how economic inequalities are generated and how they may affect psychiatric disorders.

In a recent study, we further examined the relationships between measures of social class (Wright's social class indicators, i.e., relationship to productive assets) and indicators of psychiatric disorders.[51] We tested this scheme using the Barcelona Health Interview Survey, a cross-sectional survey of 10,000 residents of the city's non-institutionalized population in 2000. Health related variables included self-perceived health (taping mostly psychiatric disorders), nicotine addiction, eating behaviours and injuries.

Findings revealed that, contrary to conventional wisdom, health indicators are often worse for employers than for managers, and that supervisors often fare more poorly than workers. Our findings highlight the potential health consequences of social class positions defined by relations of control over productive assets. They also confirm that social class taps into parts of the social variation in health that are not captured by conventional measures of social stratification. Property relations, which figure prominently in both Marxian and Weberian traditions, do not, however, exhaust the theoretical spectrum of class concepts. Another, untapped, notion is that of class exploitation.

Marxian Class Analysis: Class Exploitation and Psychiatric Disorders

Although property relations might be important predictors of psychiatric disorders,[52] they do not capture the underlying mechanism in the Marxian class tradition, namely exploitation.[53] According to that tradition, a measure of social class should not only capture property relations but the domination of the 'exploited' by the 'exploiter' and the extraction and appropriation of labour effort [54] In fact most Neo-Marxian measures of social class are exchangeable with Neo-Weberian measures of employment relations because they capture only property relations. That is, both sets of indicators tap into employment relations or labour market exchanges such as 'employer' 'employee', but do not capture the amount of labour effort extracted from the 'employee' by the 'employer', which forms the basis of 'exploitation' as a social mechanism in the classic Marxian tradition.[55] To follow that tradition, indicators of class exploitation should take into account that: (1) the material welfare of a class causally depends on the material deprivation of another; (2) this causal relation in (1) involves the asymmetrical exclusion of the exploited class from access to certain productive resources (e.g., property rights); and (3) the causal mechanism that translates the exclusion in (2) into differential welfare involves the appropriation of the fruits of labour of the exploited class by those who control the access to productive resources (i.e., the exploiter class).[56] Thus we can observe that most Neo-Marxian measures of social class measure (1) and (2) in the form of property relations, but do not capture the appropriation of labour effort. In a recent study,[57] we found an association between class exploitation and depression using organizational level indicators that capture both property relations and the extraction of labour effort (for profit ownership, managerial domination, lack of wage increases). These indicators were strong predictors of depressive symptoms in these studies. They are different from employment relations indicators in that they capture social class exploitation at the organizational level (i.e., the combination of for profit ownership, managerial pressure and lack of wage increases taps into high levels of extraction of labour effort and low compensation, or higher exploitation, as compared to the residual category).

In sum, our argument is that there are a number of class constructs that can illuminate the relation between economic inequality and psychiatric disorders. There are numerous, literally hundreds of measures of mental health and psychiatric disorders in the literature. (see Buro's Psychiatric Measurement volumes). On the other hand the social part of the equation remains vastly underdeveloped, with researchers using only a handful of measures (income, education, occupation).

The Paradox of Epidemiology, Social Psychiatry and the Sociology of Mental Disorders

In spite of their pragmatic, often non-theoretical approach to social factors, psychiatric epidemiology and social psychiatry (both part of public mental health) have now and then tackled structural inequalities. A strong concern for social justice and reducing inequalities (race, gender, poverty) could explain the strong interest in social inequalities in health among epidemiologists. The contemporary definition of public health – as organized efforts by society to improve the health of populations – implicitly acknowledges both social determinants and collective responsibility for the public's health.[58]

Public mental health is thus faced with the obligation to improve the health of groups affected by social inequality – that is, public health officials have the responsibility to improve the psychiatric disorders of populations that due to economic, political, or cultural inequalities have a high rate of psychiatric disorders. In these disciplines, it is understood that a society's unequal distribution of economic, political, or cultural resources will generate worse psychiatric disorders among the relatively poor, powerless, and with less credentials.[59]

Furthermore, it is widely recognized that inequalities in property generate an intergenerational transmission of poverty that has disproportionately affected African-Americans in the U.S.[60] Other acknowledged sources of economic inequality involve political inequalities that preclude immigrants from obtaining equal rights, while confining them to economic, political, and cultural subordination. And cultural factors such as racism, ideology, or ignorance that can lead to labour market discrimination and residential segregation with negative economic, political, and cultural consequences for people of various races and ethnicities, nationalities, religions, age groups, sexual orientations, gender, diseases or disabilities, and social classes. It is within this public health ethos of reversing inequalities associated with the social movements of the sixties and seventies that recent research focuses on the interactions between class, gender and race/ethnicity and psychiatric disorders.[61] Although generalizations are often inaccurate in social epidemiology, overall this body of research on the triad of class, gender and race tends to find worse psychiatric disorders among members of the groups exposed to the three forms of inequality.[62] Epidemiologists have also been leaders in topics that overlap with the more structural concerns traditionally associated with sociology and mainstream economics such as the study of the psychiatric disorder effects of new forms of labour market arrangements,[63] the effects of social class across the lifespan,[64] or the contextual effects of neighbourhood economic inequality on psychiatric disorders.[65] Because these studies are often published outside of psychiatry, their contributions to theories of social inequality in psychiatric disorders remain under-recognized.

There is thus a curious paradox that looms large in the literature on the sociology of psychiatric disorders. It is not uncommon to observe that (1) epidemiologists and public health researchers without a PhD in social science are those who bring a socio-structural perspective to health inequalities;[66] (2) in spite of some notable exceptions,[67] social scientists have been devoted to socio-psychological rather than socio-structural explanations.[68] Yet social scientists are leaders in psychiatric epidemiology and public mental health without bringing a particular sociological content to their work.[69] A detailed historical, professional, and institutional analysis (e.g., are health researchers trained to be critical in general so they dare to approach thorny issues such as 'class' when they shift to social inquiry? Do medicine, public health and psychiatry attract conservative social scientists? Why did social psychology have more influence on the sociology of psychiatric disorders than the socio-structural perspective?), will be needed to sort out the merit of these propositions. They suggest, however, the need for more sustained attention to structural explanations in psychiatric epidemiological research.

Given the soundness of the methods and the robustness of the findings in psychiatric epidemiology and social psychiatry, one might be tempted to conclude that deeper sociological insights are superfluous to such applied disciplines. Why not just raise the minimum wage or increase welfare assistance to the poor as primary prevention? The answer is not so simple as implicit social models permeate both psychiatric epidemiology and social psychiatry with sharp differences in their policy implications.[70] More specifically, underlying most research on economic inequality and psychiatric disorders we find competing implicit social models of what constitutes desirable social and health policies. Two opposing views of the social inequalities in psychiatric disorders are prominent.[71] The first is that behaviour is a matter of individual agency or volitional control, accounting for the disproportionate burden of psychiatric illness among workers, women, and minorities. This view holds that most social outcomes, including psychiatric disorders, reflect personal autonomous choices and that therefore there is little that society, as a whole, is obliged to do for people who are afflicted by psychiatric disorders.[72] In one study,[73] for example, educated 'liberals' respected the autonomy and individual rights of homeless persons but felt little obligation to do anything to improve their situation.

In contrast, the 'structural' view focuses on social relations of class, race, ethnicity, and gender inequality as determinants of individual behaviour and psychiatric disorders.[74] The policy implications of this view include collective responsibility for those whose psychiatric disorders are negatively affected by class, gender, and racial and ethnic inequalities in access to economic, political, and cultural resources. For example, a recent ethnographic study of African-American and white working-class men concluded that African-American men have a greater sense of collective responsibility and are less prone to use individual responsibility as an explanation for personal outcomes than are their white counterparts.[75] Western European and U.S. whites are more likely to use individualistic attributions for the outcomes of persons in social situations – personal attributes are seen as the cause of personal outcomes, as opposed to the features of the situation.[76] The implication is that unless we make social-structural inequalities explicit we cannot use social science to choose between competing policy perspectives.

Although most studies in social inequalities in psychiatric disorders[77] use stratification indicators that eschew social structure (i.e., the set of economic, political and cultural relations in a given social system),[78] there is nowadays sufficient evidence to suggest that class, gender, and racial/ethnic inequalities in psychiatric disorders stem from social structures, rather than solely from personal choices or individual attributes. Thus studies using employment relations indicators social class have been found to predict psychiatric disorders over and above mere stratification indicators.[79] The implication is that structural social class measures are useful in social psychiatry not only because they provide a social mechanism (e.g., the relation between supervisor and supervisee), but because they can be strong predictors psychiatric disorders.[80]

From Status Syndrome to Capitalist Syndrome: The Role of Class Exploitation in Social Psychiatry

The evidence on the inverse association between measures of social stratification such as income and education and common psychiatric disorders is well established. Yet little is known about the relation between the social processes that generate economic inequalities and psychiatric disorders. Recent research points to the need for social psychiatry to delve into the social relations that produce social inequalities in psychiatric disorders, not only into the micro social processes linking social interactions to psychiatric disease (e.g., service utilization, stigma). Social mechanisms generating economic inequalities such as relations of production, property relations, or exploitation are too central to social systems to be addressed exclusively by clinicians. Class analysis input will be ultimately essential to the advancement of our understanding of the relation between economic inequality and psychiatric disorders. Greater Class analytic (e.g., Neo-Marxian class exploitation) insight into research on social inequalities in psychiatric disorders would give social psychiatry more depth; would allow testing of alternative models for the social production of psychiatric illness, which now are not accessible due to focus on the outcomes of social structure (e.g., income inequalities); and would ultimately yield deeper causal models that might lead to effective policy interventions.

Notes

1. For example, see D.G. Blazer, R.C. Kessler, K.A. McGonagle, and M.S. Swartz, 'The Prevalence and Distribution of Major Depression in a National Community Sample: The National Comorbidity Survey,' 151 *American Journal of Psychiatry* (1994): 979–986; W.W. Eaton, S. Buka, A.M. Addington, J. Bass, S. Brown, and S. Cherkerzian, 'Risk Factors for Major Mental Disorders: A Review of the Epidemiologic Literature.' Retrieved January 24, 2005 from http://apps1.jhsph.edu/weaton/MDRF/main.html; F. Jacobi, H.U. Wittchen, C. Holting, M. Hofler, H. Pfister, and N. Muller, 'Prevalence, Co-morbidity and Correlates of Mental Disorders in the General Population: Results from the German Health Interview and Examination Survey (ghs),' 34(4) *Psychological Medicine* (2004): 597–611; E. Lahelma, P. Martikainen, O. Rahkonen, E. Roos, and P. Saastamoinen, 'Occupational Class Inequalities Across Key Domains of Health: Results from the Helsinki Health Study,'15(5) *European Journal of Public Health* (2005): 510; D. A. Regier, J.H. Boyd, J.D. Burke Jr., D.S. Rae, J.K. Myers, and M. Kramer, 'One-month Prevalence of Mental Disorders in the United States. Based on five epidemiologic catchment area sites,' 45(11) *Archives of General Psychiatry* (1988): 977–986; R.E. Roberts and E.S. Lee, 'Occupation and the Prevalence of Major Depression, Alcohol, and Drug Abuse in the United States,' 61(2) *Environmental Research* (1993): 266–278.

2. C. Muntaner, P. Wolyniec, P.J. McGrath, and A.E. Pulver, 'Differences in Social Class Among Psychotic Patients at Inpatient Admission,' 46(2) *Psychiatric Services* (1995): 176–178; M. Alegria, R.V. Bijl, E. Lin, E.E. Walters, and R.C. Kessler, 'Income Differences in Persons Seeking Outpatient Treatment for Mental Disorders: A Comparison of the United States with Ontario and The Netherlands' 57 *Archives of General Psychiatry* (2000): 383–391; A.C. Cohen, P.R. Houck, K. Szanto, M.A. Dew, S.E. Gilman, and C.F. Reynolds, 'Social Inequalities in Response to Antidepressant Treatment in Older Adults,' 63(1) *Archives of General Psychiatry* (2006): 50–56.

3. For example, S. Asthana, A. Gibson, G. Moon, P. Brigham, and J. Dicker, 'The Demographic and Social Class Basis of Inequality in Self Reported Morbidity: An Exploration of Using the Health Survey for England' 58(4) *Journal of Epidemiology & Community Health*, (2004): 303–307.

4. V. Navarro and C. Muntaner, *Political and Economic Determinants of Population Health and Well-being: Controversies and Developments* (Amityville, NY: The Baywood, 2004).

5. C.J. Murray and A.D. Lopez, 'Evidence-based Health Policy—Lessons From the Global Burden of Disease Study,' 274(5228) *Science* (1996): 740–743.

6. T. Fryers, D. Melzer, R. Jenkins, and T. Brugha, 'The Distribution of the Common Mental Disorders: Social Inequalities in Europe,' 1(14) *Clinical Practice and Epidemiology in Mental Health*, (2005) doi:10.1186/1745–1719-1–14; D. Melzer, T. Fryers, R. Jenkins, T. Brugha, and B. McWilliams, 'Social Position and the Common Mental Disorders with Disability: Estimates From the National Mental Survey of Great Britain,' 38(5) *Social Psychiatry and Psychiatric Epidemiology* (2003): 238–243; R. Poulton, A. Caspi, B.J. Milne, W.M. Thomson, A. Taylor, and M.R. Sears, 'Association Between Children's Experience of Socioeconomic Disadvantage and Adult Health: A Life-Course Study,' 360 *The Lancet* (2002): 1640–1645; S.A. Stansfeld, J. Head, R. Fuhrer, J. Wardle, and V. Cattell, 'Social Inequalities in Depressive Symptoms and Physical Functioning in the Whitehall ii Study: Exploring A Common Cause Explanation,' 57(5) *Journal of Epidemiology & Community Health* (2003): 361–367.

7. Michael Marmot, *The Status Syndrome: How Social Standing Affects Our Health* (London: Bloomsbury, 2004).

8. H. Chung and C. Muntaner, 'Political and Welfare State Determinants of Population Health: An Analysis of Wealthy Countries,' 63(3) *Social Science & Medicine* (2006): 829–842.

9. For example, S. Geyer, H. Haltenhof, and R. Peter, 'Social Inequality in the Utilization of In- and Outpatient Treatment of Non-Psychotic/Non-Organic Disorders: A Study with Health Insurance Data,' 36(8) *Social Psychiatry and Psychiatric Epidemiology* (2001): 373–380.

10. W.W. Eaton and C. Muntaner, 'Socioeconomic Stratification and Mental Disorder,' in *Handbook for the Study of Mental Health: Social Contexts, Theories and Systems*, ed. A.V. Horwitz and T.L. Scheid (New York: Cambridge University Press, 1999); C. Muntaner, W.W. Eaton, R. Miech, and P.O'Campo, 'Socioeconomic Position and Major Mental Disorders,' 26 *Epidemiological Review* (2004): 53–62.

11. Eaton & Muntaner, 1999, Note 10.

12. V. Lorant, D. Deliege, W.W. Eaton, A. Robert, P. Philippot, and M. Ansseau, 'Socioeconomic Inequalities in Depression: A Meta-Analysis,' 157(2) *American Journal of Epidemiology* (2003): 98–112.

13. Blazer et al., 1994, Note 1.

14. W.W. Eaton, *The Sociology of Mental Disorders*, 3rd ed. (London: Praeger, 2001).

15. Ibid.

16. C. Muntaner, W.W. Eaton, C. Diala, R.C. Kessler, and P.D. Sorlie, 'Social Class, Assets, Organizational Control and the Prevalence of Common Group Mental Disorders,' 47(12) *Social Science & Medicine* (1998): 2043–2053.

17. Roberts & Lee, 1993, Note 1.
18. Eaton et al., 2004, Note 1.
19. Ibid.
20. Ibid.
21. Eaton, 2001, Note 14; Eaton et al., 2004, Note 1; Regier et al., Note 1.
22. Regier et al., 1988, Note 1.
23. Eaton et al., 2004, Note 1; Eaton & Muntaner, 1999, Note 10.
24. Muntaner et al., 2004, Note 10; R.G. Wilkinson and K.E. Pickett 'Income Inequality and Population Health: A Review and Explanation of the Evidence,' 62(7) *Social Science & Medicine* (2006): 768–1784.
25. J.W. Lynch, G. Davey-Smith, G.A. Kaplan, and J.S. House, 'Income Inequality and Mortality: Importance to Health of Individual Income, Psychosocial Environment, or Material Conditions,' 320 *British Medical Journal* (2000): 1200–1204; C. Muntaner, 'Commentary: Social Capital, Social Class and the Slow Progress of Psychosocial Epidemiology,' 33(4) *International Journal of Epidemiology* (2004): 674–680; N. Pearce and G. Davey Smith 'Is Social Capital the Key to Inequities in Health?' 93(1) *American Journal of Public Health* (2003): 122–129.
26. Lynch et al., 2000, Note 25.
27. R. Wilkinson, *The Impact of Inequality* (New York: The New Press, 2005).
28. G. Lewis, P. Bebbington, T. Brugha, et al., 'Socioeconomic Status, Standard of Living, and Neurotic Disorder,' 352 *Lancet* (1998): 605–609; G. Lewis, P. Bebbington, T. Brugha, et al., 'Socio-economic Status, Standard of Living and Neurotic Disorder,' 15 *International Review of Psychiatry* (2003): 91–96; S. Weich and G. Lewis, 'Material Standard of Living, Social Class, and the Prevalence of the Common Mental Disorders in Great Britain,' 52(1) *Journal of Epidemiology and Community Health* (1998): 8–14.
29. Ibid.
30. Lewis et al., 1998, Note 28.
31. Eaton et al., 2001, Note 14; Weich & Lewis, 1998, Note 28.
32. Marmot, 2004, Note 7.
33. Ibid.
34. For example, R.J. Turner, B. Wheaton, and B. Lloyd, 'The Epidemiology of Social Stress,' 60 *American Sociological Review* (1995): 104–225. See the *Journal of Health and Social Behavior* for the last twenty years.
35. J. Macleod, G. Davey Smith, P. Heslop, C. Metcalfe, D. Carroll, and C. Hart, 'Psychological Stress and Cardiovascular Disease: Empirical Demonstration of Bias in a Prospective Observational Study of Scottish Men,' 324 *British Medical Journal* (2002): 1247–1251.
36. J.E. Ferrie, M.J. Shipley, S.A. Stansfeld, G. Davey Smith, and M. Marmot, 'Future Uncertainty and Socioeconomic Inequalities in Health: The Whitehall ii Study,' 57 *Social Science and Medicine* (2003): 637–646.
37. N. Krieger, D.R. Williams, and N.E. Moss, 'Measuring Social Class in U. S. Public Health Research: Concepts, Methodologies, and Guidelines,' 18 *Annual Review of Public Health* (1997): 341–378; C. Muntaner, and P.J.O'Campo, 'A Critical Appraisal of the Demand/Control Model of the Psychosocial Work Environment: Epistemological, Social, Behavioral and Class Considerations,' 36(11) *Social Science & Medicine* (1993): 1509–1517.
38. Muntaner et al., 1998, Note 16.

39. C. Muntaner and J. Lynch, 'Income Inequality, Social Cohesion, and Class Relations: A Critique of Wilkinson's Neo-Durkheimian Research Program,' 29(1) *International Journal of Health Services* (1999): 59–81.

40. M. Bartley and M. Marmot, 'Social Class and Power Relations at the Workplace,'15 *Occupational Medicine: State of the Art Reviews* (2000): 73–78.

41. For example, C. Borrell, C., Muntaner, J. Benach, and L. Artazcoz, 'Social Class and Self-Reported Health Status Among Men and Women: What is the Role of Work Organization, Household Material Standards and Household Labour?,' 58(10) *Social Science & Medicine* (2004): 1869–1887; C. Muntaner, J.C. Anthony, R.M. Crum, and W.W. Eaton, 'Psychosocial Dimensions of Work and the Risk of Drug Dependence Among Adults,' 142(2) *American Journal of Epidemiology* (1995): 183–190; C. Muntaner, C. Borrell, J. Benach, M.I. Pasarin, and E. Fernandez, 'The Associations of Social Class and Social Stratification with Patterns of General Mental Health in a Spanish Population,' 32(6) *International Journal of Epidemiology* (2003): 950–958; Muntaner et al., 1998, Note 16; C. Muntaner and P.E. Parsons, 'Income, Social Stratification, Class and Private Health Insurance: A Study of the Baltimore Metropolitan Area,' 26(4) *International Journal of Health Services* (1996): 655–671.

42. E.O. Wright, *Approaches to Class Analysis.* (Cambridge: Cambridge University Press, 2005). Most of the measures we have used in our studies do not distinguish the Neo-Marxian conceptualization of social class from the Neo-Weberian conceptualization, a framework that focuses on class as employment relations but does not contemplate exploitation as a central mechanism. We discuss the importance of adding indicators of exploitation in the next section on Marxian class analysis.

43. Muntaner et al., 2004, Note 10.

44. Eaton et al., 2004, Note 1; J.W. Lynch, and G.A. Kaplan, 'Socioeconomic Position,' in *Social Epidemiology*, ed. L. F. Berkman and I. Kawachi (New York: Oxford University Press, 2000): 76–94.

45. Muntaner and Lynch, 1999, Note 39.

46. Krieger et al., 1997, Note 37.

47. Borrell et al., 2004, Note 41; Muntaner et al., 2003, Note 41; Muntaner et al., 1998, Note 16; T. Wohlfarth, 'Socioeconomic Inequality and Psychopathology: Are Socioeconomic Status and Social class Interchangeable?' 45(3) *Social Science & Medicine* (1997): 399–410; T. Wohlfarth, and W. Van Den Brink, 'Social Class and Substance Disorders: The Value of Social Class as Distinct From Socioeconomic Status,' 47(1) *Social Science & Medicine* (1998): 51–58.

48. Wohlfarth, 1997, Note 47.

49. Muntaner et al., 2003, Note 41; Muntaner et al., 1998, Note 16.

50. E.O. Wright, *Class Counts* (Cambridge: Cambridge University Press, 1996).

51. Borrell et al., 2004, Note 41.

52. Eaton & Muntaner, 1999, Note 10; Wohlfarth, 1997, Note 47.

53. Wright, 1996, Note 50.

54. S. Resnick and R.D. Wolff, 'Classes in Marxian Theory,' 13(4) *Review of Radical Political Economics* (1982): 1–18; Wright, 1996, Note 50.

55. Muntaner et al., 1998, Note 16; Wright, 2005, Note 42.

56. Wright, 1996, Note 50.

57. Muntaner et al. 2004, Note 25; Muntaner et al. 2005.

58. J. A. Last, *Dictionary of Epidemiology* (New York: Oxford UP, 1995).
59. Navarro & Muntaner, 2004, Note 4.
60. D. Conley and N. G. Bennett, 'Birth Weight and Income: Interactions Across Generations,' 42(4) *Journal of Health & Social Behavior* (2001): 450–465.
61. L. Artazcoz, J. Benach, C. Borrell, and I. Cortes, 'Unemployment and Mental Health: Understanding the Interactions Among Gender, Family Roles, and Social Class,' 94(1) *American Journal of Public Health*, (2004): 82–88; P.O'Campo, W.W. Eaton, and C. Muntaner, 'Labor Market Experience, Work Organization, Gender Inequalities, and Health Status: Results from a Prospective Analysis of U.S. Employed Women,' 58(3) *Social Science & Medicine* (2004): 585–594; S. Outram, G.D. Mishra, and M.J. Schofield, 'Sociodemographic and Health Related Factors Associated with Poor Mental Health in Midlife Australian Women,' 39(4) *Women Health* (2004): 97–115.
62. N. Krieger, P.D. Waterman, C. Hartman, et al., 'Social Hazards on the Job: Workplace Abuse, Sexual Harassment, and Racial Discrimination—A Study of Black, Latino, and White Low-income Women and Men Workers in the United States,' 36(1) *International Journal of Health Services* (2006): 51–85.
63. L. Artazcoz, J. Benach, C. Borrell, and I. Cortes, 'Social Inequalities in the Impact of Flexible Employment on Different Domains of Psychosocial Health,' 59(9) *Journal of Epidemiology & Community Health* (2005): 761–767; I.H. Kim, C. Muntaner, Y.H. Khang, D. Paek, and S.I. Cho, 'The Relationship Between Nonstandard Working and Mental Health in a Representative Sample of the South Korean Population,' 63 *Social Science & Medicine* (2006): 566–574..
64. E. Breeze, A.E. Fletcher, D.A. Leon, M.G. Marmot, R.J. Clarke, and M.J. Shipley, 'Do Socioeconomic Disadvantages Persist into Old Age? Self-reported Morbidity in a 29-year Follow-up of the Whitehall Study,' 91(2) *Am J Public Health* (2001): 277–283.
65. C. Eibner, R. Sturn, and C.R. Gresenz, 'Does Relative Deprivation Predict the Need for Mental Health Services?' 157(4) *Journal of Mental Health Policy and Economics* (2004): 167–175; Muntaner et al., 2004, Note 10; C. Muntaner, Y. Li, X. Xue, P.O'Campo, H. J. Chung, and W. W. Eaton, 'Work Organization, Area Labor-Market Characteristics, and Depression Among U. S. Nursing Home Workers: A Cross-Classified Multilevel Analysis,' 10(4) *International Journal of Occupational & Environmental Health* (2004): 392–400; J. Schneiders, M. Drukker, J. van der Ende, F.C. Verhulst, J. van Os, and N.A. Nicolson, 'Neighbourhood Socioeconomic Disadvantage and Behavioural Problems from Late Childhood into Early Adolescence,' 57(9) *Journal of Epidemiology and Community Health* (2003): 699–703; M. Stafford and M. Marmot, 'Neighbourhood Deprivation and Health: Does it Affect Us All Equally?' 32(3) *International Journal of Epidemiology* (2003): 357–366; N. Wainwright and P.J.G. Surtees, 'Area and Individual Circumstances and Mood Disorder Prevalence,' 185 *British Journal of Psychiatry* (2004): 227–232.
66. For example, Krieger et al., 1997, Note 37; Muntaner et al., 1998, Note 16.
67. M.L. Kohn, and C. Schooler, *Work and Personality: An Inquiry into the Impact of Social Stratification* (Norwood, NJ: Ablex, 1983).
68. L.I. Pearlin, 'The Sociological Study of Stress,' 30(3) *Journal of Health & Social Behavior* (1989): 241–256; P.J.A. Thoits, 'Differential Labeling of Mental

Illness by Social Status: A New Look at an Old Problem,' 46(1) *Journal of Health & Social Behavior* (2005): 102–119.

69. R.C. Kessler, K.A. McGonagle, S. Zhao, et al., 'Lifetime and 12-Month Prevalence of DSM-Iii-R Mental Disorders in the United States,' 51 *Archives of General Psychiatry* (1994): 8–19.
70. C. Muntaner, W.W. Eaton, and C. Diala, 'Socioeconomic Inequalities in Mental Health: A Review of Concepts and Underlying Assumptions,' 4 *Health* (2000): 89–15.
71. Ibid.
72. Muntaner & Lynch, 1999, Note 39.
73. B.G. Link, S. Schwartz, R. Moore, et al., 'Public Knowledge, Attitudes, and Beliefs About Homeless People: Evidence for Compassion Fatigue,' 23(4) *American Journal of Community Psychology* (1995): 533–555.
74. Muntaner et al., 2000, Note 70.
75. M. Lamont, *The Dignity of Working Men* (New York: Russell Sage, 2000).
76. R.E. Nisbett, *The Geography of Thought* (New York: The Free Press, 2003).
77. Eaton et al., 2004, Note 1.
78. Muntaner & Lynch, 1999, Note 39.
79. See review by Muntaner et al., 2004, Note 10.
80. Ibid.

11

Beyond the Income Inequality Hypothesis: Class, Neo-Liberalism, and Health Inequalities

DAVID COBURN

Introduction

In this chapter, I take a view of the relationship between income inequality and health status which is more sociological than epidemiological. Whereas most attention has focused on the consequences of income distributions or socio-economic status (SES) for health, I discuss here the class-based production of inequalities. Doing so leads to an alternative conceptualization of the determinants of health inequalities within and between nations to that of the income inequality perspective. The political economy approach taken links study of the health effects of income inequality with social and class changes including the spread of neo-liberalism, the decline of the welfare state, differences amongst nations regarding welfare regime type, and, most generally, the relationships between class structure, economies and human well-being. This approach builds on a model developed to

This chapter is reprinted with permission from *Social Science & Medicine*, 58(1), January 2004, 41–56.
Earlier versions of this chapter were presented in the Department of Sociology, University of Western Ontario, at the International Sociological Association World Congress in Brisbane, Australia, July, 2002 and at the School of Public Health at La Trobe University, Melbourne.

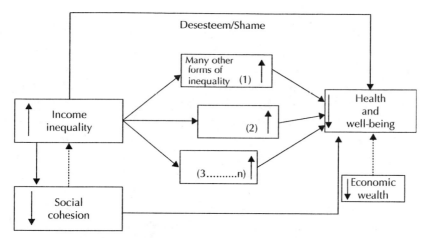

FIGURE 11.1 The Class/Welfare Regime Model.

help explain 'the rise and fall' of medical dominance[1] and on the theories and findings of a number of others – particularly Navarro[2] but also Ross and Trachte,[3] Esping-Andersen,[4] Lynch and colleagues,[5] and of course, Wilkinson[6] and the many epidemiological researchers who have focused on income inequality.[7]

After briefly describing and critiquing the income inequality hypothesis I present an alternative model (Figure 11.1) and empirically explore its usefulness using available data.

The Income Inequality Hypothesis and Its Critics

Income Inequality and Health

Analysis of the relationships between income inequalities and health has become a major focus of studies of the social determinants of health. Within-nations income inequality plays a prominent role in analyses of SES-related health inequalities. That is, it has been found that, everywhere, the rich live longer, healthier lives than do the poor. Moreover, the income inequality hypothesis is the dominant approach to discussion about health inequalities between as well as within the developed nations. Elements of the income inequality approach, such as the importance of social hierarchies, have also found their way into the health policy arena through their impact on the new paradigm of population health.[8]

In: *Unhealthy Societies: The Afflictions of Inequality*,[9] Richard Wilkinson argued that, amongst the less developed nations, GNP/capita is the most important correlate of average levels of health status. However, above about $5–$10,000 GNP/capita, the point at which chronic diseases begin to displace acute illness as the chief causes of death, Wilkinson contends that it is the degree of income inequality, rather than national wealth which is the most important determinant of national differences in health status. It is worthwhile noting that, even under the $5–$10,000 mark, there is a wide distribution of health for any particular GNP/capita level. Discussion of the health of the less developed nations cannot be dismissed as the simple product of GNP/capita.[10] However, following Wilkinson, the major focus here is on income inequality and health status within and between the 14–20 most developed nations.

Noting that high-level British civil servants show poorer health than those even higher in the hierarchy, income inequality theorists concluded that relative, rather than absolute income differences underlie the relationships between income and health. Hence, they turned their attention less to material inequalities, poverty or absolute income than to psycho-social status hierarchies. Social hierarchies are said to produce disease because of the poor self-esteem associated with lower status which, in turn, through psycho-neurobiological pathways, negatively influences health. Wilkinson, Kawachi, and others also contend that income inequality leads to loss of social cohesion which produces lower health status.[11]

Wilkinson and colleagues claim that there are two major dimensions of society, degree of hierarchy (vertical separation) and social cohesion or fragmentation (horizontal separation) which, measuring the 'quality of life', determine average national or regional health status. From an initially small collection of empirical correlations, income inequality theorists have built up an impressive edifice of findings and explanations leading to far-reaching conclusions about the nature of human societies and the fundamental characteristics of human nature and health. In that sense Wilkinson and colleagues built on, but went much beyond earlier empirical studies of the relationship between income inequality and health status by Preston[12] and Rodgers[13] (1979). The underlying income inequality model is shown in Figure 11.2.

Criticisms of the Income Inequality Thesis

There have been recent criticisms of the income inequality approach.[14] These have centred (1) on whether or not the original findings are valid or exaggerated[14] and (2) whether international income inequality-health correlations are 'artifactual' (if the relationship between income and health within nations is curvilinear rather than linear, any decrease in national or regional levels of inequality would 'automatically' lead to higher average health status.[15] However, from the perspective of this chapter, the

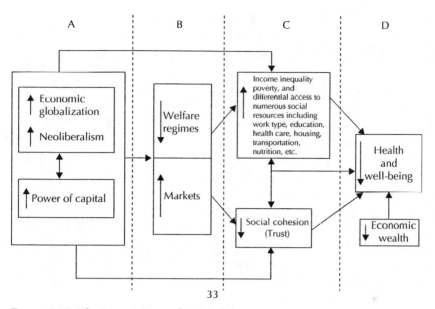

FIGURE 11.2 The Income Inequality Model.

most important criticism, noted by a wide variety of commentators is (3) whether the effects attributed to income inequality or to social cohesion are as much the consequence of the many social factors with which income inequality/social cohesion correlate as they are to income-determined relative (psycho-social) status differences.

From a sociological point of view I also note (4) that the theory is one based on status hierarchies, yet nowhere are status differences or self-esteem directly measured. There are reasons for doubting the assertion that those lower in income feel 'disesteemed', because status is not uni-dimensional, there are many social hierarchies and some may attach more esteem to some hierarchies than to others. Moreover, (5) any individual's status and income can vary quite radically over a lifetime. There may be national variations in income and status mobility.[16]

The original income studies examined international cross-sectional correlations amongst GNP/capita, measures of income inequality, and health. Yet (6) even within the theory one would expect a latency period between social conditions and their effects on health. Probably the exception is regarding infant mortality which is commonly assumed as more likely to reflect contemporary conditions than are such chronic conditions as cardiovascular disease. Disease and death are likely due to life-long cumulative influences rather than only to conditions in the immediate environment.

There are also (7) suggestions that the relationship between income inequality and health within nations is asymptotic rather than linear and that the shape of these relationships varies in different nations. The linear relationships previously found focused on such highly status-oriented groups as British civil servants.[17] A recent analysis[18] suggests that, in the United States, use of general measures of income inequality, such as the Gini index, tend to obscure the strong effects of inequalities at low income and the weak effects of income inequalities at higher income on health.[19]

I agree with those observers who now feel that income inequality may be correlated with health but that income inequality probably reflects or is a proxy for a variety of social conditions, operating through individual and collective, material and psycho-social pathways, rather than income inequality being a single main cause of poorer health. For example, in the US, Muller[20] found state educational levels more important than income inequality. Deaton suggests that state racial composition explains away the effect of state differences in relative deprivation on health status.[21] In addition, income inequality differences among US states co-vary with a series of other social factors from percentage of children in school to the availability of community resources.[22]

Rather than income inequality being the chief determinant of such societal types, I draw here on the existing literature on classes, neo-liberalism and welfare regimes to point to ways in which we can begin to understand inequalities in historical and cross-sectional perspective. In this model, income inequality is itself the consequence of fundamental changes in class structure which have produced not only income inequality but also numerous other forms of health-relevant social inequalities. Welfare measures in turn reflect basic social, political and economic institutions tied to the degree to which societies take care of their citizens or leave the fate of citizens up to the market, i.e., neo-liberalism. Income inequality is a consequence, not the determinant, of societal 'types'.[23]

In an alternative model (Figure 11.1) described below, income inequality has a place but not the central causal status given to it in the orthodox income inequality literature. This chapter is thus not simply about arguing 'against' the income inequality thesis but is an attempt to encompass it, and to go beyond it by opening up analysis of the determinants of health within a broader, more contextualized and more sociologically meaningful causal model.

An Alternative Explanation

An adequate sociological account has to help explain both historical change and contemporary variation. In what follows, I use the idea of global capitalism as a new phase of capitalism replacing earlier forms[24] to analyse historical change and welfare regime types[25] to account for national cross-sectional health inequality differences. This approach is broadly congruent with a critical realist perspective.[26]

To sketch an explanation—capitalism is viewed as moving through particular phases—entrepreneurial, monopoly, and most recently global, capitalism. Each of these phases has its own set of class, economic and political characteristics. Economic globalization, as a real force, and as ideology, brought the re-emergence of business on national and international levels to a dominant class position from the previous phase of a nationally focused monopoly capitalism in which capital and labour had arrived at various forms of accommodation. Contemporary business dominance, and its accompanying neo-liberal ideology and policies, led to attacks on working class rights in the market (e.g., by undermining unions) and to citizenship rights as expressed even in the liberal (market-dependent) version of the welfare state enacted in most of the Anglo-American nations. Labour's lessened market power and fragmentation, and the shredding of the welfare state also led to major increases in social inequality, poverty, income inequality and social fragmentation. I earlier[27] pointed out that neo-liberalism has doctrinal affinities with inequality and with lowered social cohesion. Neo-liberal philosophy and policies are either unconcerned with, or positively endorse, inequalities (as encouraging work motivation, participation in markets, etc). Moreover, they are particularly 'individualist' in attacking various forms of collective or state action—insisting that we face markets only as individuals or families—that we 'provide for ourselves'. I argue that the forceful enactment of neo-liberal ideologies and politics exacerbates differences amongst rich and poor within the market, and, at the same time, undermines those social institutions which might help reduce poverty or income inequalities or which buffer the effects of income inequalities on health.

Neo-liberal economic globalization undermined the welfare state. But there are alternative national forms of welfare regime based on varying national class and institutional structures.[28] These differentially resist international trends towards the dominance of market-based inequalities. Welfare regimes can be categorized according to the extent to which they decommodify citizens' relationships to the market. Decommodification refers to the degree to which citizens have an alternative to complete dependence on the labour market (on working for money), in order to have an acceptable standard of living.[29] Esping-Andersen notes three major types of welfare state: the Social Democratic welfare states, showing the greatest decommodification and emphasis on citizenship rights; the Liberal welfare state which is the most market-dependent and emphasizes means and income testing; and an intermediate group, the Conservative, Corporatist or Familist welfare states, which are characterized by class and status-based insurance schemes and a heavy reliance on the family to provide support.[30] These countries might be viewed as strong-, weak- and intermediate or mixed-type welfare states, respectively, although Esping-Andersen's main point was that these are fundamentally different kinds of society.

The major examples of the Social Democratic welfare states are the Scandinavian countries such as Sweden, Norway, and Finland. The Liberal welfare states include the Anglo-American nations particularly the United Kingdom and the United States (at one time the UK was close to Social Democratic status). The corporatist/familist states include such countries as Germany, France, and Italy. It is important to note that these nations represent differing ways of approaching both market and state welfare phenomena based on differing class structures and class coalitions—they constitute distinct socio-political and not only welfare state regimes.[31] For example, Social Democratic regimes tend to have higher overall labour force participation (particularly among women) and stronger labour market policies aimed at full employment. Markets and states are not separate but are mutually constituted.

Within the welfare state literature, a major explanatory stream is a class or class coalitional perspective.[32] Greater working class strength and/or upper class weakness and various combinations of class coalitions, degrees of class cohesion/organization (e.g., the formation of a working class-based political party) and degree of working class institutionalization produce stronger welfare regimes or helps preserve these in the face of attack. Welfare regimes not only have causes but they also have consequents for the class and stratification structure.

The model (Figure 11.1) is one which views neo-liberal economic globalization as a new phase of capitalism. Globalization reinforced business class power and reduced that of oppositional classes. Global neo-liberal politics and policies have increased within national inequalities—and within-nation health inequalities—partly through changes in markets (weakening unions resulting in lower negotiated pay/benefits) and partly through attacks on the welfare state. However, neo-liberalism has somewhat different effects on different nations because of national variations in class structure and in their institutionalized form of welfare regime.

Most previous analyses link factors in C (Figure 11.1) with health or well-being (D). The model described deepens the causal explanation by including the determinants (A and B) of access to a variety of social assets (whether individual e.g., income, or collective, e.g., universal health care, public transportation) and other forms of inequality or deprivation. The model can encompass the fact that the health effects of various social phenomena might have both material and symbolic dimensions. Income inequality occupies a prominent place within this model although the question of how prominent as compared with other factors (e.g., relative or absolute poverty, housing, nutrition) is left open. This analysis also leads to speculation that income inequality may be more important for health in more neo-liberal societies than in others. Families or individuals in market-oriented societies have to rely on individually acquired market-related assets (such as income) to determine the degree to which they can access health-related societal resources (private health insurance versus public provision, private education/housing, etc.). The model can also handle the possibility that the curve relating income to health may take a different form in different societies—being more curvilinear in neo-liberal societies and more linear in more Social Democratic societies. The major alternative to both income inequality and class-based models is that a region's economic wealth is the chief determinant of health and health inequalities.

I begin the empirical exploration of the class/welfare regime model by providing examples linking all four of the different areas or levels outlined in Figure 11.1(A–D). I show that the onset of global neo-liberalism and the existence of different welfare regime types are important factors — first, regarding inequalities within nations, and second, with respect to health differences amongst the developed nations. Some of the indices used relate to 1980, many of them to the more recent date of 1995—the latter chosen as a date for which a variety of measures were readily available.

Class and Welfare Regimes

As used here class refers to a structural and relational rather than an SES approach. In fact, class is seen as determining and shaping SES and income inequality. To oversimplify a complex literature: classes are conceived in relation to one another and in relationship to the means of production.[33] Thus, there are business classes (capital) and working or oppositional classes and social movements. In general, the interests of one of these are inversely related to the interests of the other. On the other hand, income inequality or SES simply refer to individuals or families who are higher or lower on some characteristic without any real social relationships between these and without any necessary antagonism among those lower or higher.

Historically, a major difference between the phases of capitalism noted above is that in the monopoly phase the working classes had greater power than they do in the contemporary global phase in which capital is overwhelmingly predominant. But, at all times, in democracies or otherwise, capital has greater inbuilt structural power because of its control over investment and the disposition of productive resources. This is not to say capital is unchallenged or has hegemonic power, simply that events are more likely to follow the interests of capital than those of oppositional classes.

TABLE 11.1. Mean Infant Mortality Rates (Deaths/1000 Live Births) 1960–1995 by Welfare Regime Type (18 Nations)

	1960	1970	1980	1990	1995[a]
Social Democratic	23.1	15.4	9.1	6.8	4.5
Christian Democratic	29.2	20.1	11.2	7.4	5.4
Liberal	26.3	19.2	11.6	8.0	6.3
Ex-Fascist	53.8	37.0	18.2	9.4	6.6
Liberal minus Social Democratic mean infant mortality rate	30.7	17.6	9.1	2.6	2.1
Liberal mean as a percentage of the Social Democratic mean (%)	114	125	127	118	140

Source: Adapted from Navarro and Shi (2001), Table 11.7.

Notes: [a]1995 from OECD Health Data 2000.

Social Democratic: Austria; Sweden; Denmark; Norway; and Finland.

Christian Democratic: Belgium; Germany; Netherlands; France; Italy; and Switzerland.

Liberal: United Kingdom; Ireland; United States; and Canada.

Ex-Fascist: Spain; Portugal; and Greece.

In the literature on welfare states some have focused on the causes, others the characteristics, and others the consequences of welfare regimes. A few analysts incorporate all of the causes, policies and their effects (there may be slippage between these) within particular societal welfare regime types. I use three ways of measuring welfare regimes. I begin with Navarro and Shi's[34] typology of welfare states in which they divide the advanced nations into Social Democratic, Christian Democratic, Liberal Anglo-Saxon and Conservative or Fascist dictatorships (for the nations included see Table 11.1). This categorization is based on the prevailing political regimes in these countries between 1945 and 1980. For example, the Social Democratic political economies had a mean of 23.5 years of Social Democratic government during 1946–1980 (the years of the building of the welfare state) as compared to a mean of 4.7 years for the Liberal Anglo-Saxon nations. The Social Democratic nations show greater well-being on a wide variety of characteristics than do the Liberal regimes.[35]

A slightly different conception of welfare regimes is described by Korpi and Palme[36] They focus on welfare state institutions and their effects in 18 OECD countries rather than on their political determinants. Their categorization includes: Encompassing, Corporatist, Basic Security and Targeted welfare regimes. The 'Encompassing' type (Finland, Norway and Sweden) approximates Social Democratic regimes and 'Basic Security' (eight nations—Canada, Denmark, the Netherlands, New Zealand, Switzerland, Ireland, the UK and the US) and 'Targeted' (Australia) approximates 'Liberal' (neo-liberal) regimes. Korpi and Palme's categories are constructed (a) for old-age pensions and (b) for sickness insurance programs. Each program is assessed on three different dimensions: (1) benefits provided on the basis of need, contributions, belonging to a specific occupational category, or on the basis simply of citizenship); (2) the extent to which benefits replace lost income; and (3) the forms for governing social insurance programs (co-operative or not between employers and employees) for 1985.

The main analytic focus in what follows is on the two contrasting types of welfare regimes, those nations exemplifying a 'strong' welfare regime (the least neo-liberal) i.e., the Social Democratic or Encompassing nations, and the most neo-liberal welfare state countries i.e., the Liberal or Basic Security nations. Hence, for some purposes results for the other types of welfare state are omitted for ease of comparison (e.g., Table 11.2).

TABLE 11.2. Rank Order of Infant Mortality Rates, 1960–1995 by Welfare Regime Type (18 Nations. Results for the Christian Democratic and Ex-Fascist Nations Omitted for Case of Comparison)

	I – LOW INFANT MORTALITY		RANK ORDER IN 1995 RELATIVE TO 1960[a]
	1960	1995	
Social Democratic			
Austria	14	8	+6
Sweden	1	2	−1
Denmark	6	5	+1
Norway	3	2	+1
Finland	4	1	+3
Christian Democratic			
Belgium, Germany, Netherlands, France, Italy, Switzerland			
Liberal			
United Kingdom	7	12	−5
Ireland	11	14	−3
United States	8	17	−9
Canada	9	11	−2
Ex-Fascist			
Spain, Portugal, Greece			

Source: Welfare Regime Classification from Navarro and Shi (2001).
Notes: [a]1995 infant mortality rates from OECD Health Data 2000.

I include as an additional measure of welfare regimes an index of 'decommodification' drawn from Esping-Andersen.[37] This index refers to the degree that citizens can have an adequate standard of living independently of their position in the market (e.g., whether they are employed or unemployed). Although decommodification is assessed only as of 1980, it does permit a more intensive examination of the relationships between the degree of welfare statism and national health status. The decommodification index was measured regarding three programs—pension, sickness and unemployment benefits and three aspects of each of these programs: ease of eligibility rules; levels of income replacement; and the range of entitlements provided[38] (Korpi and Palme's categorization of welfare regimes is based on similar criteria). The index ranges from 13.0 (Australia) to 39.1 (Sweden). On this index for 1980, the least decommodified (neo-liberal) nations are Australia, the US, New Zealand, Canada, Ireland and the UK and the most decommodified Sweden, Norway, Denmark, The Netherlands and Belgium.

The literature makes clear that income redistribution is an important facet of welfare regimes, but more as a consequence of regime type than as a characteristic or as a determinant. Also important are labour market policies and other health-relevant factors such as poverty and access to resources not dependent on income (e.g., collectively provided health care, education, housing, transportation). The chief contention of this chapter is that degree of neo-liberalism is a major factor linking global changes, class structures and within- and between-nation health inequalities. In the contemporary world welfare regime types may approximate an underlying 'degree of neo-liberalism' dimension[39] (see Hicks, 1999) i.e., Social Democratic/Encompassing regimes are less neo-liberal and Liberal/Basic Security regimes are more neo-liberal.

Income Inequality and National Wealth

National levels of income inequality are measured by the Gini index of income inequality for 1995.[40] The higher the Gini, the higher the income inequality.

The measure of economic wealth used is GDP/capita in $US measured at purchasing power parity (PPP). These data (from OECD Health Data, 2000) measure GDP/capita but adjust it for differences in purchasing power in different nations for a standard package of goods. For purposes of comparison with the index of decommodification, we use GDP/cap in $US at PPP (hereafter simply GDP/cap) for 1980, but also include a more recent measure for 1995.

Neo-Liberalism, Income Inequalities and Health Inequalities within Nations

In the developed nations, the onset of neo-liberalism has been associated with increasing within-nation inequalities. The most readily available data concern income inequalities and measures of poverty. Gottschalk and Smeeding[41] reporting on data from the Luxembourg Income Studies, show that inequality has increased in 14 of the 17 nations they examined between 1979 and 1995. Increases in inequality have been particularly pronounced in those nations adopting more stringent neo-liberal or market-oriented politics and policies. In the early 1990s the United States, Australia, Canada and the United Kingdom stood at the top of the income inequality ladder with Norway, Sweden and the Netherlands being the lowest (although by 1994 Canada had moved more towards the middle). In Table 11.3, I have indicated which countries in this list either Navarro and Shi or Korpe and Palme view as being Social Democratic/Encompassing (table footnote a) as opposed to Liberal/Basic Security (more neo-liberal welfare regimes) (table footnote b)

Two examples of increasing income and health inequalities associated with the politics of neo-liberalism are the UK and US. Beginning with the Reagan and Thatcher regimes, the United States and the United Kingdom demonstrate particularly high, and ever-increasing, rates of inequality (Figures 11.3 and 11.4—adapted from Gottschalk & Smeeding[42]). Prior to the neo-liberal era, income inequality in the United States and the United Kingdom had been relatively low and declining since the Second World War—the welfare state, such as it was in those two nations, actually did what it was supposed to do. From about 1968 in the US and 1977/78 in the UK, income inequality began a rapid rise that continued into the 1990s.

Even during times of economic expansion, inequality increased in the United States. The lowest 60 per cent of households in that country actually experienced a decrease in after-tax income between 1977 and 1999. During the same period, incomes of the top 5 per cent of households grew by 56 per cent and the top 1 per cent mushroomed by 93 per cent.[43] In fact, despite being one of the richest nations on earth, in 1991 the United States had one of the highest rates of absolute (as well as relative) poverty amongst the developed nations—of 15 countries only Italy, Ireland, Australia and the UK had higher rates.[44]

Data also indicate that welfare regimes actually did lessen poverty and inequality (links between B and C in Figure 11.1). Kenworthy's analysis demonstrates that, as of 1991, social welfare policies reduced both absolute and relative poverty.[45] The data I use also shows that different

TABLE 11.3. Ratio of the Top 10% of Income Earners to the Bottom 10% and the Gini Index of Inequality

COUNTRY	DECILE RATIO 90/10	GINI INDEX
Finland 1991[a]	2.75	0.233
Sweden 1992[a]	2.78	0.229
Belgium 1992	2.79	0.230
Norway 1995[a]	2.85	0.242
Denmark 1992[a]	2.86	0.239
Luxembourg 1994	2.93	0.235
The Netherlands 1991[b]	3.05	0.249
Italy 1991	3.14	0.255
Taiwan 1995	3.38	0.277
Switzerland 1982[b]	3.43	0.311
New Zealand 1987/88[b]	3.46	NA
Germany 1994	3.84	0.300
Canada 1994[b]	3.93	0.287
Spain 1990	4.04	0.306
France 1989	4.11	0.324
Israel 1992	4.12	0.305
Japan 1992	4.17	0.315
Ireland 1987[b]	4.18	0.328
Australia 1989[b]	4.30	0.308
United Kingdom 1995[b]	4.56	0.346
United States 1994[b]	6.44	0.368

Source: From Figure 11.2; Gottschalk and Smeeding (2000).

Notes:

[a] Social Democratic (Navarro and Shi, 2001), or Encompassing (Korpi and Palme, 1998) regimes.

[b] Liberal (Navarro and Shi, 2001) (Neo-liberal) or Basic Security (Korpi and Palme, 1998)/ Targetted regimes.

types of welfare regime are indeed associated with differing levels of income inequality and absolute and relative poverty. Even omitting the United States, by far the most unequal Liberal nation, the differences between four Social Democratic nations as measured by the Navarro and Shi categorization and three Liberal nations are large. The Liberal nations have average (1995) Gini indices of income inequality of 320 compared to 236 (the higher the Gini the higher the inequality) for the Social Democratic nations. In 1991, the Social Democratic countries had 4.3 per cent of their populations in absolute poverty and 2.8 per cent in relative poverty as compared to 17.6 and 5.2 per cent for the Liberal nations.[46] Kenworthy used '40 per cent of the median posttax/posttransfer household (size adjusted) income in the United States' for 1991 as the absolute poverty level—and 'Percentage of individuals in households with incomes (adjusted for household size) below 40 per cent of the median within each country' for 1991 to measure relative poverty. Comparing the Korpe and Palme categories of three Encompassing nations versus six Basic Security nations (Kenworthy omits New Zealand and I omit the US as an extreme case) shows similar, though slightly smaller, differences.

Interestingly, the index of decommodification (1980) shows very high correlations (using either Pearson correlations or a more conservative measure of rank-order correlations—Spearman's rho) with the Gini (1995) and with absolute and relative poverty (1991) (Spearman's rho's of 0.75, 0.69 and 0.83, respectively—14 nations). On the other hand, GDP/cap 1980 is not very highly related either to the Gini or to the two measures of poverty. In fact, the relationships between GDP/cap (1980) income inequality and absolute and relative poverty are somewhat curvilinear. It is nations in the middle range of GDP/cap (rather than those highest in GDP) that show the lowest inequality and the lowest absolute and relative poverty. The importance of welfare regime type is indicated by the fact that it is precisely this group of 'middle GDP/cap' nations which shows the highest levels of decommodification. The lack of a linear GDP/cap—inequality/poverty correlation is one consequence of the power of welfare regime effects.

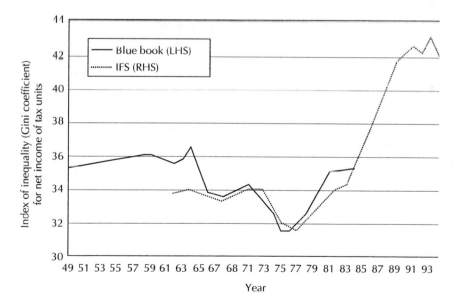

FIGURE 11.3 Change in Income Inequality in the UK from 1949 to 1994.
NOTES: (LHS) The Blue Book is an annual publication of the office of National Statistics National Accounts in the UK; (RHS) refers to the Institute for Fiscal studies, an independent research organization located in London.

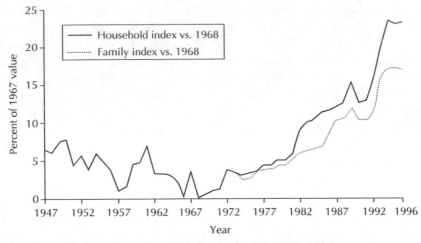

FIGURE 11.4 Change in Income Inequality in the US, 1947–1996.

Most relevant for this analysis, different welfare regimes and rising inequalities of various kinds have important implications for health
inequalities within nations since social inequalities of many kinds are
related to health status differences. In general, the higher a group's SES
or income, and, it is assumed the lower the other forms of inequality, the
higher its health status. And, income and other forms of inequality tend to
be greater in precisely those nations which also have fewer social welfare
'buffers' which might meliorate the effect of income and other inequalities
on health status.

Within nations, SES differences in health (however measured) are substantial and have been widely reported. I simply provide some illustrative
comparisons from the United States and the UK. In a comparison of US
Metropolitan Areas, the health differences between high- and low-SES
areas were equivalent to: 'The combined loss of life from lung cancer,
diabetes, motor vehicle crashes, HIV infections, suicide and homicide.'[47]
Mortality would be reduced by 139.8 deaths per 100,000 if the SES differences noted were eliminated. In the US people in the very poorest households were 4–5 times more likely to die in the next 10 years than were
those in the richest.[48]

In Britain in 1996, the differences in longevity between the highest SES
group and the lowest (of five groups) were 9.5 years for men and 6.4 years
for women. In Canada there are similar, but perhaps a little less extreme,
health differences between those high and low in income.[49]

Despite 'expanding economies', health inequalities have increased. A recent study showed all-cause inequalities in mortality between low- and high-SES areas to have increased amongst adults in the US by from 50 to 58 per cent (for males and females, respectively) from 1969 to 1998.[50] A commentator on Britain, a nation that experienced a prolonged period of neo-liberal politics, noted that: 'The inequalities in health between social classes are now the greatest yet recorded in British history.'[51] Another British study shows an increasing gap 'between social classes 1 (high) and V (low) (which) widened from 2.1:1 in 1970–72 to 3.3 in 1991–93.'[52] For the first time in decades in 1992 some sex/age groups (males aged 25–40) actually began to exhibit increasing mortality rates per 100,000 as compared to a decade earlier (*The Economist*, 11 January 1997). One recent study reported that simply reducing current wealth inequalities in Britain to their 1983 level would save 7,500 deaths among people younger than 65.[53]

What about the central focus of many Income Inequality studies—differences in health status amongst nations?

Differences in Health Status in the US, the UK and Canada

Before Examining the Welfare Regime thesis regarding between-nation differences more closely the United States, the UK, and Canada will be specially considered. The United States is a striking outlier in respect to income inequalities and national health status. Whereas the US is one of the highest ranked nations in the world in terms of GNP/capita, it displays a dismal inequality and health record. That country ranks well below other, much poorer nations regarding health status. For example, in 1999 the United States ranked 23rd in the world and the United Kingdom 20th in longevity. These two countries thus ranked below, e.g., Italy, Greece, Spain and Ireland. Using another measure of health, Potential Years of Life Lost (PYLL), measuring the number of years death occurs before age 70, amongst 21 developed nations the US ranks 20th, just above Portugal. Regarding the probability of dying before age five, the US ranks 23rd in the world regarding males and 33rd regarding females. The corresponding ranks for the UK on death before age five are 15th for males (tied with six countries) and 14th for females (tied with 10 countries).

Canada provides an interesting comparison with the United States because in many respects the two countries are alike, while Canada still has somewhat better welfare measures (including national health insurance). Canada shows lower income inequality than does the United States[54] but higher inequality than many European countries. And, concomitantly,

Canada can boast of relatively high longevity rates, lower infant mortality rates, better rates of PYLL, and lower SES or income-related health differences than the United States or the UK In fact, in 1996 the infant mortality rates in the poorest neighbourhoods in Canada were better than the national rate of infant mortality in the US yet the rates in the richest Canadian neighbourhoods were not much better than the national average rates in Sweden.[55] There is speculation that Canada's remaining social support programs, from medicare to education and social infrastructure, generally mediate or reduce the effect of income inequality on health in Canada more so than in the US. There are fears, however, that recent government cutbacks (e.g., in the proportion of the unemployed receiving Employment Insurance) will soon begin to have their health effects.

Lynch et al.[56] indicate that including or excluding the United States in international analyses makes a huge difference to the size of correlations of the relationships between income inequality and health. For example, omitting the United States reduced the original correlations between income inequality and female infant mortality from r ¼ 0:69 to 0:26.[57] In what follows, any key relationships found are checked by repeating the analysis excluding the US.

Welfare State Regimes and Health Differences

Infant Mortality

Table 11.1 indicates that regime type[58] is highly related to infant mortality (the number of deaths under one year/1,000 live births). The Social Democratic nations show better infant mortality rates than do the Liberal nations. Moreover, while all nations show decreasing infant mortality rates between 1960 and 1995, the percentage differences between the mean infant mortality rates for the two contrasting regime types, the Social Democratic and the Liberal, are substantial. Using Korpi and Palme's categorization of welfare regimes produces similar results (not shown).

If welfare regime arguments are correct, one might expect increasing differences over time in the relative standing of nations regarding infant mortality. Given greater movements towards neo-liberalism shown by the Liberal nations, one would expect them to drop in the World League Tables of infant mortality as compared to the Social Democratic countries. Indeed, that is what the rank order of infant mortality rates does show (Table 11.2). For example, while in 1960 the UK and the US were ranked 7th and 8th in infant mortality (of 18 nations, with one being the

TABLE 11.4. Correlations between the Index of Decommodification, GDP/Capita and Infant Mortality (1980, 1995)

	INFANT MORTALITY[a]	DECOMMODIFICATION[b] (1980)	GDP/CAP[b] (1980)	GDP/CAP[c] (1995)
1980		−0.58 (−0.57)[d]	−0.18	NA
1995		−0.52 (−0.50)[d]	−0.25	−0.10

Notes:

[a] Infant mortality. OECD health data 2000.

[b] Index of Decommodification (Esping-Andersen, 1990 in Kenworthy, 1999).

[c] GNP/cap in SUS at purchasing power parity OECD health data 2000.

[d] Partial correlation controlling for GDP/cap 1980.

nation with the best infant mortality rate), by 1995 they were 13th and 17th out of the same 18 nations. In Table 11.2, the Christian Democratic and Ex-Fascist nations are omitted for ease of direct comparison between the Social Democratic versus Liberal welfare regime nations.

The most direct 'competitor' to welfare regime effects is GDP/cap rather than income inequality. This is because model 2 assumes that income inequality is part of the causal chain linking class/welfare regime types with health. Table 11.4 shows that the index of decommodification (1980) has higher correlations with infant mortality for 1980 and for 1995 than does GDP/cap at PPP for either 1980 or 1995. The correlations between decommodification and infant mortality remain high even when GDP/cap is statistically controlled for, and whether the US is included or excluded from the calculations.

Incidentally, though not central to this chapter, examining the influence of income inequality we find that the Gini (1995) correlates r = 0:31 with infant mortality (1995) (14 nations—omitting the US), which is much lower than the correlation of decommodification with the same infant mortality rate (r = 0:52). Controlling for GDP/cap (1995) does not materially reduce the size of the correlation between the Gini index and infant mortality (partial correlation of r = 0:30). However, controlling for decommodification (1980) totally eliminates the correlation of the Gini (1995) with infant mortality (1995) from a zero-order correlation of r = 0:31 to a partial correlation of r = 0:05. But, conversely, controlling for the Gini (1995) reduces the correlation of decommodification (1980) with infant mortality (1995) only slightly from r = 0:52 to a partial correlation of r = 0:44 (n = 14).

Overall, the data on infant mortality indicate that since the 1960s, there has been a general and widespread international decrease in absolute levels while there are continuing substantial national differences. Comparing extreme cases the United States has about twice the infant mortality rates of such countries as Sweden and Norway. There is a telling loss of life between the best and worst case scenarios.

Mortality rates, number of people alive at ages 45/65 and PYLL

What about other measures of health status? Most to some degree reflect infant mortality and there is great overlap amongst measures; they are not independent estimates of health. The relationships may also be highly influenced by latency or lag effects. Nevertheless, to permit comparison with previous studies I report here on the class/welfare regime hypothesis and a variety of measures of national health status.

Examining regime types as categorized by Navarro and Shi or Korpi and Palme (data not shown)—there are small but consistent mean differences in favour of the Social Democratic as opposed lo the Liberal nations in over-all age-adjusted mortality rates (1980 and 1995—from OECD Health Data, 2000) and in the number of males and females still alive at ages 45 and 65 (1995) per 100,000 population born (standardized to a common population), for both females and for males (from WHO World Health Statistics Annual, 1996). However, omitting the US generally greatly reduces even these differences.

More substantial mean differences between the two major contrasting regime types are shown regarding PYLL. PYLL is a measure which empha-sizes the presumably more preventable deaths at younger ages and is calcu-lated by adjusting mortality rates for the number of years the person died before age 70. Using data from OECD Health Data 2000—in all cases the Social Democratic/Encompassing nations show better PYLL levels than do the Liberal/Basic Security nations.

Turning to the decommodification index and comparing the correlations of this index with the various measures of health status for 1980 and 1995 with the corresponding correlations for GDP/cap in $US PPP with the same health measures reveals a mixed pattern (Table 11.5). The index is related in the expected direction in all instances except for overall mortality rates in 1995. As expected, it is much more highly related to PYLL than to the other measures (because PYLL partly reflects infant mortality rates). Most strik-ingly, however, GDP/cap shows much higher correlations with overall age-ad-justed mortality rates than does the decommodification index. Though much of these latter correlations are due to only two outliers—the low mortality of high GDP Switzerland and the high mortality of low GDP Ireland—the mor-tality indices bear further investigation for reasons discussed in Lobmayer and Wilkinson[59] and Lynch et al.[60] Both of these studies reported that mor-tality was related differentially to GNP/cap and to income inequality at dif-ferent ages. This finding is also supported here by the negative (opposite to the direction expected) correlations between GDP/cap and number of people alive at age 45 yet the expected positive correlations for those 65+.

TABLE 11.5. Correlations between the Index of Decommodification, Gdp/Cap at Purchasing Power Parity and Health Status, 1980 and 1995

		DECOMMODIFICATION[a] (1980)	GDP/CAP AT PPP[b] (1980)
No. people alive (1995)[c]			
Age 45	F	0.22	−0.17
	M	0.18	−0.26
Age 65	F	0.30	0.53
	M	0.22	0.25
PYLL			
1980	F	−0.46	−0.27
	M	−0.51	−0.06
1995	F	−0.27	−0.25
	M	−0.03	−0.30
Overall mortality rates			
1980	F	−0.23	−0.56
	M	−0.38	−0.61
1995	F	0.03	−0.64
	M	0.08	−0.65

Notes:
[a] Index of decommodification (Esping-Andersen, 1990) from Kenworthy (1999).
[b] GDP/cap at purchasing power parity from OECD health data 2000.
[c] Health data from OECD health data 2000 except for number of people alive from World Health Statistics Annual, 1996.

Age/Sex Specific Mortality Rates

Correlations between decommodification and GDP/cap and mortality rates for different age groups indicate why regime types or decommodification do not show high relationships with such measures as overall mortality rates. Under the age of 35, the higher the decommodification the better the mortality rates, but above that age, the higher the decommodification the worse the mortality rates. In exploring this relationship, the relationships for specific ages: under 1, 1–34, 35–64, 65+, for the Korpi and Palme categories generally show consistent relationships between regime type and mortality rates across the age groups in favour of the Encompassing regime type (results not shown). The Navarro and Shi categorizations show a somewhat similar but not quite as consistent a pattern.

The correlations between the decommodification index and the GDP/cap 1980 in $US at PPP with the age/sex clustered mortality rates are shown in Table 11.6. The pattern is clear—decommodification is related in the expected direction with under-35 mortality rates but in the opposite direction for the above-35 age groups. GDP/cap shows the opposite

TABLE 11.6. Correlations between the Index of Decommodification, GDP/Cap at Purchasing Power Parity and Age/Sex Specific Mortality Rates, 1995 (14 Nations)

AGE IN YEARS[a]	DECOMMODIFICATION[b] (1980)		GDP/CAP[c] (1980)	
	FEMALES	MALES	FEMALES	MALES
Less than 1 year	−0.44	−0.36	−0.32	−0.24
1–34 years of age	−0.54	−0.43	0.13	0.19
35–64 years	0.25	0.22	−0.35	−0.27
65+ years	0.24	0.30	−0.66	−0.69

Notes:
[a] Age-specific mortality rates from WHO Statistics Annual, 1996, Table 11.1.
[b] From Esping-Andersen (1990) in Kenworthy (1999).
[c] OECD health data 2000.

pattern—positive, rather than the expected negative relationships for the 1–35 age group but negative correlations with the 65+ age category. The reason why GDP/cap is highly related to overall mortality rates appears to be, as Lobmayer and Wilkinson note,[61] that most deaths occur in the older age groups and these death rates heavily weigh overall mortality rates. The lesser number (but perhaps more important/preventable) deaths at younger age groups for nations high in decommodification is overwhelmed by the far larger number of 'older' deaths in the same countries.

It is puzzling that across nations some countries with better mortality rates at younger ages show worse mortality rates at older ages and vice versa. For example, the United States and Greece both show poor infant mortality rates yet low-mortality rates for those 65 and over. Finland and Denmark, on the other hand, show the opposite tendency. Belgium and Ireland show higher rates for both younger and older ages while Sweden and France show low-mortality rates for both under 1 year and for those 65 and over. The top three countries with high infant mortality rates but lower 65+ mortality rates are Liberal and those showing the opposite pattern tend to be Social Democratic. It seems that mortality rates at older ages are higher because the 'preventive' (Social Democratic) countries have a greater number of 'fragile' people surviving to 65+ than do the more neo-liberal nations. The very success of less neo-liberal regimes at preserving life at younger ages militates against these nations showing low overall mortality rates.

The difference in proportions of people alive at age 65 are considerable. For example, in 1994 the United States had an estimated 74,710 males and 85,460 females per 100,000 population born still alive at age 65 but Sweden 83,525 males and 90,075 females. Interestingly, Canada is closer to Sweden than to the US; Costa Rica shows better rates than the US and Cuba about the same as the US.

TABLE 11.7. Correlations between the Index of Decommodification (1980) and Health Status for 8 High GDP/Capita Nations

		DECOMMODIFICATION[a]
Infant Mortality		
1980		−0.76
1995		−0.85
Mortality		
1980	F	−0.35
	M	−0.67
1995	F	−0.25
	M	−0.08
Number of People Alive (1995)		
Age 45	F	0.68
	M	0.64
Age 65	F	0.57
	M	0.49
PYLL		
1980	F	−0.86
	M	−0.78
1995	F	−0.70
	M	−0.36
Age-Specific Mortality	**Female**	**Male**
Under 1 year	−0.87	−0.83
1–34	−0.76	−0.73
35–64	−0.49	−0.36
65 and over	0.22	0.46

Notes:
[a] Nations with GDP/capita over $9,000 US at purchasing power parity in 1980: Australia, Canada, France, Germany, Norway, Sweden, Switzerland, and United States.

What about sub-groups i.e., those groups which show particularly low or high correlations between welfare regime status and health? In earlier examination of the associations amongst GDP/cap, decommodification, income inequality and poverty we noted the curvilinear relationships between GDP/cap and decommodification. Nations highest in decommodification were at medium-high rather than at the highest levels of GDP/cap. This suggested possible interaction effects between GDP/cap and decommodification. In exploring these interactions, it was found that for those eight countries of the 15 nations included in the decommodification index (1980) whose GDP/cap (1980) was over US$9,000 (i.e., high-GDP nations), the decommodification index is related in the expected direction for females and for males to all of the mortality and longevity indicators: number of people alive at ages 45 and 65, PYLL and mortality rates—the latter up to age 65 (Table 11.7).

For the seven nations under $9,000 GDP/capita, the relationships remain high for infant mortality but are much lower and not consistent in direction for the other measures. This suggests that GDP/cap is a necessary cause of improved health, and decommodification is a sufficient cause. There are, however, reasons to doubt this initial explanation as discussed below.

Conclusions

A class-based model of the relationships between inequalities in health within and between nations has been described by setting income inequality and health linkages within a broader conceptual framework. This model places income inequality and social cohesion within a radically different causal sequence to the orthodox income inequality approach and suggests that many other material factors, and their interpretation or imputed meaning, rather than simply income inequality, are central determinants of health inequalities. However, both models emphasize the social nature of inequalities in health within and between nations and cast doubt on purely economic growth interpretations of the determinants of human health. Moreover, as the products of human actions the social and economic determinants of health are open to change.

The examples given indicate that neo-liberal economic globalization is associated with increasing inequalities within the developed nations. Social inequalities can be expected to have corresponding effects on health inequalities within countries. Much more data needs to be reported, however, regarding trends in within-nation inequalities.

On differences amongst the most developed countries the evidence was very strong for the influence of categorical regime type on infant mortality and mortality rates at younger ages and somewhat less so for PYLL and number of people alive at ages 45/65. The relationship between decommodification and overall mortality rates was generally opposite to that expected. However, the reason for higher overall mortality rates amongst nations higher in decommodification appears to be because these nations keep more people alive to older ages and the larger number of deaths after these ages heavily weight overall mortality rates. Moreover, among the highest GDP countries decommodification does have substantial effects on mortality.

There are hints in the data that welfare regimes provide the link between GDP and health and well-being. There are also studies which show an increasing divergence between growth in GNP and improvements in well-being in both Canada and the United States beginning in the 1970s which also point to social and state actions as linking economies and well-being.[62] These interactive effects require further exploration. Yet the United States shows that economic wealth is not a sufficient cause of better national health. The instances of Kerala, Costa Rica, Cuba, Finland, and The Netherlands at various levels of GDP/cap suggests that economic wealth is not even a necessary condition for health. In these instances, government or collective action of some kind is important. Indeed, even amongst the advanced nations Esping-Andersen's[63] examples indicate that what Swedish citizens pay through taxes for various services, citizens of the United States pay about the same through markets. The difference seems to be that market provision of many services (particularly health care)[64] is inefficient and ineffective.

In this chapter, the connections explored were largely between the areas B–D in Figure 11.2. However, the numerous linkages between forms of inequality noted in C and health need to be described. Many of the influences of class and welfare regime may be indirect—through the influence of these on a whole series of market or welfare-related forms of inequality—and some of these may be reflected in income and others not. It is also likely that the effects of neo-liberalism are not all channeled through its effects on the welfare state. A more explicit test of the influence of neo-liberalism is possible using direct measures of neo-liberalism, e.g., as indicated by low taxes and 'small' governments, rather than using welfare regimes measures as the more indirect measure.

Medical care has been largely ignored in studies of national differences in health because it is assumed that social factors are more important determinants of overall health status than are health care systems. Most developed nations have forms of national systems which help ensure lower income groups access to care. However, there are still differences in medical care[65] such as the quality of primary care, which deserve study[66] and which might help explain international health differences. In addition, more qualitative or historical case studies may help provide a more causally oriented view of changes in national socio-political structures and health status. It would be worthwhile focusing on the historical experience of countries increasing (the UK and New Zealand) or resisting (Norway, Sweden) the application of neo-liberal policies. More detailed study of contrasting cases such as Canada and the United States, or the examination of theoretical and empirical 'anomalies' i.e., countries with higher or lower health than their GDP or welfare regimes status would predict, would also prove fruitful. For example, Australia and Canada both have increasingly adopted neo-liberal policies yet they do show relatively low overall mortality rates. In these nations, immigration rates may be important since immigrants tend to have better health status than do indigenous populations and these two nations have the highest percentage of foreign born citizens in the developed world. There are also suggestions that Canada in particular but perhaps also Australia (see Castles, 2001) have, or had, more egalitarian or less purely neo-liberal policies than an initial estimate of their welfare regime status would allow.

What is clear from the data presented is that countries pursuing neo-liberal policies display far greater social inequalities and show more people in absolute or relative poverty than do more social democratic nations—an indictment in itself. Furthermore, these inequalities have implications for both within- and between-nation health inequalities and cast doubt on the economic globalization paradigm that neo-liberal forms of free trade are automatically related to improved human well-being.

The class/welfare regime model thus provides an approach which can help encompass both within- and between-nation health inequalities, it can help account for a number of previous arguments regarding the possible multi-factor nature of the determinants of health amongst nations, and it aids in theoretically contextualizing and broadening in a more sociological direction the provocative findings produced by social epidemiologists.

Acknowledgements

The Social Sciences and Humanities Research Council Grant No. 410–1998-0838 helped support this project. The School of Public Health and the Department of Sociology at La Trobe University, Melbourne, sponsored me for a Visiting Fellowship June–July, 2002. Some of the ideas in the chapter had their origins in discussions within the Critical Social Science and Health Group at the University of Toronto. Many thanks are due to Bessie Gorospe and Larry Nieva for help in the numerous revisions of this chapter.

Notes

1. D. Coburn, "Phases of Capitalism, Welfare States, Medical Dominance, and Health Care in Ontario," 29(4) *International Journal of Health Services* (1999): 833–851; D. Coburn, "Health, Health Care and Neoliberalism," in *The Political Economy of Health and Health Care in Canada*, ed. P. Armstrong, H. Armstrong, and D. Coburn (Toronto: Oxford University Press, 2001).
2. V. Navarro, "Neoliberalism, Globalization, Unemployment, Inequalities, and the Welfare State," 28(4) *International Journal of Health Services* (1998): 607–682; V. Navarro, "The Political Economy of the Welfare State in Developed Capitalist Countries," 29(1) *International Journal of Health Services* (1999): 1–50; V. Navarro, "Health and Equity in the World in the Era of Globalization," 29(2) *International Journal of Health Services* (1999): 215–226; V. Navarro, & L. Shi, "The Political Context of Social Inequalities and Health," 52 *Social Science & Medicine* (2001): 481–491.

3. R.J.S. Ross and K.C. Trachte, *Global Capitalism: The New Leviathan* (Albany, NY: State University of New York, 1990).

4. G. Esping-Andersen, *The Three Worlds of Welfare Capitalism* (Princeton, NJ: Princeton University Press, 1990); G. Esping-Andersen, *Social Foundations of Postindustrial Economies* (Oxford: Oxford University Press, 1999).

5. J.W. Lynch, G.A. Kaplan, E.R. Pamuk, et al., "Income Inequality and Mortality in Metropolitan Areas of the United States," 88(7) *American Journal of Public Health* (1998): 1074–1080; J.W. Lynch, G. Davey-Smith, G.A. Kaplan, and J.S. House, "Income Inequality and Mortality: Importance to Health of Individual Income, Psychosocial Environment, or Material Conditions," 320 *British Medical Journal* (2000): 1200–1204; J. Lynch, G. Davey-Smith, M. Hillemeier, M. Shaw, M.T. Raghunathan, and G. Kaplan, "Income Inequality, the Psychosocial Environment, and Health: Comparisons of Wealthy Nations," 358 *The Lancet* (2001): 194–200; C. Muntaner and J. Lynch, "Income Inequality, Social Cohesion and Class Relations: A Critique of Wilkinson's Neo-Durkheimian Research Program," 29(1) *International Journal of Health Services* (1999): 59–81; J.W. Lynch and G.A. Kaplan, "Understanding How Inequality in the Distribution of Income Affects Health," in *The Society and Population Health Reader: Income Inequality and Health*, ed. I. Kawachi, B. Kennedy, and R.G. Wilkinson (New York: The New Press, 1999).

6. R.G. Wilkinson, *Unhealthy Societies: The Afflictions of Inequality* (London: Routledge, 1996).

7. See I. Kawachi, B. Kennedy, and R.G. Wilkinson, eds., *The Society and Population Health Reader: Income Inequality and Health* (New York: The New Press, 1999).

8. B. Poland, D. Coburn, J. Eakin, A. Robertson, and Members of the Critical Social Science and Health Group, "Wealth, Equity and Health Care: A Critique of a 'Population Health' Perspective on the Determinants of Health," 46(7) *Social Science & Medicine* (1998): 785–798.

9. Wilkinson (1996), Note 6.

10. A. Sen, *Inequality Reexamined* (New York: Russell Sage Foundation, Cambridge, MA: Harvard University Press, 1992); A. Sen, "Social Justice and the Distribution of Income," in *Handbook of Income Distribution*, ed. A.B. Atkinson, and F. Bourguignon, Vol. 1., (Amsterdam: Elsevier, 2000).

11. Kawachi et al. (1999), Note 7; I. Kawachi, B.P. Kennedy, K. Lochner, and D. Prothrow-Stith, "Social Capital, Income Inequality and Mortality," 87 *American Journal of Public Health* (1997): 1491–1499; R.G. Wilkinson, "Comment: Income Inequality and Social Cohesion," 89(9) *American Journal of Public Health* (1997): 1504–1506.

12. S.H. Preston, "The Changing Relationship Between Mortality and Level of Economic Development," 29(2) *Population Studies* (1975): 231–248.

13. G.G. Rodgers, (1979) "Income and Inequality as Determinants of Mortality: An International Cross-section Analysis," 33 *Population Studies* (1979): 343–351. See also special section of the *International Journal of Epidemiology*, 2002, 31(3).

14. See A. Forbes and S.P. Wainwright, "On the Methodological, Theoretical and Philosophical Context of Health Inequalities Research," 51 *Social Science & Medicine* (2001): 801–816. On whether original findings are valid or exaggerated see A. Deaton, *Health, Inequality, and Economic Development*. Paper

prepared for working group 1 of the WHO Commission on Macroeconomics and Health. Research Program in Development Studies and Center for Health and Wellbeing, (Princeton, NJ: Princeton University, May, 2001); A. Deaton, *Relative Deprivation, Inequality, and Mortality* (Princeton, NJ: Center for Health and Wellbeing, Princeton University, 2001); K. Judge, "Income Distribution and Life Expectancy: A Critical Appraisal," 311 *British Medical Journal* (1995): 1282–1285; K. Judge, "Income and Mortality in the United States," [Letter in response to Kaplan et al.] 313 *British Medical Journal* (1996): 1206–1207 (see responses in the same issue); K. Judge, J.-A. Milligan, and M. Benzeval, "Income Inequality and Population Health," 46(4–5) *Social Science & Medicine* (1998): 567–579; Lynch et al., (2001), Note 5; J.M. Mellor and J. Milyo, "Reexamining the Evidence of an Ecological Association Between Income Inequality and Health," 26(3) *Journal of Health Politics, Policy and Law* (2001): 487–522.

15. G.T.H. Ellinson, "Letting the Gini Out of the Bottle? Challenges Facing the Relative Income Hypothesis," 54(4) *Social Science & Medicine* (2002): 561–576; H. Gravelle, "How Much of the Relation between Population Mortality and Unequal Distribution of Income is a Statistical Artifact?" 316 *British Medical Journal* (1998): 382–1385 (and responses); H. Gravelle, J. Wildman, and M. Sutton, "Income, Inequality and Health: What Can We Learn from Aggregate Data?" 54(4) *Social Science & Medicine* (2002): 577–589.

16. P. McDonough and P. Berglund, *Histories of Poverty and Self-rated Health Trajectories*. Department of Public Health Sciences (Toronto: University of Toronto, 2002); P. McDonough, G.J. Duncan, D. Williams, and J. House, "Income Dynamics and Adult Mortality in the United States, 1972 through 1989," 87(9) *American Journal of Public Health*, (1997): 1476–1483.

17. Deaton 2001, Note 14; M.G. Marmot, "Social Differences in Health Within and between Populations," 123 *Daedalus* (1994): 197–216.

18. A. Laporte, "A Note on the Use of a Single Inequality Index in Testing the Effect of Income Distribution on Mortality," 55(9) *Social Science & Medicine* (2002): 1561–1570.

19. cf. B.P. Kennedy, I. Kawachi, and D. Prothrow-Stith, "Income Distribution and Mortality: Cross Sectional Ecological Study of the Robin Hood Index in the United States," 312 *British Medical Journal* (1996): 1004–1007.

20. A. Muller, "Education, Income Inequality, and Mortality: A Multiple Regression Analysis," 324 *British Medical Journal* (2002): 23.

21. Deaton, "Relative Deprivation," Note 14.

22. G.A. Kaplan, E.R. Pamuk, J.W. Lynch, R.D. Cohen, and J.L. Balfour, "Inequality in Income and Mortality in the United States: Analysis of Mortality and Potential Pathways," 312 *British Medical Journal* (1996): 999–1003, (erratum 31, 1253).

23. cf. V. Navarro, ed., *The Political Economy of Social Inequalities* (Amityville, NY: Baywood, 2002).

24. From Ross & Trachte (1990), Note 3.

25. From Esping-Andersen (1990, 1999), Note 4.

26. M. Archer, R. Bhaskar, A. Collier, T. Lawson, and A. Norrie, *Critical Realism: Essential Readings* (London and New York: Routledge, 1998).

27. D. Coburn, "Income Inequality, Social Cohesion and the Health Status of Populations: The Role of Neoliberalism," 51 *Social Science & Medicine* (2000): 135–146.

28. Esping-Andersen (1990, 1999), Note 4.
29. J.S. O'Connor and G.M. Olsen, eds., *Power Resources Theory and the Welfare State: A Critical Approach* (Toronto: University of Toronto Press, 1998).
30. Esping-Andersen (1990, 1999), Note 4.
31. O'Connor and Olsen (1998), Note 29.
32. A. Hicks, *Social Democracy and Welfare Capitalism* (London and Ithaca, NY: Cornell University Press, 1999); W. Korpi, "Power Politics and State Autonomy in the Development of Social Citizenship: Social Rights During Sickness in Eighteen OECD Countries Since 1930," 54 *American Sociological Review* (1989): 309–328; O'Connor and Olsen (1998), Note 29.
33. Re: class and health see: Muntaner and Lynch (1999), Note 5; G. Scambler and P. Higgs, "Stratification, Class and Health: Class Relations and Health Inequalities in High Modernity," 33(2) *Sociology* (1999): 275–296 or the writings of Navarro, e.g., Note 2 and 23.
34. Navarro and Shi (2001), Note 2.
35. Ibid.
36. W. Korpi and J. Palme, "The Paradox of Redistribution and Strategies of Equality: Welfare State Institutions, Inequality, and Poverty in the Western Countries," 63(5) *American Sociological Review* (1998): 661–687.
37. Esping-Andersen (1990), Note 4; L. Kenworthy, "Do Social-Welfare Policies Reduce Poverty? A Cross-national Assessment," 77(3) *Social Forces* (1999): 1119–1139.
38. See Esping-Andersen (1990), Note 4, chapter 2.
39. See Hicks (1999), Note 32.
40. From P. Gottschalk and T.M. Smeeding, "Empirical Evidence of Income Inequality in Industrialized Countries," in *The Handbook of Income Distribution*, ed. A.B. Atkinson and F. Bourguignon, Vol. 1 (Amsterdam and New York: Elsevier, 2000): 261–307.
41. Ibid.
42. Ibid.
43. J. Bernstein, L. Mishel and C. Brocht, "Anyway You Cut It: Income Inequality on the Rise Regardless of How It's Measured," (Washington, DC: Economic Policy Institute, 2001): 7. Briefing Paper, http://epinet.org.
44. Kenworthy (1999), Note 37, p.1125.
45. Ibid.
46. Ibid.
47. Lynch et al. (1998), Note 5.
48. G.A. Kaplan, *Economic Policy is Health Policy*. Paper presented at the income inequality, socioeconomic status and health conference. (Washington, DC, April, 2000).
49. K.H. Humphries and E. van Doorslaer, "Income-related Health Inequality in Canada," 50 *Social Science & Medicine* (2000): 663–671.
50. G.K. Singh and M. Siahpush, "Increasing Inequalities in All-cause and Cardiovascular Mortality among US Adults Aged 25–64 Years by Area Socioeconomic Status, 1969–1998," 31(3) *International Journal of Epidemiology* (2002): 600–613.
51. G. Yamey, "Study Shows Growing Inequalities in Health in Britain," 319 *British Medical Journal* (1999): 1453; D. Dorling, *Death in Britain: How Local Mortality Rates Have Changed: 1950s to 1990s* (Joseph Rowntree

Foundation, 1997). See http://www.jrf.org.uk; M. Shaw, D. Dorling, D. Gordon, and G. Davey Smith, *The Widening Gap: Health Inequalities and Policy in Britian* (Bristol: The Policy Press, 1999).

52. D. Blane and F. Drever, "Inequality among Men in Standardized Years of Potential Life Lost 1970–93," 317 *British Medical Journal* (1998): 255–260.

53. Dorling (1997), Note 51; R. Mitchell, M. Shaw, and D. Dorling, *Inequalities in Life and Death: What if Britain Were More Equal?* (Great Britain: The Joseph Rowntree Foundation, The Polity Press, 2000). See also: http://www.jrf.org.uk.

54. N.A. Ross, M.C. Wolfson, J.R. Dunn, J.-M. Berthelot, G.A. Kaplan, and J.W. Lynch, "Relations Between Income Inequality and Mortality in Canada and in the United States," 320(1) *British Medical Journal* (2000): 898–902.

55. Statistics Canada, "Health Reports: How Healthy are Canadians?" *The Daily*. Statistics Canada (March 31, 2000) Statistics Canada Cat. No. 11–001E

56. Note 5.

57. Ibid.

58. Navarro and Shi (2001), Note 2.

59. P. Lobmayer and R. Wilkinson, "Income, Inequality and Mortality in 14 Developed Countries," 22(4) *Sociology of Health and Illness* (2000): 401–414.

60. Note 5.

61. Note 59.

62. S. Brink and A. Zeesman, "Measuring Social Well-being: An Index of Social Health for Canada," Research paper series, Paper R-97–9E, Applied Research Branch, Strategic Policy, Human Resources Development Canada, 1997.

63. Esping-Andersen (1990, 1999), Note 4.

64. See D. Drache and T. Sullivan, eds., *Health Reform: Public Success, Private Failure* (London and New York: Routledge, 1999).

65. See A. Deaton and C. Paxson, *Mortality, Income and Income Inequality Over Time in Britian and the United States* (Princeton, NJ: Center for Health and Wellbeing, Princeton University, 2001).

66. B. Starfield, "Improving Equity in Health: A Research Agenda," 31(3) *International Journal of Health Services* (2001): 545–566.

67. F.G. Castles, "A Farewell to Australia's Welfare State," 31(3) *International Journal of Health Services*, (2001): 537–544.

12

Gender Inequity in Health: Why It Exists and How We Can Change It

GITA SEN AND PIROSKA OSTLIN

Background

Gender inequality damages the health of millions of girls and women across the globe. It can also be harmful to men's health, despite the many tangible benefits it gives men through resources, power, authority, and control. These benefits to men do not come without a cost to their own emotional and psychological health, often translated in to risky and unhealthy behaviours and reduced longevity. Taking action to improve gender equity

This chapter is reprinted with permission from *Global Public Health* 3(1), Suppl. 1, 2008, 1–12. This chapter was the introduction to a Special Supplement of Global Public Health that brought together the short versions of eight reviews, written in 2007, as part of the work of the Women and Gender Equity Knowledge Network(WGEKN) of the World Health Organization (WHO) Commission on Social Determinants of Health (CSDH). The authors of this introduction were coordinators of the WGEKN, which was established in 2006 and funded by the Swedish Ministry for Foreign Affairs through WHO, the Swedish National Institute of Public Health (SNIPH), and the Foundation Open Society Institute (Zug). The task of the WGEKN was to synthesize knowledge and to develop recommendations about the mechanisms, processes, and actions that can be taken to reduce gender-based inequities in health. The recommendations of the WGEKN are included in the journal issue as an appendix. The Final Report of the WGEKN was submitted to the CSD in September 2007.

in health, and to address women's rights to health, is one of the most direct and potent ways to reduce health inequities overall, and to ensure effective use of health resources. Deepening and consistently implementing human rights instruments can be a powerful mechanism to motivate and mobilize governments, people, and, especially, women themselves.

Gender relations of power constitute the root causes of gender inequality, and are among the most influential of the social determinants of health. They determine whether people's health needs are acknowledged, whether they have a voice or a modicum of control over their lives and health, and whether they can realize their rights. Addressing the problem of gender inequality requires actions both outside and within the health sector, because gender power relations operate across such a wide spectrum of human life and in such inter-related ways. Taking such actions is good for the health of all people: girls and boys, women and men. In particular, inter-sectoral action to address gender inequality is critical to the realization of the Millennium Development Goals (MDGs).[1]

Like other social relations, gender relations, as experienced in daily life, and in the everyday business of feeling well or ill, are based on core structures that govern how power is embedded in social hierarchy. The structures that govern gender systems have basic commonalities and similarities across different societies, although how they manifest through beliefs, norms, organizations, behaviours, and practices can vary. Gender inequality and equity in health are socially governed and, therefore, actionable. Sex and society interact to determine who is well or ill, who is treated or not, who is exposed or vulnerable to ill health and how, whose behaviour is risk-prone or risk-averse, and whose health needs are acknowledged or dismissed.

However, gender intersects with economic inequality, racial or ethnic hierarchy, caste domination, differences based on sexual orientation, and a number of other social markers. Only focusing on economic inequalities across households can seriously distort our understanding of how inequality works, and who actually bears much of its burdens. Health gradients can be significantly different for men and women; medical poverty may not trap women and men to the same extent or in the same way. Discussion of gradients, gaps, and medical poverty traps typically focus on differences between rich and poor countries, households, or people. Our trawling of the literature found that the bulk of the work on health equity, in both high- and lower-income countries, has this bias. Because income/wealth is only one source, however powerful, of social inequality, a proper understanding of its impact on health means that we must look into how it interacts with other sources of social inequality, such as gender, race, or caste.

The right to health is affirmed in the Universal Declaration of Human Rights, and is part of the WHO's core principles. The affirmation of equal and universal rights to health for all people, irrespective of economic class, gender, race, ethnicity, caste, sexual orientation, disability, age, or location, can only be beneficial to people when it is translated into practical changes in policies, organizational frames, and institutional norms.

Framework for the Role of Gender as a Social Determinant of Health

The conceptual framework, developed within the WGEKN, proposes several pathways to explain how different factors interact, at the individual and collective levels, to generate inequalities that influence the health status of women and men in a given population. The pathways from the gendered structural determinants (see explanation below), to the intermediary factors that determine inequitable health outcomes, are multiple and can be complex. The intermediary factors are broadly four-fold: (1) discriminatory values, norms, practices, and behaviours, in relation to health within households and communities; (2) differential exposures and vulnerabilities to disease, disability, and injuries; (3) biases in health systems; and (4) biased health research. These intermediary factors result in biased and inequitable health outcomes, which, in turn, can have serious economic and social consequences for girls and boys, women and men, their families and communities, and their countries. Feedback effects, from outcomes and consequences to the structural determinants or to intermediary factors, can also be important. Figure 12.1 summarizes these relationships.

Gendered Structural Determinants of Health

Gender systems have a variety of different features, not all of which are the same across different societies. Women may have less land, wealth, and property in almost all societies; yet have higher burdens of work in the economy of 'care', ensuring the survival, reproduction, and security of people, including young and old. Girls, in some contexts, are fed less, educated less, and more physically restricted; women are typically employed and segregated in lower-paid, less secure, and 'informal' occupations. Gender hierarchy governs how people live, and what they believe, and claim to know, about what it means to be a girl or a boy, a woman or a man. Girls and women are often viewed as less capable or able, and in some regions are seen as repositories of male or family honour and the self-respect of communities.[2] Restrictions on their physical mobility, sexuality, and reproductive capacity are perceived

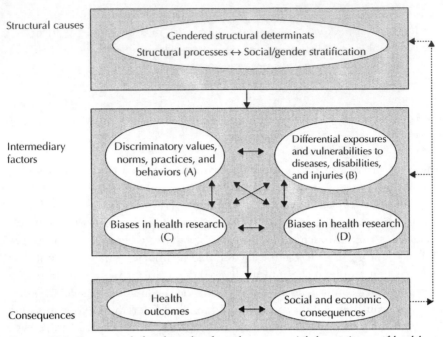

Structural causes

Intermediary factors

Consequences

FIGURE 12.1 Framework for the role of gender as a social determinant of health.
NOTE: The dashed units represent feedback effets.
SOURCE: Sen, Östlin, and George 2007.

to be natural; and, in many instances, accepted codes of social conduct and legal systems condone, and even reward, violence against them.[3]

Women are thus seen as objects rather than subjects (or agents) in their own homes and communities, and this is reflected in norms of behaviour, codes of conduct, and laws that perpetuate their status as lower beings and second-class citizens. Even in places where extreme gender inequality may not exist, women often have less access to political power, and lower participation in political institutions, from the local municipal council or village to the national parliament and the international arena. While the above is true for women as a whole vis-à-vis men, there can be significant differences among women themselves based on age or life cycle status, as well as on the basis of economic class, race, caste, and ethnicity. Iyer, Sen, and Östlin, for example, highlight the importance of a methodological approach based on the concept of intersectionality.[4] They suggest that intersecting stratification processes can significantly alter the impacts of any one dimension of inequality taken by itself. Insufficient attention to intersectionality in much of the health literature has significant human costs because those affected most negatively tend to be those who are poorest and most oppressed by gender and other forms of social inequality.

Much of the above also holds for transgender and intersex persons, who are often forced to live on the margins of mainstream society with few material assets, who face extreme labour market exclusion leaving them little other than sex-work as a means of survival, and who are often ostracized, discriminated against, and brutalized.[5]

The other side of women's subordinate position is that men typically have greater wealth, better jobs, more education, greater political clout, and fewer restrictions on behaviour. Moreover, men in many parts of the world exercise power over women, making decisions on their behalf, regulating and constraining their access to resources and personal agency, and sanctioning and policing their behaviour through socially condoned violence or the threat of violence. Again, not all men exercise power over all women; gender power relations are intersected by age and lifecycle, as well as the other social stratifiers such as economic class, race, or caste. The impact of gender power for physical and mental health (of girls, women, and transgender/intersex people, and also of boys and men) can be profound. Furthermore, the extent to which the needs of young populations, as well as older populations, have to be met through the unpaid 'care' work of women is exacerbated by crumbling health services and vanishing paid health staff. Women become the shock-absorbers in the system, expected to act as such in both normal economic and health times, and during the bumps caused by health crises and emergencies.

Together, gender systems, structural processes, and their interplay constitute the gendered structural determinants of health. What determines the pace or pattern of change in gender systems, and how do they affect people's health? The interplay between gender systems and structural processes, such as rising literacy and education, demographic transitions in birth and death rates and in family structures, globalization (including its effects on labour forces, policy space, health systems, and violence), and the strengthening of human rights discourse, all work to weaken or strengthen gender hierarchies and their effects on people's health.

In some instances, however, these changes also set off backlashes, as those who wield gender power in families, communities, and religious structures attempt to control and discipline (especially) young women. Trying to hold on to power has led to attempts to roll back internationally agreed upon norms on gender equality and sexual and reproductive health and rights in particular. Such attempts have had serious implications for the health and human rights of women and men and of young people.

Three implications of globalization are of particular significance for our focus on gender relations. The first is how it has transformed the composition of workforces, and the implications for women's health. Feminization of workforces has gone hand in hand within increased casualization, and continuing unequal burdens for unpaid work in the household, with serious implications for women's health, both their occupational health and the consequences of insufficient rest and leisure.[6] A second gendered consequence of globalization is through its narrowing of national policy space, that has resulted in reducing funds for health and education, with negative impacts on girls' and women's access.[7] A third aspect of globalization of importance for health is the rise in violence linked to the changing political economy of nation states in the international order. Laurie and Petchesky apply the political theory of Agambenon 'states of exception' as a way of understanding current gender dynamics in reproductive health, militarization, and camps for refugees and internally displaced persons.[8] It argues that a human rights approach to gender and health equity is essential in such sites of exclusion. Importantly, gendered violence does not only affect girls and women, but also includes violence against boys and men, as well as transgender and intersex persons, and all those who do not meet heterosexual norms.

Some of the negative consequences of globalization contrast with the deepening, during recent decades, of the normative framework of human rights. This deepening has been important in altering values, beliefs, and knowledge about gender systems and their implications for health and human rights. The first action priority is, therefore, to protect and promote women's human rights that are key parts of the normative framework for health. This, in turn, requires strengthening women's hands, and empowering them so that they can actually claim and realize their human rights. This points to the next two action priorities: cushioning women who act as the 'shock absorbers' through key structural reforms, including gender-sensitive infrastructure, and expanding women's opportunities and capabilities.

Intermediary Factors

Discriminatory values, norms, practices, and behaviours in relation to health within households and communities (A). Gendered norms in health, manifest in households and communities on the basis of values and attitudes about the relative worth, or importance, of girls versus boys and men versus women; about who has responsibility for different household/community needs and roles; about masculinity and femininity; who has the right to make different decisions; who ensures that household/community order is maintained and deviance is appropriately sanctioned or punished; and who has final authority in relation to the inner world of the family/community and its outer relations with society.[9] Norms around masculinity not only affect the health of girls and women but also of boys and men themselves.[10] Direct causal relationships, linking cultural biases against girls and women to health outcomes, vary widely across regions and cultures, and over time. These biases include differential access to nutrition and healthcare for boys versus girls, and women versus men. Unequal control over income and productive resources, such as land and credit, can affect the value given to women's lives and health and, hence, to health practices, health-seeking behaviours, and health access.

Unequal burdens of work and responsibility, for the care of young and old, often means that women are expected to sacrifice their own rest, leisure, and health; women themselves internalize these values, which often mark who is seen to be a 'good' woman. Norms of masculinity vary, as do models of what represents perfect femininity. Idealized women in different cultures may be virgins, goddesses, sacrificing mothers, even sexual temptresses, but, ubiquitously, the sexuality and reproductive capacity of the good woman is the property of her husband, family, clan, or community. Men, similarly, may be expected to be aloof, unemotional, aggressive, more emotional, but, everywhere, they are also expected to look after their female property and keep it in good order. The threat of violence, and violence itself, are central to the maintenance of the masculine–feminine order. This has obvious and serious consequences for the physical, emotional, and psychological health of women and of men themselves.

Challenging gender norms, especially in the areas of sexuality and reproduction, touch the most intimate personal relationships, as well as one's sense of self and identity. No single or simple action or policy intervention can be expected, therefore, to provide a panacea for the problem. Targeting women and girls is a sound investment, but outcomes are dependent on integrated approaches and the protective umbrella of policy and legislative actions.[11] Multi-level interventions are needed. We identify three sets of actions: (1) creating formal agreements, codes, and laws, to change norms that violate women's human rights, and then implementing them; (2) adopting multi-level strategies to change norms, including supporting women's organizations; and (3) working with boys and men to transform masculinist values and behaviours that harm women's health and their own.

Differential exposures and vulnerabilities to disease, disability, and injuries (B).Gender differentials in exposure and vulnerability to health risks can arise for two main reasons: the interplay of biological sex with the social construction of gender, and the direct impacts of structural gender inequalities. Differently from some other social determinants, it is impossible to ignore biology when considering why health outcomes for women and men may be different. The complex interplay between sex (as a biological factor) and gender (as socially shaped) has to be disentangled in tracing causality. For example, how much of women's vulnerability to HIV infection is due to female biology, and how much can be attributed to girls' and women's lack of power in sexual relationships?

Snow highlights the dynamic and changeable nature of gendered health vulnerabilities, underscoring how they differ across time and space.[12] She argues that analyses of gender and health are currently undermined by conflation of sex and gender in much of the epidemiological and clinical literature, thus, precluding any meaningful reflection on the contributions of genetics versus gendered socialization to health vulnerabilities.

In addition, structural gender inequalities in legal frameworks governing control over resources, and women's status and autonomy as subjects and citizens, the functioning of labour and other markets, access to social services, health care, education, and inter alia, can have a powerful impact on differences in health risks for women and men. The consequences of gender inequality can be experienced by women as: differential vulnerability and exposure to illness, poor acknowledgement of women-specific health needs, and inequitable treatment of health problems across a wide spectrum of health (reproductive, occupational, environmental, infectious disease). Women's health has been beset by 'resounding silences' and 'misdirected or partial approaches'.[13] These have affected such problems as: kitchen air pollution, risks of heart disease, mental health, reproductive tract infections, breast and cervical cancers, and depression, to give just a few examples. Where biological sex differences interact with social determinants, to define different needs for women and men in health, policy efforts must address these different needs. Significant advocacy is required to raise attention and sustain support for other services that address the specific health needs of poor women, and those in low-income countries, thereby reducing their exposure and vulnerability to unfavourable health outcomes. Not only must neglected sex-specific health conditions be addressed but also sex-specific needs in health conditions, that affect both women and men, must be considered, so that treatment can be accessed by both women and men without bias. Two intertwined strategies to address social bias are: tackling the social context of individual behaviour, and empowering individuals and communities for positive change. Strategies that aim at changing high risk life-styles would be more effective if combined with measures that could tackle the negative social and economic circumstances (e.g., unemployment, sudden income loss) in which the health damaging life-styles are embedded. Individual empowerment, linked to community level dynamics, is also critical in fostering transformation of gendered vulnerabilities. For strategies to succeed they must provide positive alternatives that support individuals and communities to take action against the status quo.

Biases in health systems(C).While the traditional approach to health care systems tends to be management oriented, with focus on issues such as infrastructure, technology, logistics, and financing, the WGEKN looked at the human component of health care systems, and the social relationships that characterize service delivery. Evidence shows the different ways in which the health care system may fail gender equity from the perspective of women, as both consumers (users) and producers (carers) of health care services. Action priorities include, supporting improvements in (especially poor) women's access to services, recognition of women's role as health care providers, and building accountability for gender equality and equity into health systems, and especially in ongoing health reform programmes and mechanisms.

Lack of awareness (knowledge of women, their families, and health care providers about the existence of a health problem), and acknowledgement (recognition that something should and can be done about the health problem), are important barriers to women's access to and use of health services.[14] Access depends, therefore, both on factors affecting the demand side (how families treat women who may be potential users, and how women see themselves) and the supply side (including different aspects on the side of providers). Health systems also tend to ignore women's crucial role as health providers, both within the formal health system (at its lower levels) and as informal providers and unpaid carers in the home. George examined the experiences of nurses, community health workers, and home carers in health systems.[15] She found that these female frontline health workers compensate for the shortcomings of health systems through individual adjustments, at times to the detriment of their own health and livelihoods.

Absence of effective accountability mechanisms for available, affordable, acceptable, and high-quality health services and facilities may seriously hinder women and their families in holding government and other actors accountable for violations of their human rights to health. Govender and Penn-Kekana argue that gender biases and discrimination occur at many levels of the health care delivery environment, and affect the patient–provider interaction.[16] Ensuring good interpersonal relationships between patients and providers (an important marker of quality of care) requires a broader approach of gender-sensitive interventions at multiple levels of policies and programmes.

Health sector reforms can have fundamental consequences for gender equality and for people's life and well-being, as patients, in both formal and informal health care as paid and unpaid care providers, as health care administrators, and as decision makers. However, health sector reforms that have been implemented in many countries have tended to focus on their implications for the poor and their consequences for gender equity in general and, particularly, in health care have seldom been discussed or taken into consideration in planning.[17] Health sector reform strategies, policies, and interventions, introduced during the last two decades, have had limited success in achieving improved gender equity in health. Minimizing gender bias in health systems requires systematic approaches to building awareness and transforming values among service providers, and requires steps to improve access to health services and developing mechanisms for accountability.

Biased health research (D). Gender discrimination and bias not only affect differentials in health needs, health-seeking behaviour, treatment, and outcomes, but also permeate the content and process of health research.[18] Gender imbalances in research content include the following dimensions: slow recognition of health problems that particularly affect women; misdirected or partial approaches to women's and men's health needs in different fields of health research; and lack of recognition of the interaction between gender and other social factors. Gender imbalances in the research process include: non-collection of sex-disaggregated data in individual research projects or larger data systems; research methodologies are not sensitive to the different dimensions of disparity; methods used in medical research and clinical trials for new drugs, that lack a gender perspective and exclude female subjects from study populations; gender imbalance in ethical committees, research funding, and advisory bodies; and differential treatment of women scientists. Mechanisms and policies need to be developed to ensure that gender imbalances in both the content and processes of health research are avoided and corrected.

The importance of having good quality data and indicators for health status, disaggregated by sex and age from infancy through old age, cannot be overstated. Gender-sensitive and human-rights-sensitive country level indicators are essential to guide policies, programmes, and service delivery; without them, interventions to change behaviours, or increase participation rates, will operate in a vacuum.

Removing Organizational Plaque

Many of the organizational structures of government, and other social and private institutions, through which gender norms have to be challenged and practices altered, have been in existence for decades, even centuries. Thickly encrusted with traditional (usually male dominated) values, relationships, and methods of work, it has been a serious challenge to expect these same structures to deliver gender equality and equity. Working towards gender equality challenges long-standing male dominated power structures and patriarchal social capital (old boys' networks) within organizations. It crosses the boundaries of people's comfort zones by threatening to shake up existing lines of control over material resources, authority, and prestige. It requires people to learn new ways of doing things about which they may not be very convinced, and from which they see little benefit to themselves, and to unlearn old habits and practices. Resistance to gender-equal policies may take the form of trivialization, dilution, subversion, or outright resistance, and can lead to the evaporation of gender equitable laws, policies, or programmes.

Tackling this requires effective political leadership, well-designed organizational mandates, structures, incentives, and accountability mechanisms with teeth. It also requires actions to empower women and women's organizations, so that they can collectively press for greater accountability for gender equality and equity. Murthy, for example, observes that four kinds of human rights instruments, legislation, structures, and tools have been used by citizens to press for accountability to gender and health.[19] Among other things, she recommends that accountability strategies should be extended to the private health sector and donors, that resources should be earmarked to respond to gender specific health needs, and that mechanisms for enforcement of policies should be improved. Ravindran and Kelkar-Khambete argue that the gap between intention and practice is large.[20] This can be attributed to depoliticization and delinking of gender mainstreaming from social justice agendas; top-down approaches; hostility within the global policy environment to justice and equity concerns; as well as privatization and retraction of the state's role in health.

The Way Forward

Gender relations of power exist both within and outside the health sector, and exercise a pernicious influence on the health of people. A rapidly growing body of evidence identifies and explains what gender inequality and inequity mean, in terms of differential exposures and vulnerabilities for women versus men, and also, how health care systems, and health research, reproduce these inequalities and inequities instead of resolving them. The consequences for people's health are not only unequal and unjust, but also ineffective and inefficient.

At the same time, a growing number of actions, by non-governmental and governmental actors and agencies, seeks to challenge these injustices and to transform beliefs and practices within and outside the health sector, in order to generate sustained changes that can improve people's health and lives. In particular, women's organizations have been critical to ensuring that women have a voice and the ability to insist that all actors be accountable. Despite the courage and creativity of these organizations in putting forward innovative approaches, their access to funds has been declining in recent years. This trend must be halted and reversed.

Notes

1. C. Grown, G.R. Gupta, and R. Pande, 'Taking Action to Improve Women's Health through Gender Equality and Women's Empowerment', 365 *The Lancet* (2005): 541–543.
2. I. Fazio, 'The Family, Honour and Gender in Sicily: Models and New Research', 9 *Modern Italy* (2004): 263–280.
3. C. Garcia-Moreno, H. Jansen, M. Ellesberg, L. Heise, and C.H. Watts, On behalf of the WHO Multi-Country Study on Women's Health and Domestic Violence against Women Study Team, 'Prevalence of Intimate Partner Violence: Findings from the WHO Multi-Country Study on Women's Health and Domestic Violence', 368 *The Lancet* (2006): 1260–1269.
4. A. Iyer, G. Sen, and P. Östlin, 'The Intersections of Gender and Class in Health Status and Health Care', 3(Suppl. 1) *Global Public Health* (2008): 13–24.
5. Institute of Development Studies Bridge, 'Cutting Edge Pack on Gender and Sexuality' (2007), available at www.bridge.ids.ac.uk/reports_gend_CEP.html# Sexuality (accessed February 14, 2008).
6. S. Joekes, 'Gender and Livelihoods in Northern Pakistan', 26 *IDS Bulletin* (1995): 66–74; H. Standing, 'Gender and Equity in Health Sector Reform Programmes: A Review', 12 *Health Policy Plan*, (1997): 1–18; K. Messing and. P. Ostlin, *Gender Equality, Work and Health: A Review of the Evidence* (Geneva: World Health Organization, 2006).
7. B. Herz and D. Sperling, *What Works in Girl's Education: Evidence and Policies from the Developing World* (New York: Council on Foreign Relations Press, 2004); J.E. Stiglitz and A. Charlton, *Fair Trade for All. How Trade Can Promote Development* (New York: Oxford University Press, 2005).
8. M. Laurie and R.P. Petchesky, 'Gender, Health, and Human Rights in Sites of Political Exclusion', 3(Suppl. 1) *Global Public Health* (2008): 25–41.
9. A.R. Quisumbing and J.A. Maluccio, *Intrahousehold Allocation and Gender Relations: New Empirical Evidence*. Policy Research Report on Gender and Development (Working Paper Series, No. 2, Development Research Group/ Poverty Reduction and Economic Management Network, The World Bank, 1999).
10. B. Barker and C. Ricardo, 'Young men and the Construction of Masculinity in Sub-Saharan Africa: Implications for HIV/AIDS, Conflict, and Violence' (Washington, DC: World Bank, Social Development Department (Social Development Papers: Conflict Prevention and Reconstruction Paper No. 26; Social Development Paper No. 84, 2005).
11. H. Keleher and L. Franklin, 'Changing Gendered Norms about Women and Girls at the Level of Household and Community: A Review of the Evidence', 3(Suppl. 1) *Global Public Health* (2008): 42–57.
12. R.C. Snow, 'Sex, Gender, and Vulnerability', 3(Suppl. 1) *Global Public Health* (2008): 58–74.

13. G. Sen, A. George, and P. Östlin, 'Engendering Health Equity: A review of Research and Policy', in *Engendering International Health: The Challenge of Equity*, ed. G. Sen, A. George, and P. Östlin (Cambridge: The MIT Press, 2002): 1–34.

14. A. George, The Outrageous as Ordinary: Primary Health Care Workers' Perspectives on Accountability in Koppal District, Karnataka State, India. Institute of Development Studies. Brighton Sussex University (2007). Doctoral thesis.

15. A. George, 'Nurses, Community Health Workers and Home Carers: Gendered Human Resources Compensating for Skewed Health', 3(Suppl. 1) *Global Public Health* (2008): 73–89.

16. V. Govender and L. Penn-Kekana, 'Gender biases and discrimination: a review of health care interpersonal interactions', 3(Suppl. 1) *Global Public Health* (2008): 90–103.

17. PAHO, *Evaluating the Impact of Health Reforms on Gender Equity. A PAHO Guide* (Washington, DC: Pan American Health Organization, 2001).

18. M. Eichler, A.L. Reisman, and E.M. Borins, 'Gender Bias in Medical Research', 12 *Women & Therapy* (1992): 61–70.; Sen et al. 2002, Note 16; P. Östlin, G. Sen, and A. George, 'Paying Attention to Gender and Poverty in Health Research: Content and Process Issues', 82 *Bulletin of the World Health Organization* (2004): 740–745. [Editorial11]; S. Theobald, B. Nhlema Simwaka, and B. Klugman, 'Gender, Health and Development III: Engendering Health Research', 6 *Progress in Development Studies* (2006): 1–5.

19. R.K. Murthy, 'Strengthening Accountability to Citizens on Gender and Health', 3(Suppl. 1) *Global Public Health* (2008): 104–120.

20. T.K.S. Ravindran and A. Kelkar-Khambete, 'Gender mainstreaming in health: looking back, looking forward', 3(Suppl. 1) *Global Public Health* (2008): 121–142.

PART III

Practitioners Take Action: Strategies for Organizational Change and Working with Communities

13

Initiating Social Justice Action through Dialogue in a Local Health Department: The Ingham County Experience

DOAK BLOSS

Introduction

By their nature, bureaucracies do not welcome change. They do not invite transformation, and often their normal response to the threat of change is to resist it, reject it, or, worst of all, assimilate it in a way that blunts any real impact on the status quo. If local health departments are bureaucratic institutions—and in my experience they are—then any quick and deliberate attempt to transform their practice to focus on the elimination of the root causes of health inequity will quickly and predictably fail. The call for change must come from within, from the occupants of the bureaucracy itself—public health workers—and from the community the department serves. Furthermore, it must come as a consequence of accrued evidence and realization that what we are doing now to "preserve and protect the public health" is inadequate, because the social forces that advantage one group of people over another in our society are too deeply entrenched ever to be undone by conventional public health programming and regulation.

Public health needs a new frame for its work—one that does more than simply adjust or recast the statutory mandates and programmatic objectives of the current frame. Local health departments must adopt as a core goal the identification and elimination of policies that maintain an uneven playing field on the basis of class, race, gender, and other forms of differ-ence. The Ingham County experience was an attempt to explore whether a dialogue process—sustained, applied, and conjoined with other dialogue processes occurring in the community—could be a vehicle for creating this new frame.

In this chapter, I seek to assist those who are considering a similar use of facilitated dialogue to bring about a transformation of public health prac-tice within local health departments. This should not be seen as a "how to" course in facilitation techniques or a curriculum for raising awareness of social justice issues, although I briefly describe both the dialogue method-ology and the educational content used in the process. Most importantly, I hope to illuminate the likely road ahead for local health departments interested in using dialogue in this way. I begin with an overview of the Social Justice Project and dialogue process that was used to move it for-ward. Then I focus on three specific challenges that shaped the next phase of work, which I describe as a predictable incubation period many depart-ments may need to go through before change at the institutional level can begin. Finally, I describe the most recent efforts to institutionalize change within the department—specifically, change that instills in our daily prac-tice new responsiveness to the root causes of health inequity—and offer some preliminary conclusions about the role dialogue played in bringing them about.

Overview

In January 2005, the Ingham County Health Department initiated its Social Justice Project. The project's objectives were to illuminate the ways in which the department's policies and practices had a bearing on the root causes of health inequity—the systematic and unjust differences in the distribution of illness and disease—in Ingham County, either positive or negative, and to create and implement an Action Plan for improving the department's responsiveness to those root causes. The engine for this work was an internal dialogue process that the department had previously used, with great success, in efforts to engage and mobilize neighborhood residents around self-defined community health improvement goals, and to develop community support for an "organized system of care" for the uninsured. The Social Justice Project was the department's first attempt to use this dialogue method to engage and mobilize its own employees around an initiative intended to change the department's internal practice.

The Action Plan that resulted from this initial dialogue process did not immediately transform the department's practice. Senior staff reviewed the plan's five broad goals, detailed objectives, and specific action steps but did not implement them in any tangible or concrete way. Rather, for the next year and a half, participants in the original process continued to promote dialogue—formally and informally, within the health department and in the community—raising the central questions addressed in the Action Plan: what are the root causes of health inequity, and what should the local health department do to address them? This 18-month "incubation" period, though neither intended nor predicted, set the stage for a change process within the department that was intentional indeed, and which is now moving forward with the explicit intention of changing the way the department frames its core functions.

The process that occurred in Ingham County between 2005 and 2008 illuminates the practical challenges involved in attempting to change a local health department's approach to social justice issues from the ground up. These challenges include overcoming the modern mindset of what public health workers do, defining the appropriate leadership role a local health department should play in its community, and finding an effective balance between *facilitating* and *promoting* change in a bureaucratic institution.

Dialogue means different things to different people, and certainly not all forms of dialogue will serve as a successful vehicle for change. In Ingham County, *dialogue* was defined as a facilitated process designed to elicit, gather, and synthesize the collective wisdom of a group of people in answering a specific question, through the broadest possible participation and achieving the broadest possible ownership of the resulting decisions. Students of the Brazilian educationalist Paolo Freire may find resonance with this definition, in that it at least implies consistency with some of the dialogic methods advanced by Freire. (See Box 13.1.)

Box 13.1 What is a Dialogue?—Strands of Paulo Freire

Some characteristics of Freirean dialogue that are consistent with the dialogue process applied in Ingham County are as follows:

1. **Eliciting knowledge from participants rather than "dispensing" it to them.** Freire espoused a conversational rather than didactic approach to education, one that developed critical thinking, reflection, and learning through questioning rather than inculcation or a transference of existing knowledge.
2. **Aiming toward informed action and social change.** Freire emphasized social transformation and enablement within a process of illumination, rather than method and technique.

(Continued)

3. **Naming the world to reveal the power of consciousness to change it.** Freire explored the implications of the relationship between knowledge, meaning, and power within the process of interaction and engagement. Social imagination and risk taking are seen as part of the process.
4. **Focusing on lived experience.** Freire incorporated thinking, feeling, and action into the learning process, which was framed as a process of discovery and experience, not training.
5. **Transcending the educator's unilateral role.** Freire stressed creative exploration and the exchange of ideas; learners were to be encouraged, not led. A fundamental assumption of the learning process is that no knowledge is value free.

Background: The Legacy of Community Voices

Although the term "social justice" was not used to describe it, Ingham County's social justice work began as early as in 1998, with the implementation of its *Community Voices* initiative. Funded primarily by a grant from the W.K. Kellogg Foundation and a smaller grant from the Robert Wood Johnson Foundation, this initiative stressed active community engagement as a means to improving access to health and health care. The dialogue method described in this chapter was used both at the grassroots level and at the systems level to establish consensus and action planning for improved community health and an organized system of care for the uninsured in Ingham County.

Many tangible outcomes resulted from these dialogue initiatives. At the grassroots level, work groups succeeded in organizing and implementing a wide range of health improvement projects through neighborhood network centers,[1] all grounded in the notion that *social connection* was the key ingredient to community health. At the institutional level, the Ingham Health Plan gained traction and support as a coverage model that eventually enrolled over 16,000 uninsured adults.

Changed Thinking about Assets and Resources

An initiative that connects the dots between social injustice and health disparities must seek a new framework for the work of public health. It requires a transformation in the way public health workers think and act in their communities. In Ingham County, this change in thinking clearly began with the dialogue processes that occurred through *Community Voices*.

Attempts to portray this transformation can be found in conceptual diagrams created in 2004, after community dialogue processes were completed and their action plans implemented. Figures 13.1a and 13.1b

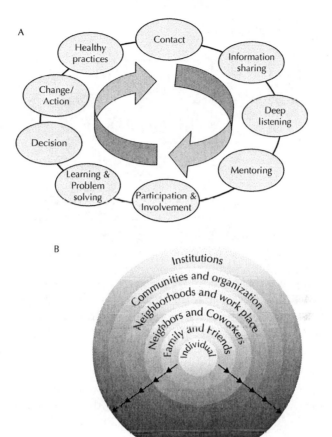

FIGURE 13.1a and 13.1b Allen Neighborhood Center's Conceptual Model for "Spiraling toward Health."
NOTE: Conceptual model developed by Ann Francis, Allen Neighborhood Center, Lansing, Michigan.

illustrate the way residents and grassroots workers turned conventional thinking on its head after their 2001 neighborhood health summit. Improved health is not the result of institutions injecting their expertise into communities, they have told us; rather, it is the product of persistent, person-to-person interaction moving outward through concentric rings of engagement. Organized individuals change institutions, not vice versa.[2]

Also as a consequence of *Community Voices*, the health department as an institution began to rethink its strategy for allocating and using resources. At the programmatic level, the department gained a new appreciation of the value of having neighborhood residents actively working to achieve the department's community health goals in such areas as smoking cessation, enrollment in coverage, and cancer prevention and detection. More

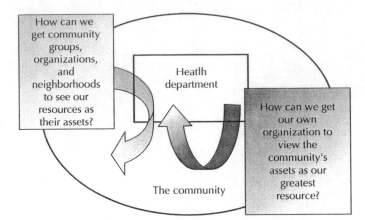

FIGURE 13.2 Rethinking Assets and Resources.

fundamentally, department administrators began to ask the following two questions of themselves, and to urge other institutions to do likewise: 1) How can we get community groups, organizations, and neighborhoods to see our resources as their assets?; and 2) How can we get our own organization to view the community's assets as our greatest resources? (Figure 13.2).

The Ingham County Health Department launched its Social Justice Project in this context of changed institutional thinking. As with these earlier initiatives, facilitated dialogue was to serve as a catalyst for transformation, this time within the department itself.

The Social Justice Project

The Social Justice Project was the first substantial attempt to apply the *Community Voices* dialogue process internally within the health department. Leadership for the effort was provided by myself, in my role as Access to Health Coordinator—a position created specifically to coordinate the various activities of the *Community Voices* initiative in 1998. My hiring in itself was somewhat unusual: I possessed no formal training in public health, and became involved with the health department through my facilitation of community and interagency processes throughout the 1990s. Once hired, I reported directly to the Health Officer, in effect occupying a position outside the conventional boxes of the department's organizational chart. This remained true until 2007, when a departmental reorganization made health equity and social justice a formal component of the organizational structure for the first time.

Recruitment and Participation

The original Social Justice Project convened a team of 20 Health Department employees, who would explore through dialogue the root causes of health inequity. This Social Justice Team would generate recommendations during a 5-month process, and then, in collaboration with the department's senior staff, formulate an Action Plan to guide departmental and community action to address the root causes of health inequity.[3]

To recruit the members of the team, I issued a call for participants to approximately 40 managers within the department, inviting them to nominate people to be on the team. In addition to describing the project's objectives and process, the invitation detailed the time commitment team members would be expected to make and a list of characteristics that were desired for the team (e.g., independence of thought, respect, and influence among colleagues, creativity, etc.).

For the first phase of the project (the dialogue process), senior staff were intentionally excluded from participation in the team, although each was invited to observe team meetings and received team reports. The primary reason was a concern that the participation of senior managers would inhibit the team's candor in discussing issues of race, class, and gender discrimination, especially as they might be experienced within the department itself.

All 21 employees nominated for the team agreed to participate. These included three nurses, three health analysts, two program coordinators, two middle managers, two communications specialists, two accounting staff, two clerical staff, one nurse practitioner, one health educator, one outreach specialist, one medical assistant, and one sanitarian. Demographically, the team was composed of 17 women and 4 men; 11 Caucasians, 7 African Americans, 2 Latinas, and 1 Native American.

Timeline and Products

The initial phase of the dialogue process consisted of eight meetings of the Social Justice Team between February 28 and July 8, 2005. Two meetings each were dedicated to three root causes of health inequity: (1) socioeconomic or class exploitation; (2) institutionalized racism; and (3) gender discrimination and exploitation. Each of the dialogues yielded preliminary recommendations for how the health department might respond, in the form of actions it could take or strategies it could apply. In June, the members of the Social Justice Team joined senior staff for a 2-day retreat to strengthen relationships around the issues that the team had been wrestling with for the previous 5 months. In July and August, the team and senior staff met 4 times to translate the preliminary recommendations into five overarching goals, with objectives and action steps for each.

The five overarching goals of the Social Justice Action Plan (September 2005)

Policy reform: Illuminate for the community barriers to economic freedom for women, immigrants, people of low socioeconomic status, and people of color that are embedded in public and institutional policy. Encourage a coordinated community effort to eliminate these barriers.

Information and communication: Ensure community access to accurate information on health inequity, responsible media coverage of health equity issues, and the inclusion of historically underserved groups in community dialogue.

Community engagement and mobilization: Establish the community will to create a "Culture of Equity" in Ingham County.

Partnerships for economic justice and equal opportunity: Motivate recognition across public systems of their responsibility to end inequities in access to education and economic resources.

Public health workforce mobilization: Ensure that the workforce of Ingham County Health Department (ICHD) is (1) aware of the many ways in which conditions that lead to health inequity are rooted in social injustice; (2) accountable for the department's responsibility to work for social justice and health equity in daily practice; and (3) comprised of people at all levels of the organization whose identities, experience, and demographics reflect the diversity of the populations we serve.

The Dialogues

The structure for each dialogue was built around a specific sequence of inquiry—activities and questions leading to a Focus Question to which the group generated multiple answers. The facilitator translated these answers into recommendations for action, which were then reviewed, revised, and validated by the group at a shorter follow-up session. The dialogue methodology was modeled on techniques taught in the Technologies of Participation (ToP) training developed by the Institute for Cultural Affairs (ICA).[4] Anyone interested in learning more about this facilitation methodology is urged to visit the ICA web site at www.ica-usa.org and consider attending a ToP training.

What follows is a general description of the dialogue process that led to the ICHD Action Plan. Returning to the characteristics of Paolo Freire's dialogic approach (see Figure 13.1a), note that the methodology we used in Ingham County was not intrinsically Freirean, although we used it to undertake a process that Freire might have recognized. In retrospect, the more deeply we delved into health equity and social justice as driving concepts for our department, the more our process took on the characteristics ascribed to Freirean dialogue; but this was more a function of the questions we asked than the dialogue methodology we adopted.

The Focus Question

Each dialogue was built around the task of answering a single question related to one of the root causes, which was presented at the start of the session. The Focus Questions for the three dialogues were as follows:

Socioeconomic or class exploitation: "In terms of policy or practice, what actions or strategies by ICHD would reduce the impact of class or socioeconomic status as a root cause of health inequity?"

Institutionalized racism: "What are some ways ICHD can reduce the impact of racism as a root cause of health inequity?"

Gender exploitation and discrimination: "What are some 'upstream' ways ICHD can work toward the elimination of gender exploitation and discrimination as a root cause of health inequity?"

Each of these Focus Questions could have been expressed more simply and transparently: "As a local health department, what do we need to do to eliminate _____ as a root cause of health inequity?" The Focus Questions we used reflect an evolving intention to balance two opposite concerns. The first was that the team, overwhelmed by the enormity of the goal of eliminating something as huge as class prejudice, racism, or gender discrimination, would retreat to minor adjustments in practice (changing the way we schedule patients in our health centers, etc.). The second was that the team, taking the challenge truly to heart, would set lofty goals for itself with no specific strategies for how to achieve them (e.g., "reform welfare"). This balancing act is the core challenge of creating an effective Focus Question for a social justice dialogue; ideally, it should aim dialogue participants directly at root causes while still focusing on tangible, achievable changes in policy or practice. To the extent that it is strategically wise to do so, the Focus Question should also make the goal of transforming practice explicit. In our department in 2005, it was not.

Trigger Information

Over the course of the three dialogues, we used several different types of trigger information to stimulate the group's exploration of root causes of health inequity. These included written materials and data, summary presentations, experiential exercises, and the sharing of team members' personal experiences. The goal was to provide a balance of factual and experiential stimulation to the team members.

- **Written materials and data.** Examples: papers on public health's historical focus on human rights and social justice (as an orientation to core concepts); local statistics on health and social factors such as early death, correlation between physical and emotional health; national reports correlating such factors.
- **Summary presentations of written material.** Each dialogue included custom-made graphic representations of the major ideas discussed in the readings. Lasting no more than 20 minutes, they were important in assuring that all team members (including those who failed to read the advance materials) were starting from the same place.
- **Experiential exercises.** Examples: the "Ten Chairs" exercise developed by Teaching Economics as if it Mattered,[5] which simulates the disproportionate accumulation of wealth in the United States; the "Privilege Walk," several versions of which are available from organizations that train on multicultural awareness; a candid interview with a grassroots community outreach worker who had sought assistance from a social service agency for other people, and experienced sharply different attitudes from the agency when seeking assistance for herself; short documentary films, most notably the two series form California Newsreel, *Race, the Power of an Illusion,* and *Unnatural Causes—Is Inequality Making Us Sick?*[6]
- **Visioning/personal reflection.** At the start of the race dialogue, participants were asked to recall one of their earliest experiences of noticing racial difference, and then, on a voluntary basis, to share it with the group. This was one of the most evocative and powerful trigger experiences of the entire dialogue series, particularly for the striking differences between the recollections of whites and people of color.

Open Dialogue

Following the trigger information, the facilitator prompted an "open dialogue" about what the team had just seen and heard. The facilitator tracked this conversation by writing down key points made by each speaker on index cards and affixing them in threads on an adhesive board.[7] This produced a literal picture of the group's collective thinking, while allowing individuals to move back and forth between topics throughout. The facilitator's job at this point, in addition to capturing what is being shared, is to elicit the diverse experience and insights of the participants so that they can inform the process of answering the Focus Question. In the written reports on each session, discussion points made during the Open Dialogue often helped to explain the thinking behind the recommendations the team produced.

Summary Questions

The next step in the dialogue process was to ask a series of short-answer questions of the participants that would help them summarize all of the information they needed to consider in answering the Focus Question. A number of variations in the "summary question" sequence were applied in the three Social Justice dialogues. Probably the clearest and most effective was the one below, which was used when the team addressed institutionalized racism as a root cause of health inequity:

Summary questions—race dialogue

1. Of everything that you've seen and heard this far this morning, what stands out for you as particularly surprising or important?
2. What if any new thoughts about racism have you had in the past few hours?
3. What fears or concerns prevent ICHD from responding directly to racism?
4. If Ingham County were to address racism in a meaningful way, internally or externally, what would it look like?
5. Who are the community change agents—people, groups, or institutions—that might accelerate a meaningful strategy for eliminating racism?
6. What are the potential rewards to the community for addressing racism more directly?
7. What can ICHD do to engage those change agents or realize those rewards?

An important function of the summary questions is to create a bridge between the random, free-flowing responses of the Open Dialogue and the more focused, intentional nature of the final exercise to answer the Focus Question. By limiting team members to short answers to specific, sequenced questions, the group naturally falls into a more concentrated, thoughtful attitude—one characterized by periods of silence and deep listening.

Answering the Focus Question

The exercise used to answer the Focus Question consisted of three parts:

1. *Individual brainstorm.* Each participant writes out answers to the focus question.
2. *Group sharing of answers.* Two or more team members compare their lists, and decide upon a set number of answers they can support together.

3. *Pairing, clustering, and naming answers.* The facilitator places answers on the adhesive board and arranges them into pairs, then clusters, at the direction of the participants. Through additional dialogue, the facilitator clarifies what each cluster means as an action or strategy for change.[8]

Using this method, the three dialogues of the Social Justice Project produced a total of 20 recommendations (seven each from the Class and Gender dialogues, and six from the Race dialogue). Even though the resulting recommendations were framed as an end product for each of three dialogues, the team understood that these recommendations would be further translated into an Action Plan, in collaboration with senior staff. The next section of this chapter discusses the dynamics of this phase, where I describe three important challenges the team faced.

Three Challenges

Challenge 1: Shifting from Consequences to Root Causes

In addition to confronting difficult issues of prejudice and privilege in their organization and their community, the Social Justice Team struggled through the dialogue process with two underlying concepts of the Social Justice Project: (1) that the health department had a responsibility to address root causes of health inequity in its daily practice, and (2) that it could have a meaningful impact on social forces that were so pervasive and overwhelming in our society.

This challenge actually emerged during the orientation itself, when, after an hour or so of general concurrence with the idea that unearned power and privilege based on class, race, or gender greatly influenced health outcomes, one member of the team had the courage to voice a different perspective. In her work helping people to quit smoking, she said, one critical factor was helping them accept personal responsibility for change. While, as a Latina, she knew firsthand the experience of prejudice in our society, she expressed concern that a new focus on issues like racism could very well work against her goals as a health educator. Ultimately, aren't we all responsible for own choices?

The conversation that followed was the beginning of an important internal debate within the team. In the moment, virtually everyone in the room tried to dissuade this one dissenter from her viewpoint, pointing out how "personal responsibility" was often used as a means of denying prejudice and reinforcing racial and ethnic stereotypes. If we pretend the playing field is level when it is not, we only maintain the status quo and fall into the trap of blaming the victim. However, in the weeks that followed it became clear that the concern expressed by this health educator was not hers alone. In numerous water cooler conversations, team members expressed anxiety and confusion about the feasibility of the team's work. Since their focus had traditionally been so exclusively on responding to the consequences of health inequity—smoking, infant mortality, lead paint— some began to feel a dissonance between the ideas of the Social Justice Project and their normal work roles. Besides, did we really think that our department alone would be able to meaningfully change the underlying conditions we were talking about?

To help the team members wrestle with their internal conflicts about the shift from consequences to root causes, I developed exercises to augment the dialogue process, three of them described below in sequence.

1. Changing the questions

At the second meeting of the team, the facilitator introduced the idea that, in our traditional roles as public health workers, our work is shaped by questions that focus on health outcomes. To make clearer to ourselves what it means to shift toward a focus on root causes, perhaps we need to reframe these questions that guide our work. Four examples were offered, as shown in Table 13.1.

The following assignment was then given to the team members: "Construct a question that your unit of the Health Department currently

TABLE 13.1. "Changing the Questions" Examples

INSTEAD OF ONLY ASKING...	PERHAPS WE SHOULD ALSO ASK...
Why do people smoke?	What social conditions and economic policies predispose people to the stress that encourages smoking?
Who lacks health care coverage, and why?	What policy changes would redistribute health care resources more equitably in our community?
How do we connect isolated individuals to a social network?	What institutional policies and practices maintain rather than counteract people's isolation from social supports?
How can we create more green space, bike paths, and farmer's markets in vulnerable neighborhoods?	What policies and practices by government and commerce discourage access to transportation, recreational resources, and nutritious food in neighborhoods where health is poorest?

TABLE 13.2. Points of View for Role-play Dialogue

PERSON "A"	PERSON "B"
Changing behaviors is the best way to improve health. Focusing on things like racism just distracts people from taking personal responsibility for their behaviors. We cannot end racism—it is too big and too pervasive.	Our mission is to preserve and protect the public health. If racism prevents people from having a good education, a good job, and good health, we have to address racism. We have a responsibility to look at underlying social forces that predispose people to ill health.

asks as a routine part of its work, and create an alternative question that reframes it in a social justice context." The assignment proved to be difficult for many team members, who at the next meeting talked more about the struggle itself than an actual reframed question they had designed. It did, however, illuminate the fundamental difference in approach that a social justice orientation entailed: the difference between addressing *causes* rather than the *consequences* of inequity.

2. Role-play dialogue

At the fourth meeting, team members were paired off and asked to role-play a conversation about the issue of addressing a root cause of health inequity (racism), versus addressing the behaviors that contribute to poor health. The following points of view were assigned to the two players in each conversation:

In several of the pairs in Table 13.2 , the person playing the "A" role found it difficult to maintain the pretense of resistance, because it did not match their own point of view. It was also common for pairs to move to a middle-ground position rather than resolve the difference of opinion, probably to avoid conflict. The exercise served as a rehearsal for many conversations the team would engage in as the rest of the department began to hear of the team's work. The team needed to find ways to explain that a focus on root causes does *not* negate all of the work we do to help people adopt healthy behaviors.

3. "How far upstream?" exercise

This exercise was introduced during the seventh meeting to explore the team's understanding of activities that are truly *upstream*, that is, addressing the root causes rather than the consequences of health inequity. Four levels of "upstream-ness" were proposed, and three groups of five

TABLE 13.3. "Levels of Upstream-ness" for the "How Far Upstream?" Exercise

Level 1: "Upstream"	An activity that attempts to eliminate those things in the social structure that deny certain people voice, power, and political influence in society (such as class exploitation, racism, and gender discrimination)
Level 2: "Moderately Upstream"	An activity that directly attempts to give people access to the things that will help them obtain an equal footing with those who are currently privileged (such as quality education, low-interest loans, inclusion in social networks)
Level 3: "A Little Upstream"	An activity that moves people from conditions that impede health into conditions that support health (such as secure and good-paying jobs, quality and affordable housing, access to transportation)
Level 4: "Downstream"	An activity that relieves stress or changes unhealthy behaviors (such as support groups, smoking cessation campaigns, family planning education)

participants each then talked about ten proposed activities, attempting to determine which level the activity represented. The definitions of the four levels are shown in Table 13.3.[9]

The team found this exercise extremely helpful in revealing and challenging ideas about what activities will really impact root causes. One common discovery was that certain activities, such as "publishing a report," "convening a dialogue," or "disseminating the findings of focus groups" on issues pertinent to class, race, and gender discrimination *could* be Level 1, but only if they were followed up with corrective action. A report that exposed health inequities would not necessarily eliminate the causes of inequity, participants asserted, *unless it was intentionally used to that end.*

In some cases, individuals believed that activities most people considered Level 3 or 4—for instance, a safe sex pamphlet in Spanish—could be considered more upstream because they were targeted to people who were otherwise denied access to information. The prevailing view, however, was that the only acceptable norm was to provide such information to all, and that the pamphlet's purpose was clearly downstream, that is, changing an unhealthy behavior.

"Placing an ad for a vacant administrative position in publications targeted to communities of color" was also considered Level 1 by many, but not all. Again, the key considerations were (1) whether this was undoing an existing failure of the organization to adequately recruit qualified minority candidates for positions, and (2) whether the activity actually resulted in attracting people of color to apply for positions of power in the organization.

Challenge 2: The Leadership Role of the Health Department

As mentioned earlier, throughout the dialogue process tension arose over just how much the health department—and the Social Justice Team—could be expected to do to address the root causes of health inequity. At one end of the spectrum, some team members tended to focus on situational concerns that they noticed, either in the department or the community. Others were quite willing to recommend broad, sweeping policy changes, many of which were well beyond the power of the health department alone to effect. Over the course of the three dialogues, the team moved gradually toward a middle ground: recommendations that placed the health department in a catalytic role, helping to move both ourselves and other institutions toward changes in policy and practice.

This tension resurfaced when the Social Justice Team began meeting with senior staff in July 2005 to translate the 20 preliminary recommendations into an Action Plan. During the beginning of these sessions, some of the comments by team members again focused on very specific incidences of social injustice that they believed were occurring in our community, and implied that it was the department's responsibility to call attention to them. This alarmed some senior staff, who expressed concern that the Social Justice Team now intended for the health department to respond immediately to every incident of social injustice that anyone in the health department detected, rather than systematically laying out strategies for addressing the root causes of health inequity. In turn, some members of the team interpreted this to mean that top administration was ignoring the hard work of the team, and considered abandoning the project as a consequence.

Two things were happening, both predictable. In a hierarchical environment, any bottom-up rather than top-down process will likely produce tension when senior administration enters into a dialogue that has heretofore involved only midlevel and front line staff. Until senior administrators in our department could be more fully exposed to the information, feelings, and insights that had emerged from the team's process, they viewed its findings with understandable skepticism. At the team's request, after the first joint session, the Health Officer met with members of the team who explained to them the developmental nature of the recommendations and the team's concern that they were being prematurely dismissed by senior staff. At the next session, the Health Officer and other administrators clarified both their position on the scope of the recommendations, and their support for the team's work. No one resigned from the team, and the remainder of the initial action-planning process proceeded smoothly. This was the first but certainly not the last time the Social Justice Team found itself in a tense relationship with senior administration over the nature of its work; in each case dialogue has been critical to resolving the tension.

Secondly—and more critically—our department was just beginning to wrestle with a thornier question: what *is* the leadership role for a health department to play in addressing class oppression, institutional racism, and gender discrimination in its community? Regionally and across the state of Michigan, ICHD enjoys a well-earned reputation for creatively brokering resources and fostering collaborative responses to community problems. It does this primarily by convening and facilitating, not by asserting or demanding action. The uncomfortable question behind many of the action-planning dialogues was whether, in the name of health equity, we would suddenly be doing more. Would the health department, as some members of the Social Justice Team clearly believed, carry a brighter banner for others to follow? Would we become more activist in our pursuit of social and environmental justice? How would this diminish our reputation as a neutral convener and facilitator of collaborative action?

And who, ultimately, decides? One of the clear lessons of the *Community Voices* initiative was that neighborhoods and communities are their own best advocates for change. Empowerment of grassroots partners through dialogue led to new, bottom-up infrastructure aimed at creating social cohesion in vulnerable parts of our community, and new support for covering the uninsured. Through the Social Justice Project, public health workers were similarly empowered by dialogue to recommend action to improve community health by attacking the root causes of health inequity. If we asked community members the same questions we had asked ourselves about health equity and social justice, would they come up with the same answers? This would be revealed in subsequent phases of the project, which I describe in the next section.

Given the wide differences that exist between local health departments and the way they function in their communities, it may be useful to think of the department's "change agent" role on a continuum (Figure 13.3). In some instances, under certain circumstances, ICHD's most appropriate role may be to aid others in community planning by providing accurate information. In other cases, it may be to engage the community by facilitating dialogue, or mobilizing the community around catalytic action. In cases

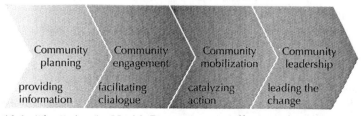

FIGURE 13.3   The Role of a Health Department in Effecting Change: A Continuum.

where no other role will be effective in impacting a problem—structural racism, for example—it may indeed need to lead because no one else will do so.

Challenge 3: How Explicitly "Transforming" Can Dialogue Be?

On its surface, dialogue facilitation appears to be a passive function. Its goal is to enable a diverse group of people to share insights, listen deeply, and generate recommendations derived from its collective intelligence. A central premise of this book is that local health departments need to *transform their policy and practice* in order to create health equity through social justice. Can such a passive enterprise as facilitated dialogue possibly do this? Two dilemmas of facilitation are entwined in that question: the supposed neutrality of a good facilitator of dialogue, and the temptation to predetermine the outcome of the dialogue.

As facilitator of each of the dialogues described in this chapter, I found it very difficult to facilitate questions of social justice in quite the same way I have facilitated hundreds of other dialogues over the past decade. Throughout the process, I adopted a much more assertive role than I normally do, overtly advancing social justice concepts rather than patiently eliciting them from the group. The first meeting's conversation about personal responsibility was a good example of this. Normally, when faced with a situation where one member of the group holds an outlier position, my course of action is to help that person be heard and understood by others. In this case, when the health educator asserted that a focus on root causes might undermine her clients' struggle to take personal responsibility for their health, I overtly challenged the opinion, leaving her to fend for herself against the tide of contrary opinion already present in the room. While a more facilitative approach would probably have been more effective in this case, I have a growing conviction that one cannot facilitate issues of social justice from an assumed stance of neutrality because neutrality is so often the stance that allows members of privileged groups to discount their privilege and maintain the status quo ("I don't see color," "I treat all people the same"). I must reveal my belief that social injustice is real and at the root of health inequity if I am to facilitate *this* dialogue effectively.

Still, I believe that effective dialogue is premised on what James Surowiecki has termed, in the title of his intriguing book, *The Wisdom of Crowds*.[10] According to Suroweicki, if certain conditions are in place— namely diversity, independence, and decentralization—any random group of people will be smarter in addressing a problem than a group of certified experts. The basic reason for this is that the random group brings an abundance of knowledge, experience, and insight to the problem-solving process, whereas, in most cases, the experts each bring essentially the same knowledge, experience, and insight: conventional expertise. This should be equally true when the focus of dialogue is on exposing and eliminating something as pervasive as institutional racism. Conventional experts will reveal conventional paths to change that very often only serve to maintain the status quo. Only through the voices of those who experience oppression and exploitation in all its modern, veiled forms can we hope to reach consensus on the need to transform institutional policy and practice. The facilitator's job must be to empower those voices. The very concept of unearned privilege on the basis of race, class, or gender predicts that, unless the voices of the oppressed are heard and validated, those in privilege will discount, deny, and ultimately suppress them.

A well-facilitated dialogue can be seen as an attempt to set the conditions for applying Suroweicki's premise. Facilitators present information. Participants share impressions and experiences, and collectively identify their insights. Everyone together produces promising actions and strategies, which they then systematically collect, articulate, and validate. But how can these conditions be met if the entire enterprise has an explicit expectation that we must transform public health practice? The assumption that current conditions are inherently wrong or inferior (public health's abandonment of its historic role in advancing social justice) automatically skews the dialogue toward predetermined outcomes, and could very well in the process disenfranchise the contribution of some participants. This is a challenge that anyone attempting to facilitate dialogue on social justice must confront.

In trying to resolve this challenge for myself, I was frequently drawn back to my experience with the *Community Voices* initiative—in particular, the comparative ease with which change occurred when the questions we asked avoided an *assumption* that change was necessary.

Prior to the *Community Voices* dialogues in 1999 and 2000, most health care stakeholders in Ingham County actively opposed the pursuit of universal health care as a goal. The dialogue process that followed therefore framed the question instead around a less daunting proposition—"organized systems of care for the uninsured"—which virtually all stakeholders had an interest in achieving. The recommendations from the dialogue process were instrumental in rallying community support for a new, collaboratively managed health care plan that achieved coverage of 62% of the county's uninsured within four years. Similarly, local policy makers opposed the concept of neighborhood network centers because they anticipated a competition for the resources needed to create them. But the *Community Voices* summit dialogues asked a more universal question: how do we create health in our community? The summits resulted in the funding of neighborhood hubs for grassroots-driven health initiatives throughout the city of Lansing.

What does this tell us about the use of dialogue in addressing social justice? I do not mean to suggest that we must avoid words like "transformation" or "fundamental change in the social structure" just to avoid alarming those who are invested in maintaining the (inequitable) status quo. But timing matters, as the next three years of our project demonstrated. In the first phase of the work, we sensed that an explicit goal of transforming our practice would put too many in our workforce on the defensive, so we found other, more innocuous words, for example, "improving our effectiveness by confronting health inequities." This did not fully calm the anxieties of managers and front line workers who openly worried about what our agenda was. But it did allow us enough time to let the fundamental ideas of social justice and health inequity to percolate in the hearts and minds of our organization. Transformation, we trusted, would come later.

From Action to Traction

Is talk action?

This was the simple question posed to the 250 people gathered for a "Community Conversation on Health and Social Justice" in Lansing in June 2006. Community members and health and human service providers convened to hear the findings of the Social Justice Project, and to add their voices to the experience and insights that had contributed to its Action Plan.

Typical of the next phase of Ingham County's Social Justice Project, this event involved sharing many things—data, experiences, preliminary recommendations for action—but it did not provide a clear pathway toward community or departmental change. Agencies, grassroots organizations, and young people praised the health department for confronting the root causes of poor health outcomes. People of all ages and walks of life made personal declarations of their commitment to continue the work on an individual basis. But the Action Plan that had been developed did not make any concrete progress toward implementation.

Nor did it make much progress over the next year of health department activity. Between the fall of 2005 and the summer of 2007, the original team continued to meet, though less frequently, and to discuss ways to pursue recommendations of the Action Plan. On two occasions, team members met again with senior staff to gain approval for its next proposed activities. These meetings ended with an understanding that management would pursue certain action steps in the plan, but none in a way that would substantially reorient the department from business as usual. Over time, the team increasingly believed that senior administrators were reluctant to do any more than continue *talking* about the need for change.

Two inhibiting factors surfaced during this period. The first was the team's lack of confidence in the administration's support for pursuing a visible social justice agenda, as reflected in its suggestion that the department should not overreach its sphere of influence by responding to nonhealth concerns. Although Ingham County is known to be socially progressive within Michigan, clearly our own department was not comfortable shifting our focus toward root causes such as institutional racism. Team members consequently approached such areas of its action plan as Policy Reform with caution. Rather than charging forward with evidence intended to revise local housing or economic policy, we proposed a series of presentations to area consortia. While well received and conspicuously praised in the community, these sessions were hardly transformative; they would best be characterized as community conscious raising.

The second inhibiting factor had more to do with what the team had discovered about our own department in its initial dialogues in 2005. During that 5-month process, the team's internal analysis of ICHD and its organizational culture revealed a deep sense of denial—a "cultural of politeness," according to one participant—that racism, classism, and sexism existed to any significant degree in our own agency. Beneath our reputation as a progressive and enlightened organization, the Social Justice Team discovered another reality: an almost reflexive dismissal of perceived discrimination within our own workplace. While examples of overt racism or other forms of discrimination in the workplace were rare, employees were quick to recall isolated examples of racist, classist, or sexist behavior or language—and, more importantly, the unwillingness of supervisors to accept or investigate them. Within the organization, it appeared that an entirely unprogressive message had been learned, especially by people of color: if you see racism, keep it to yourself or risk being labeled as "playing the race card." For the Social Justice Team, this implied a certain hypocrisy in our Action Plan. Who were we to educate the community about health and social inequity when we had not yet taken steps to put our own house in order?

Consequently, rather than directly transforming either policy or practice, this interim phase of social justice work focused on considerably lower-hanging fruit:

- *Policy reform*: By making the case for the root causes of health inequity, ICHD persuaded a major multipurpose community collaborative, the Power of We Consortium to add health inequity as an indicator in its triennial report on community well-being. Labeled as "under construction," the indicator lacked hard data in the 2007 report, but included two pages describing health inequity, its importance in addressing community health, and the challenges of measurement. A work group led by the health department is attempting to construct a measure of health inequity to be included in the 2010 edition.

- *Information and communication*: While no formal change occurred in the department's information and communications function, the staff person tasked with managing department communications, as well as the Medical Examiner, consciously attempted to incorporate health equity and social justice themes into their public responses to disease outbreaks and in columns for local newspapers.
- *Community engagement and mobilization*: The Social Justice Project coordinator's job expectations were formally changed to allow him to facilitate planning processes for outside organizations on topics whose work affected the social determinants of health: housing and foreclosure policy, land use, the elimination of food deserts, neighborhood empowerment, and so forth. While this exemplified the department deploying its resources in a new way, it only affected one employee's practice—the one whose job assignment specifically included work on social justice issues.
- *Partnerships:* ICHD regularly presented its dialogue and action-planning process to other organizations and community groups, and was frequently invited to do so from groups that at least gave lip service to their intentions of tackling root causes. These presentations created important connections to individuals within organizations; they did not however result in strategic alliances across organizations to confront health inequity.
- *Public health workforce*: From 2005 to 2007, the Social Justice Team sponsored informal, voluntary lunchtime dialogue sessions with department staff, usually in conjunction with video discussion triggers such as the three episodes of California Newsreel's series, *Race: The Power of an Illusion*. These sessions, attended by 30–60 staff, evoked franker conversations about race, class, and gender than had heretofore been the norm for the department.

More than anything, it was the lunchtime dialogues that created an opportunity for internal traction for the ideas of health equity and social justice. Although a frequent complaint of those who attended the sessions was that "the people who really need to hear this aren't coming," the sessions enabled senior staff to get a different view of the department's comfort level with issues of race, class, and gender. The department leadership began to gain a new appreciation of the need to reorient our workforce, our policies, and our practice, and of the challenges involved in doing so. With the appointment of a new Health Officer in January 2007—the former Medical Examiner, who had been consistently attentive to the project from the beginning—a new opportunity for traction emerged. This involved both a reorganization of the department, the intentional hiring of administrative staff who would champion the transformative nature of the Social Justice Project, and a reexamination of the organization's core values.

From Traction to Transformation: Expanding the Dialogue

Following the incubation period, the next phase of activity might be called Learning to Walk. In June 2008, ICHD's commitment to transforming its practice as well as the community's consciousness of the health implications of racism, class oppression, and gender discrimination has never been more visible or intentional. It has also never been more rooted in the primacy of dialogue as a vehicle for the transformation.

In the fall of 2007, several months prior to his appointment, our new Health Officer began actively recruiting people to the department who would support and sustain a more substantial effort to transform the department's focus. Six months after becoming the Health Officer, he completed a departmental reorganization that notably changed the organization. What had for decades been a top tier of 10 or 11 senior staff, all but 2 of whom were white males, was replaced by a team of 3 Deputy Health Officers, one of whom had been explicitly recruited because of her experience and expertise on issues of health inequity. This new administrator, in charge of approximately one-third of the organization, included nearly all of the work units classified as traditional public health (Communicable Disease Control, Public Health Nursing, etc.) as well as those with the strongest ties to the community and interagency collaboration (Community Health Assessment, Health Promotion, etc.). The Social Justice Project coordinator, who had previously reported to the Health Officer while remaining formally disconnected to other parts of the organization, now had an organizational home within this division.

Within this new environment, the remaining core of the original Social Justice team quickly proposed to use a large portion of the limited Social Justice budget[11] to launch a train-the-facilitators program. The purpose of the program was to create the capacity within the department *and within the community* to facilitate both training and dialogue that would advance people's understanding of the root causes of health inequity. All health department staff would subsequently be trained by the new team, and would, upon completion of training, be able to:

- Describe modern forms of discrimination, and appropriate responses to these forms of discrimination when they are encountered in the community or the workplace.

- Explain the principles of social justice and health equity, their relevance to public health practice, and their primacy as values of the Ingham County Health Department.
- Specify in concrete terms changes in their own behavior or work practice that they are committed to making as a result of participation in training.

Thirty people were recruited to be a part of the "Social Justice Facilitator Training," which consisted of 12 full days of in-depth exploration of the personal, interpersonal, institutional, and cultural levels at which oppression and change occur. These training days occurred over the course of 5 months, with the expectation that at least 20 participants would successfully complete the program and be able to begin facilitating in-house trainings for the ICHD staff. Trainees, recruited both from the department's workforce and the community, included grassroots, neighborhood, and religious groups as well as other institutional partners. As of 2008, 28 of the trainees have completed the training, including 15 ICHD employees and 13 community members. Staff training for the department's 310 employees will begin in the fall of 2008.

Every stage of the train-the-facilitator program was intentionally rooted in dialogue, including the recruitment process.[12] The training cadre included highly educated professionals from many disciplines as well as front line staff and community members whose struggles to overcome personal and institutional discrimination were ever present. The training itself provided abundant opportunities for trainees to share personal examples of their experience of oppression and privilege across many forms of difference, and in so doing create a common language for framing that experience at four levels: the *personal* (individual thoughts, beliefs, values); *interpersonal* (behavior, action, language), *institutional* (rules, policies, procedures), and *cultural* (collective ideas of what is normal, right, true, or beautiful).[13] In retrospect, this concept of four levels of oppression and change was fundamental to the course that the original Social Justice Team had charted for ICHD. Based upon the early reluctance of administrators to consciously change practice and the frustration felt by employees when raising issues of race, class, and gender within the department, we concluded that change at the *institutional* level would not be possible until changes at the *personal* and *interpersonal* levels had occurred for a critical mass of our workforce.

The resulting cadre of trainee/trainers has proved remarkably adept in challenging each other and the group as a whole in assumptions about personal and cultural values, the multiple dimensions across which power and privilege operate, and what it takes to become comfortable with discomfort in addressing all levels of oppression and change in the community.

Several team members have also described this as a "new line of account-ability," that is, a mutual responsibility to remain in authentic relationship across differences through the tools provided in the training.

Future staff trainings will also be rooted in learning through dialogue rather than imposing the concepts of equity and justice didactically. Each training will involve a maximum of 15 employees drawn from across the department's organizational units, and up to five members of the community who have expressed an interest in the project. By facilitating small numbers of people in viewing public health through the lens of social justice, we believe the transformation of the institution and its culture will become possible and, with the clear endorsement of our senior managers, inevitable.

The 28 facilitators-in-training will engage in facilitating this transformation in other ways as well. Recognizing that not all of those who completed the training would feel comfortable with the function of facilitating full-scale trainings, two other functions have been proposed. One will focus on resurrecting and implementing the Action Plan. The other will sustain and support those in the department and the community who wish to continue participating in dialogue on their experience of the four levels of oppression and change through a resource that team members have informally dubbed the "Healing Circle."

Conclusion

Although it is too soon to judge the ultimate success of the Social Justice Project in transforming public health practice in Ingham County, three preliminary conclusions can be drawn about the use of dialogue as a means toward that end.

1. Dialogue processes of this nature must be sustained over time, with consistent participation and decision making by a core group that eventually expands to include others.

For many local health departments, resource limitations are likely to discourage embarking on an extended dialogue process like the one initiated in Ingham County. Rather than dedicate 20 or so staff to the effort over several months, a more short-term or incremental approach may be favored: a 2-day retreat, perhaps, or a single session to outline options for the department. While such short-term efforts will not necessarily diminish a department's ability to address the root causes of health inequity, they are not likely to improve it unless the department is willing to invest in a more extensive process—one that truly challenges its participants' assumptions and eventually the assumptions of the department itself.

If the participants in the Ingham County team are at all representative, ideas about the appropriate role of public health workers are deeply ingrained. So is a sense of helplessness in the face of social forces that seem beyond their power to undo. Many of the participants in this 8-month process vacillated regularly between extremes of hope and despair about the team's potential to bring about real change. Interestingly, team members did not simply settle into these attitudes and stay there; the most doubtful participant one week might well become the leading proponent of perseverance in the next. This to me is one hallmark of a team committed and mutually supportive—qualities that can only be created through sustained and intensive collaboration.

Any local health department that empowers a team of public health workers to tackle social justice issues through dialogue needs to be clear and consistent in its support of their struggle. Specifically, it should not interpret the team's early vagueness or inconsistency as a sign that the process is faltering. It is very difficult to rethink one's institutional role and the core practices of one's profession and this is exactly what we are asking public health workers to do. Moreover, we should fully expect that the struggle will begin anew as each new set of participants joins the process. The Action Planning phase of the Ingham County process, during which senior staff interacted directly with the team for the first time, brought with it a whole new wave of doubt about administration's sincerity in supporting the team's work. Over the course of four facilitated meetings, this settled into a new, common understanding of how and why the team's recommendations would be implemented. As each successive training group is introduced to these issues through our new training program, we expect to encounter new skepticism and resistance, which will only erode after sustained exposure to the link between social injustice and health inequity.

2. Dialogue facilitators (and participants) should anticipate and accept that conflict, resistance, and tension are natural and inevitable elements of the process.

Opportunities for miscommunication and misunderstanding are abundant in the course of a dialogue or training process that focuses on class exploitation, institutionalized racism, and gender discrimination as root causes of health inequity. I have described some of these: the tensions that arise over personal responsibility, the cynicism workers in any bureaucratic environment are likely to feel toward organizational change, and the perception that it is the health department's job to correct every incident of social injustice that occurs in the community. An even more obvious source of potential conflict exists: differing outlooks on race and racism, and the different ways team members are likely to express themselves on these issues. No facilitator of the kind of process described in this chapter should expect to avoid conflict, resistance, and tension when race is the topic of discussion.

Excellent resources are available in communities for helping personnel become more adept and graceful in addressing race and racism, both in the workplace and in life. In the initial phase of our project, ICHD called on one such resource to help establish a relationship between the Social Justice Team and senior administrators through a 2-day workshop on "The Culture of Power and Privilege."[14] In our most recent phase of activity, we have recognized the need to develop the internal capacity to provide similar trainings to all our employees. The latter trainings will have a distinct difference, however. While we expect them to do much to improve multicultural understanding and enable our employees to engage in difficult conversation about race and racism, this is not their *primary* objective. Their primary objective is to change how our health department addresses the root causes of health inequity. We will not end racism in our own organization, let alone in our community. We will, however, be better equipped to identify it, name it, and mute its power to oppress communities of color.

I am hoping to dispel the notion that everyone must be in consensus about the need and value of refocusing public health practice before the work can move forward. I question whether such consensus has ever existed, and certainly would not advise anyone to strive to achieve it before launching a dialogue on health equity and social justice. In the case of Ingham's Social Justice Team, many troubled conversations occurred before and after team meetings, especially in the early weeks of the project. Several team members believed that others on the team were not "getting" social justice, or understanding the appropriate role of the health department, or acknowledging their own subtle prejudices toward a particular target group. Were they correct? In some cases, probably yes. Did it matter? In the long view, no. These tensions were part of a mutual learning process that required us to go through challenging self-reflection at the personal, interpersonal, and institutional levels.

The facilitator's tasks in this type of dialogue are to get people to think and talk as honestly as they can; to articulate the *collective* wisdom of the group as it emerges; and to assure continuous forward motion toward action. With regard to the problem of participants being at differing levels of understanding during the dialogue, the facilitator's task is not to remedy the dissonance but rather to identify it, move beyond it as efficiently as possible without diminishing its importance, and return to the work at hand: how do we, as a health department, address the root causes of

health inequity? In answering that question, it is important that participants bring differing and even conflicting experiences and insights to the
process.

3. The goal of critically examining public health practice should be
explicitly understood at the outset by key actors in the process.

Often, people, groups, and institutions do not like change. Therefore, they
are more likely to transform when they do not know that a transformation
is occurring. In practical terms, what does this mean for someone contem-
plating a sustained dialogue process intended to transform a local health
department's practice as it relates to the root causes of health inequity?
How much does one tip one's hand to the department at large that the
intent of the Social Justice Project is to change how we all do our work?

For any individual health department, of course, the exact answer to
those questions will depend upon its unique organizational culture, top
administrators' level of commitment to tackling social justice issues, and
the values and attitudes of the community the department serves. The chief
lesson to be drawn from the Ingham County experience as it has unfolded
thus far is that department administrators (the Health Officer, at least)
should know that a goal of the project is the critical examination of the
department's practice in relation to its mission. Without this understanding, any work by the facilitator or the team will run the risk of appearing
to overstep its boundaries as soon as anything that smacks of transformation emerges from the team's work. If our intent is to make a fundamental
difference in the way public health workers think and work, we must do
it with administrative permission to bring about that level of change. We
must also do it under a banner that acknowledges *social justice* as a concern of the health department (as opposed to less fundamental terms such
as "diversity," "disparity," or "cultural competency").

But we must resolve a larger question: what does transformed public
health practice look like? Although no one can absolutely describe the
elements of a local health department that has successfully reclaimed its
social justice legacy, Chapter 1 of this book offers broad suggestions.
Transformed public health practice is self critical and examined; it builds
capacity based on evaluation and assessment; it adapts; it is mission
driven not program focused. Transformed public health practice will likely
require changes in workforce development and education, public policy
development and analysis, addressing health inequity through the essential
services of public health, and so forth. If that is so, then why we do not
simply focus on those features of our practice? Why do we need a dialogue
process that engages public health workers in an examination of the local
impact of racism on health inequity?

Returning to the problem outlined at the beginning of this chapter, a facilitated dialogue process has the potential to create a unique impulse for change that moves outward from the ranks of the organization, and outward from grassroots community partners. That impulse, unlike one that is top-down in nature, fosters change from the inside-out—change that is less susceptible to the change-resistance mechanisms of bureaucratic institutions. Such a process will only have meaning if those who empower it in the first place know its potential to generate great changes in practice. Ironically, such a process will also likely be sabotaged if its goal is too widely portrayed as undoing the status quo too early in the process.

In Ingham County, the Social Justice Project was initiated by the Health Officer and assigned to me in my role as the department's facilitator-at-large. Early communications about the project deliberately avoided any references to transforming public health practice. Rather, they described more innocuous goals such as "improving our responsiveness" to the root causes of health inequity. I believe the mildness of such terminology was important to the initial phase of work. It allowed the team to operate for at least a while without provoking objections from middle managers and others who might fear the team's objective.

The project now enters a new phase of transformation, one that will expose every member of our workforce to information and experience explicitly designed to change how he or she sees the world and the work of public health. This would not have been possible in 2005. The very idea of putting all of our employees through such a training would have been questioned and challenged by nearly every manager in the organization. In 2008, such training is seen by senior administration as critical to our mission and our values. The community is not only applauding, it is actively joining in the work of training our workforce. Individual employees continue to question the wisdom of our department's shift toward a social justice orientation, but they do so with a sense that the shift has already been made, as reflected in our organizational values.

Is talk—dialogue—action? This much seems clear. In Ingham County, dialogue begun in 2005 was the catalyst between successive collective actions that made the reality of 2008 imaginable.

Notes

1. In keeping with the Action Plans generated by their summits, the activities taken by grassroots workers displayed a broad interpretation of what constituted "health." While some projects addressed conventional health promotion targets such as smoking cessation and breast cancer prevention, others aimed

more toward the social determinants of health: home ownership and improvement, GED acquisition, assistance in filing for Earned Income Tax Credits, and so forth. Most of these projects have only grown and proliferated in subsequent years, as new sponsoring partners become aware of their success and neighborhood groups modify and replicate each others' ideas.

2. This sentiment on health though community empowerment and action was clearly expressed in the 1986 WHO Ottawa Charter for Health Promotion. See Vol. 1(4) *Health Promotion International* (1986): 405.

3. Ingham County Health Department employs approximately 310 people, which is considerably large for a county health department in Michigan. Major divisions include Environmental Health, Public Health Nursing, Disease Control, Health Plan Management, Community Health Clinical Services, Emergency Preparedness, Community Health Assessment, Communicable Disease Control, and Financial Services. As configured in 2005, "senior staff" refers to the heads of these divisions, along with the Health Officer and Medical Examiner. In 2007, the department was reorganized under a new Health Officer. This reorganization and its positive impact on the project is discussed later in the chapter.

4. Although the facilitation method and dialogue process used in Ingham County is not identical to that taught in the Technologies of Participation training, it is unquestionably grounded in the core ideas of that training, particularly the sequence of questions asked, which ICA labels as "Objective, Reflective, Interpretive, and Decisional" or "ORID." Readers of this chapter should not regard the process described here as reflecting the content of the ToP training, and should certainly not view it as a substitute for enrolling in ICA's excellent training course—more information about which can be found at www.ica-usa. org.

5. Visit www.teachingeconomics.org

6. California Newsreel, San Francisco, CA; www.newsreel.org

7. The adhesive board or curtain is an important tool for anyone using Institute for Cultural Affairs' Technologies of Participation methodology. Essentially a portable, plastic surface sprayed with artist's spray mount, it provides a viewing area for ideas and thoughts to be arranged and rearranged during the course of a facilitated dialogue.

8. Again, readers are urged to consult the Institute for Cultural Affairs' Technologies of Participation training for guidance in applying this group facilitation method.

9. Metaphoric use of the terms "upstream" and "downstream" have recently been challenged as inaccurate and inappropriate in conveying the way in which social change is accomplished. As has been pointed out by Nancy Krieger ("Proximal, Distal, and the Politics of Causation: What's Level Got to Do with It," 98(2) *American Journal of Public Health* (February, 2008): 221–330), the consequences of oppression do not necessarily unfold as a cascading series of causes and effects. Rather, in some instances, a single policy event (for example, the Supreme Court's decision in *Roe vs. Wade*) can have instantaneous social repercussions throughout the metaphoric "stream." Caution is therefore advised in the use of this exercise as it is framed here.

10. James Surowiecki, *The Wisdom of Crowds: Why the Many Are Smarter Than the Few and How Collective Wisdom Shapes Business, Economies, Societies and Nations* (New York: Doubleday, 2004).

11. Ingham County received two successive grants from the W.K. Kellogg Foundation to advance this work. In both cases, however, the overwhelming majority of funding was contracted out to other entities (NACCHO and other local health agencies' initiating dialogue-based social justice work), with ICHD acting as fiduciary. Approximately $40,000 per year was retained by ICHD, none of which was applied to personnel. All funds were instead applied to capacity building, education/awareness tools, or meeting costs to support community dialogue.

12. Rather than participate in a conventional interview, applicants convened in groups of 4–7 to engage in a free-flowing conversation about their personal experience and reflections on multiculturalism, health equity, and social justice. Applicants were encouraged to ask as well as answer questions that emerged in the hour-long dialogue, and were assessed not only on their current knowledge and skills, but also on their curiosity and potential to grow in their understanding of core concepts.

13. This model for describing Levels of Oppression and Change was created by VISIONS Inc., Roxbury, MA; see web site at www.vision-inc.org.

14. Michigan State University Extension Multicultural Education Programming. Michigan State University Extension offers a number of multicultural education programs. Interested parties may contact Karen Pace at pace@msue.msu. edu. for more information.

14

The Metro Louisville Center for Health Equity: Expanding the Circle of Engagement

ADEWALE TROUTMAN

In the winter of 2006, the Metro Louisville Health Department established the Center for Health Equity. This was one of the first such centers operating as an independent division within a local health department. This chapter presents briefly the Center's historical context and goals and earliest actions. It is organized to combine community-based research, education, advocacy, services, staff training, and communication strategies toward the elimination of health inequity within a social justice perspective.

Introduction: The Historical Context

The necessity for action to address the shortened quantity of life and the inferior quality of life on the nation's communities of color and poor, particularly the racial and ethnic groups most severely impacted by these phenomena, is inescapable. We know through the work of Drs Michael Byrd and Linda Clayton that differences in health access and outcomes was institutionalized in the African American community through the wretched institution of slavery.[1] The health of the Asian American immigrants who toiled on the nations railroad is profiled in California Newsreel's "Race the Power of an Illusion."[2] Tragic circumstances have befallen the Native American/

American Indian population, including genocide, centuries of broken treaties, raging infectious diseases, and the destruction of social structure, traditions, and community capacity. W.E.B. Dubois' *The Philadelphia Negro*, published in 1899, documented in a landmark study that the African American community indeed suffered from worse health than the white community in America.[3]

The Negro Health Week that has morphed into National Minority Health Month was a decade-long effort to raise awareness of these health differences, build coalitions to address these issues, and sponsor programs to bring an action agenda to the work. In spite of the community center movement of the mid-60s, the release of the Heckler Report, "The Task Force Report on Black and Minority Health," was the first single set of data, analysis, and recommendations that the nation had, which concentrated on the health and excess death of its "Minority" residents.[4] It raised awareness within a certain sector of the community but never reached the masses of American society. It elevated the discussion about health among the professions but never became a national priority.

Healthy People began a process of bringing these "revelations" into the planning process with goals and objectives meant to improve the nation's health. Of course Healthy People 2000 had two sets of objectives, one for communities of color and one for the majority population in the United States. It was not until Healthy People 2010 that the nation eliminated separate objectives by populations and recognized the elimination of health disparities by 2010 as one of two overarching goals for the nation's health plan for that decade.[5]

The increasing awareness and focus on the role of social determinants of health has led to recognition of a need to reframe our thinking and thus our action. We argue that occupation, education, income, housing, discrimination, stress, social isolation, addiction, and many other factors play a key role in determining the health of populations in America and indeed around the world. It is an awareness that has led to the use of more universal terms like equity and inequity and connecting them to the principles of human rights and social justice. Many of the forces at play in determining the health of populations in America have their roots in the global community. Issues such as free trade and globalization do indeed impact health. Our awareness of the role of social determinants has of course been elevated by the work of the WHO Commission on the Social Determinants of Health.[6]

It is out of this consciousness that the Center for Health Equity was created to take local action to eliminate health inequities. As one of the first such institutional endeavors within a local health department in the nation, the Center has had to develop its own model of work and has faced many obstacles. Its experiences may serve as a model for other cities to examine for its explicability in their locales.

Louisville's Historical Legacy

Louisville is by far the largest metropolitan area in the state of Kentucky. In this state of greater than four million people, over 700,000 call Louisville home. Of that number, approximately 19% are African American with about 5% Latino and other. It sits on the banks of the Ohio River and is home to Muhammad Ali and the recently completed Ali Center for Peace and Justice. It is also the home of the Kentucky Derby. The state theme song, until recently, included the words "it's summer, the darkies are gay." Under the newly merged government, it is the 16th largest city in the nation. However, this growing city by the river is in fact two cities—one East, white, prosperous, and healthy; one West, economically deprived, African American, and a poster child for negative outcomes on measures of the social determinants of health.

Research and Planning in the Local Health Department

In Louisville, in 2006, a departmental strategic planning process resulted in the development of seven strategic goals. One of the goals mirrored that of Healthy People 2010, simply stating that the health department would improve the health and wellness of the Louisville community. The second, however, stated that the department would create *Health Equity through Social Justice in Louisville*.

At the beginning, the language of health inequities was foreign to much of the Louisville community. We began by making the clear and strong case that a data-driven health department should focus on inequities. This action recognized that local public health departments had three core functions: assessment, assurance, and policy development. That was the starting point to the assessment of health status. The data and the language of equity had to be familiar to the department, the Metro Council, the Mayor, and even the community. In order to move ahead, we needed to develop funding for efforts aimed at establishing a viable database to document the existence of health inequities. The next step would be to create a funding stream for the creation of a response to that data—namely the Center for Health Equity.

Reorganization efforts within the department led to the creation of the Office of Policy Planning and Evaluation. With this move, a locus of activity to meet the needs of community assessment and policy development was now a reality. Responding to calls to bring health assessment efforts up to national standards, the Metro Council allocated funding for a comprehensive Community Health Status Assessment Report. The results of the funded report were presented to the Council, the Mayor, and the Board of Health as well as the press. The following results made it painfully evident to all that there were in fact two Louisvilles.

1. The age-adjusted death rate from all causes for African Americans was 1209.5/100,000 compared to 941.3/100,000 for whites.
2. African Americans had higher death rates for four of the six leading causes of death in Louisville.
3. Age-adjusted death rates for diseases of the heart for African Americans was 357.6 compared to 297.4 for whites.
4. The diabetes death rate for African Americans was 74% higher than for whites.
5. The infant mortality rate was twice the rate for African American babies as compared to whites.
6. The homicide rate for African Americans was six times the rate of homicides among whites.
7. African Americans demonstrated significantly higher rates for HIV/AIDS, syphilis, gonorrhea, and Chlamydia.
8. In the public school system, 82% of African American children come from single parent households.
9. The rates of uninsured were disproportionate among African Americans and Latinos.
10. Age-adjusted death rates from cancer among African Americans was almost twice the rate of whites at 92.8/100,000 versus 55.9/100,000.
11. African American men in Louisville, in a state with the highest smoking rate in the nation, had the highest smoking rate.

The release of the report raised significant interest in many segments of the community, and the process of community education swung into high gear. Presentations at churches, political meetings, civic groups, and policy maker gatherings all focused on the presentation and discussions of the data and the condition of the African American community in particular. The language of health equity and the association of inequity with the absence of social justice were being spread throughout Louisville. The following definition of health inequities became the foundation of the departmental and community conversation on this issue, and placed human rights, social justice, and the right to health in the forefront of any discussion of the health status of excluded populations.

> *Health Inequities* are systemic, avoidable, unfair and unjust differences in health status and mortality rates and in the distribution of disease and illness across population groups. Sustained over time and generations, they remain beyond the control of individuals.[7]

Armed with the funded Community Health Status Report, we implemented mandatory staff training in *health equity through social justice,* the second strategic goal of the department. We envisioned health equity to be a major focus of the department in all its dealings that should influence all the work of the agency. Its placement as a cross-cutting goal allows us to cut across traditional silos and recognize the multidisciplinary nature of this work. Each section of the organization gets to see its connection and its place in this work.

The Center for Health Equity

The next budget cycle allowed the Center for Health Equity to become a reality. With the data collected, the Metro Council allocated the second-year budget of $250,000 to found the Center. The Center's first action was to develop the following mission statement:

> The Center for Health Equity serves as a catalyst for collaboration between public health, communities, and organizations that work to eliminate the social and economic barriers to good health. Through policy change, evidence-based interventions, and education, the Center builds new coalitions that reshape the public health landscape to assist communities in addressing barriers to health equity.

Integrating Health within Local Government Institutions

The Center focused on both internal and external strategies. One of the key strategies of the Center is to bring health equity needs and goals to the forefront of policy discussions in local government. The Louisville Metro Government is based on a cabinet arrangement of departments. As such, Metro Health is linked with Human Services, Workforce Development, Community Action, and the Family Health Centers (a Federally Qualified Health Center with multiple sites). These departments serve the population around many of the social determinants critical to creating health equity.

The structure represented an opportunity to integrate the goals of health equity across multiple departments. For example, the multisector structure allowed us to explore how to link job development strategies to those aimed at increasing access to health insurance, an opportunity not previously considered.

The same kind of integration is called for within the metro health department. The Center Director is one of several high-level administrators that reports directly to the Department Director that work as an administrative team. This structure similarly allows the department to integrate the principles of health equity to all aspects of its work and to evaluate programs' impacts on health equity. Departmental performance measures are being developed to measure this integration of equity principles and practice into our work. Working with the training officer, they will facilitate ongoing training in these principles for the entire workforce of the department.

Collaborating to Communicate the Language of Health Equity

Externally, the Center strives to change the paradigm of health in Louisville to focus on rights, equity, social determinants, and justice as foundations of health. In large part, this will be accomplished through collaborations with academic and community partners. The Center aims to partner with academic institutions, including the Morehouse School of Medicine Prevention Research Center, to conduct community-based participatory research and applied research to define the local causes of health inequities. The Center will expand general and specific community awareness of the existence of inequities and their negative effect on Metro Louisville through reporting of health status data, focus groups, and other epidemiologic research. The Center will also forge new partnerships and coalitions with agencies and organizations not traditionally associated with public/community health efforts, such as human rights organizations and groups traditionally seen as social justice advocates.

The Center will also serve as a primary source of education for metro staff and training for health professions students and policy makers regarding the dynamics of health and health inequities. We hope to influence curriculum change at our academic institutions—undergraduate, graduate, and professional—to better educate students on the links between health, equity, and social justice and the role of health in economic development. An undergraduate course, "Health Issues in the African American Community," has been developed entirely on the basis of the principles of health equity and social justice and focusing on the work of established national authorities in this field.

The Center has already become a place for policy makers to seek advice and direction on related issues. To date, two state legislators have requested our assistance in crafting legislation around the health of the state's populations of color; we are advising them on the inclusion of principles and language of health equity and social justice. We have also received funding to create a model for the policy education of local public health departments. This will be another source of education and influence on these vital themes. Plans are under way for our first conference on equity, social justice, social determinants, and health.

Health Equity Grants

The Center for Health Equity makes grants available to a diverse group of applicants including community-based organizations, nonprofit organizations, and academic researchers. The intended outcome of these community grants is policy recommendations that will make a significant improvement in a neighborhood and in the lives of its residents. The grants are meant to demonstrate the use of civic capacity building to address the social and economic macro-level policy issues that impact population health outcomes. The Center seeks to support community-based organizations that use civic capacity building efforts to engage communities in the policy process through advocacy activities that raise awareness of issues and educate policy makers.

The Center funded five awards in the first year to community-based organizations, not for profit groups and university partners. Included among the accomplishments of year one are the following: the convening of the first "Poverty Summit: Conversations with Residents," the publication of "Housing Insecurity: Neighborhood Conversations on Health Care Costs" in March, 2008, and the development of a technical assistance strategy for awardees that provides ongoing support and capacity building through mentoring and training.

The Center facilitated the development of a food security task force that evaluated access to affordable high-quality wholesome foods in the West End of Louisville (the section where the majority of residents are African American and where life expectancy is the shortest). It is also the area of town with the highest concentration of poverty, high school drop out rates, and the most dramatic health inequities in the entire city. These negative outcomes led to the creation of the Healthier Corner Store Initiative with grant funds from a partnership with the Metro YMCA. Its purpose was to increase the capacity of a corner store located within a food desert in the West End to carry and successfully market fresh fruits and vegetables to neighborhood residents and to establish a business model that can be replicated at other stores in underserved areas.

Community Organizing Training

Because the traditional public health workforce may not be equipped to work in communities at the level needed to address social determinants and facilitate community capacity building and community civic engagement, we recognized a need to train the workforce in new skills, particularly those who spend most of their time in the community. Through collaboration with a nationally known advocacy group, departmental outreach workers have been trained in community organizing and are applying lessons learned to their interaction with our constituents.

The Interdisciplinary Health Equity Assessment and Educational Training Project

The Center for Health Equity was selected as a subcontractor for a W.K. Kellogg Foundation grant to the Ingham County Health Department in Michigan. The grant's intent is to develop a dialogue process designed to move the public health workforce toward an understanding of the principles of health equity and social justice and incorporate these principles into workforce training and the practice of public health. Among the goals of our project is the development of an interdisciplinary and multidimensional health equity assessment survey instrument to measure the level of understanding of equity principles among the public health workforce. The results of the survey and subsequent group processes will be used to develop a curriculum that will be included in the training of all current and future employees of our department. Hopefully, this curriculum will also be adapted for training of all Metro Louisville employees. This process has resulted in numerous focus group sessions and early work on identifying potential leaders for the next level of work.

The West Louisville Visioning Process

Out of recognition of the need to expand the level of civic engagement in West Louisville, the Center sought to develop a method to engage community members in the development of policy advocacy and community capacity building. Its goal was to facilitate convening the residents, community leaders, nonprofit organizations, public officials, the private sector, religious leaders, and others to create long-term policy-based solutions to West Louisville's challenges. Of importance, like any viable process that requires community support, the community identified challenges. Subsequent involvement has focused on access to resources, analysis of issues, and supporting policy development.

Social Marketing Development

We recognize that the success of propagating the philosophy of health equity and its importance as a measure of social justice and the success of eliminating health inequities depends on the involvement of the entire community. As such, a key component of our strategy has been to develop a social marketing strategy focusing on heath equity, social justice, and human rights. In that regard, we engaged the support of a consultant organization to identify community perceptions around these principles as a first step in developing messages and methods of communication to advance the agenda of health equity. A lesson in this work is that our communities, those at immediate risk as well as those whose risk is not quite as clear at the moment, do not necessarily agree with the expert view that causation is upstream and that the existing health status of the population is not necessarily unfair. Moreover the overwhelming belief is that "It's all about choice." The success of the public health community in pushing personal behavior change as a primary determinant of good health has resulted in a significant barrier in communicating the structural roles of social factors and social justice. A new initiative of the University of Louisville will focus on "Creating Human Equity in the West End" with a focus on health, economic development, education, and human services. This systems change approach could expand our ability to discuss health in a holistic view and expand community support for the mission of public health.

Faith and Health Initiative

The department opened the Office of Faith and Health three years ago. For its early life, it has primarily emphasized more traditional public health programming (downstream) like addressing the Heart Association's "Search Your Heart" curriculum, which looks to decrease cardiovascular risk factors among African American congregations, adapting the Cardiopulmonary Resusitation (CPR) home training kit to use in churches for introducing the "Power to End Stroke" program in approximately 50 local African American churches. Now that we have established a relationship with them, we are focusing our attention to working with the faith community as an agent of social change. We know that our success in creating health equity must be the focus of a social justice movement. The African American church has a deep history in that regard going back to the abolition of slavery and continuing through the civil rights movement. It is therefore logical to move in this direction.

Unnatural Causes: Is Inequality Making Us Sick?

Through our participation with National Association of County and City Health Officials' (NACCHO) health equity advisory group, we were introduced to California Newsreel and participated in discussions around the development of a segment of the Public Broadcasting Service (PBS) documentary series *Unnatural Causes: Is Inequality Making Us Sick?* This highly successful project led to our hosting a town hall meeting on the social determinants of health, hosted by our Mayor, with the participation of three of the four principles in the first episode, "In Sickness and in Wealth," drawing 500 people. The session was recorded and aired on our local PBS station. We are now training community facilitators with a more community-based tool kit to use the series throughout the community to move the dialogue on social determinants to the streets and generate movement around these principles.

Challenges

The Center has enjoyed much success in its short life. New collaborations have been built, the local media has reported on the principles of health equity, community organizations are starting to recognize the role of social injustice in producing negative health outcomes, and our administration has made dramatic movement in accepting the Center's principles. We also recognize the challenges mentioned below.

Although the Center is firmly fixed in our Department of Public Health and Wellness and the Mayor accepts its mission, no legal mandate requires its existence and therefore it is subject to the demands of the budget processes and discretion of political leadership. Guaranteeing continuous sources of funding, resourceful grant seeking and effective management is critical for expansion and long-term survivability. This speaks to the need to develop a community constituency for the effort. A strong community that has seen the value of this work can be a force in assuring that as long as the need is there the work will continue. Keeping community residents engaged and supporting coalitions to address health equity will be a long-term challenge.

Retaining Center leadership with the needed skills of understanding the principles of social justice, being able to work within the government environment, and being able to work with community groups, academic institutions, granting agencies, and manage staff is a rare quality and another ongoing challenge.

The work of the Center challenges the status quo by its very nature. Those protecting the status quo could be expected to impede the work of the Center.

We have established the need for a community-wide social marketing strategy to raise consciousness about the issues that we are concerned about. A major challenge is to develop messages that will resonate with different communities and move them to action.

Each of the initiatives that we are and will undertake has and will have their own challenges specific to that project. We face these everyday and seek to meet them. We are driven by knowing that this is the right work at the right time and are confident of success. The Center continues to grow and will expand its availability as a community resource to Metro Louisville.

Notes

1. M. Byrd and L.A. Clayton, *An American Health Dilemma. Volume 1. A Medical History of African Americans and the Problem of Race: Beginnings to 1900* (New York: Routledge, 2000); M. Byrd and L.A. Clayton. *An American Health Dilemma. Volume 2. Race, Medicine, and Health Care in the United States: From 1900 to the Dawn of the New Millennium* (New York: Routledge, 2002).
2. California Newsreel (San Francisco, CA, 2003).
3. *The Philadelphia Negro: A Social Study* (New York: Schocken, 1967 [1899]).
4. U.S. Department of Health and Human Services, *The Task Force Report on Black and Minority Health*, (Washington, DC: U.S. Department of Health and Human Services, 1984).
5. U.S. Department of Health and Human Services, *Healthy People 2010* (Washington, DC, 2000).
6. WHO, Commission on Social Determinants of Health, *Closing the Gap in a Generation: Health Equity through Action on the Social Determinants of Health* (Geneva: WHO, 2008).
7. Margaret Whitehead, "The Concepts and Principles of Equity and Health," 22 (3) *International Journal of Health Services* (1992): 430.

15

Exploring the Intersection of Public Health and Social Justice: The Bay Area Regional Health Inequities Initiative

BOB PRENTICE AND NJOKE THOMAS

Health Equity and the Challenge to Local Health Departments

The organization of local health departments in California typically reflects their origins in the nineteenth and early twentieth centuries, with the largest program areas focused on infectious disease control and the health of women and children.[1] The workforce has been trained mostly in biomedical disciplines, or disciplines based on a biomedical understanding of disease.[2] Yet over three-quarters of preventable illness and premature death is now associated with chronic disease, much of which is social in origin, and the distribution of disease often reflects patterns of underlying social inequalities.[3]

How can we reconcile the inconsistencies between the way local health departments are organized and staffed with a contemporary understanding of the social etiology of disease and the inequitable distribution of disease burden that reflects underlying patterns of social inequalities? More particularly, how can local health departments not only understand, but define a public health practice, that can address the underlying causes of

This is an updated and substantially revised version of an article that originally appeared in the *NACCHO Exchange* 7(1), (Winter 2008).

health inequities? Those are questions that public health officials from local health departments in the San Francisco Bay Area decided to struggle with together, as they attempt to redefine public health practice for the purpose of eliminating health inequities, and to develop the capacity of their health departments to carry out that practice.

This chapter describes the history, organization, and trajectory of the Bay Area Regional Health Inequities Initiative (BARHII), a collaboration of eleven local health departments in the San Francisco Bay Area and beyond. The description provides an opportunity to reflect more generally on the implications of health inequities for public health practice, and for the future direction of public health building on, among others, the reports of the Institute of Medicine and the World Health Organization.[4]

Brief History of the Bay Area Regional Health Inequities Initiative (BARHII)

In the mid-1990s, a small group of public health directors and a health officer from San Francisco, Alameda, and Contra Costa counties, who had been working in the field for decades, convened to discuss how they might benefit from each other's counsel. Although they began with familiar topics, such as whether it might make sense to regionalize public health laboratories, they quickly concluded that the real potential of regional collaboration was in rethinking the vision for public health. In particular, they had been troubled by the evidence that the distribution of preventable illness and premature death pointed clearly toward the need for a confrontation with issues of social justice, yet their respective health departments were poorly prepared for such an effort.

While the conversations were episodic at first, they became monthly meetings by the late 1990s to discuss how the group might clarify its purpose and begin to make progress toward some well-defined practical ends. Colleagues from other jurisdictions, first the City of Berkeley and San Mateo County, then Marin County, asked if they could join, since they were grappling with the same issues. As with many similar undertakings launched with good intentions, the discussions were valuable but periodically led to frustrations over the lack of concrete progress. The frustrations were further compounded by the absence of staff support. At one particularly contentious gathering, when some questioned the value of continuing, one participant countered by saying, "I know why I am here. It is to transform public health practice." Not unlike a jazz improvisation, others added riffs that eventually produced not only the name—Bay Area Regional Health Inequities Initiative (BARHII)—but its mission " ... to transform public health practice for the purpose of eliminating health ineq-uities using a broad spectrum of approaches that create healthy communi-ties." Rather than the more commonly used (in the United States) "health disparities," which implies mere difference, the term "health inequities" was chosen to emphasize the relationship between patterns of disease and underlying social inequalities.

At the same time, a contingent of public health officials met with a similar regional grouping of community foundation CEOs to discuss how they might develop a collaboration to advance their common missions and regional focus. As a result, the community foundations agreed to each award small grants to help build a basic infrastructure, and a three-year grant from a large California health foundation provided operating costs sufficient to hire a full-time staff person and a part-time director in the fall of 2005. The staff person was able to help the group develop an organizational structure and work plan, which was a major step for-ward in establishing greater clarity of purpose and the actions that could be taken. Public health officials from five additional counties—Santa Clara, Solano, Napa, Santa Cruz and Sonoma—subsequently began to participate.

Why a Regional Collaboration?

Besides the advantages of consulting with public health colleagues and asserting a collective regional voice, there were other reasons to explore a regional approach. In California, for example, some regulatory func-tions, such as water and air quality, are carried out by regional bodies. Some planning functions, most notably transportation, have regional com-missions, and even those that are fundamentally local, such as land use or redevelopment, have obvious regional implications. More generally, the regional implications of economic development, labor markets, urban sprawl, and changing demographic composition demand that public health no longer confine itself to its historical, but increasingly outmoded, city and county boundaries. In addition, media markets, which are essential for policy advocacy, are mostly regional.

Building an Organization

A principle of membership in BARHII is that a public health director and/ or health officer must be willing to participate in order to commit the health department as a whole.[5] The health official then determines which senior managers best represent their own organization's work on health inequities and who should therefore attend the BARHII regular monthly meetings.

A system of committees, described later, was created to allow staff at varying levels in their health department to collectively consider the issues that confront them in their daily work. BARHII has also been a vehicle for collective trainings and presentations on various aspects of public health and health equity, including special sessions on structural racism, land use, transportation, redevelopment, climate change, and media advocacy.

While BARHII is an important forum for people from different health departments to consult with one another, it also embodies the potential for collective action, particularly related to policy advocacy. Sometimes it is more effective to represent the collective voice of senior public health officials in the Bay Area, including some situations in which a collective voice can speak to issues too risky for individual officials accountable to local governing bodies to tackle. BARHII has retained a consultant on media and policy advocacy to help make more thoughtful decisions about messages and strategies.

Organizing the Work

BARHII's work is divided among standing committees where health department managers and staff attempt to define a public health practice that can address health inequities, and define the organizational structure, culture, and staff requirements to support that practice. The committees make it possible for staff at all levels of the health departments to become active participants in BARHII, so it is no longer a top-down organization made up entirely of senior officials.

Data Committee

Establishing the evidence base for work on health inequities emerged as an immediate priority. Epidemiologists from each health department formed the Data Committee to help guide the evolving practice. The committee's first undertaking was the development of a conceptual framework (see Figure 15.1) that defines the path from mortality, morbidity, and risk behaviors—the common focus of local health department programs—to neighborhood conditions, institutional power, and social inequalities, which challenge health departments to shift their attention farther upstream. This framework has been adopted across the region as

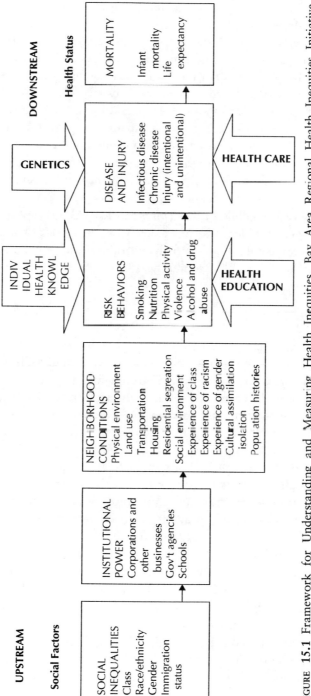

FIGURE 15.1 Framework for Understanding and Measuring Health Inequities. Bay Area Regional Health Inequities Initiative (BARHII).

an instrument for provoking dialogue about the value of a socioecological approach to addressing health inequities.

The committee's next endeavor was an analysis of the inequality in health outcomes manifested in the San Francisco Bay Area. Using regional mortality data by census tract, a report, Health Inequities in the Bay Area (www.barhii.org), documented a persistent inverse relationship between neighborhoods with a high rate of poverty and life expectancy across all Bay Area counties. A distinct social gradient was apparent for all of these factors both in the region as a whole and in individual counties. A more complex relationship between race/ethnicity and life expectancy suggested the need for a deeper exploration of the influence of racism, immigration, and culture on health. The report, released in April 2008 to coincide with the airing of the Public Broadcasting Service (PBS) series, *Unnatural Causes: Is Inequality Making Us Sick?* (see Chapter 25), garnered significant media coverage and, at least briefly, introduced into public discourse a very different way of thinking about health.

Community Committee

A Community Committee was formed to establish the basis on which health departments' work with communities on a multitude of issues over time to address the social and environmental conditions that contribute to poor health. From their earliest discussions, BARHII members acknowledged an inherent dissonance in the prevalent practice of parsing whole communities into discrete populations, diseases, and risk factors. This approach, driven largely by categorical funding, frequently resulted in duplication of effort with little attention to the underlying social factors that were culminating in a disproportionate burden of disease in some areas. To address more effectively the root causes of health inequities, local health departments are trying to adopt a broader perspective on work in communities, looking at the neighborhood conditions that contribute to poor health. Accordingly, BARHII provides a forum in which member health departments are attempting to forge new strategies for community engagement and capacity building to address these neighborhood conditions, and to establish relationships that can be sustained over time and across diseases and risk factors. The group consists of key staff from each health department who contributes their thinking and experience in crafting a shared definition of community work. The ultimate goal will be to create a clearinghouse of promising practices of health departments working with communities on the social and environmental determinants of health inequities.

Built Environment Committee

A recognition of the importance of physical conditions in neighborhoods, buttressed by a burgeoning movement linking public health to land use planning in California,[6] led to the creation of a Built Environment Committee. The conceptual framework emphasized the pathway through which social inequality manifests itself in unhealthy neighborhood conditions. While BARHII recognizes that this is not the only mechanism, the centrality of place was made abundantly clear by the regional social gradient analysis conducted by the Data Committee. The Built Environment Committee was established to identify a role for public health departments in influencing the land use and transportation planning decisions that affect neighborhood conditions. Until recently, there has been limited recognition of the health effects of built environment issues like urban sprawl and the resultant dependence on automobiles, decayed urban cores, lack of open space and accessible public transportation.[7] Several public health departments within BARHII have worked independently to raise awareness of these issues with varying levels of success. The Built Environment Committee has provided an opportunity for local health departments to consolidate their efforts, share promising practices and generate a regional forum for discussion of these issues that seldom restrict themselves to county boundaries. At this early stage, the work has focused on establishing a mutually beneficial, cross-disciplinary exchange between planning and public health, articulating to planning and transportation professionals the health consequences of their policies and practices and helping public health professionals to consider the best strategies for influencing the planning processes. The ultimate goal of this work will be to make health equity a fixture in land use and transportation planning. BARHII has also developed an initiative to expand the focus of work on the built environment beyond land use and transportation planning to include economic development and redevelopment and more explicitly focus on social and health equity.

Internal Capacity Committee

Recognizing that the organization and culture of local health departments have a major influence on their ability to effectively address health inequities, the Internal Capacity Committee was charged with developing strategies for increasing the capacity of the local health departments to engage in a new kind of public health practice. The committee has emphasized a participatory approach to understanding and addressing these issues. The first of these strategies, facilitating staff dialogues on the topic of social justice arose out of our partnership with the National Association of County and City Health Officials' (NACCHO) Health Equity and Social Justice Strategic Direction Team. Early in BARHII's development, members were introduced to a new process to shape the health equities dialogue developed at the Ingham County (Michigan) Public Health Department (see Chapter 13).[8] The broadly representative and participatory process systematically examines the influence that race, class, and gender have on population health. Ingham County's chief architect of the process facilitated an all-day training to introduce a wide cross-section of regional health department staff to the process. Widespread enthusiasm prompted several departments to select a core group of staff to receive additional training in the use of these specific facilitation methods. Through the work of the Internal Capacity Committee, this corps of trained facilitators will implement a series of dialogues throughout the region within BARHII health departments. Future work will include trainings to develop public health workforce skills to work effectively on data, community engagement and capacity building, built environment and social determinants of health inequity.

The Internal Capacity Committee has also taken a macro approach to organizational development, engaging in critical thinking about competencies, policies and standards that are essential for eliminating health inequities. These consensus-building discussions helped to define what committee members believed are the most critical elements of public health

TABLE 15.1. Public Health Standards and Competencies for Eliminating Health Inequities

WORKFORCE COMPETENCIES	ORGANIZATIONAL STANDARDS AND POLICIES
Knowledge of public health framework	Institutional commitment to address health inequities
Understand the social, environmental, and structural determinants of health	Hiring to address health inequities
Community knowledge	Structure that supports true community partnerships
Leadership skills	Support staff to address health inequities
Collaboration skills	Transparent and inclusive communication (community, staff, partners etc.)
Community organizing skills	Institutional support for innovation
Problem solving ability	Creative use of categorical funds
Cultural competency/cultural humility	Community accessible data and planning
Specific personal attributes	Streamlined administrative process

departments as social change organizations. The group ultimately categorized their outcomes into a "matrix" of nine workforce competencies and nine organizational standards and policies (see Table 15.1).

During this process, the committee also outlined a theory of change for using organizational development as a strategy for addressing health inequities. Local health departments need specific tools and processes to support systematic change. Organizational self-assessment was identified as an effective tool for gauging where health departments are already making headway in these issues and underscoring areas for improvement. This information could then be used to develop processes to increase institutional capacity. The committee retained an organizational development consulting group to weave together public health expertise and organizational development theory into a comprehensive tool, the Organizational Self Assessment Tool for Addressing Health Inequities. The tool, completed in the spring of 2008, was piloted in the City of Berkeley health department. The pilot experience and outcomes will be used to further refine the tool both in terms of content and methods of administration. The tool and a companion guide for implementation will be available for wider dissemination and to influence national processes for accreditation of local health departments.

Social Determinants of Health Ad Hoc Work Group

While the Built Environment Committee appropriately focuses on the physical environment, no one lives in a purely physical environment—it is mediated by family, community, culture, and so forth. In addition, the physical environment itself is a social construct, with decisions about what type of development will occur in which communities made by public and private institutions. Moreover, forms of social power shape the priorities that govern those decisions.

Nonetheless, public health's grasp of the social environment—or social determinants of health—is limited and, just as importantly, the role that public health can play in influencing their effects on health is unclear. As a result, BARHII created an ad hoc work group on the social determinants of health to explore research and conceptual frameworks that can help public health practitioners analyze more effectively the social environment and related strategies for public health practice.

Future Opportunities

While BARHII has been a valuable forum for local health officials and staff to explore new ways of thinking about data, community work, and strategies for organizational change, it has only begun to realize the

potential of using the collective voice of Bay Area health officials to influence policy or the standards of public health practice. Some of the early
signs, however, are encouraging.

In December, 2006, for example, BARHII hosted a forum of over
100 city and county planning directors and public health officials from
the nine-county region to review the evidence linking health to the built
environment. While individual health departments had made overtures
to planning departments in their jurisdictions, the BARHII forum established legitimacy to the public health/planning connection which greatly
improved the environment for working together. Since the forum, the
extent of joint work has expanded substantially.

The release of BARHII's report, Health Inequities in the Bay Area, in
April, 2008 provided a basis on which to expand that work. The report
documented that people who live in poor neighborhoods in the Bay Area
can expect to live on average a decade less than people who live in affluent neighborhoods. The analysis made it clear that neighborhood conditions are both about the physical environment and social factors such as
income and wealth, race/ethnicity, immigration and education. The future
trajectory of BARHII's work, then, must not only expand the focus on the
built environment beyond land use planning to include transportation,
economic development, and redevelopment, but must also define a public
health practice that can address issues like the distribution of income and
wealth, or the role that racism plays in health.

This broader perspective was the context for Bay Area health officials
weighing in collectively on a regional transportation plan being considered
before the Metropolitan Transportation Commission, and issuing a statement condemning raids by the Immigration and Customs Enforcement
(ICE) branch of the Department of Homeland Security that were intended
to provoke fear and intimidation in communities with high percentages
of Latino immigrants. More recently, BARHII has become involved in a
regional planning forum mandated by state legislation to meet regional
targets for reductions in greenhouse gas emissions in order to articulate
public health co-benefits and health equity implications of climate change
mitigation activities.

BARHII is also attempting to influence standards of public health practice beyond the Bay Area. BARHII members and staff, for example, are
in the leadership of a statewide campaign to make prevention of chronic
disease by focusing on social determinants of health a greater priority
among local and state health departments. BARHII is represented on the
NACCHO National Health Equity Work Group, and active in NACCHO's
Health Equity and Social Justice Strategic Direction Team. Particularly,
with the prospects of national efforts to accredit local health departments

and credential the workforce, BARHII and its partners will attempt to translate an evolving public health practice focused on health equity into national standards.

While the progress to date has been encouraging, major challenges still lie ahead. What does it mean, for example, for a group of local health departments to publish a report documenting the profound influence of class, race, and place on health, yet do little to actually address them in our public health practice? It is very common to hear people in the field concede that the distribution of income and wealth, or the history of racism in the United States, have a major influence on health, but counter that public health can do nothing about such large, intractable forces. How, though, do we reconcile that view with the principles of evidence-based public health? If we know these larger forces are major influences on the health of populations, it is our obligation to discover ways to address them. The burden is on public health to redefine itself, not for population health to fit into what public health is prepared to do.[9]

This challenge seems to have two broad components. One is that public health is an evidence-based discipline. Evidence is not only what guides our practice, it is what gives us the credibility to speak or act, and also gives us some reason to believe that others will take us seriously. Public health cannot compromise that credibility by appearing to be just another group of political activists, even though we are entering political territory. The other is that the territory we are entering is not, by and large, part of our training or experience, so we are obligated to figure it out as we go along. What are these "social determinants of health," and how do we develop a public health practice and the competencies to address them?

Public health's commitment to evidence-based approaches might be its greatest asset in confronting the larger forces that influence health. Documenting the association between health and the distribution of income and wealth, race/ethnicity or neighborhood conditions at least raises the issues that need to be addressed. The promising tool of Health Impact Assessments (HIAs) allows public health agencies to use evidence to consider the impact of policy decisions that affect those forces. HIAs, for example, are being used in land use, and they have been applied to local living wage ordinances.[10] The health impacts of education policies, residential segregation, or tax policies are other areas in which HIAs might be applied.

The redefinition of public health practice that includes new ways of working with communities, and learning how to work with other public agencies on land use, transportation, redevelopment, education, and the other dimensions of our social and physical environments, will require a reexamination of the public health workforce, as well as the financing and organization of local health departments. It will also challenge current national processes to credential the workforce and accredit local health departments. Pushing boundaries while others are trying to achieve consensus definitions will make for interesting times.

While much of this work is exploratory and outside conventional practice, that has been the tradition of public health. From pump handles to AIDS, public health practitioners have had to act before they fully understood the nature of their interventions. The evolving practice generates the experience and research that will become the basis of future evidence-based practice, as well as the competencies that public health will need to carry it out.

These are the challenges that public health officials are trying to confront through BARHII.

Notes

1. See Bob Prentice and George Flores, "Local Health Departments and the Challenge of Chronic Disease: Lessons From California, in Preventing Chronic Disease," 4(1) CDC online (January 2007). California has 58 county and 3 city health departments.
2. Los Angeles County Department of Health Services, UCLA Center for Health Policy Research, *The burden of Disease in Los Angeles County* (Los Angeles: Los Angeles County Department of Health Services; 2000).
3. See, for example, John D. and Catherine T. MacArthur Foundation Research Network on Socioeconomic Status and Health, *Reaching for a Healthier America: Facts on Socioeconomic Status and Health*, 2008, www.macses.edu; Bay Area Regional Health Inequities Initiative, Health Inequities in the Bay Area, 2008, www.barhii.org.
4. See, for example, Institute of Medicine, *The Future of the Public's Health in the 21st Century* (Washington, DC: National Academies Press, 2002). See, also, *Closing the Gap in a Generation: Health Equity through Action on the Social Determinants of Health*, Final Report of the Commission on Social Determinants of Health, World Health Organization, Geneva, Switzerland.
5. The leadership of local health departments in California does not conform to a single pattern. While all 61 local health departments have statutorily mandated physician health officers, the role of the health officer varies. In a few counties, the health officer is also the director of a combined health services agency; in some counties, the health officer is also the public health director; in other counties, the health officer reports to a public health director who is an administrator; particularly in smaller, more rural jurisdictions, the health officer might be a physician in private practice under contract to perform the duties of a health officer, most commonly focused on communicable disease control. The BARHII membership principle is designed to accommodate the variations in the bay area.

6. For resources in California that link health to the built environment, see web sites for Planning for Healthy Places, a project of Public Health Law & Policy at the Public Health Institute, www.healthyplanning.org; the Local Government Commission, which has promoted smart growth principles as a foundation for health, www.lgc.org; the Center for Civic Partnerships, which has sponsored Healthy Cities initiatives for decades, www.civicpartnerships.org; and PolicyLink, which has framed land use and health within the context of equitable development, www.policylink.org; Dick Jackson, M.D., former Director of the National Center for Environmental Health, former California Public Health Officer and coauthor of the influential book, *Urban Sprawl and Health*, played a major throughout the state promoting the renaissance of public health and planning. The California Endowment, www.calendow.org, has funded many local and state initiatives on land use and health, particularly associated with obesity prevention.

7. See, for example, H. Frumkin, L. Frank, and R. Jackson, *Urban Sprawl and Health* (Washington, DC: Island Press, 2004).

8. Doak Bloss, "Initiating Social Justice Action through Dialogue in a Local Health Department: The Ingham County Experience and Beyond," this volume, Chapter 13.

9. See, for example, Anthony B. Iton, "The Ethics of the Medical Model in Addressing the Root Causes of Health Disparities in Local Public Health Practice," this volume, Chapter 28.

10. See, for example, A.L. Dannenberg, R. Bhatia, B.L. Cole, et al., "Growing the Field of Health Impact Assessment in the United States: An Agenda for Research and Practice," 96(2) *American Journal of Public Health*, (February 1, 2006): 262–270; B.L. Cole, R. Shimkada, H. Morgenstern, G. Kominski, J.E. Fielding, and S. Wu, "Projected Impact of the Los Angeles City Living Wage Ordinance," 59(8) *Journal of Epidemiology and Community Health* (August 1, 2005): 645–650; R. Bhatia and M. Katz, "Estimation of Benefits from a Local Living Wage Ordinance," this volume, Chapter 17.

16

Using Our Voice: Forging a Public Health Practice for Social Justice

RAJIV BHATIA, JUNE WEINTRAUB, LILI FARHANG, KAREN YU, AND PAULA JONES

Introduction

The toll of social disadvantage on health is undisputed. Cumulatively and collectively, poverty, substandard housing, hunger and food insecurity, environmental stressors, social isolation, and political exclusion result in avoidable injury, disability, disease, and death.[1,2,3] Public health institutions have recognized equitable social conditions as prerequisites for healthy societies and have established clear goals for the elimination of health inequities. For example, in its Ottawa Charter for Health Promotion, the World Health Organization, acknowledged that social justice and equity were "fundamental conditions and resources for health," along with food, income, education, and shelter, and stated that "Health promotion action aims at reducing differences in current health status and ensuring equal opportunities and resources to enable all people to achieve their fullest health potential."[4] In the United States in 1999, the United States Department of Health and Human Services for the first time made the elimination of health inequities a national public health goal.[5]

While society appears to place significant value on both the protection of health and social equity, there remains a vast gulf between public health knowledge of health inequities and the necessary institutional and societal actions to address their root causes.[6] Do public institutions lack the capacity, tools, and strategies to translate their evidence on health inequities into meaningful policy or social change? Or, are health inequities simply symptomatic of a culture that tolerates inequities, regardless of their human consequences?

This chapter argues that local public health institutions, working collectively with other constituencies, have untapped capacity to effect change in the conditions and institutions underlying health inequities. Using public health's voice to change social conditions requires learning the terrain of diverse social institutions outside of the public health discipline, developing relationships and coalitions with actors already engaged in social justice struggles, and a willingness to challenge unjust institutional actions. The chapter presents five related strategies that can collectively guide health equity practice. Using examples from practice at the Program on Health, Equity and Sustainability and the San Francisco Department of Public Health, the chapter illustrates how these strategies can be employed by a local public health institution and can effectively eliminate sources of health inequity. The practice stories underscore the complementary nature of health equity strategies, the necessity of participation in coalitions for social justice, and the iterative and adaptive nature of transformative practice. The chapter concludes by identifying specific actions, based on the practice examples, that may help public health institutions to surmount traditional barriers to an interdisciplinary and an equity-focused practice.

Five Strategies for Local Health Equity Practice

The idea that public health institutions should act to improve societal conditions required for health and health equity is not new. The 1986 Ottawa Charter outlined a comprehensive approach for the promotion of population health, including: putting health on the agenda of policy makers in all sectors; joint action among public sectors; systematic assessment of the health impacts of environmental change; care for each other and our environment; and the reorientation of health services. Importantly, the Charter recognized that health promotion was not simply a task for experts and bureaucrats but, rather that "At the heart of this process is the empowerment of communities—their ownership and control of their own endeavors and destinies."[4]

Local public health institutions have relationships with and responsibilities for communities and populations burdened by health inequities, and the charter suggests important roles for public health institutions in changing structural conditions responsible for health inequities. We believe that local public health roles can involve five related strategies: (1) establishing a collective responsibility for health and health equity; (2) translating research into policy change; (3) forging relationships with social movements; (4) monitoring institutional accountability; and (5) facilitating a consensus for change. As explained in the sections below and as illustrated in the practice examples that follow, the five strategies are complementary and component elements of strategic practice to eliminate health inequities.

Not surprisingly, the pursuit of health equity strategies in local public health institutions confronts diverse challenges—namely, narrow public and political expectations, disciplinary boundaries, established organizational culture and practices, and conflicting social interests, including some that benefit from the current distribution of wealth and privilege. In the following section, we also elaborate on these institutional and social barriers.

Establishing a Collective Responsibility for Health and Health Equity

Public health efforts have documented inequalities in health conditions at many levels.[5, 7, 8] Yet, this descriptive analysis does not assign the cause or responsibility for health inequities. Society may not deliberately maintain health inequities; however, health inequities result from social choices and people must act collectively as a society to dismantle inequities. To do so, people must first acknowledge that society has failed to provide healthful conditions for all its members, and that this inequity is unfair.[9]

The social principles of fairness are critical to addressing health inequities because fairness is a shared value that can help motivate collective action. Health equity advocates can attempt to make a claim upon the need for fairness (for equal opportunity for health); however, it is not yet universally accepted that health inequities are the result of unfair circumstances, much less a failure of society to provide healthful conditions for all its members. For example, the view that health is individually and behaviorally determined and a commodity to be purchased or provided by health professionals is dominant in our society.[10,11] This view limits how problems of health inequities get framed and placed on the policy and political agenda.

Because they are society's health experts, public health institutions have the ability to redefine and reframe the causes of good or poor health. One way to do this is to use public concerns about poor health outcomes as an opportunity to advance understanding of social and environmental determinants of health and the political decisions affecting these determinants. For example, concerns about high rates of asthma symptoms in a neighborhood create an opportunity to draw attention to problems of indoor and outdoor air quality and how policy decisions regarding housing, transportation, and environmental quality affect air quality. Partnership with opinion leaders, artists, and the media organizations can also support this kind of reframing. For example, in 2008, producers of *Unnatural Causes: Is Inequality Making Us Sick?* used documentary film to translate a scientific understanding of health inequities to a wider public audience.

Translating Research into Policy Change

Many policies, rules, and laws have broad impacts on population health and health equity. For example, occupational regulations protect worker safety, environmental quality standards limit exposure to chemical hazards, and zoning and land use regulations affect community access to parks, transportation, and other public services. Presumably, public health research should serve to inform and shape all public policies that impact human health, yet public health evidence on the causes and consequences of health inequities are not routinely integrated into policy deliberation and action.

Effective translation of public health research by public health institutions requires communicating research findings in ways that are sensitive to and complementary of political interests, contexts, and dynamics. Unfortunately, public health practitioners have few mechanisms to introduce health considerations into policies outside their institutional domains. The fragmentation of public institutions by sector or discipline and poor communication among disciplines means that the health consequences of public policy are often overlooked, inadequately analyzed, or diminished.

One approach to addressing disciplinary fragmentation and lack of communication is through the practice of health impact assessment (HIA) which aims to make the consideration of health effects of social decisions more routine and transparent in the policy-making process.[12] Health evidence, organized through HIA, may lead to a more thorough evaluation of trade-offs in situations of policy conflict. Health evidence can establish the status of socially vulnerable populations, identify health sensitivities or hazards from cumulative exposures, and trigger existing legal or regulatory requirements protective of health.[13] Public health evidence may also add weight to the force of arguments on one side of a policy debate, may legitimize policy positions raised by advocates for equity, and may mobilize equity-oriented constituencies to engage in policy coalitions. As discussed in the example of a living wage law below, HIA can provide a counterweight to a monetary calculus in policy making.

Ideally, decision makers are open and attentive to the needs of health, recognize their limited capacity to understand health needs, and seek or welcome public health evidence that supports policy design and implementation. However, policy making is not simply a rational, evidence-based process, and the production and translation of health evidence does not ensure healthy policy.[14] Multiple instances exist where policy makers have not implemented interventions that could protect health even when ample evidence of benefits exists (e.g., Head Start, national air quality standards, gun control, needle exchange). Thus, public health institutions advocating evidence in policy contexts need to be attentive to both the limits of evidence as well as to the political and economic factors at play in the decision-making process.

Forging Relationships with Social Movements

The limitations to the role of public health institutions in policy processes underscore the need for public health to address health inequities in the context of coalitions. Indeed, no single organization or interest group has either the knowledge or the influence to undo social inequities in their totality. The goals of health equity reflect the shared values of social justice advocates working to advance a more equitable distribution of societal benefits and burdens. Social justice actors for example include those representing the interests of labor and economic rights, the environment and environmental justice, civil rights, corporate accountability, and political reform.

Despite shared goals, few public health agencies are openly engaged in social justice coalitions or campaigns. Yet, in the past, public health workers have been valuable and active participants in social movements addressing housing, poverty, occupational safety, environmental hazards, and community development. For example, in the 1960s, the United States Office of Economic Opportunity supported a model of community-oriented primary care where rural health centers worked with community members to provide not only medical care but to address environmental problems, provide mentorship and tutoring for young people, and facilitate loans to build community infrastructure and assets.[15]

When public health develops meaningful relationships with civil society organizations engaged with social justice struggles all sides can benefit. First, social movements that are rooted in developed coalitions help public health actors understand the political requirements for change. In many cases, coalitions have already determined community priorities through outreach and organizing and have engaged with political actors and institutions around multilevel policy agendas. Working with coalitions helps to ground public health action in what is politically viable and also provides built-in advocacy resources for public health goals. Second, public health institutions can strengthen social justice constituencies by providing technical assistance to community organizations to develop grant-writing capacity, to collect data, to research interventions, to develop or manage programs, to conduct strategic planning, or to evaluate programs.

Public health practitioners engaged in partnerships must be mindful that their voices represent elites in policy process. Members of the public health community may have an incomplete understanding of the needs and challenges of those facing social disadvantage, in part because they themselves may not face adverse social conditions on a daily basis. In contrast, participatory knowledge-building envisions all participants as actors for change and involves mutual respect, shared power, and trust.[16] Effective and inclusive community participation in design and implementation of research and policy helps to ensure that interventions address priority needs, are holistic and culturally appropriate, and are likely to benefit those with the least advantage.[17] In the field of public health, community-based participatory research (CBPR) is emerging as a recognized means to gain a shared understanding of a problem and to implement social change.[18, 19]

Monitoring Institutional Accountability

Establishing equity-oriented public policy even through a broad-based collaboration does not ensure its implementation. For example, school desegregation laws promised more equal opportunities for childhood education but were undermined by racism and other social forces that produced white flight from urban areas, subsequent urban disinvestment, and entrenched residential segregation.

When failure to implement or enforce policies, rules, and laws results in public health consequences, public health agencies have a responsibility to raise attention to such failures and seek action on the part of sister institutions, either directly or indirectly. Public health and health care practitioners are often on the front lines of recognizing the human consequences of failures to enforce health-protective policies and regulations. Pointing out the failures of sister agencies, if not done sensitively, may risk alienating colleagues or undermining progress. However, public health practitioners who objectively identify consequences for public health, provide constructive solutions, and work collaboratively to mobilize the actions of external interests, can influence outcomes. For example, when the Seattle Housing Authority embarked upon a process to develop new mixed-income housing in West Seattle's High Point neighborhood, Public Health Seattle and

King County worked in partnership with community organizations to improve design features such as ventilation systems to address asthma triggers among low-income children.[20]

Facilitating a Consensus for Change

While targeted policy goals and interventions may remedy the consequences of inequity, they do not address the historical forces that created the unfair conditions in the first place.[6] Imbalances of power in a collective decision-making process and conflicting interests among social groups are two more fundamental barriers to health inequities.

Where subpopulations do not have the ability to access or effectively use information, public health can be a resource on the decision-making process and its outcomes and impacts, helping people explore available alternatives to a particular course of action. By providing expert testimony on behalf of groups whose perspectives may not be otherwise represented, public health can give marginalized stakeholders the tools and legitimacy needed to ensure their perspectives are considered in a decision-making process.

Marginalized communities are not the only stakeholders in health equity practice. Policies addressing social inequalities often involve conflicts between social groups with diametrically opposed positions of privilege, power, or political capital. While strategies to address social inequality often aim to improve the circumstances of those at the bottom of social hierarchies—the disadvantaged—strategies must also take into account the privilege and interests of those at the top of social hierarchies. Furthermore, there is rarely one community voice or position and public health activities must acknowledge diversity among community needs.

Advancing a health equity agenda involves not only helping marginalized social groups "win" better conditions and a more equitable stake in society but also helping move all people towards a common vision and commitment to equity. Such action requires a dialogue with diverse audiences including those that may "lose" in the short term from actions that reduce inequities. In some cases, public health institutions may have sufficient trust as neutral and objective bodies to help mediate conflicts among competing interests. This convening ability might be successfully applied to building consensus about the collective value of reducing inequities. For example, in recognizing that race-based disparities in health were related to institutional and interpersonal racism, Boston's Public Health Commission developed policies to build community partnerships, promote an antiracist work environment, and realign external activities to address racism. In so doing, the Commission acknowledged the historical and structural forces at play in generating health inequities, and was able to realign its work both internally and externally to account for the role of racism in health practice.[21]

Obstacles to Local Public Health Action for Health Equity

As argued above, the institution of public health has a legitimate stake in the public and political processes that affect health equity and has assets that it can bring to struggles for social change. However, relatively few public health agencies are openly engaged in social justice movements, coalitions, or campaigns, and it is often not apparent to actors working to change health-relevant policies and laws (e.g., minimum wage, affordable housing) that they have an available partner in public health.

Not surprisingly, the place of a local public health department within governmental institutional arrangements presents formidable barriers to extending public health practice to health equity. Like most other public institutions, public health is accountable formally to political leadership. Public health does not always have a clear mandate to work across disciplinary and institutional boundaries to act on health equity. Furthermore, public health programs are generally organized categorically, either by diseases (e.g., AIDS, cancer), risk factors (e.g., lead, mold) or services (nutrition, vaccination), and administrators, funding agencies, and political leaders often expect public health practitioners to demonstrate the impact of interventions quantitatively and in relatively short time frames. Few funding organizations provide resources or incentives for public health institutions to undertake initiatives on responsible social and environmental determinants of health, outside of institutional boundaries, or across disciplines (e.g., with transportation or parks agencies).

Disciplinary culture within public health creates an additional obstacle to taking action on health inequities. The institution of public health tends to frame public health problems and solutions in terms familiar to its own discipline and focused on its own institutional mandates. This specificity constrains the role of public health evidence in contexts outside of public health. However, if public health practitioners increase their willingness to work on problems identified by a wider range of communities, institutions and disciplines (e.g., education, employment, or housing), and apply health evidence to relate to those identified concerns, greater opportunities present themselves to target conditions and forces that effect population level health outcomes and to connect health to other institutional sectors. Acknowledging community partners' perspectives, being willing to play a supportive role, supporting priorities regardless of direct and immediate connections to health outcomes, and willingness to try community-originated strategies are all necessary to address health inequity.

San Francisco's Program on Health, Equity, and Sustainability

Beginning in the 1990s, the San Francisco Department of Public Health (SFDPH) began to recognize the necessity to work on health equity through strategies that lay outside of its formal mandates, and began to reorganize its capacity to invest in actions that improve the social determinants of health and eliminate health inequities.[22] Environmental justice advocates in particular made strong demands on SFDPH to take action on health in some of the City's most impoverished neighborhoods.[23]

In 2002, SFDPH created a new organizational division—the Program on Health, Equity, and Sustainability (PHES) within its Environmental Health Division. Not constrained by traditional organizational mandates, PHES had explicit goals to improve urban environmental, social, and economic conditions through policy-relevant applied research and collaboration. At the outset, PHES staff expressed their vision to advance "health equity through effective, sustained social participation." The work of PHES sought to bring together community organizations and government agencies, to examine the relationships between health and living and working conditions, and to take collective action on these conditions (see Box 16.1).

For PHES, the emphasis on external collaboration recognized that health expertise and evidence, while a powerful tool, was most useful when made relevant by those with power and influence in political contexts. Partners outside the institution were often in better positions to identify high-priority policy discourses and strategically to translate public health facts in political processes. Finally, community members, who often defined problems in a more holistic way, might be a catalyst for transdisciplinary approaches in public health practice.

As illustrated in the practice stories below, the work of PHES focused on both traditional as well as emerging environmental health and justice issues, including noise and air quality, employment conditions, food security, housing adequacy, and land use and transportation systems. The practice stories do not reflect the depth and complexity of the tasks and interaction involved in each of the initiatives. However, the stories do illustrate how the five strategies described earlier—defining health issues as a collective responsibility, translating evidence into policy, participating in social movements, building institutional accountability for health, and facilitating a consensus for equity—collectively helped steer the initiatives towards sustainability and meaningful outcomes.

Box 16.1 San Francisco Department of Public Health
Occupational and Environmental Health
Program on Health, Equity and Sustainability
Statement of Mission, Vision and Guiding Principles

The Program on Health, Equity and Sustainability supports San Franciscans working together to advance urban health and social and environmental justice. Through ongoing integration of local government and community efforts and through valuing the needs, experiences, and knowledge of diverse San Francisco residents, we accomplish this by:

- Initiating and facilitating dialogue and collaboration among public agencies and community organizations;
- Expanding public understanding of the relationships between the natural, built, and social environments and human health;
- Supporting local capacity for participation in public policy;
- Conducting and supporting local and regional research;
- Developing and evaluating new methods for interdisciplinary and inclusive involvement in public policy;
- Documenting and disseminating our strategies.

In our vision of San Francisco, communities are engaged in democracy and committed to equality and diversity. We believe this will create and maintain sustainable and healthy places for all San Franciscans to live, work, learn, and play. Guiding Principles and Core Values:

- **Healthful Environments** Healthy people reflect healthful environments. Following the 1986 WHO Charter on Health Promotion, we define the basic conditions and resources needed for health to be peace, shelter, education, food, income, stable ecosystems, sustainable resources, social justice, and equity;
- **Inter-connectedness** The natural and built environments, human activities, and human relationships are connected;
- **Equity** A fair distribution of economic, political, social and natural resources and opportunities improves individual livelihood and the overall health of society;
- **Sustainability** Conserving and improving economic, social and environmental systems so that present and future community members can lead healthy, productive and enjoyable lives;
- **Public Access and Accountability** The process for making public choices must be open and involve the people most affected. Good public policy decisions ensures that all participants have access to relevant information, including an understanding of underlying conflicts and competing interests;

(Continued)

- **Meaningful Participation** Ensuring meaningful public participation in policy-making requires sincere actions to support people's involvement, the valuing of local knowledge and experiences, and incorporating the perspectives and needs of communities into decision-making.

Source: Program on Health, Equity and Sustainability web site. Available at: www.sfphes.org

The Genesis of PHES: Securing a Floor for Wages and Benefits

Secure employment and sufficient income are well-established determinants of health, yet labor conditions are typically not considered health policy. Unemployment means a shortened life expectancy and higher rates of cardiovascular disease, hypertension, depression, and suicide.[24, 25, 26] Compared to those with higher incomes, people with lower incomes have higher risks for poor health and premature mortality at every point on the distribution; furthermore, poverty is associated with giving birth to low birth weight babies, for suffering injuries or violence, for getting most cancers, and for getting chronic conditions.[27, 28]

In 1999, in the context of an emerging nationwide movement, the San Francisco legislature proposed a local living wage law. Staff at SFDPH recognized that documenting the human health benefits of the living wage in a public process might provide a compelling counterweight to opposition to the living wage law by business interests. SFDPH offered the idea to a legislator who subsequently commissioned SFDPH to conduct a quantitative analysis that would estimate the health and human development benefits of changes to wage rules.[29] (See Chapter 17) That same year, San Francisco adopted the living wage ordinance for workers of employers under city contracts and employers leasing city properties.

Demonstrating that public health research could support labor policy connected SFDPH to a wider social movement fighting for living wages. Over the following years, community constituencies requested PHES staff to remain engaged in labor policy. For example, in 2003, San Francisco residents passed Proposition L increasing the minimum wage from $6.75 to $8.50 for over 50,000 workers in San Francisco. Community organizations and city legislators invited PHES staff to testify on the laws health impacts at public hearings.

In 2006, a coalition of labor and social justice advocates requested PHES to support the passage of a local Paid Sick Days Ordinance. PHES subsequently mobilized a substantial evidence-based case for the paid sick days policy focusing on three likely health outcomes: (1) reducing illness duration and severity by enabling workers to take the time off needed to manage and/or recover from an illness and care for ill family members; (2) limiting exposure to coworkers and the public due to communicable infectious disease; (3) reducing the social and economic costs of avoidable hospitalizations by facilitating use of primary care. City legislators called on PHES to give public testimony on these benefits, complementing and validating numerous personal stories and addressing business concerns about adverse economic impacts. Following the passage of the law, PHES staff remained engaged with state and national paid sick day campaigns and continued to support and evaluate the law's implementation in San Francisco.

In sum, health analysis of employment policies in San Francisco began to raise awareness among city leaders of a constructive role for public health institutions in policy research, and relationships with local legislators and advocacy coalition helped bring public health evidence into the political process. These lessons were seminal in the genesis of PHES.

Advancing Health and Safety for Day Laborers

PHES engagement with day laborers exemplifies how traditional public health roles can evolve into ones that address health inequities. "Day laborers" find work and get paid on a daily or very short-term basis, have multiple employers, and are usually paid in cash. Working in many high risk industrial sectors, day laborers meet an employer's needs for flexible labor demands allowing circumvention of rules that require they document workers, pay payroll taxes, or provide nonwage benefits.[30] In many of their occupations, neither day laborers nor their employers are familiar with occupational hazards and controls. Yet when hazards become apparent to these workers, their dependence on daily wages, the temporary and informal nature of their work agreements, their limited English skills, and their immigration status make them reluctant to raise concerns about workplace conditions and invisible to responsible federal and state labor and occupational safety agencies.[31, 32, 33]

SFDPH staff initially encountered day laborers through an educational campaign to reduce childhood lead poisoning. Work commonly done by day laborers in San Francisco—the renovation of old housing stock containing lead-based paint—is a risk factor in occupational and environmental lead poisoning. Cognizant of the limited ability of day laborers to take action to protect themselves, in 2000, the staff began to conduct occupational health and safety training for the San Francisco Day Labor Program (DLP), which included the provision of protective equipment. What became apparent through dialogue with day laborers was that the day laborers' primary concern was finding a job and that their willingness to accept dangerous jobs was, in part, due to job insecurity. Furthermore, laborers desired vocational but not health and safety training.

In 2003, SFDPH and La Raza Centro Legal (La Raza), the nonprofit legal assistance agency that operates the DLP, received a grant from the National Institute of Environmental Health Sciences (NIEHS) to conduct community-based participatory research to improve day laborer's working conditions. The project explicitly confronted the separate goals of occupational health and job security. For example, the research collaboration included a local private construction company which helped staff to develop a vocational training program, ultimately run by day laborers, to skills in both construction and injury and illness prevention. The project also funded a community economic development agency to create a business plan to market the services of the DLP more effectively.

The NIEHS funded partnership was also successful in engaging in local occupational health policy. For example, La Raza's work to help immigrant workers recover unpaid wages and workers' compensation benefits revealed that many employers did not provide legally required workers' compensation benefits to day laborers. Consequently, PHES and La Raza began exploring local legislation to ensure that employers in industries like construction maintained adequate workers' compensation insurance.

Developing a partnership with a legal services agency working for social justice forced PHES to reframe occupational health goals in terms of workers' rights and human rights in order to relate better to the principles and values of La Raza. The combined public health, economic security, and workers' rights agenda not only enabled La Raza and SFDPH to work more effectively together but also became a model shared through La Raza's and the DLP's relationships with national coalitions working for immigrant labor rights, including the National Day Labor Network.

While it was easy to recognize the mutual benefits of the partnership with La Raza, many of its challenges were unfamiliar to PHES staff. Chief among these challenges were community agencies and day laborers' distrust of government officials. At the first meeting of the Unidos partnership, one of the community agency's staff commented: "We hate the government."

Another challenge for PHES arose from day laborers' advocacy for public restrooms at hiring locations. Many residents in the neighborhood opposed public restrooms, claiming that they would attract unlawful activities such as drug dealing. Acknowledging this concern, PHES staff promised to conduct community meetings to discuss this and other environmental hazards in the neighborhood. Since the DLP had been at odds with antirestroom residents for many years, the DLP staff could not understand how PHES could simultaneously acknowledge the health needs of the day laborers and the concerns of the residents. PHES learned that public health practitioners must effectively communicate their own institutional constraints to community partners. Despite these challenges, La Raza and PHES continued to effectively collaborate through the course of the project, demonstrating the value attributed to the public health contribution.

Building an Urban Collaboration for Food Equity

Access to nutritious food resources varies considerably by place and economic means, making it an important contributor to health inequities, yet public health agencies have only recently become attuned to the importance of the food environment and food security. For example, federal studies document the widespread prevalence of hunger and food insecurity among the poor.[34] The presence of a supermarket in a neighborhood predicts higher fruit and vegetable consumption and reduced prevalence of overweight and obesity.[35, 36]

In San Francisco, as elsewhere, responsibilities for urban food policies and programs are fragmented across agencies, including SFDPH, the San Francisco Unified School District (SFUSD), the County Agriculture Commissioner, and human services, land use planning and redevelopment agencies. To begin to address the need for coordinated municipal food policies, in 2002, PHES created a public–private partnership, the San Francisco Food Systems (SFFS), with a local nonprofit fiscal sponsor to: (1) integrate food system planning into city and county government; (2) ensure access to healthy food for all San Francisco's residents; and (3) open urban markets for local and regional sustainable agriculture. The initiative used a "food systems" framework which integrated a number of related goals: improving access to healthy foods for all residents; supporting regional markets for agriculture; reducing food transportation costs; reducing chemical inputs in agriculture and food processing; providing urban markets for family farms; recirculating financial capital in the community; and greening the urban environment.

An initial PHES and the SFFS action was to convene an interdisciplinary group, the San Francisco Food Alliance, to conduct a food systems assessment in order to generate data for local food related policy and decision making. Partners involved represented food distributors, food banks, community gardeners, child care agencies, restaurateurs, free dining rooms, and other city agencies. The assessment offered a holistic overview of the local food system with current data and statistics for measures and indicators of food access and equity.[37]

The assessment highlighted critical equity issues, including the underutilization of federal nutrition programs and the poor-quality food options for those relying on these programs. For example, few food pantries or sites serving free and low-cost meals were located in parts of San Francisco where poor seniors lived. The assessment also found that while farmers' markets sold low-cost nutritious fruits and vegetables, few farmers' markets accepted federally funded food program vouchers or Electronic Benefits Transfer (EBT) cards, depriving lower income families of the benefits of high quality, regionally grown produce. In response, PHES and the SFFS researched barriers to the use of EBT at markets in San Francisco and secured technical support and equipment for markets with commitments to increasing federal food program participation. By 2005, six markets were accepting EBT, and ultimately, the City enacted legislation to require acceptance of food stamps and all federal nutrition benefits at all markets.

School nutrition programs were another equity focus of the PHES–SFFS collaboration. Public school nutrition services in San Francisco had been long neglected, in part because of competing educational priorities and declining public support for public schools. The food systems assessment also revealed a disturbing progressive decline in student participation in school breakfasts. Working with the SFUSD Student Nutrition Service department, the collaboration initiated a farm-to-school initiative to increase the amount and quality of locally grown, fresh produce offered through the federally subsidized school lunch program. This effort was an opportunity to support regional food procurement, higher quality food, and nutritional and environmental education, potentially achieving multiple system goals simultaneously.

Work within the public school system quickly revealed the structural barriers to providing high-quality food, including low federal reimbursement rates, complex procurement rules, and high labor costs. Acknowledging these external constraints and developing allies within the school nutrition services programs was essential to secure the support of school nutrition program staff, and subsequent work focused on identifying external resources for public school nutrition. For example, with short-term grant funds from USDA, partners were able to pilot test salad bars. Later, the partnership leveraged the results from the successful model to secure long-term resources from the City General Fund for salad bars.

Through their assessment of the school food environment, PHES also recognized inequities in food choices within the public school nutrition programs. In San Francisco's middle and high schools, students relying on federally subsidized lunches received a different standard of food service, with different meal choices, than students paying cash in a separate *a la carte* line. While the initial objective of the *a la carte* system had been to increase revenues for school nutrition programs by selling snacks and beverages, the *a la carte* system had evolved into a system where the food choices offered to cash paying students were different and more numerous than the choices offered to students using vouchers.

The two-tier system was overtly discriminatory, created a potent and unnecessary stigma for students without higher economic means, reduced participation in the federally subsidized lunch program, and appeared to violate legal standards for equal access to school food (42 U.S.C. 1758(b) (10)). PHES confirmed these practices through observations at school sites and interviewed students who indicated that they preferred to spend their own money in the *a la carte* line or forego lunch entirely, rather than stand in the separate line for the subsidized meal. Potential impacts on student health included hunger and challenges to learning. With documentation from several school sites and best practice evidence on feasible alternatives, PHES advocated with responsible school officials for the creation of a single standard of meal service and later shared this research with external stakeholders who were able to bring legal opinions and national media public attention to the issue.[38] Ultimately, the SFUSD committed to investing in the technological infrastructure and programmatic and policy changes to replace the two-tier system with the ongoing participation of PHES.[38]

The constituency created by the SFFS and PHES for a comprehensive food policy agenda has grown to include advocates for public health, the environment, schools, and economic vitality. The initiative maintains focus on equity concerns such as hunger, food security, and nutrition by working with and in low-income communities, drawing on participatory assessments, supporting community food resources including supermarkets, farmers' markets, and community gardens, and building understanding between farming and consumers. Today the initiative is advancing public policy strategies, such as chain restaurant menu labeling, to create a more equitable and healthy food landscape for San Francisco.[39]

Planning the Healthy City

Historically, urban conditions including pollution, crowding, child labor, and dangerous work have been recognized as harmful to the health and the underprivileged.[40] In the twentieth century, housing, land use, and transportation policy combined "exclusionary zoning" with the interstate highway system, tax subsidies for home mortgages, and urban "renewal" programs and condemned central city neighborhoods to disinvestment, poverty, and environmental risks,[41, 42] created sprawl, and contributed to physical inactivity, air pollution, and global warming.[43]

Today, globalization and urbanization are reshaping urban physical and social landscapes, creating new vulnerabilities for health. In some urban areas, gentrification has led to increased land values and rents and the involuntary displacement of tenants out of their homes.[44] High housing costs force households to choose between rent, food, clothing, transportation, and medical care or to accept unsafe or crowded housing.[45] Displacement of people or businesses resulting from redevelopment or gentrification results in the loss of economic security and health-protective social networks.[46] The deindustrialization of our economy has also shifted work towards the retail and service sectors, widening the distribution of income and wealth.[47]

By the end of 2000, gentrification struggles in San Francisco had become a center of political and organizing activity.[44] Antidisplacement activists were successful in getting representation on the city's Planning Commission and in advancing new regulations (e.g., inclusionary zoning) to protect and create affordable housing. Most importantly a shift from citywide to district legislative elections opened the way for representation of neighborhood concerns at the city level.

In 2002, the San Francisco Planning Department (SF Planning) launched the Eastern Neighborhoods Community Planning Process to respond to recognized land use conflicts in several neighborhoods: the Mission, South of Market (SoMa), Showplace Square/Potrero Hill, and Bayview/Hunters Point. Many stakeholders in these neighborhoods viewed the planning process, which was primarily focused on the rezoning of historically industrial lands for new residential uses, as unresponsive to neighborhood concerns of unaffordable housing, residential and job displacement, gentrification, public safety, and inadequate open space.

At the same time, PHES had begun to introduce the practice of HIA locally as a tool to raise attention to the health impacts of public policy.[23] Working closely with community organizations, PHES conducted workshops in which participants collectively identified and described potential pathways between health, environmental, economic, and cultural conditions and public policies. For instance, youth working on food access described how farmers' markets might lead to a family sharing home-cooked meals more frequently, improving family cohesion and providing greater interpersonal support. Most participants readily understood that factors such as adequate housing, work security, and supportive social relationships impacted health and that political decisions either created or eliminated such health resources.

Participants in the HIA workshops appropriately questioned whether a science-based tool like HIA would be effective in achieving social change. Many believed that comprehensively describing the impacts of policy on urban conditions could be a powerful advocacy tool, yet others indicated the limitations of scientific evidence alone in changing public policy. One participant remarked, "...we already know this, how do we get [the legislators] to know this?" Others suggested that HIA must be conducted with both proponents and opponents of a particular policy position. Overall, participants appeared ready to commit the time and resources to participate in a HIA, particularly if decision makers could be held accountable to the findings.

Following these initial workshops, one community organization, People Organized in Defense of Environmental and Economic Rights (PODER), asked PHES staff how HIA might advance their neighborhood goals in land use planning. PODER, part of the Mission Anti-Displacement Coalition (MAC) a coalition of neighborhood organizations organizing community residents in response to displacement, had argued for greater consideration of health, social, and economic impacts in the regulatory process for conducting environmental impact assessments (EIA). EIA was an established regulatory process designed to assess adverse environmental effects of public decisions, including effects on human health.[13] However, community residents were typically at the receiving end of the analysis and did not have the opportunity to articulate values, define problems, or identify goals. As one MAC community organizer complained, "... [Planning officials] kept saying that we could only talk about issues they could address [in the Environmental Impact Report] but, we were just talking about bread and butter issues." MAC believed the exclusion of community and economic issues was symptomatic of the more general exclusion of residents from the planning process and viewed HIA as a vehicle to voice resident experiences and perspectives in a more inclusive and responsive EIA process.

One of the first opportunities to test the value of HIA in San Francisco came in 2003 when soon-to-be-evicted tenants challenged an environmental impact assessment on a proposed development project which would have demolished 377 rent-controlled housing units and replaced them with new market-rate condominiums. Tenants vocally testified to the health and social impacts of the demolition. PHES conducted an HIA on the project, and corroborating the testimony of tenants, provided empirical evidence of the likely health impacts of unaffordable housing and displacement[48] (see Chapter 18). Ultimately, in response to community demands, the project developer promised to offer lifetime leases in the new building to existing tenants, to maintain rents at present rates, and to delay demolition until sufficient replacement units were located.

In November 2004, PHES embarked on a more ambitious effort to evaluate all of the community planning efforts in the Eastern Neighborhoods.[49]

Combining principles found in HIA, planning, and deliberative democratic experiments, PHES recruited and convened a Community Council comprised of more than 20 diverse community organizations to oversee the Eastern Neighborhoods Community Health Impact Assessment (ENCHIA). Conducted over a period of 18 months, ENCHIA produced a vision of and objectives for a healthy city; community health indicators to measure progress towards this vision; and quantitative targets and policy strategies for healthy urban development.[49] At the end of the process, ENCHIA developed the *Healthy Development Measurement Tool* (HDMT) as a comprehensive metric to evaluate land use plans and projects.[8, 50]

To advance the ENCHIA's vision of a healthy city, the Community Council asked PHES to institutionalize the use of the HDMT in local development-related decision making. In 2007, after development of the HDMT, pilot tests and peer review, PHES successfully used the metric to evaluate the Eastern Neighborhoods Area Plans, the original target for the ENCHIA process. The evaluation, conducted in partnership with the Planning Department, resulted in the addition of plan policies and implementation strategies to protect residents from poor environmental quality, increase childcare options, and improve housing conditions.[50]

Beyond its impacts on the planning process, ENCHIA increased awareness among community organizations of the relationships between human health and land use development. Some San Francisco organizations were readily able to use and translate health research conducted by PHES through ENCHIA in the policy process to achieve social change goals. For example, the South of Market Community Action Network (SOMCAN), a former member of the ENCHIA Council, used ENCHIA research to justify and negotiate a community impact fee from a luxury condominium development to build neighborhood infrastructure and prevent displacement.[48, 51]

The ENCHIA process did not occur without substantial challenges for PHES. Many Council members had strong expectations that PHES would use the ENCHIA process to influence the Planning Department to meet community demands. PHES had a strong interest in promoting health through land use policy but did not have established relationships and influence with responsible sister agencies. The limited power of PHES in the planning process meant that it could not assure Council stakeholders the adoption of the Council's findings or recommendations. Furthermore, land use planning decision making was highly contested. PHES staff aimed to have the Council play an objective role, believing that the explicit inclusion and dissemination of public health evidence in the decision-making process would best protect community health interests. PHES staff attempted to steer Council away from adopting positions on specific development projects, knowing that these would engender the greatest controversy.[49]

PHES has established a long-term program at SFDPH to maintain and apply the HDMT and to conduct applications of city plans and projects. To help ensure its long-term sustainability, PHES trained several local organizations to use the HDMT, and The California Endowment, a health-oriented philanthropy, has funded Council organizations to apply the HDMT in their engagement with land use. In addition, in 2007, the San Francisco legislature appointed PHES staff to participate on the Western South of Market Citizens' Planning Task Force, a neighborhood-based comprehensive planning effort, to provide health-based technical support for their community plan. Collectively, the diverse users and applications helped build a constituency and legitimacy for public health analysis of land use policy and planning in San Francisco.

Learning from the PHES Experience

The evolution of PHES at SFDPH demonstrates the implementation of the strategies presented at the beginning of this chapter and the possibility of an equity-oriented public health practice within a governmental institution. As illustrated in the practice stories, health equity has become an issue on the public and institutional agendas of San Francisco and has created new roles for the Department in City policy making. The efforts resulted in impacts on local environmental conditions and institutional practices; greater capacity of people to influence the conditions of their lives; more examples of interdisciplinary institutional practices; and a deeper understanding by the public and policy makers of needs of health. Most critically, PHES has forged new relationships among health interests and diverse stakeholders, institutions, interests, and agendas outside of public health.

Such work did not occur without challenges. PHES had to mobilize and organize resources to conduct this work. Many stakeholders challenged the appropriateness of public health engagement in policy beyond the traditional mandates of "public health." Taking an active role in monitoring institutional accountability resulted in criticism from sister public institutions. Nevertheless, PHES was able to navigate these challenges by working in a flexible and adaptive way.

San Francisco may be thought of as an exceptional place for such public health activism, but the work suggests that all public health institutions have potential power to address health inequities. Below we identify and summarize the characteristics of our work that we believe contributed to establishing a health equity practice and that may be applicable to other public health institutions. Specifically, we argue that the following tactics enabled us to develop an effective health equity practice:

- Mobilizing evidence and taking positions on current policy debates
- Actively engaging constituencies working for social justice
- Using resources and funding creatively
- Allowing individual and organizational flexibility
- Working with and being responsive to critics

Mobilizing Evidence and Taking Positions on Current Policy Debates

The work of PHES did not begin with a new set of health equity policy goals but leveraged the existing engagement of many residents and community organizations in policy making. Many local groups were working to protect and promote healthy communities without an explicit recognition of the health costs or benefits of their struggles. PHES took advantage of available policy struggles and engaged constituencies to bring health evidence into the public discourse. This helped both to raise attention to determinants of health inequities and also to build relationships with ongoing social activists. For example, when San Francisco was considering its living wage policy, SFDPH responded to the demand for a public health analysis of the policy and made a clear connection between the effect of income on health and inequity. This approach recognized that evidence is more likely to be translated and used if linked to issues already on the public agenda. It also showed that social justice activists could call upon health practitioners to support their objectives in contested policy settings. In these examples, the use of public health evidence created through practice of HIA also helped PHES avoid the label of the "biased advocate." Overall, by engaging in contemporary policy debates using evidence, PHES developed an identity as a potential partner in efforts for social change.

Actively Engaging Constituencies Working for Social Justice

Public health aims to respond to the demands and needs of its constituencies. The impact, sustainability, and legitimacy of PHES required creating a new constituency for its health equity activities. Its primary method was to form strategic partnerships with established social movements who shared a health equity agenda with public health.

In some cases, it was not difficult to find partners and demonstrate shared agendas. For example, in San Francisco, housing managed by the Public Housing Authority has been plagued by structural deficiencies (e.g., broken windows, stairs) and poor-quality conditions in the homes (e.g., lead, mold). Low-income tenants living in such housing experienced a higher incidence of preventable injuries and hospitalizations. In this case, the local public health department was able to bring both expertise and regulatory authority to a coalition organized around asthma prevention for low-income residents to improve habitability and safety standards in the Housing Authority properties.[52]

In other cases, particularly around land use planning, community social justice struggles were not yet organized around health objectives. In these cases, it was not appropriate for PHES to introduce a new agenda into the landscape; however, it was possible to explore how the expertise or position of a public health agency could contribute to existing agendas of community groups. This often meant attending and participating in processes such as community meetings and public hearings and as an observer and listener. Over time, translating evidence on social conditions and health equity in the context of political struggles catalyzed demand for public health engagement and expanded the constituencies for health equity practice.

Using Resources and Funding Creatively

The SFDPH mission statement and strategic plan provided legitimacy for work on social conditions; still, at the outset, no funding, resource, or high-level political commitment existed in San Francisco to create PHES. In 2001, PHES established its two funded positions specifically for HIA through a reorganization and consolidation of more traditional environmental health and regulatory functions. Generating additional staff resources to the program required writing grants and appealing to staff interests. PHES management invited environmental health inspectors, who were able to efficiently complete their day-to-day duties, to identify and pursue work on issues of equity and environmental improvement as part of their jobs. Many staff took this opportunity even though it required additional effort beyond their mandated regulatory duties. When hiring vacant positions, PHES similarly recruited applicants who had commitments to health equity and interests in working outside of traditional organizational roles. Today, PHES has grown beyond its first two initial positions to the current team of nine full- and part-time staff.

Allowing Individual and Organizational Flexibility

PHES began as an experimental approach, being organized around flexible goals, issues, and strategies, and evolved organically without any significant long range planning. Yet it has been critical to develop an organizational structure to support and evaluate the work. An early group activity was the creation of a mission statement and identification of group values (see Box 16.1). Staff also committed to working collectively in teams, improving overall accountability for projects, and allowing for debate in project decision making. The larger PHES group provided a place to support collective staff needs such as peer review and links to potential collaborators. Staffs now brings new situations to the attention of the team for consideration of opportunities and direction. Evaluation occurs on an adaptive ongoing basis, work progresses iteratively and adapts to changing conditions. As a group, PHES commits to using a single set of performance metrics, producing an annual report of its activities, and to communicating its work and accomplishments as examples of a unified approach.[53]

Working with and Being Responsive to Critics

Listening and responding to criticism from sister public agencies was necessary for PHES to work beyond traditional institutional boundaries. For example, officials in the Planning Department understood the nexus between health and land use development but initially expressed skepticism about the value of collaboration with a public health agency. Some city officials criticized the ENCHIA process as duplicative or competitive with the formal planning process. They also believed that the practice of HIA may potentially expose failures of city planning, identify additional impact of development requiring mitigations, or provide fuel for antidevelopment interests.

PHES did not respond defensively to such challenges, but maintained a commitment to public health concerns and to working in a way that acknowledged the limitations and concerns of the Planning Department. PHES was particularly attentive to developing better ways to analyze health effects and to identifying strategies that were both feasible economically and consistent with the planning department's goals. For example, in order to provide objective ways to assess health impacts of planning policy, PHES developed tools and techniques to analyze traffic and vehicle emissions data and to predict impacts on diverse pollutant-related health effects.[54] Similarly, PHES used available data on the transportation network, land uses, and demographics to develop a forecasting model to predict vehicle–pedestrian collisions. Today, with the support of constituencies built through the above practice stories, these tools are being integrated into the city's planning and regulatory practices. By the end of the ENCHIA process, consideration of health goals had increased the requirements placed on urban development, but through sustained dialogue, the sharing of evidence, and consistent presence in community planning contexts, the Planning Department came to understand the necessity and value of those additional development requirements.

Conclusion

Despite broad recognition of health inequities, a comprehensive public health institutional strategy for their elimination does not exist. Many public health practitioners are questioning the limits of contemporary public health practice, recognizing the need for a holistic framework for health, and arguing for greater advocacy to improve social and environmental conditions. These calls echo those sounded more than two decades ago in the 1986 Ottawa Charter for Health Promotion.

Public health fulfills a narrow role in a system of fragmented institutions. By acknowledging the inseparability of health from other human needs and aspirations, health equity practices can fundamentally challenge popular definitions of public health, as well as the traditional roles of public health institutions. But to do this, public health will need to work to a much greater degree outside institutional boundaries and integrate diverse voices and skills. Fortunately, commitments to social justice exist in other institutions and disciplines and public health can cultivate partnerships across disciplines. Partnering with those most affected by health inequities and with those who witness and personally experience the consequences of health inequities provides a way to describe qualitatively stories that embody the facts, reframe the problem of social inequality, legitimize new roles for public health, and generate collective commitments to eliminating health inequities.

Effective action requires acknowledging the contested political contexts of social justice struggles and leveraging public health expertise and standing to influence these struggles in the interest of health. Using public health's power also requires recognition of the privileged institutional position of public health and a readiness to risk that privileged position.

Working on practices to address health inequities demands a strong personal commitment from the public health practitioner. Simultaneously, playing agency insider and health advocate requires relinquishing several traditional disciplinary values and doctrines. For many, work on health inequities also makes it possible to align that work with personal values, to develop knowledge and skills beyond a singular discipline, and to develop meaningful relationships with community members and other professionals.

Practitioners acting to address underlying social and physical environmental conditions will be challenged to demonstrate the value of their efforts to political leaders. Activities that extend beyond traditional institutional practices may even be censored. Yet, public health practitioners who build their reputations can establish legitimacy to be representatives of people's interests and to work outside their traditional roles.

Ultimately, the achievement of health equity transcends the responsibility of public health practitioners and institutions alone. Ensuring that those with the least resources actually benefit from health inequity interventions requires institutional accountability in all sectors. Achieving health equity demands a strong consensus to equity and the willingness to forego social privilege. This will indeed be an enduring challenge for all of society.

References

1. M. Marmot, R.G. Wilkinson, *Social Determinants of Health*. 2nd ed. (Oxford: Oxford University Press, 2006).
2. D.P. Keating and C. Hertzman, eds., *Developmental Health and the Wealth of Nations* (New York: The Guilford Press, 1999).
3. I. Kawachi and L.F. Berkman, eds., *Neighborhoods and Health* (New York: Oxford University Press, 2003).
4. WHO (World Health Organization). *Ottawa Charter for Health Promotion.* First International Conference on Health Promotion, Ottawa. November 21, 1986.
5. USDHHS (U.S. Department of Health and Human Services). *Healthy People 2010: Understanding and Improving Health.* 2nd ed. (Washington, DC: U.S. Government Printing Office, November 2000).
6. A.T. Geronimus, "To Mitigate, Resist, or Undo: Addressing Structural Influences on the Health of Urban Populations," 90 *American Journal of Public Health* (2000): 867–872.
7. Communities Count 2002. http://www.communitiescount.org/ (accessed August 6, 2008)
8. SFDPH (San Francisco Department of Public Health). *Healthy Development Measurement Tool.* www.thehdmt.org (accessed May 12, 2008)
9. A. Sen, *Inequality Reexamined* (New York: Oxford University Press, 1992).
10. A. Scott-Samuel, "The Politics of Health," 1 *Journal of Public Health* (1979): 123–126.
11. S.N. Tesh, *Hidden Arguments: Political Ideology & Disease Prevention Policy* (New Brunswick, NJ: Rutgers University Press, 1998).
12. J. Kemm, J. Parry, and S. Palmer, *Health Impact Assessment: Concepts, Techniques and Applications* (New York: Oxford University Press, 2004).
13. R. Bhatia R and A. Wernham, "Integrating Human Health Into Environmental Impact Assessment: An Unrealized Opportunity for Environmental Health and Justice,"116 *Environmental Health Perspectives* (2008): 991–1000.
14. J. Keeley and I. Scoones, *Understanding Environmental Policy Processes: A Review. Institute of Development Studies*, Working Paper 89. University of Sussex, 1999.
15. H.J. Geiger, "Community-oriented primary care: A path to community development," 92 *American Journal of Public Health* (2002): 1713–1716.
16. P. Freire, *Pedagogy of the Oppressed* (New York: Continuum, 1970).
17. A.M. Goetz and J.J. Gaventa, *Bringing Citizen Voice and Client Focus into Service Delivery. Institute of Development Studies*, Working Paper 138. University of Sussex, 2001.

18. M. Minkler and N. Wallerstein, eds., *Community-Based Participatory Research for Health* (San Francisco, CA: Jossey-Bass, 2003).
19. NIEHS (National Institute of Environmental Health Sciences). *Environmental Justice and Community Based Participatory Research.* http://www.niehs.nih.gov/research/supported/programs/justice/index.cfm (accessed May 12, 2008)
20. E. Hood, "Dwelling disparities: How poor housing leads to poor health," 113 *Environmental Health Perspectives* (2005): A290–A291.
21. J. Brewer, *Public Health Responses to Racism and Domestic Violence.* Family Violence Prevention Fund. http://www.endabuse.org/health/ejournal/archive/1–4/responses_to_racism.php (accessed May 12, 2008)
22. SFDPH (San Francisco Department of Public Health). *Strategic Plan* (San Francisco, CA: San Francisco Department of Public Health, 2000).
23. R. Bhatia, "Swimming Upstream in a Swift Current: Public Health Institutions and Inequality," in *Health and Social Justice: Politics, Ideology, and Inequity in the Distribution and Disease,* ed. Richard Hofrichter (San Francisco, CA: Jossey-Bass, 2003).
24. R.L. Jin, C.P. Shah, and T.J. Svoboda, "The Impact of Unemployment on Health: A Review of the Evidence," 153 *Canadian Medical Association Journal* (1995): 529–540.
25. F. McKee-Ryan, Z. Song, C.R. Wanberg, and A.J. Kinicki, "Psychological and Physical Well-Being during Unemployment: a Meta-Analytic Study," 90(1) *Journal of Applied Psychology* 2005: 53–76.
26. M. Voss, L. Nylén, M. Floderus, F. Diderichsen, and P. Terry, "Unemployment and Early Cause-Specific Mortality: a Study Based on the Swedish Twin Registry," 94(12) *American Journal of Public Health* (2004): 2155–2161.
27. J.S. Feinstein, "The relationship between socioeconomic status and health: A review of the literature," 71 *Milbank Quarterly* (1993): 279–322.
28. I.H. Yen and S.L. Syme, "The Social Environment and Health: A Discussion of the Epidemiologic Literature," 20 *Annual Review of Public Health* (1999): 287–308.
29. R. Bhatia and M.H. Katz, "Estimation of health benefits from a local living wage ordinance," 91 *American Journal of Public Health* (2001): 1398–1402.
30. A. Valenzuela, "Day Labor Work," 29 *Annual Review of Sociology* (2003): 307–333.
31. N. Walter, P. Bourgois, and H.M. Loinaz, "Social Context of Work Injury among Undocumented Day Laborers in San Francisco," 17(6) *Journal of General Internal Medicine* (2002): 121–229.
32. P. Worby, *Pride and daily survival: Latino Migrant Day Laborers and Occupational Health.* Master's Thesis (Berkeley, CA: University of California, 2002).
33. GAO (General Accountability Office). *Worker Protection: Labors' efforts to enforce protections for day laborers could benefit from better data and guidance.* Report to the Honorable Luis V. Guitierrez, US House of Representatives. September, 2002. General Accounting Office. http://www.gao.gov/cgi-bin/getrpt?GAO-02–925 (accessed May 12, 2008)
34. M. Nord, M. Andrews, and S. Carlson, Household Food Security in the United States, 2006. ERR-49, U.S. Dept. of Agriculture, Econ. Res. Serv. November 2007.

35. K. Morland, A.V. Diez Roux, and S. Wing, "Supermarkets, other food stores, and obesity: the atherosclerosis risk in communities study," 30(4) *American Journal of Preventive Medicine* (2006): 333–339.

36. S. Inagami, D.A. Cohen, B.K. Finch, and S.M. Asch, "You are where you shop: Grocery store locations, weight, and neighborhoods," 31(1) *American Journal of Preventive Medicine* (2006):10–17.

37. SFFS (San Francisco Food Systems). *San Francisco Collaborative Food System Assessment* (San Francisco, CA: San Francisco Food Systems, 2005). http://www.sffoodsystems.org/pdf/FSA-online.pdf (accessed August 6, 2008)

38. C. Pogash, "Free Lunch Isn't Cool, So Some Students Go Hungry," *New York Times* (March 1, 2008).

39. E.S.F. Allday, "Supes Require Posting of Nutrition Info," *San Francisco Chronicle* (March 12, 2008).

40. J. Corburn, "Confronting the challenges in reconnecting urban planning and public health," 94 *American Journal of Public Health* (2004): 541–546.

41. J. Jacobs, *The Death and Life of American Cities* (New York: Random House, 1961).

42. D.R. Williams and C. Collins, "Racial residential segregation: a fundamental cause of racial disparities in health," 116 *Public Health Reports* (2001): 404–416.

43. H. Frumkin, L. Frank, and R. Jackson, *Urban Sprawl and Public Health: Designing, Planning, and Building for Healthy Communities* (Washington, DC: Island Press, 2004).

44. S.V. Alejandrino, *Gentrification in San Francisco's Mission District: Indicators and Policy Recommendations* (San Francisco, CA: Mission Economic Development Agency, 2000).

45. J. Krieger and D.L. Higgins, "Housing and health: time again for public health action," 92 *American Journal of Public Health* (2002): 758–768.

46. San Francisco Department of Public Health (SFDPH), *The Case for Housing Impacts Assessment: the Human Health and Social Impacts of Inadequate Housing and Their Consideration in Ceqa Policy and Practice.* PHES Technical Research Report, 2004. http://www.sfphes.org/publications/reports/HIAR May 2004.pdf (accessed July 31, 2008)

47. W. Curran, "Gentrification and the nature of work: Exploring the links in Williamsburg, Brooklyn," 36 *Environment and Planning A* (2004): 1243–1258.

48. R. Bhatia, "Protecting health using an environmental impact assessment: A case study of San Francisco land use decision-making," 97(3) *American Journal of Public Health* (2007): 406–413.

49. San Francisco Department of Public Health (SFDPH), *Eastern Neighborhoods Community Health Impact Assessment (ENCHIA) Final Report*, September 2007. http://www.sfphes.org/publications/PHES_publications.htm (accessed May 12, 2008)

50. L. Farhang, R. Bhatia, C.C. Scully, J. Corburn, M. Gaydos, and S. Malekafzali, "Creating tools for healthy development: Case study of San Francisco's Eastern Neighborhoods Community Health Impact Assessment," 14(3) *Journal of Public Health Management and Practice* (2008): 255–265.

51. S.T. Jones, "From lightning rod to love fest: How Rincon Towers got so popular and what it says about urban planning in San Francisco," *San Francisco Bay Guardian*. (February 4, 2004).

52. San Francisco Asthma Task Force (SFATF), *San Francisco Asthma Task Force website*. http://www.sfgov.org/site/asthmatf_index.asp (accessed July 2, 2008)

53. San Francisco Department of Public Health (SFDPH), *Program on Health, Equity and Sustainability: Annual Report 2007* (San Francisco, CA: SFDPH, 2008).   http://www.sfphes.org/publications/PHES_2007_Annual_Report.pdf (accessed May 12, 2008)

54. R. Bhatia and T. Rivard, *Assessment and Mitigation of Air Pollutant Health Effects from Intra-urban Roadways: Guidance for Land Use Planning and Environmental Review* (San Francisco, CA: San Francisco Department of Public Health, 2008). http://www.sfphes.org/publications/PHES_publications. htm (accessed August 6, 2008)

17

Estimation of Health Benefits from a Local Living Wage Ordinance

RAJIV BHATIA AND MITCHELL KATZ

The inverse relationship between socioeconomic status (SES) and health, which has been extensively documented,[1–6] may be mediated by material, behavioral, psychosocial, or physiologic pathways.[2,7–9] Income is a widely used dimension of SES that at lower levels predicts poor health and premature death, whether measured at the individual or at the aggregate level.[10–13] Increasing the federal minimum wage is one means of limiting income poverty in the United States. Indeed, many municipalities in the United States have increased the minimum wage for certain sectors of the local labor force by establishing local "living wage" laws. In contrast to the national minimum wage, a living wage generates an income sufficient to meet subsistence needs such as food, shelter, clothing, transportation, and child care.[14,15] San Francisco's legislative board recently considered adopting a living wage of $11 per hour for workers of the city's contractors and property leaseholders. We estimated the magnitude of the anticipated health improvement associated with this legislation.

This chapter is reprinted with permission from *American Journal of Public Health*, 91(2001): 1398–1402. Copyright 2001 American Public Health Association.

Methods

Data

In 1999, the city and county of San Francisco commissioned an economic analysis by San Francisco State University to examine the implications of a proposal to require that all workers of city contractors and property lease-holders receive a minimum hourly wage of $11.00. The analysis relied on 2 principal sources of information: (1) surveys mailed to city contractors and property leaseholders and (2) administrative data on contractor budgets provided by city departments.[16] The response rate to the 2 parts of the mailed survey was low (approximately 24% and 26%, respectively), and the administrative data from city departments was often of limited quality and completeness. The analysis assessed the number of part-time and full-time workers in designated wage ranges and their benefits and provided estimates of the aggregate income gains for these workers that the proposed minimum hourly wage of $11 would bring about. The average income benefit was calculated by dividing the aggregate gain by the number of affected workers separately for full-time and part-time workers in each of 4 sectors: city contractors, airport leaseholders, port leaseholders, and other leaseholders. Confidence intervals for the number of workers affected and the average wage gain were not provided.

Because the San Francisco State University analysis did not directly assess the social or economic characteristics of the affected workers, we used 3 years of Bureau of Labor Statistics data for the San Francisco Bay area (1997–1999 Annual March Current Population Survey) to characterize workers aged 18 to 64 years who earned $5.75 to $11 per hour and currently worked in occupational and industry categories likely to be affected by the city ordinance. We adjusted income data to current dollars by using the urban consumer price index. Estimated proportions were pooled across the 3 survey years, and standard errors were calculated by methods supplied by the Bureau of Labor Statistics.

Estimates were based on peer-reviewed published studies of income's effect on health. Health outcomes of interest were premature mortality, preventable hospitalizations, and emergency room visits. We identified relevant literature on health outcomes by using Melvyn Medline (available at: http://www.library.ucsf.edu/db/medline/medframe) and by searching for English language articles that matched the subject-heading search terms "income" and "United States" (and "mortality," "hospitalization," or "health status indicators") and that were published between 1990 and 1998. A priori, we developed the following 6 criteria for study inclusion: (1) subjects representative of the US general population; (2) income measured at the individual, family, or household level; (3) longitudinal design; (4) statistical adjustment for age and sex; (5) year of income ascertainment provided; and (6) income applied as a continuous variable. When several analytic models were used in a single study, we selected those models that assessed nonlinear effects of income and adjusted for other correlates of social position, such as education.

We identified 8 general population studies of income's effects on all-cause mortality. All of these studies observed an inverse association between income and premature mortality. Four of the prospective national studies categorized income.[17–20] Two analyses were cross-sectional,[21,22] and one used a ratio of income to the poverty level as the independent variable and limited the analyses to whites and African Americans.[23] Only one study of income and mortality, a reanalysis of the Current Population Survey data, met all 6 of our criteria.[24] The investigators stratified the analysis by 3 age categories and by sex and additionally adjusted for age, household size, education, and marital status. The model that used a logarithmic transformation of income resulted in the best fit to the risk of mortality. One nationally representative study of income and hospital utilization was identified; however, income was assessed at the zip code level, and this predictor was not available in our analysis.

We identified 4 studies of the relationship between individual income and health status indicators in representative US populations.[13,25–27] All 4 studies were cross-sectional; however, one study, by Ettner,[27] used a 2-stage instrumental variable approach that allowed assessment of temporal relationships, so we included it in our analysis. The Ettner study assessed several health status indicators by using 3 data sets: the 1987 National Survey of Families and Households, the 1986–1987 panels of the Survey of Income and Program Participation, and the 1988 National Health Interview Survey. Outcomes were modeled as a function of log-transformed income, and the analyses were adjusted for sex, household size, marital status, race/ethnicity, age, education, and metropolitan area of residence. The analysis demonstrated a statistically significant exogenous relationship between income and 3 continuous health outcomes—the Center for Epidemiologic Studies scale of depressive symptoms, the number of days sick in bed in the past 4 months, and average daily alcohol consumption—as well as 3 discrete outcomes—self-rated health, work limitations, and limitations in activities of daily living.

We were also interested in the relationship between income and childhood development because of the importance of child development to lifelong social position and because of its potential intervening role in the relationship of income to health. We estimated the effect of increased wages on educational attainment and on early childbearing out of marriage by using an analysis from the Panel Study of Income Dynamics.[28] We selected this study because it illustrated the contribution of family income to childhood educational achievement and met all of our a priori inclusion criteria. For our analysis, we used the coefficients derived from models that used a log transformation of income and that adjusted for race/ethnicity, sex, number of siblings, family structure, and maternal age, schooling, and employment.

Analytic Approach

Effect measures and their standard errors were abstracted from the selected studies or were obtained from the study authors. The urban consumer price index was used to adjust the expected gain in income due to the proposed wage increase and the current income of earners to the year of income valuation reported in the studies. We estimated expected changes in health outcomes for full-time and part-time workers by applying the current estimated family income and the expected income gain to the study model. Given a specified annual income gain, this approach produced a value for each point on the current income distribution of the target population of workers. Depending on the study outcome and model used, the benefit of the living wage was expressed as either a difference, a ratio, or a percentage change.

Results

The San Francisco State University economic analysis estimated that 42,118 full-time and part-time earners working in 4 economic sectors would be affected by the proposed $11-per-hour living wage.[16] Estimated annual income gains varied by sector but averaged (in current dollars) $2668 for affected part-time workers and $4822 for full-time workers.

Table 17.1 describes selected characteristics of currently employed workers in the San Francisco Bay area aged 18 to 64 who worked at least 26 weeks a year as well as characteristics of those whose wages, industries, and occupations were most similar to those affected by the living wage. Of those affected by the living wage, 32.1% (90% confidence interval [CI] = 27.0, 37.1) were members of families with annual incomes less than $25,000. Compared with all current workers, workers targeted by the ordinance were more likely to be female, young, less educated, unmarried, without children, and working part time.

Wage gains predicted mortality risk reductions and improvements in health status for both men and women and for both part-time and full-time workers. The average magnitudes of these benefits for adult workers aged 24 to 44 with a current family income of $20,000 are presented in Table 17.2. The estimated reduction in mortality risk (relative hazard) for a full-time worker decreases with increasing current income,

TABLE 17.1. Selected Characteristics of Workers: San Francisco Bay Region[a], California, 1997–1999

CHARACTERISTIC	ALL WORKERS (n = 2667), % (90% CI)	WORKERS TARGETED BY ORDINANCE (n = 377), % (90% CI)
Female	43.3 (41.2, 45.3)	56.2 (50.8, 61.6)
Age, year		
18–23	8.3 (7.2, 9.4)	24.9 (20.2, 29.5)
24–44	58.0 (56.0, 60.0)	50.4 (44.9, 55.8)
45–64	33.7 (31.8, 35.6)	24.8 (20.1, 29.5)
Race/ethnicity		
White	74.7 (72.9, 76.4)	70.5 (65.5, 75.5)
Black	6.0 (5.1, 7.0)	5.9 (3.4, 8.4)
Asian/Pacific Islander	18.4 (16.8, 19.9)	23.0 (18.4, 27.6)
Native American	0.9 (0.6, 1.3)	0.6 (0, 1.3)
Marital status		
Married	56.7 (54.7, 58.7)	43.2 (37.8, 48.5)
Widowed, divorced, or separated	27.4 (25.8, 29.0)	9.9 (6.7, 13.1)
Unmarried	29.0 (27.2, 30.8)	46.9 (41.5, 52.3)
Family size		
1	26.5 (24.8, 28.3)	25.8 (21.1, 30.5)
2	23.9 (22.2, 25.6)	21.9 (17.4, 26.4)
3–4	38.0 (36.1, 40.0)	38.6 (33.4, 43.9)
>4	11.5 (10.3, 12.8)	13.6 (9.9, 17.3)
Any children <18 y	37.2 (35.2, 39.1)	28.2 (23.3, 33.1)
Any children <6 y	16.7 (15.2, 18.2)	12.7 (9.0, 16.3)
College graduate	41.8 (39.8, 43.7)	16.2 (12.3, 20.2)
Working full time	86.3 (85.0, 87.7)	72.8 (68.0, 77.6)
Earning >50% of family income	60.4 (58.4, 62.3)	45.0 (39.6, 50.4)
Family annual income <$25 000	9.6 (8.4, 10.8)	32.1 (27.0, 37.1)

Note: CI – confidence interval

[a]These estimates were derived from Bureau of Labor Statistics Annual March Current Population Survey data for the San Francisco Bay area (1997–1999). "Current workers" indicates currently employed workers aged 18 to 64 years who were working at least 26 weeks per year. "Workers targeted by ordinance" refers to the subset of current workers earning $5.75 to $11 per hour in occupational and industry categories who would probably be affected by adoption of a proposed living wage of $11 per hour for workers of the city's contractors and property leaseholders.

from 0.93 (95% CI = 0.90, 0.96) for men and 0.95 (95% CI = 0.93, 0.97) for women with a family annual income of $15,000 to 0.98 (95% CI = 0.977, 0.990) for men and 0.99 (95% CI = 0.985, 0.994) for women with a family income of $75 000 (Figure 17.1). The number of days sick

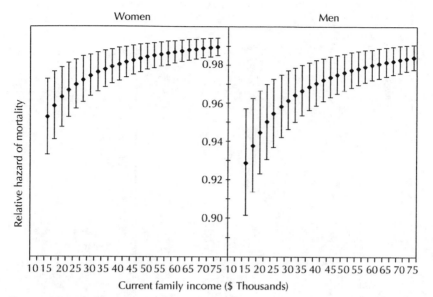

FIGURE 17.1 Estimated mortality risk reduction among full-time workers aged 24 to 44 years benefiting from the proposed San Francisco, CA, living wage ordinance.

NOTE: Bars represent 95% confidence intervals.

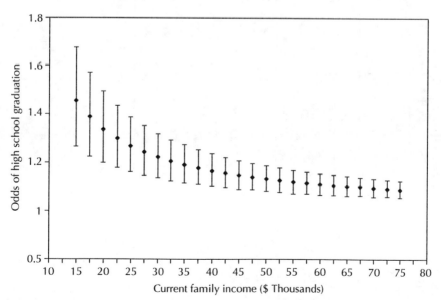

FIGURE 17.2 Estimated change in the likelihood of high school graduation among children from birth to 15 years of age in families with full-time workers benefiting from the proposed San Francisco, CA, living wage ordinance.

NOTE: Bars represent 95% confidence intervals.

TABLE 17.2. Estimated Health and Educational Effects on Workers and Their Children Resulting from Adoption of a Living Wage for Families with Incomes of $20000: San Francisco Bay Region, California. 1997–1999

STUDY/OUTCOME	MODEL	EFFECT MEASURE	ESTIMATE FOR FULL-TIME WORKERS (95% CI)	ESTIMATE FOR PART-TIME WORKERS (95% CI)
Backlund et al.[24]				
Mortality–male	Proportional hazards[a]	Hazard ratio	0.94 (0.92, 0.97)	0.97 (0.96, 0.98)
Mortality–female	Proportional hazards	Hazard ratio	0.96 (0.95, 0.98)	0.98 (0.97, 0.99)
Ettner[27]				
Health status	Ordered probit[b]	Relative risk	0.94 (0.93, 0.96)	0.97 (0.96, 0.98)
ADL limitations	Probit	Relative risk	0.96 (0.95, 0.98)	0.98 (0.97, 0.99)
Work limitations	Probit	Relative risk	0.94 (0.92, 0.96)	0.97 (0.95, 0.98)
CES-Depression scale	2-part[c]	Elasticity	-1.9%	-1.1%
No. of sick days	2-part	Elasticity	-5.8%	-3.2%
Alcohol consumption	2-part	Elasticity	+2.4%	+1.3%
Duncan et al.[28]				
Completed schooling	OLS regression	Years of schooling	0.25 (0.20, 0.30)	0.15 (0.12, 0.17)
Completed high school	Logistic regression	Odds ratio	1.34 (1.20, 1.49)	1.18 (1.11, 1.26)
Nonmarital childbirth	Proportional hazards	Hazard ratio	0.78 (0.69, 0.86)	0.86 (0.81, 0.92)

Note. CI – confidence interval; ADL – activities of daily living; CES – Center for Epidemiologic Studies; OLS – ordinary least squares.

[a]Effect measures for the 24- to 44-year age groups were used.

[b]The probit models required specifying the values of all the model covariates; the values given above were calculated for a married 30-year-old white female with 2 children living in a metropolitan area.

[c]The 2-part model used least squares regression on a log transformation of the dependent variable, with a conditional sample of subjects with positive values used for the outcome. The effect measure, elasticity, did not enable us to calculate confidence intervals.

in bed, depressive symptoms, the risks of limitations in work or activities of daily living, and being in the poorest subjective health would all be expected to be modestly reduced for full-time workers with current family incomes of $20,000; however, daily alcohol consumption would modestly increase (Table 17.2). For the children of workers benefiting from a living wage, the chances of completing high school would increase (Figure 17.2), as would the number of years of completed education. For girls, the risk of childbirth outside of marriage would be expected to fall.

Discussion

Estimating the magnitude of societal benefits resulting from a living wage is crucial because of the sizable costs of implementing this policy. Policymakers must be able to weigh the relative benefits and costs of a living wage compared with alternative means of achieving similar benefits.

Our analysis demonstrates that a modest gain in income resulting from a living wage would be associated with substantial health benefits. In addition, the educational attainment of workers' children would be improved and the risk of premarital childbirth among offspring would be lower with these modest income gains. Although our analysis predicted an increase in alcohol consumption, which may negatively affect health, the higher consumption of alcohol predicted by the applied study was attributed to a greater prevalence of drinking among wealthier persons.[27]

The major limitation of our analysis is the assumption of both a causal and a dynamic relationship between income and health. Since all available studies of the influence of income on health are observational, the apparent association could be due to confounding. Although all of the studies we applied adjusted for age, sex, race/ethnicity, education, and marital status, other unmeasured individual factors may explain the relationship between income and health. We were not able to account for neighborhood poverty, institutional racism, and inequalities in regional income distributions, which may also influence health outcomes independently of individual income.[8,11,29-33]

Reverse causality (i.e., poor health leads to poverty) is commonly raised as an alternative explanation of the association between SES and health. However, the evidence from prospective studies and the evidence for relationships between education and health and between spousal SES and health refute this hypothesis.[6] As childhood development is unlikely to influence parental income, reverse causality should not be an issue for these outcomes. Recent experience with welfare reform also provides compelling experimental evidence for the causal effect of income supplementation on childhood educational performance.[34]

Even if a causal relationship between income and health exists, we cannot be certain that an increase in income during adulthood will result in a prospective change in adult health. SES in childhood has been shown to predict health status in adult life, indicating that socioeconomic influences may be cumulative, have latent effects, or set an individual on a particular health trajectory.[9,35-38] However, longitudinal studies have demonstrated higher mortality rates among individuals in the middle income range whose incomes drop by more than 50%.[19]Also, significant effects of changes in family income on early childhood IQ and young adult achievement within families have been demonstrated.[28,39]

The application of observational studies in this policy analysis was constrained by the way the study data were reported and analyzed. While many of the reviewed mortality studies were prospective and statistically adjusted for potential confounders, few used continuous measures of income. For studies to be useful for estimating the health benefits accruing from modest income gains, researchers should retain income as a continuous measure and model nonlinear effects. Our analysis was not intended to capture all of the possible economic effects, and their implications for health, of a living wage ordinance. Secondary economic benefits of a living wage would be "wage push" (resulting in increasing wages for persons just above a living wage), "wage ripples" (increases in prevailing wages for persons doing similar work on noncity contracts), and local "multiplier" effects (due to the workforce spending additional income in the local economy). A potential negative effect of the living wage would be displacement of workers on city contracts due to competition from higher-paid or higher-skilled workers. Over the short term, the program would not be expected to result in displacement. However, even if displacements occurred, the ordinance would still increase the number of jobs in the community that paid a living wage. Our study demonstrates that a more egalitarian distribution of income may have long-term positive effects on individual and community health. However, attempts to modify the distribution of wealth are likely to face significant social, scientific, and economic challenges.[7,40-43]

Acknowledgments

Jennifer Mann and Randy Reiter shared in developing the original concept for this project. Susan Ettner provided invaluable assistance in applying the data from her original research.

Notes

1. M.G. Marmot, M. Kogevinas, and M.A. Elston, "Social/Economic Status and Disease," 8 *Annual Review of Public Health* (1987): 111–135.
2. J.S. Feinstein, "The Relationship Between Socioeconomic Status and Health A Review of the Literature," 71 *Milbank Quarterly* (1993): 279–322.
3. N. Krieger and E. Fee, "Measuring Social Inequalities in Health in the United States: A Historical Review, 1900–1950," 26 *International Journal of Health Services* (1996): 391–418.
4. S. Macintyre, "The Black Report and Beyond: What are the Issues?" 44 *Social Science & Medicine* (1997): 723–745.
5. M. Marmot and R.G. Wilkinson, eds., *Social Determinants of Health* (New York: Oxford University Press, 1999).
6. I.H. Yen and S.L. Syme, "The Social Environment and Health: A Discussion of the Epidemiologic Literature," 20 *Annual Review of Public Health* (1999): 287–308.
7. R.G. Evans and G.L. Stoddart, "Producing Health, Consuming Health Care," 31 *Social Science & Medicine* (1990): 1347–1363.
8. D.R. Williams, "Race and Health: Basic Questions, Emerging Directions" 7 *Annals of Epidemiology* (1997):322–333.
9. D.P. Keating and C. Hertzman, eds., *Developmental Health and the Wealth of Nations* (New York: Guilford Press, 1999).
10. E.M. Kitagawa and P.M. Hauser, *Differential Mortality in the United States: A Study in Socioeconomic Epidemiology* (Cambridge, MA: Harvard University Press, 1973).
11. M. Haan, G.A. Kaplan, and T. Camacho, "Poverty and Health: Prospective Evidence from the Alameda County Study," 125 *American Journal of Epidemiology* (1987): 989–998.
12. N.J. Waitzman and K.R. Smith, "Phantom of the Area: Poverty-area Residence and Mortality in the United States," 88 *American Journal of Public Health* (1998): 973–976.
13. A.T. Geronimus and J. Bound, "Use of Census-based Aggregate Variables to Proxy for Socioeconomic Group: Evidence from National Samples," 148 *American Journal of Epidemiology* (1998): 475–486.
14. California Budget Project, *Making Ends Meet: How Much Does It Cost to Raise a Family in California?* (Sacramento: California Budget Project, 1999).
15. J. Morris, A. Donkin, D. Wonderling, P. Wilkinson, and E. Dowler, "A Minimum Income for Healthy Living," 54 *Journal of Epidemiology and Community Health* (2000): 885–889.
16. S. Alunan, L. Blash, R.B. Murphy, M. Poetepan, H. Roff, and O. Sidime-Brazier, *The Living Wage in San Francisco: Analysis of Economic Impact, Administrative, and Policy Issues* (San Francisco, CA: San Francisco Urban Institute, 1999).
17. K. Fiscella and P. Franks, "Poverty or Income Inequality as Predictor of Mortality: Longitudinal Cohort Study," 314 *British Medical Journal* (1997): 1724–1727.
18. P.D. Sorlie, E. Backlund, and J.B. Keller, "US Mortality by Economic, Demographic, and Social Characteristics: The National Longitudinal Mortality Study," 85 *American Journal of Public Health* (1995): 949–956.

19. P. McDonough, G.J. Duncan, D. Williams, and J. House, "Income Dynamics and Adult Mortality in the United States, 1972 through 1989," 87 *American Journal of Public Health* (1997): 1476–1483.
20. P.M. Lantz, J.S. House, J.M. Lepkowski, D.R.Williams, R.P. Mero, and J. Chen, "Socioeconomic Factors, Health Behaviors, and Mortality: Results from a Nationally Representative Prospective Study of US Adults," 279 *Journal of the American Medical Association* (1998): 1703–1708.
21. G. Pappas, S. Queen, W. Hadden, and G. Fisher, "The Increasing Disparity in Mortality between Socioeconomic Groups in the United States, 1960 and 1986," 329 *New England Journal of Medicine* (1993): 103–109.
22. R.G. Rogers, "Living and Dying in the USA: Sociodemographic Determinants of Death Among Blacks and Whites," 29 *Demography* (1992): 287–303.
23. J.S. Kaufman, A.E. Long, Y. Liao, R.S. Cooper, and D.L. McGee, "The Relation Between Income and Mortality in US Blacks and Whites," 9 *Epidemiology* (1998): 147–155.
24. E. Backlund, P. Sorlie, and N. Johnson, "The Shape of the Relationship Between Income and Mortality in the United States: Evidence from the National Longitudinal Mortality Study," 6 *Annals of Epidemiology* (1996): 12–20.
25. M.G. Marmot, R. Fuhrer, S.L. Ettner, N.F. Marks, L.L. Bumpass, and C.D. Ryff, "Contribution of Psychosocial Factors to Socioeconomic Differences in Health," 76 *Milbank Quarterly* (1998): 403–448, 305.
26. B.P. Kennedy, I. Kawachi, R. Glass, and D. Prothrow-Stith, "Income Distribution, Socioeconomic Status, and Self Rated Health in the United States: Multilevel Analysis," 317 *British Medical Journal* (1998): 917–921.
27. S.L. Ettner, "New Evidence on the Relationship Between Income and Health," 15 *Journal of Health Economics* (1996): 67–85.
28. G.J. Duncan, W. Yeung, J. Brooks-Gunn, and J.R. Smith, "How Much Does Childhood Poverty Affect the Life Chances of Children?," 63 *American Sociological Review* (1998): 406–424.
29. N. Krieger and S. Sidney, "Racial Discrimination and Blood Pressure: the CARDIA Study of Young Black and White Adults," 86 *American Journal of Public Health* (1996): 1370–1378.
30. G.A. Kaplan, E.R. Pamuk, J.W. Lynch, R.D. Cohen, and J.L. Balfour, "Inequality in Income and Mortality in the United States: Analysis of Mortality and Potential Pathways," 312 *British Medical Journal* (1996): 999–1003.
31. I. Kawachi and B.P. Kennedy, "Income Inequality and Health: Pathways and Mechanisms," 34 *Health Services Research* (1999): 215–227.
32. R.G. Wilkinson, "Health, Hierarchy, and Social Anxiety," 896 *Annals of the New York Academy of Science* (1999): 48–63.
33. J.W. Lynch, G.D. Smith, G.A. Kaplan, and J.A. House, "Income Inequality and Mortality: Importance to Health of Individual Income, Psychosocial Environment, or Material Conditions," 320 *British Medical Journal* (2000): 1200–1204.
34. P.A. Morris, A.C. Huston, G.J. Duncan, D.A. Crosby, and J.M. Bos, *How Welfare and Work Policies Affect Children: A Synthesis of Research* (New York: Manpower Research Development Corporation, 2001).
35. D.J. Kuh and M.E. Wadsworth, "Physical Health Status at 36 Years in a British National Birth Cohort," 37 *Social Science & Medicine* (1993): 905–916.

36. G.D. Smith, C. Hart, D. Blane, and D. Hole, "Adverse Socioeconomic Conditions in Childhood and Cause Specific Adult Mortality: Prospective Observational Study," 316 *British Medical Journal* (1998): 1631–1635.

37. P. Holland, L. Berney, D. Blane, G.D. Smith, D.J. Gunnell and S.M. Montgomery, "Life Course Accumulation of Disadvantage: Childhood Health and Hazard Exposure During Adulthood," 50 *Social Science & Medicine* (2000): 1285–1295.

38. G. Duncan and J. Brooks-Gunn, eds., *Consequences of Growing Up Poor* (New York: Russell Sage Foundation, 1997).

39. G. Duncan, J. Brooks-Gunn, and P.K. Klebanov, "Economic Deprivation and Early Childhood Development," 65 *Child Development* (1994): 296–318.

40. H.L. Wilensky, "Social Science and the Public Agenda: Reflections on the Relation of Knowledge to Policy in the United States and Abroad," 22 *Journal of Health Politics & Policy Law* (1997): 1241–1265.

41. S.N. Tesh, *Hidden Arguments* (New Brunswick, NJ: Rutgers University Press, 1990).

42. J.B. McKinlay and L.D. Marceau, "To Boldly Go..." 90 *American Journal of Public Health* (2000): 25–33.

43. A.T. Geronimus, "To Mitigate, Resist, or Undo: Addressing Structural Influences on the Health of Urban Populations," 90 *American Journal of Public Health* (2000): 867–872.

18

Protecting Health with Environmental Impact Assessment: A Case Study of San Francisco Land Use Decision Making

RAJIV BHATIA

The 1969 National Environmental Policy Act requires federal agencies to identify and analyze potentially adverse environmental effects of public agency-approved policies, programs, plans, and projects. Furthermore, when indicated, federal agencies are required to prepare a "detailed statement" of effects and related mitigations, i.e., an environmental impact statement.[1,2] So far, US public health professionals have not used the environmental impact assessment (EIA) to provide the public and policymakers with a systematic analysis of health consequences from effects on such factors as housing quality; land use density, design, and diversity; public infrastructure; and residential segregation.[3-5]

The health impact assessment (HIA) is an emerging practice that is closely related to the EIA and aims to inform policymakers about potential direct and indirect health effects in institutional contexts as diverse as urban planning, agriculture, energy, and economics.[6] Some countries, including Australia and Canada, integrate the HIA within an EIA; in other

This chapter is reprinted with permission from *American Journal of Public Health*. 97(2007): 406–417. Copyright 2007, American Public Health Association.

countries, such as the United Kingdom and Sweden, practitioners conduct the HIA as an independent appraisal.[7-10] With a growing understanding of the associations between social determinants, the built environment, and health in the United States, public health professionals have new opportunities for participating in land use and transportation policymaking and planning,[11-16] and the EIA is a vehicle for this engagement.[17,18] The National Environmental Policy Act and its related federal guidelines have explicit language that requires the evaluation of both direct and indirect effects on health as well as health effects on low-income and minority populations.[19,20] At the state level, the California Environmental Quality Act mandates environmental impact reports whenever "the environmental effects of a project will cause substantial adverse effects on human beings, either directly or indirectly,"[21] and Hawaii requires an EIA to consider changes in economics and social welfare, impacts on public health, and effects on cultural beliefs, practices, and resources.[22]

In this case study, I describe the use of EIA procedural requirements by the San Francisco Department of Public Health (SFDPH) to account for potential indirect health effects of land use development. This case study shows how the identification of potential health effects within the EIA process can influence policy decisions and legitimize needs raised by marginal stakeholders. I have evaluated this health appraisal approach as a form of an HIA and make recommendations for law, research, and practice that could enable its further development.

Context and Approach

In San Francisco, during the 1990s, high housing costs, low-wage jobs, gentrification, contaminated landfills, air pollution, and substandard housing emerged as public health and environmental justice concerns.[23,24] San Francisco residents, business owners, and community organizations mobilized to demand that the city's Department of City Planning act to (1) prevent gentrification and displacement, (2) promote affordable housing, (3) preserve light industry, and (4) ensure greater community oversight with respect to real estate development.[25] Through several community health partnerships, community objectives (e.g., displacement prevention) became health objectives;[26] subsequently, community groups encouraged me, as a representative of SFDPH, to conduct health effects analyses on land use plans and projects.

In San Francisco, the Department of City Planning implements land-use planning and zoning and provides oversight for all local public agency environmental impact reports. The SFDPH routinely reviews these environmental impact reports to ensure there has been adequate study of the impacts on air quality, noise, and chemical hazards. In 2003, the SFDPH began to appraise selected land-use and transportation planning and policy proposals with a more comprehensive set of criteria. Community stakeholders, such as the South of Market Community Action Network, legislators, or public agencies requested or solicited these reviews; however, the requests occurred in the context of the agency—the aforementioned community partnerships.

This health appraisal approach, which became part of my routine practice as one of the deputy public health officers, assembles a rapid or desktop approach to an HIA, generally done in a short period of time (weeks) without community oversight and typically without original data collection or quantitative research.

Box 18.1 shows the general sequence of steps that guided the SFDPH's reviews. When proposals for review were screened, the following criteria were considered: the objectives of the project, the potential pathways between decision outcome and health outcomes, the incidence of related health outcomes among the population, the potential magnitude and distribution of effects, the consideration of health issues during the decision-making process, the existence of health evidence, and the associations between evidence and stakeholder positions. Literature on the social determinants of health, health disparities, place and health, and the concept of social change processes guided the identification of pathways between the proposed action and health effects[27] (Table 18.1). The appraisal involved mapping pathways, assessing relevant empirical research, conducting secondary data analysis, and in some cases, conducting focus groups, monitoring exposure, or quantifying impacts with empirical models. Testimony at public hearings, informal presentations, and formal agency comment on environmental impact reports informed decisions. Evaluation of the practice included monitoring changes in decision outcomes and using health-based arguments by stakeholders.

I examined 2 residential development projects that were the first 2 local applications of approach described in Table 18.1. Table 18.2 shows the subsequent experience that the SFDPH and I had when we used this approach.

Trinity Plaza and Residential Displacement

The first review concerned the demolition of Trinity Plaza Apartments, which comprised 360 rent-controlled units, and the reconstruction of 1400 new condominiums. Officials from the Department of City Planning initially concluded that redevelopment of the site would not have adverse housing impacts, because the proposal increased the total number of dwelling units.

Box 18.1 Rapid Healthy Appraisal Approach for Land Use Projects, Plans, and Policies

Screening

What is the problem or need that the project addresses?

Has the evaluation of the project considered significant potential pathways between the decision's outcomes and health outcomes?

Does public health evidence exist to support these pathways?

Do community/lay positions or concerns about the project relate to these pathways

Are the health impacts potentially of significant magnitude?

Can the project result in disparate effects to different social or economic groups

Is the decision-making process open or closed?

Are decision makers considering all feasible alternatives to address the problem or need?

Analysis

Document existing data on health outcomes logically related to the decision (e.g., baseline incidence of pedestrian injuries, asthma rates)

Document empirical peer-reviewed and "grey" literature relevant to the health impacts you have identified for analysis

Document existing environmental conditions in the project setting related to these health impacts (e.g., traffic volumes, noise measurements, unmet housing needs)

Apply existing environmental data to effect measures, where appropriate, to forecast health impacts

Informing the decision

Summarize the background information, logic model, literature review, secondary data review, and forecasting in a report or letter to decision makers or a comment letter on the EIR

Informally present findings to decision makers, agency staff, and community stakeholders

Testify on the findings at a public hearing

Evaluation

Review response to comments on EIR, comments and questions by legislators,

Document changes in the content of the EIR

Document changes in the final or proposed plan or action

Residents and tenant advocates challenged the city's determination in public testimony by arguing that displacement of people would physically impact the residents, leading to mental stress and the destruction of a cohesive community. The SFDPH review subsequently identified several health consequences of the redevelopment proposal: psychological stress,

TABLE 18.1. Health Determinants Potentially Affected by Land Use Planning in Urban Areas

CATEGORY	EXAMPLES OF HEALTH DETERMINANTS WITHIN CATEGORY
Housing	Housing adequacy and affordability Stable housing tenure Housing quality and safety
Livelihood	Security of employment Adequacy of wages, income, benefits, and leave Job hazards Job autonomy Economic diversity Locally owned businesses
Nutrition	Food cost Food quality and safety Proximity of retail food resources
Air Quality	Contaminants/pollutants in outdoor air Contaminants/pollutants in indoor air Exposure to environmental tobacco smoke
Water Quality	Contaminants or infectious agents in drinking water Safety of the recreational waters
Noise	Intensity and frequency of environmental noise
Safety	Rate of violent crime Rate of property crime Rate of structural fires Pedestrians hazards and injuries
Transportation	Access to jobs, goods, services, and educational resources Proportion of trips walking and bicycling Total miles traveled using personal vehicles
Education	Quality, proximity, and capacity of schools
Parks and Open Space	Quality, proximity, and capacity of parks
Private Goods	Quality and proximity of financial institutions Quality and proximity of childcare services Quality and proximity of health services
Public services	Quality and proximity of health services Capacity of safety net resources for housing and welfare

(Continued)

TABLE 18.1. (Continued)

CATEGORY	EXAMPLES OF HEALTH DETERMINANTS WITHIN CATEGORY
Social Networks	Number and quality of contacts with friends and families Participation in voluntary organizations Quality of informal interactions
Social Inclusion	Population living in relative poverty Attitudes towards or stereotypes of minority racial, social, and ethnic groups Residential segregation by race, ethnicity, religion, or class Degree of inequality in income or wealth
Political Participation	Degree and quality of participation in public decision-making Responsiveness of government to popular needs

fear, and insecurity caused by eviction; crowding or substandard living conditions because of limited affordable replacement housing; food insecurity or hunger caused by increased rent burdens; and loss of supportive social networks owing to displacement.[28-32] Furthermore, the SFDPH qualitatively assessed the health impacts of eviction through focus groups with affected tenants.

Providing evidence that associated the demolition with adverse health impacts met the California Environmental Quality Act threshold requirement to study any environmental change that may be adverse to humans. Officials from the Department of City Planning acknowledged this requirement but challenged the SFDPH to show how adverse consequences could be analyzed.

How could one estimate the socioeconomic status of displaced tenants and their future housing choices, level of crowding, commute lengths, and relationships with family or friends? Officials also worried that requiring a health analysis within an environmental impact report would demand greater agency time and resources and would invite legal challenges and controversy.

Department of City Planning officials ultimately revised their determination for the Trinity Plaza proposal and required the project's environmental impact report to analyze residential displacement and any indirect impacts on health. The developer—who was facing tenant organizing, public criticism, the potential for adverse environmental impact report findings, and a possible citywide legislative moratorium on demolition—ultimately agreed to negotiate with tenants. In 2005, a revised proposal called for the replacement of the 360 rent-controlled units, continued leases for existing tenants, a 1000-square-foot meeting space, and a children's play structure.[33]

The Rincon Hill Special Use District and Smart Growth

Soon after the Trinity Plaza review, community organizations asked the SFDPH to review 2 high-rise condominium projects in the proposed Rincon Hill Special Use District. The Rincon Hill District is south of the downtown area and is adjacent to the South of Market neighborhoods, where community organizations were working to prevent displacement. Department of City Planning staff also encouraged SFDPH to document the associations between real estate development and health, because they believed that documenting the health benefits of neighborhood schools, pedestrian-friendly streets, and community centers would support requirements for developer funding of these improvements.

Developers had already promoted the environmental benefits of building housing near public transit and jobs.[34] However, in its review, the SFDPH raised concerns about the costs of housing (a studio apartment had an estimated cost of approximately $700,000) and argued that although housing for people who worked nearby was needed, only a small proportion of workers would be able to take advantage of housing that was prohibitively expensive.[35] The mismatch between income and housing costs thus missed an important opportunity for reducing commutes, energy consumption, and pollution. The SFDPH recommended that a jobs–housing balance analysis disaggregated by income be conducted as part of a revised environmental impact report.[36]

Officials from the Department of City Planning responded that housing affordability was a social concern not associated with environmental quality. They further claimed that it was speculative to predict the environmental effects of changes in housing affordability by stating that people choose residence on the basis of not only job location and housing costs but also amenities, location of family and friends, and quality of schools.

The SFDPH review also criticized the project for potentially reinforcing segregation. San Francisco law required the project developer to ensure 12% of the developed units were affordable to households with moderate incomes. However, some developers elected to build these required units in a high-poverty neighborhood outside the Rincon Hill planning area. The SFDPH review suggested that adverse impacts of segregation,

TABLE 18.2. Project and Plan Health Reviews Conducted Using the Rapid Appraisal Approach

	DESCRIPTION OF PROJECT, POLICY, OR PLAN	YEAR OF REVIEW	REQUEST BY PUBLIC AGENCY	REQUEST BY COMMUNITY STAKEHOLDERS	CATEGORIES OF HEALTH DETERMINANTS AFFECTED	APPRAISAL METHODS	COMMUNICATION TO DECISION MAKERS
Trinity Plaza Redevelopment	Demolition and reconstruction of multi-family residential development	2003		X	Housing Social networks	Lit review Focus group Local data review	Written report Public testimony EIR comment
Spear/Folsom Development	Development of new mixed use multi-family residential and commercial development	2003	X		Housing Social integration Parks Community schools Air quality	Lit review Local data review	Written report Public testimony EIR comment
Rincon Hill Plan	Land use plan for new residential and commercial mixed use neighborhood	2004	X	X	Housing Social integration Parks Community schools Air quality	Lit review Local data review	Written report Public testimony EIR comment
Housing Element of the San Francisco General Plan	State required plan for housing including statements of policy, objectives, and implementation activities	2004	X		Housing Social integration Air quality	Lit review Local data review	Written report Public testimony

(Continued)

TABLE 18.2. (Continued)

DESCRIPTION OF PROJECT, POLICY, OR PLAN	YEAR OF REVIEW	REQUEST BY PUBLIC AGENCY	REQUEST BY COMMUNITY STAKEHOLDERS	CATEGORIES OF HEALTH DETERMINANTS AFFECTED	APPRAISAL METHODS	COMMUNICATION TO DECISION MAKERS
Redevelopment of University of California Family Housing Redevelopment	Demolition and reconstruction of university family housing	2004		X	Housing Social integration Social networks	Lit review Local data review	EIR comment
Central Station Redevelopment	New market-rate residential development within redevelopment area at site of historic train station	2005		X	Housing Social integration Social networks Air quality	Lit review Local data review	EIR comment
Oak to Ninth Avenue Development	New 3500 unit market-rate residential development on industrial waterfront land	2006		X	Housing Air quality Noise Pedestrian safety	Lit review Local data review Pedestrian injury forecasting	EIR comment

Note: EIR = Environmental impact report.

including higher rates of mortality and violent injury and lower opportunity for educational and economic success, could indirectly result from building an exclusive high income neighborhood. Finally, the project did not provide for a neighborhood school, which raised the potential of negative impacts on traffic air pollution, physical activity, and children's educational success.[37]

The Department of City Planning approved the environmental impact report for the project without any further environmental study; however, questions about the project's affordability, its effects on social integration, and its demands on public infrastructure remained. Community organizations appealed the approval of the environmental impact report to the city's board of supervisors, and 1 legislator, who used findings from the SFDPH review, negotiated a higher proportion of affordable units. Zoning rules subsequently approved for the Rincon Hill planning area in 2005 required all below-market-rate units to be constructed within the adjacent South of Market planning district and included developer fees for street improvements, parks, and a community center and "community stabilization" funds for affordable housing and community economic development.

Lessons Learned

The Trinity Plaza and Rincon Hill case studies illustrate how land-use development projects along with their associated EIAs can be informed and influenced by HIA. Parry and Kemm suggested that the diverse approaches to an HIA all share 3 interrelated objectives: "To predict impacts in a robust manner and to judge both their magnitude and importance [predicting effects]; to involve people affected in the assessment process [stakeholder participation]; and to inform the decision-making process [informing decisions]."[38] (p1123)

I considered the SFDPH practice against these 3 objectives. There was no formal external evaluation of this approach, and these reflections are mine alone.

Predicting Effects

These health appraisals did not quantify health effects; nevertheless, evidence, including empirical research and local data, provided the basis for potential pathways between the project and health outcomes and showed the direction and the relative magnitude of these health effects as well as their local significance. Some decision makers and Department of City Planning staff challenged the validity of predictions not substantiated by quantitative methods and estimates; however, the suggestion of specific tools to support estimation (e.g., jobs–housing balance analysis) did not lead to their implementation.

Stakeholder Participation

External participation was limited within the appraisal, but it was evident in both the screening and informing decisions. The reviews supported the interests of both community organizational stakeholders and public health; however, they would not have occurred without the community organizations' understanding of the potential policy contribution of a local health agency, which highlights the instrumental role of community partnerships. Community members were involved in the focus group but were not involved in other appraisal activities. The SFDPH shared documents, data, and other findings with community stakeholders and the Department of City Planning in advance of public testimony staff to support the dissemination and influence of the appraisals.

Informing Decisions

Policy decisions on the Trinity and Rincon Hill developments occurred in the context of a vigorous public debate, and it is not possible to attribute changes in the developments exclusively to the health appraisals. However, changes to the scope of environmental analysis required by Department of City Planning for the EIA of the Trinity Plaza project, the negotiated changes in affordability requirements for the Spear and Folsom projects (Table 18.2), and the final zoning rules for the Rincon Hill planning area all suggest that the SFDPH reviews influenced policy.

Some of the issues raised in the health reviews (e.g., housing affordability) were already high on the public agenda. In these cases, a key contribution of the health appraisal was the enumeration of causal pathways between the project decision, social and environmental conditions, and human health outcomes. Several stakeholders and legislators took public positions, in part, on the basis of health-related arguments. The SFDPH understood how reviews would legitimatize particular community interests. Not surprisingly, the actions taken by the SFDPH were met with criticism and even hostility by those who took alternative positions.

Directly communicating our findings to Department of City Planning staff who were responsible for staff reports and recommendations to the planning commission also created awareness and concern. For example, staff at the Department of City Planning changed their position on the need for studying displacement in the context of demolition, and they also expressed interest in learning how design changes could mitigate health impacts. The health impacts of residential segregation appeared to have contributed to the agency changing its position on requiring that below-market-rate units be built near market-rated housing developments.

Finally, the SFDPH contributed new data to the planning process. Community stakeholders used maps that showed locations and sizes of city parks, locations of pedestrian injuries, and locations of overcrowding and segregation to successfully argue for development impact fees for the new neighborhoods.

Recommendations for Practice, Research, and Law

Although these development projects show the potential of a health analysis within an EIA, application in more diverse contexts is necessary before the value of health analysis approach can be fully appraised. The following are recommendations for supporting the development and application of an HIA within an EIA.

Use an Environmental Impact Assessment Process

The first recommendation is simple: practitioners should use existing procedures and laws for an EIA whenever possible to promote public and decision maker awareness about the potential health effects of public decisions. Although some believe that an HIA should occur as a voluntary process without the procedural and legal limitations of an EIA—as the case studies illustrate—the regulatory standing of an EIA is in part responsible for its influence on policymakers and project proponents.[39,40]

Public health practitioners also can use an EIA in some cases to promote awareness and analysis of the social and economic determinants of health. An EIA is triggered by decisions that lead to physical environmental changes; nevertheless, the National Environmental Policy Act requires an environmental impact statement to include all effects on the human environment whenever economic or social and natural or physical environmental effects are interrelated.[41] More specifically, California law requires agencies to analyze economic or social effects if these effects are on a causal pathway that leads to environmental effects.[42]

Despite federal guidelines for a social analysis within an EIA,[43-45] these analyses occur sporadically.[46] The practice of community impact assessment with transportation planning suggests some recent shifts in attitudes about a social analysis within an EIA, and planning for recent roadway projects has included mitigations of impacts on health and community cohesion.[47,48] Public health practitioners should capitalize on both federal guidelines and more recent developments.

Build Tools for Forecasting Health Effects

Although EIA regulations legally enable a health and social analysis, they provide no guidance on how that analysis should occur. An HIA needs new analytic methods that forecast the effects of changes in social and environmental measures on traditional human health outcomes (e.g., life expectancy, hospitalization rates, disease incidence). Evidence-based causal diagrams should be the starting point for forecasting efforts. Such diagrams also should be recognized as tools in themselves for building community and policymaker understanding.

Existing research within planning and health disciplines often provides a solid basis for forecasting health effects. For example, on the basis of numbers and types of jobs that are the result of a project, a health analysis may be able to estimate effects on income, health insurance benefits, and vacation and sick leave and subsequent effects on effects on health-related outcomes such as life expectancy, injury and illness rates, avoidable hospitalization, and childhood development.[49] Changes in tax revenue might be similarly associated with the availability of public health, public safety, and other social services. Ecosystem health concepts and models of climate change can provide other templates for mapping diverse and interrelated human environments and health pathways.[50,51]

Recent research has begun to associate land use, urban design, and transportation system characteristics with outcomes such as physical activity, air pollution, environmental noise, body mass index, and social cohesion.[52-55] This research could be used with existing EIA metrics. For example, health effects analysis can associate changes in motor vehicle traffic volumes with health-related outcomes such as injuries, sleep disturbance, noise-related stress, diabetes, respiratory disease, and social cohesion. In a review of the Oak to Ninth project (Table 18.2), I used an empirically derived road facility safety performance function and the environmental impact report's estimates of changes in roadway volumes to quantitatively forecast changes in pedestrian injuries.

Adopt Supportive Rules and Standards

Broader application of this health appraisal approach might require changes to laws that require an EIA to include more explicit requirements for an HIA. Regulatory changes also should enable the assessment of beneficial environmental effects because current laws for an EIA mandate only the study of adverse impacts. For example, in the case of the Rincon Hill project, the environmental impact report included a detailed analysis of the increase in local traffic but did not consider the benefits conferred by reducing regional traffic. Furthermore, making the case for community health assets, such as neighborhood schools, grocery stores, parks and recreational centers, and pedestrian and bicycle facilities (e.g., sidewalks, benches, enhanced crosswalks, bicycle lanes and parking), requires the inclusion of a benefits analysis.

An EIA involves making a determination about the significance of effects, where significance is often judged against existing regulatory standards. Thus, there exists a need to create, reference, or adopt more health-based standards associated with social and environmental conditions. In California, agencies are permitted to develop locally specific significance thresholds for an EIA through a legislative or administrative process.[56] Local standards that are based on empirical associations with health outcomes might include those for proximity to and accessibility of parks or open space, transit service frequency, pedestrian safety, and housing quality.

Several federal and state agencies already publish measures and targets that are potentially adaptable to a health analysis. For example, the US Housing and Urban Development's 2000–2006 Strategic Plan identifies the decline of residential segregation by race/ethnicity or income as a measurable performance objective, and the US Census Bureau collects measures of housing quality, such as overcrowding.[57] Healthy People 2010 objectives associated with community design include the reduction of violence, pedestrian injuries, and substandard housing; improved air quality; and increased daily physical activity.[58]

Integrate New Practices for Inclusive Participation

Similar to the National Environmental Policy Act, the California Environmental Quality Act provides rules for information transparency and allows the public to inform the scope and the methods of the analysis. In practice, lay stakeholders, such as residents, who attempt to participate in policy analysis processes are usually forced to discuss technical issues isolated from the broader public agenda, moral and political questions, and issues of institutional legitimacy and public trust.[59-62] In San Francisco, community groups frequently claimed that the environmental impact report analysis ignored day-to-day social, health, and economic impacts of environmental planning decisions. As Oscar Grande of the People Organized to Demand Environmental and Economic Rights explained during testimony given to the San Francisco Board of Supervisors Land Use Subcommittee, "[Planning officials] kept saying that we could only talk about issues they could address [in the EIA], but we were simply talking about bread-and-butter issues."

Without meaningful public participation, a technical analysis of the health effects within an EIA might not effectively serve as a proxy for health needs. Effective public participation in a public agency decision-making process is necessary not only because it identifies problems hidden to experts but also because it contributes ideas for more effective solutions, it makes explicit competing values and interests, it creates opportunities for articulating and advancing a common interest, and it generates the buy-in necessary for effective policy implementation.[63,64] New methods for public involvement, such as consensus conferences and habitat conservation planning, also show how scientific analysis and public deliberation can complement each other in a policy analysis.[65-67] Methods for participatory action research, including community-based participatory research, call for the democratization of research and technical practice and attempts to link the production of new theory and knowledge with social action.[68] Community-based participatory research may provide a more inclusive way for developing HIA processes and health analysis tools for impact assessment.[69] The Eastern Neighborhoods HIA in San Francisco is an early example of joining participatory and deliberative methods with empirical health research in a land use HIA.[70]

Conclusions

The National Environmental Policy Act envisioned the environmental impact statement to be prepared "using an inter-disciplinary approach which will insure the integrated use of the natural and social sciences and the environmental design arts."[71] Although this vision remains unrealized, the SFDPH experience suggests that the public health community has significant opportunities for using the existing procedural framework of an EIA—at least in land use policy settings—to gain knowledge about several social and environmental determinants of health. Practice can begin in an experimental and adaptive mode that is sensitive to context and political limitations and that builds on experiences and lessons learned. Institutionalizing practice will require building interdisciplinary collaborations and supportive constituencies, developing analytic methods, revising regulations, and demonstrating the value of an HIA within the EIA process.

Acknowledgments

This work reflects the collective efforts of the author, SFDPH staff, and local community organizations, including the Mission Housing Development Corporation, the Mission Economic Developmental Agenda, People Organized To Demand Environmental and Economic Rights, the Mission Agenda, St. Peter's Housing, and the South of Market Community Action Network. Jason Corburn, PhD, June Weintraub, PhD, and the Journal's anonymous reviewers provided invaluable direction on the manuscript.

Notes

1. National Environmental Policy Act. Title 42 USC §4331(b)(2), 2005.
2. B.C. Karkkainen, "Towards a Smarter NEPA: Monitoring and Managing Government's Environmental Performance," 102 *Columbia Law Review* (2002): 903–972.
3. M.C. Arquiaga, L.W. Canter, and D.I. Nelson, "Integration of Health Impact Considerations in Environmental Impact Studies," 12 *Impact Assessment* (1994): 175–197.
4. A. Steinemann, "Rethinking Human Health Impact Assessment," 20 *Environmental Impact Assessment Review* (2000): 627–645.
5. K. Davies and B. Sadler, *Environmental Assessment and Human Health: Perspectives, Approaches, and Future Directions* (Ottawa, Ontario: Health Canada, 1997).
6. J. Kemm, J. Parry, and S. Palmer, *Health Impact Assessment: Concepts, Techniques and Applications* (Oxford: Oxford University Press, 2004).
7. E. Ison, *Resource for Health Impact Assessment* (London: London's Health, 2000).
8. J. Lehto and A. Ritsatakis, *Health Impact Assessment as a Tool for Intersectoral Health Policy: A Discussion Paper for a Seminar at Gothenburg, Sweden* (Brussels: European Center for Health Policy, 1999).
9. R.E. Kwiatkowski and M. Ooi, "Integrated Environmental Impact Assessment: a Canadian Example," 81 *Bulletin of the World Health Organization* (2003): 434–438.
10. National Health and Medical Research Council, *National Framework for Environmental and Health Impact Assessment* (Canberra, Australia: Australian Government Publishing Service, 1994).
11. H. Frumkin, L. Frank, and R. Jackson, *Urban Sprawl and Public Health: Designing, Planning, and Building for Healthy Communities* (Washington, DC: Island Press, 2004).
12. I. Kawachi and L.F. Berkman, *Neighborhoods and Health* (New York: Oxford University Press, 2003).
13. J. Maantay, "Zoning, Equity, and Public Health," 91 *American Journal of Public Health* (2001): 1033–1041.

14. A.L. Dannenberg, R. Jackson, H. Frumkin H et al., "The Impact of Community Design and Land-Use on Public Health: A Scientific Research Agenda," 93 *American Journal of Public Health* (2003): 1500–1508.

15. D.R. Williams and C. Collins, "Racial Residential Segregation: a Fundamental Cause of Racial Disparities in Health," 116 *Public Health Reports* (2001): 404–416.

16. J. Corburn, "Confronting the Challenges in Reconnecting Urban Planning and Public Health," 94 *American Journal of Public Health* (2004): 541–546.

17. R. Banken, *Strategies for Institutionalizing HIA* (Brussels: European Center for Health Policy, 2001).

18. R. Rattle and R.E. Kwiatkowski, "Integrating Health and Social Impact Assessment," in *The International Handbook of Social Impact Assessment: Conceptual and Methodological Advances*, ed. H.A. Becker and F. Vanclay (Cheltenham: Edward Elgar, 2003) 92–107.

19. Regulations for Implementing NEPA. 40 CFR §1508.8; 1978.

20. Council on Environmental Quality, *Environmental Justice: Guidance Under the National Environmental Health Policy Act* (Washington, DC: Executive Office of the President, 1997).

21. Guidelines for Implementation of the California Environmental Quality Act. California Code of Regulations. §15065(a)(4).

22. *A Guidebook for the State Environmental Review Process* (Honolulu, Hawaii: Office of Environmental Quality Control, 1997).

23. S.V. Alejandrino, *Gentrification in San Francisco's Mission District: Indicators and Policy Recommendations* (San Francisco, CA: Mission Economic Development Agenda, 2000).

24. *Report on the Census of Families with Children Living in Single-Room Occupancy Hotels in San Francisco* (San Francisco, CA: Citywide Families in SROs Collaborative, 2001).

25. *Mission Zoning Interim Controls,* (San Francisco, CA: Department of City Planning, 2001).

26. R. Bhatia, "Swimming Upstream in a Swift Current: Public Health Institutions and Inequality," in *Health and Social Justice: Politics, Ideology, and Inequity in the Distribution and Disease,* ed. R. Hofrichter (San Francisco, CA: Jossey-Bass, 2003) 557–578.

27. M. Van Schooten, R. Vanclay, and R. Slootweg, "Conceptualizing Social Change Processes and Social Impacts," in *The International Handbook of Social Impact Assessment: Conceptual and Methodological Advances,* ed. H.A. Beker and F. Vanclay (Cheltenham: Edward Elgar, 2003) 74–91.

28. R. Bhatia and C. Guzman, *The Case for Housing Impacts Assessment* (San Francisco, CA: Department of Public Health, 2004).

29. J. Krieger and D.L. Higgins, "Housing and Health: Time Again for Public Health Action," 92 *American Journal of Public Health* (2002): 758–768.

30. M. Cooper, *Housing Affordability: A Children's Issue* (Ottawa, Ontario: Canadian Policy Research Network, 2001).

31. A. Meyers, D. Frank, N. Roos, and K.E. Peterson, "Housing Subsidies and Pediatric Nutrition," 148 *Archive of Pediatric Adolescence* (1995): 1079–1084.

32. L.F. Berkman and S.L. Syme, "Social Networks, Host Resistance and Mortality: A Nine Year Follow-up Study of Alameda County Residents," 109 *American Journal of Epidemiology* (1979): 186–204.

33. R. Shaw, "Historic Trinity Plaza Deal Finalized," *Beyond Chronicle* (June 9, 2005). Available at http://www.beyondchron.org/news/index.php?itemid=358. (accessed December 11, 2006).

34. S.T. Jones, "From Lightning Rod to Love Fest How Rincon Towers Got So Popular and What it Says About Urban Planning in San Francisco," *San Francisco Bay Guardian* (February 4, 2004).

35. M. Baldassare, *PIC Statewide Survey: Special Survey on Californians and Their Housing* (San Francisco, CA: Public Policy Institute of California, 2004).

36. R. Cervero, "Jobs-Housing Balance Revisited: Trends and Impacts in the San Francisco Bay Area," 62 *American Planning Association Journal* (1996): 492–511.

37. *Schools for Successful Communities: An Element of Smart Growth* (Scottsdale, Arizona: Council of Educational Facility Planners International, 2004).

38. J.M. Parry and J. Kemm, "Criteria for Use in the Evaluation of Health Impact Assessments," 119 *Public Health* (2005): 1122–1129.

39. B.L. Cole, M. Wilhelm, P.V. Long, J.E. Fielding, G. Kominski, and H. Morgenstern, Prospects for Health Impact Assessment in the United States: New and Improved Environmental Impact Assessment or Something Different?" 29 *Journal of Health Policy & Law* (2004): 1153–1186.

40. A.L. Danneberg, R. Bhatia, B.L. Cole, et al., "Growing the Field of Health Impact Assessment in the United States: An Agenda for Research and Practice," 96 *American Journal of Public Health* (2006): 262–270.

41. Regulations for Implementing NEPA. 40 CFR §1508.14, 1978.

42. Guidelines for Implementation of the California Environmental Quality Act. California Code of Regulations. §15131.

43. Inter organizational Committee on Guidelines and Principles for Social Impact Assessment, *Guidelines and Principles for Social Impact Assessment* (Washington, DC: US Dept of Commerce, 1994).

44. Federal Highway Administration, Community Impact Assessment: A Quick Reference for Transportation. Available at http://www.ciatrans.net/cia_quick_reference/purpose.html. (accessed December 11, 2006).

45. California Department of Transportation, Community Impact Assessment, CalTrans Environmental Handbook. Available at: http://www.dot.ca.gov/ser/envhand.htm. (accessed June 8, 2005).

46. R.J. Burdge, *A Conceptual Approach to Social Impact Assessment* (Madison, WI: Social Ecology Press, 1998).

47. Community Impact Assessment in the 21st Century: Making Connections and Building Relationships. Third National Community Impact Assessment Conference. (Madison, Wisconsin August 19–21, 2002).

48. Federal Highway Administration. Community Impact Mitigations Case Studies. Available at: http://www. ciatrans.net/community_impact_mitigation/cim_introduction.html. (accessed December 11, 2006).

49. R. Bhatia and M. Katz, "Estimation of Health Benefits Accruing From a Living Wage Ordinance," 91 *American Journal of Public Health* (2001): 1398–1402.

50. D.J. Rappaport, G. Bohm, D. Buckingham, et al., "Ecosystem Health: The Concept, the ISEH, and the Important Tasks Ahead," 5 *Ecosystem Health* (1999): 82–90.

51. J.A. Patz, M.A. McGechin, S.M. Bernard, et al., "Workshop Summary: the Potential Health Impacts of Climate Variability and Change for the United

States: Executive Summary of the Report of the Health Sector of the U.S. National Assessment," 108 *Environmental Health Perspectives* (2000): 367–376.

52. L.D. Frank, J.F. Sallis, T.L. Conway, J.E. Chapman, B.E. Saelens, and W. Bachmand, "Many Pathways from Land Use to Health," 72 *Journal of the American Planning Association* (2006): 75–87.

53. R. Cervero and M. Duncan, "Walking, Bicycling, and Urban Landscapes: Evidence from the San Francisco Bay Area," 93 *American Journal of Public Health* (2003): 1478–1483.

54. K.M. Leyden, "Social Capital and the Built Environment: the Importance of Walkable Neighborhoods," 93 *American Journal of Public Health* (2003): 1546–1551.

55. D.S. Morrison, H. Thomson, and M. Petticrew, "Evaluation of the Health Effects of a Neighborhood Traffic Calming Scheme," 58 *Journal of Epidemiology & Community Health* (2004): 837–840.

56. *Thresholds of Significance: Criteria or Defining Environmental Significance, CEQA Technical Advice Series* (Sacramento, CA: Office of Planning and Research, 1994).

57. US Department of Housing and Urban Development, *Strategic Plan FY2005–FY2006.* 2nd ed. (Washington, DC: US Government Printing Office, 2000).

58. US Department of Health and Human Services, *Healthy People 2010: Understanding and Improving Health,* 2nd ed. (Washington, DC: US Government Printing Office, 2000).

59. S. Arnstein, "A Ladder of Citizen Participation," 35 *Journal of the American Planning Association* (1969): 216–224.

60. J. Keeley and I. Scoones, *Understanding Environmental Policy Processes: A Review* (Sussex: Institute of Development Studies, 1999).

61. C. Shore and S. Wright, "Policy: A New field of Anthropology," in *An Anthropology of Policy: Critical Perspectives on Governance and Power,* ed. C. Shore and S. Wright (New York: Routledge, 1997) 3–39.

62. B. Wynne, "May the Sheep Safely Graze?: A Reflexive View of the Expert-lay Knowledge Divide," in *Risk, Environment, and Modernity: Towards a New Ecology,* ed. S. Lash, B. Szerynski, and B.Wynne (Newbury Park, CA: Sage, 1996) 44–83.

63. A. Fung and E.O. Wright, "Deepening Democracy: Innovations in Empowered Participatory Governance," 29 *Politics & Society* (2001): 5–41.

64. T. Dietz, "What is a Good Decision? Criteria for Environmental Decision making," 10 *Human Ecology Forum* (2003): 33–39.

65. F. Fischer, *Citizens, Experts and the Environment: The Politics of Local Knowledge* (Durham, NC: Duke University Press, 2000).

66. C. Sabel, A. Fung, and B. Karkkainen, *Beyond Backyard Environmentalism* (Boston, MA: Beacon Press, 2000).

67. I.A. Anderson and B. Jaeger, "Scenario Workshops and Consensus Conferences: Towards a More Democratic Decision-making," 26 *Science & Public Policy* (1999): 331–340.

68. J. Corburn, *Street Science: Community Knowledge and Environmental Health Justice* (Cambridge, MA: MIT Press, 2005).

69. L.R. O'Fallon and A. Dearry, "Community-based Participatory Research as a Tool to Advance Environmental Health Sciences," 110 (Suppl. 2) *Environmental Health Perspectives* (2002): 155–159.
70. San Francisco Department of Public Health, Eastern Neighborhoods Community Health Impact Assessment. Available at: http://www.sfdph.org/phes/enchia.htm. (accessed March 23, 2006).
71. Regulations for Implementing NEPA. 40 CFR §1502.6; 1978.

19

The Community Action Model in a Public Health Department Setting Case Study: Tobacco Divestment on College Campuses

MELE LAU SMITH, ALMA AVILA-ESPARZA, ALYONIK HRUSHOW, SUSANA HENNESSEY LAVERY, DIANE REED, AND MELINDA MOORE

Introduction

Inequities in social systems—whether the political system, health care system, economic system or justice system—contribute to health inequities. However, public health solutions frequently focus on getting people to change their "unhealthy" behaviors or to make "healthier" lifestyle decisions. Unfortunately, this approach places the onus on the individual and does not challenge the social structures that shape many of our "choices" and "decisions." Health status cannot be improved through individual behavior change alone—rather any solution to improve health must focus on changes in social systems. Socioeconomic status appears to be an indicator of health status such that there is mounting evidence that the gap between rich and poor contributes to health inequities between the "haves" and "have nots."[1] Because race and ethnicity are major determinants of socioeconomic status, communities of color are more likely to have poor health and to die early due to disparities in health.[2] Tobacco

This chapter is reprinted with permission from *American Journal of Public Health* 95(2005): 611–616. Copyright 2005 American Public Health Association.

related illness is no exception as communities of color and low socio-economic status groups have higher prevalence of tobacco use.[3] African Americans have the highest lung cancer incidence and mortality rates. American Indians and specific AAPI communities have the highest prevalence of tobacco use. Lung cancer is the leading cause of cancer deaths for Latinos.[4]

The Tobacco Epidemic as a Social Justice Issue

In California's tobacco control program, the tobacco industry is seen as the vector of tobacco-related diseases. The tobacco industry has a long history of deceit, deception, and duplicity in its pursuit of ever growing profits. Through manipulative and targeted advertising, disinformation campaigns refuting the health consequences of smoking, and political lobbying, the tobacco industry has grown and prospered over the years. And as the tobacco industry has prospered, the number of people who die due to tobacco-related diseases has increased. Any discussion of addressing the disparities in tobacco-related illnesses must analyze these disparities in the context of the market-based global economic structure and the tools that promote this structure such as privatization (turning public entities such as health care into private, for-profit entities), deregulation (eliminating laws and regulations that, often times, protect health and the environment), and free trade (the free movement of products and services across borders).

Utilizing these tools, the tobacco industry engages in aggressive marketing and promotion targeted at communities of color, women, youth, the lesbian, gay, bisexual, and transgender (LGBT) community, and communities of low socioeconomic status resulting in higher prevalence rates in these communities and subsequent disproportionate rates of tobacco-related diseases.

A Health Department Takes a Social Justice Approach

In response to these inequities, the San Francisco Tobacco Free Project (SFTFP) of the Community Health Promotion and Prevention section of the San Francisco Department of Public Health, has viewed the tobacco epidemic as a social injustice issue and has moved away from projects that focus solely on changing individual lifestyle and behavior (helping smokers quit or educating teens not to start) to projects that mobilize community members and agencies to change environmental factors such as tobacco advertising, promotion, and tobacco product access for minors that promote health inequity. As part of the comprehensive tobacco control plan for San Francisco, the SFTFP has funded community-based agencies to implement the Community Action Model (CAM), a five-step model focused on environmental change through policy development or change in organizational practices rather than individual behavior change. The intent of the CAM is to work in collaboration with communities and provide a framework for community members to acquire the skills and resources to investigate the health of the place where they live and then plan, implement, and evaluate actions that change the environment to promote health.

As part of the CAM process, SFTFP staffs provide interactive trainings and technical assistance to community-based organizations to facilitate a sharing of existing skills and community strengths so that the actions are community driven. It is the Tobacco Free Project's intention that community groups will find that these skills are transferable to community issues other than tobacco control, such as violence prevention, and are encouraged to integrate other community health issues into their work.

Between 1995 and 2004, the SFTFP has funded thirty-seven projects to implement the Community Action Model. SFTFP funds community-based organizations (CBOs) in San Francisco who, in turn, work with community advocates (community members) to implement the five steps of the CAM (see Figure 19.1). The CAM has successfully mobilized community members and agencies to change environmental factors that promote unhealthy behavior such as tobacco advertising, promotion, and access for minors.

As part of funding the CAM process, SFDPH staff meets regularly with project staff and advocates to problem solve how to implement each step of the CAM process, to develop appropriate activities to use with advocates and come up with lists of potential "Actions" in each issue area. Additionally SFDPH staff often provide guidance to project staff who often times do not get support from their agency due to lack of resources for staff development. The SFTFP also funds an evaluation contractor and sets aside funds for media consultants to provide assistance to the funded projects. This approach provides for collaboration and linkages between the CAM project's focus, tobacco control, and other issues of deep concern to the community such as immigrant rights, housing issues, environmental justice, and food security. For example, one project concerned with food security issues in a low-income community of color in San Francisco is promoting a Good Neighbor corner store policy to promote inner city access to healthy food alternatives to tobacco subsidiary food products.

The CAM model draws from long history of indigenous peoples struggles to overcome oppression and disparities through community organizing. The CAM provides a framework to fund environmental change projects at the community level; allowing health departments to partner with community to make change. Central to this funding approach is a social justice analysis and a commitment to the community-driven process as well as a commitment by DPH staff to work in partnership with the community and act as a resource for the community.

The CAM is consistent with the public health model and provides a structured process for achieving sustainable outcomes. The CAM is designed to achieve this type of change through community capacity building rather than individual behavior change. By addressing the root causes of a problem, environmental change through the adoption of policies has a lasting impact and creates changes in social norms.

For example, having policies and laws that prohibit smoking in workplaces has had a lasting impact on reducing exposure to secondhand smoke. Focusing only on educating the public about the hazards of second hand smoke would not have achieved the permanent reduction in exposure and it also changed the public's norms or view of what is socially acceptable as far as smoking in workplaces including restaurants and bars.

The Community Action Model

Based on the theory of Paulo Freire, the CAM is a five-step model focused on environmental change through policy development or change in organizational practices rather than individual behavior change. Freire, a Brazilian educationalist, who integrated educational practice and liberation, emphasized dialogue, praxis, situating education in the lived experience of the participants and "consientizacion" or developing consciousness to have the power to transform reality, specifically with respect to addressing oppression. The CAM involves participatory action research approaches, and is asset based (builds on the strengths of a community to create change from within). Its intent is to create change by building community capacity, work in collaboration with communities, and provide a framework for community members to acquire the skills and resources to investigate the health of the place they live and then plan, implement and evaluate actions that change the environment to promote and improve health. The goals of the CAM are twofold:

1. Environmental change: by moving away from projects that focus solely on changing individual lifestyle and behavior to mobilizing community members and agencies to change environmental factors that promote economic and environmental inequalities.

2. People acquire the skills to do it themselves: through asset-based action research, the CAM provides a framework for community members to acquire the skills and resources to investigate the health of the place where they live and then plan, implement, and evaluate actions that change the environment to promote and improve health.

The five-step process of the CAM: (1) skill-based trainings where advocates choose an area of focus; (2) action research where advocates define, design, and do a community diagnosis (action research); (3) analysis where advocates analyze the results of the diagnosis and prepare findings; (4) organizing where advocates select, plan, and implement an "Action" for environmental change and educational "Activities" to support it; and (5) implementation where advocates ensure that the policy outcome is enforced and maintained. A curriculum has been developed in English and Spanish to implement the model and includes specific curricula activities to assist advocates in implementing the steps. To further facilitate the transferability of the CAM to other health issues, a "facilitator guide" to accompany the CAM has been developed. The curriculum and facilitator guide can be found at: http://sftfc.globalink.org/capacity.html.

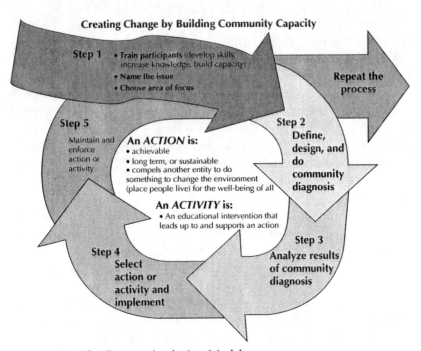

Creating Change by Building Community Capacity

Step 1
• Train participants (develop skills, increase knowledge, build capacity)
• Name the issue
• Choose area of focus

Repeat the process

Step 5
Maintain and enforce action or activity

An ACTION is:
• achievable
• long term, or sustainable
• compels another entity to do something to change the environment (place people live) for the well-being of all

An ACTIVITY is:
• An educational intervention that leads up to and supports an action

Step 2
Define, design, and do community diagnosis

Step 4
Select action or activity and implement

Step 3
Analyze results of community diagnosis

FIGURE 19.1 The Community Action Model.

How Did the SFDPH Operationalize Implementation of the CAM?

Most SFTFP CAM projects are funded at the $50K–100K/year level; however, other CAM projects are funded from between $10–25K/year level. Aside from the following budget requirements, much of the same support goes into a $10K CAM as a $50K CAM.

- Funded a fiscal sponsor contractor—activist-oriented CBOs tend to be fairly small oftentimes making it difficult for them to me the requirements for a city government contract, the SFTFP funded a fiscal sponsor organization with the infrastructure to meet the requirements for a city government contract. This enabled smaller CBOs to be a subcontractor on a larger contract. In addition, this structure allowed SFTFP staff to streamline the application process. The original application was lengthy and bureaucratic while more recent applications have been reduced to 4–6 pages.
- Funded CBOs as subcontracts to the fiscal sponsor contract to complete the five-step CAM process with emphasis on selecting an "Action" (that meets the three criteria) and completion of an action plan to achieve it. This is a requirement for funding that is included in the MOU, work plan, deliverables etc. Provided technical assistance, training, and consultation to ensure that the CBO will identify an "Action" and develop an action plan to achieve it.
- Identified three criteria to maximize a CBO's ability to successfully implement the CAM: (1) must be community based, (2) must demonstrate a history or interest in activism (not just service oriented), (3) must have infrastructure to support staff to implement a system change focused project. These criteria were integrated into the application and evaluation criteria. The application specifically stated that the funded CBO would be required to implement the CAM, choose an action meeting the criteria, and implement a community organizing action plan to work towards successful completion of the action.
- Included in the Request of Funding Application (RFA) a list of potential actions for applicants to respond to that gave them an idea of the types of projects that would be funded.
- Included non-direct-service-based CBOs in the outreach mailing lists for the release of the application.
- Developed simple work plans, budgets, budget revision, and invoice processes to alleviate some of the administrative burden of implementing a CAM. Other guidelines required a minimum of .50 FTE project coordinator, funds for stipends for community advocates, and budgets for

incentives for program participants. Projects could use their budget to purchase computers and pay for access to the Internet.

- Integrated an analysis of the root causes and solutions to the health issues into trainings in the case of tobacco, the role of the transnational tobacco companies, the elements of the corporate led global economy and related issues. Funded CAM projects partner with CBOs in countries with fewer resources, participate in "intercambio" exchange meetings and collaborate on joint environmental change actions.
- Provide data training for agencies funded to implement the CAM that addresses how to set up the necessary infrastructure, administrative support (budgets, work plans, staffing, computer, email), and methods to compensate advocates (stipends/pay/incentives) etc.
- Provided an orientation training for project staff and advocates to "walk" them through the five-step process of the CAM. Sample trainings are in the CAM curriculum.
- Coordinated regular meetings of all funded project staff to collectively brainstorm and collaborate as well as regular meetings between specific funded project staff and SFTFP staff to enhance ongoing collaboration and the potential for success.
- Initiated regular meetings with agency staff to problem solve, brainstorm, and share resources.
- Provided ongoing, as-needed trainings for skill development at specific steps in the process.
- Funded an evaluation contractor to provided technical assistance and consultation in design of diagnosis, data analysis, and training in evaluation methodology. SFTFP staff and evaluators are not community based and may not have in-depth knowledge of a community's issues and concerns; thus ongoing collaboration is essential and must involve mutual information sharing and respect for the community-driven aspect of the process. During the diagnosis (step 2) phase, the evaluator works closely with advocates as they define, design and implement the research.
- Provided funds to each funded project to identify a culturally competent media consultant to support advocacy efforts.

Case Study: Tobacco Divestment on College Campuses

Since 1995 the SFTFP has committed to fund community-based organizations to implement the CAM as part of its comprehensive tobacco control plan and budget. During the most recent three year plan (2001–2004), six CAM projects were funded from January 2002 through June

2004. Following is a case study of one of those projects, the Latino Issues Forum (LIF). LIF was funded to implement the CAM at San Francisco State University (SFSU) and City College of San Francisco (CCSF).

Get Ready, Get Set, Go

The Request for Application was released in October 2001 and the submitted proposals were reviewed by an independent review team who selected LIF as the successful applicant. There were six other projects funded at the same time. Once the projects were staffed and ready to go, the SFTFP provided a full-day training on the CAM. This training included interactive activities that moved training participants through the five-steps of the CAM. During the course of the 2.5 year project, SFTFP staff worked closely with the project coordinator through regular meetings, telephone calls, and review of project related documents as well as supporting the project by attending rallies, board of director meetings, and providing and coordinating trainings and presentations for the student advocates. The Project Coordinator was extremely organized and had the skills to successfully implement the project with technical assistance and consultation from SFTFP staff.

Step 1: Recruitment and training and selecting the focus area

At both campuses a core group of student advocates were recruited and trained to carry out and lead the tobacco-free education and policy advocacy campaign. The student advocates researched tobacco-related issues and policies on each campus, educated the campus community, developed concrete, permanent tobacco control policies at each campus, and worked for their passage, implementation, and enforcement. The advocates were expected to accomplish a variety of complex and demanding tasks:

- Research global issues of tobacco control;
- Conduct a diagnosis of campus and community tobacco policies and identify campus and community policymaking agencies;
- Research opinions and awareness of tobacco control issues and policies;
- Organize support for an educational campaign around tobacco control and passage of tobacco-free policies on both campuses;
- Implement a tobacco-free educational and media campaign to raise awareness of tobacco control issues;

- Advocate for the adoption of the chosen tobacco-free policy or policies by policymaking bodies; and
- Design a plan to enforce the policy after its passage.

To ensure that student advocates were prepared to meet the demands of the project, LIF provided extensive training during the first year of the project. The advocates learned about tobacco control issues and policy. They were given articles to read and were assigned additional research. The areas covered included: tobacco advertising; tobacco stock divestment; tobacco economics and profits; marketing to people of color, youth, and in foreign countries; environmental tobacco smoke; tobacco litigation; subsidiary products; tobacco and campaign finance; tobacco and individual health; tobacco and international trade/global economy; tobacco and agriculture/pesticides; and tobacco smuggling.

The student advocates on both campuses chose similar goals: permanently banning the sale of all tobacco products on campus and permanent divestment of all tobacco stocks owned by the Foundations on each campus. This case study will focus on the advocacy campaign related to divestment of tobacco stocks. During the recruitment and training stage, SFTFP staff provided on going consultation via both telephone and in person including suggesting materials and activities for the training, reviewing training plans, and offering suggestions and consultation on where, how and how many students to recruit and train. Recruited student advocates also participated in monthly SFTFP-sponsored provider meetings to provide a time for information sharing and joint problem solving. The SFTFP staff established a collegial relationship with both the project coordinator and student advocates by being available and attending project sponsored events.

Step 2: Designing and doing the diagnosis

The first task for the advocates was to conduct a community diagnosis of the tobacco environment on their respective campuses. Each group documented the following information:

- Current tobacco-related campus policies;
- The decision-making bodies and process on each campus;
- The extent of tobacco availability on each campus;
- The extent of tobacco sponsorship at college events; and
- The extent of tobacco stock in the investment portfolios of each campus.

The advocates used key informant interviews and surveys to collect information gathered from each project site as part of the community diagnosis. During this phase, the SFTFP staff and evaluator continued to be available to project staff and advocates to meet with them to discuss the design of the diagnosis—to review key informant interview questions and to brain storm how to complete the diagnosis.

Step 3: Analyzing results of community diagnosis

SFSU advocates sent an initial informational letter about the campaign and its policy objectives on the campus to all SFSU Foundation Board members in late October to determine if SFSU had tobacco investments. There was some initial confusion about whether or not SFSU had tobacco holdings. The financial manager of the Foundation was "fairly certain" the Foundation did invest in some tobacco stocks, but was uncertain about how to go about checking on it. The advocates were later informed that investments are confidential and board members, even if they know about specific investments, are not permitted to share this information with the public. One of the board members told the advocates that SFSU did not have tobacco investments and agreed to work with the advocates to get a statement in writing and begin working towards a permanent moratorium on tobacco investment.

The CCSF advocates were initially told that the school itself had no tobacco investments and that CCSF faculty and employees are part of the San Francisco retirement fund that had already divested. However, the student advocates discovered that the Foundation had investments in mutual funds that might include tobacco stocks in their portfolios. No formal written policy existed that prohibited the CCSF Foundation from investing in tobacco stocks. During this step, support from SFTFP staff and evaluator consisted of researching and providing information on divestment, brainstorming on ways to "compel" the college foundations to disclose their investment information, and participating in campus rallies to garner support for their advocacy campaigns.

Step 4: Designing and implementing the action plan

The advocates describe the project approach as "influencing and educating people," "networking," and "being persistent" to accomplish their goals of tobacco divestment and banning on-campus sale of tobacco and subsidiary products. One student thought having students involved in a high-profile way on campus made it easier to attract other students.

A large part of the work of the project entailed educating students, faculty, administrators, and policy makers about tobacco control issues, and organizing the campus community to rally around policy changes championed by the project. While few had prior community organizing experience, the student advocates on both campuses did form broad-based and effective coalitions to organize for those changes. The student advocates on each campus aggressively targeted campus policy-making bodies to advocate for policy changes to counter pro-tobacco influences.

On June 17, 2003, the SFSU Foundation Board of Directors unanimously updated the Foundation's list of restricted investments officially prohibiting the Foundation to invest in tobacco companies and in September 2003. The CCSF Foundation Board agreed to pass a policy permanently prohibiting tobacco investments if it was determined that the Board had no tobacco holdings.

This is generally the most labor intensive part of the CAM process. During this step, support from SFTFP continued in the same manner—monthly meetings, ongoing telephone conversations, participation in rallies and other support garnering events, attendance at hearings and review of materials, and strategy discussions. During this time, SFTFP staff met with student advocates to provide trainings on the global economy.

Step 5: Maintaining/enforcing the action

The Tobacco-Free College Campuses Project was successful in meeting most of its goals. The project educated the SFSU and CCSF campuses about the tobacco industry and its harmful practices, mobilized the campus community to support tobacco-free policies on both campuses, and successfully advocated adoption of administrative policies to permanently end financial ties between both colleges and tobacco corporations.

- On June 17, 2003, after 8 months of advocacy by TACTIC, the SFSU Foundation Board of Directors unanimously passed a written policy updating its restricted investments to permanently prohibit investment in tobacco companies. The Board also passed an SRI policy that, while not specifically mentioning tobacco or other industries as prohibited investments, represents a step in the right direction. The student advocates were unsuccessful in convincing the Foundation's board to adopt a stronger SRI policy but were able to get the Associated Students (AS) to agree to incorporate tobacco as part of its agenda for the following year. The student advocates felt that incorporating the tobacco agenda into the larger Associated Students agenda that would provide the best chance to institutionalize ongoing tobacco prevention work at SFSU.
- City College advocates continued to work with the City College Foundation to divest the small amount of money it has invested in

tobacco companies over a period of time and/or ensuring that all new funds are invested into a socially screened portfolio.

- NO BI advocated the successful passage of "Proposition A" on the April 2004 student trustee election ballot. Proposition A asked: "Does the student body recommend that the CCSF Foundation establish a socially responsible investment mutual fund to invest their capital?" The measure passed with 64% of the vote.
- NO BI contacted other community colleges in California to build a coalition for a blanket socially responsible investment policy among all community college foundations. The original project coordinator left at the end of two years to purse educational opportunities and a new coordinator was hired for the last six-months of the project. Therefore, technical assistance from SFTFP staff included overall orientation and review of the project's activities as well as technical assistance and consultation on current project activities. During this time, SFTFP staff arranged for a number of consultations with investment experts and attorneys to discuss possible avenues of interest to the student advocates. SFTFP acted as liaison for student advocates to set up meetings and get information from sources.

Beyond the CAM

The CAM is designed to have a lasting impact both in developing an individual and organization's capacity to continue social justice work by creating environmental change through policies. As the root of health disparities is social inequities in systems, empowering those members of the community most impacted to acquire the skills to change the social structures and inequities through environmental change will address health disparities. While the CAMs funded by the SFTFP are, by necessity, focused on tobacco-related issues, the skills and capacities developed are transferable to other issues affecting the community and preventing them from being healthy. The advocates felt a strong connection to the project and their work in large part because they were given leadership roles and liked having "a lot of say in what they were doing."

The student advocates also had opportunities to be involved in local, statewide, national, and global tobacco control events, which helped keep them, focused, stimulated, and aware of the connections between global tobacco control issues and their work on campus. Over the course of the project the advocates:

- Testified before the San Francisco Board of Supervisors in support of a citywide tobacco permit ordinance.

- Testified before the U.S. delegation to the Framework Convention on Tobacco Control (FCTC) in Nashville, Tennessee in September 2002 in support of stricter standards for worldwide tobacco marketing and advertising giving advocates an opportunity to practice their public speaking and presentation skills.
- Regularly attended meetings of the Global Action Task Force (GATF) and participated in GATF's November 2002 Intercambio in San Francisco that hosted tobacco control advocates from Africa, Latin America, and India.
- Traveled to the WTO meeting in Cancun in September 2003 and the FTA meeting in Miami in November 2003 to protest liberal trade policies that put multinational corporate profits over public health.
- Traveled to Ecuador to hold an intercambio (educational exchange) with Ecuadorian high school and college students on tobacco control issues, share tools for policy advocacy, and work together in the growing youth-led tobacco control movement.

Most of the advocates saw the project as an opportunity to learn or improve their skills in research, communication, public speaking, writing, community organizing, and decision-making. The challenge of working on a long-term basis trying to convince high-level policymakers to change existing policies helped them to fine tune all of those skills and be constantly learning and challenged, even though some of the work involved doing things some weren't comfortable with, like public speaking. One advocate also mentioned that at times there has been a lot of pressure trying to balance demanding extracurricular activities *and* schoolwork.

The project director fostered positive relationships and a family-like support system with the advocates through meetings, get-togethers, and special lunches and dinners. The project used other ways to foster positive interactions for the advocates that made the project less of a job and more of a student-run club or project where all members give equally of their time, commitment, and ideas. These included: providing lunch at events and meetings,

Conclusions

The SFTFP began funding community-based organizations to implement the CAM process in 1995. By 2004, thirty-seven projects had been funded in six funding cycles. Thirty of these projects implemented an action plan towards the accomplishment of an "Action" (that meets the three criteria)

and twenty-eight of them successfully accomplished the "Action" itself. The CAM is designed to have a lasting impact both in developing an individual and organization's capacity to continue social justice work by creating environmental change through policies. Empowering those members of the community most impacted to acquire the skills to change the social structures and inequities through environmental change will address health inequities. The CAM is one concrete model for Departments of Public Health to draw from in funding environmental change projects. All it takes is the will and commitment.

Notes

1. R.T. Anderson, P. Sorlie, E. Backlund, et al., "Mortality Effects of Community Socioeconomic Status," 8 *Epidemiology* (1997): 42–47.
2. M. Haan, G.A. Kaplan, and T. Camacho, "Poverty and Health: Prospective Evidence from the Alameda County Study," 125 *American Journal of Epidemiology* (1987): 989–998.
3. N.E. Adler, T. Boyce, and M.A. Chesney, "Socioeconomic Status and Health: The Challenge of the Gradient," 49 *American Psychology* (1994): 15–24.
4. Center for Disease Control and Prevention, *Tobacco Use among U.S. Racial/Ethnic Minority Groups—African Americans, American Indians and Alaska Natives, Asian Americans and Pacific Islanders, and Hispanics: A Report of the Surgeon General*. A Report of the Surgeon General (Washington, DC: US Dept of Health and Human Services, 1998).

20

Tackling the Root Causes of Health Disparities through Community Capacity Building

ANTHONY B. ITON, SANDRA WITT, ALEXANDRA DESAUTELS, KATHERINE SCHAFF, MIA LULUQUISEN, LIZ MAKER, KATHRYN HORSLEY, AND MATT BEYERS

Health, disease, and death are not randomly distributed in a society. Poor health concentrates among low-income people and people of color residing in certain places. Access to proven health protective resources like clean air, healthy food, and recreational space, as well as opportunities for high-quality education, living wage employment, and decent housing, is highly dependent on the neighborhood where one lives, which is ultimately a reflection of the relative social, political, and economic power of the residents of these communities. These social inequities cluster and accumulate over people's lives, and over time, successfully conspire to diminish the ultimate quality and length of human life in these places.

This chapter highlights the relationship between health inequities and social inequities and how one local public health department is employing an explicit community power-building strategy to achieve social and health equity through institutional change, community capacity building, and strategic local policy interventions. By building social, political, and economic power in low-income communities of color, Alameda County's practice intends that community residents can achieve a higher degree of control over their neighborhood environments and be better able to advocate with local institutions and in the policy-making arena for a more equitable distribution of health protective resources. Public health practice as a social justice enterprise must be cognizant of the pervasive influence of persistent social, political, and economic forces that create and maintain striking patterns of inequitable wealth distribution, residential racial segregation, and educational disparities in the United States. Ultimately, changing the status quo and eliminating health disparities will require a public health practice that sustainably changes the power equilibrium at the local level.

Why We Have Health *Disparities* in the United States

Wealth: A Fundamental Determinant of Health

In the United States, wealth is the strongest determinant of health. While this phenomenon is by no means unique to the United States, the strength of the relationship in this country is profound and increasing. *In the United States, wealth equals health.*[1-6] In addition to the direct link from wealth to health, wealth also impacts other factors that also affect health. Two critical pathways include neighborhood residential segregation and education, both of which are affected by wealth and in turn, impact wealth accumulation.

Wealth confers a number of important social benefits that are strongly associated with positive health outcomes. These benefits include access to a variety of social goods, such as high-quality education, employment, housing, child care, recreational opportunities, nutrition, medical care, and safer and cleaner neighborhoods. While this general relationship has been demonstrated in many developed countries, the extent to which wealth controls access to these social goods varies substantially across the developed world. Generally speaking, in countries with a well-developed social safety net, formal mechanisms facilitate access to key social goods for all economic strata within the society. These mechanisms often include substantial government investments and subsidies for housing, child care, education, vocational training, employment, medical care, and food access. A direct and intended consequence of these investments is the reduction of the powerful influence of wealth as a determinant of health. Conferring independent access to these critical social benefits reduces the strength of the relationship between wealth and health.

In order to invest in critical social benefits, governments generally tax income and effectively redistribute resources in the form of greater access to social benefits for lower income groups. Where these investments are in place, inequality in the distribution of income is often reduced. Substantial evidence shows that life expectancy increases and other health indicators improve as the distribution of income and resources in developed countries becomes more egalitarian.[7,8]

In the United States wealth is the primary portal through which one accesses a variety of critical social benefits. Further complicating this issue in the United States is the enormous disparity in wealth between various racial and ethnic groups and the profound legacy of racial discrimination that is inextricably embedded in this country's history and political practices, past and present. African American and Latino households have less than ten cents for every dollar in wealth owned by white households. Approximately one-third of African American households and one-quarter of Latino households have zero or negative net worth. Nationwide, the percentage of whites who own their homes is about 75%, whereas homeownership rates for African Americans and Latinos is about 47%.[9] These racialized patterns of wealth distribution are consistent from community to community across the United States. Furthermore, no substantial evidence suggests that this racial wealth disparity is narrowing; in fact, the opposite is occurring.

Thus, in the U.S. context, wealth equals health. As wealth is strongly correlated with race, it follows that a strong relationship would exist between health and race. In this way, large inequities in wealth translate to large racial health inequities in the United States. Without understanding this fundamental relationship, health inequities are often simply construed as "health disparities" divorced from the powerful social context in which they arise (see Box 20.1).

Box 20.1 Health Disparities and Health Inequities

The National Institutes of Health defines *health disparities* as "differences in the incidence, prevalence, mortality, and burden of diseases and other adverse health conditions that exist among specific population groups in the United States."[10] *Health inequities* are "differences in health which are not only unnecessary and avoidable but, in addition, are considered unfair and unjust."[11] Thus, equity and inequity are value-based, normative concepts based on the ideas and principles of social justice whereas "disparity" is a descriptive term that refers to measurable quantities but does not imply whether this disparity arises from an unjust root cause.[12,13] For the purposes of this article, the term "inequity" is used when the referenced differences in health outcomes have been produced by historic and systemic social inequities.

Neighborhood Residential Segregation and Health: Concentrations of Race and Poverty

In addition to racialized patterns of wealth distribution that lead to a relative concentration of poverty in certain racial groups, the *spatial* concentration of poverty has also increased sharply in the United States, enhancing a de facto residential apartheid. The direct link between wealth and health, neighborhood segregation and the concentration of poverty into spatial areas provides another pathway from wealth to health. As racial and wealth-based segregation increases, so do the negative health consequences. Between 1970 and 1990, the percentage of urban poor in the United States living in nonpoor neighborhoods (defined as fewer than 20% of households living below the poverty level) declined from 45% to 31%, while the percentage living in poor neighborhoods (between 20% and 40% of households in poverty) increased from 38% to 41%. The proportion living in very poor neighborhoods (over 40% in poverty) grew from 17% to 28%. While this trend reversed itself somewhat between 1990 and the boom year of 2000, there was still much higher concentrated poverty in 2000 than in 1970 or 1980.[14] As a consequence, many U.S. neighborhoods are becoming poorer and more segregated.

Segregation by race and income causes a concentration of disadvantage in neighborhoods, including a greater concentration of risk factors for disease and injury. Generally, in many of these neighborhoods, poorly performing schools are the norm and school dropout rates are exceptionally high. Access to transportation, quality affordable housing, adequate parks and recreational opportunities, and grocery stores is often very limited. Furthermore, these neighborhoods tend to be in closer proximity to sources of environmental pollution. These inequitable neighborhood conditions affect individual and community health. Two pathways through which the neighborhood social and physical environment may produce health disparities are:

- *Shaping individual behaviors*: Characteristics of the physical environment such as availability of parks, grocery stores, and community centers, create the context in which individual behavioral choices are made concerning physical activity, nutrition, tobacco and alcohol use, and other health-related behaviors. In low-income communities, these neighborhood physical conditions may be operating in a manner that increases the likelihood that certain adverse risk behaviors will be adopted.
- *Increasing individual risk factors*: Characteristics of the social environment may produce certain physiological changes in individuals that directly increase their risk of disease. A robust literature base has developed around several proposed theories to explain this including

Weathering, and *Allostatic Load*.[15] These hypotheses generally propose a link between the cumulative impact of various social and environmental stressors and human physiological response. In this way, neighborhood-level poverty, racism, crime, lack of education, unemployment, and social isolation act synergistically to produce detrimental physiologic changes (hypertension, increased free radical activity, elevated cortisol, impaired immune system responsiveness, etc.).

Protective or resiliency factors in neighborhood social environment are also relevant. These factors include high educational attainment, stable family relationships, positive relationships between youth and adults, meaningful opportunities for civic participation, positive race/ethnic intergroup relations, protective cultural factors, and timely access to appropriate health and social services, and high expectations for career/employment. These factors are theorized to act as buffers against poverty, crime, racism, and other negative exposures, and thus reduce the impact of weathering and allostatic load, ultimately resulting in improved health outcomes for those individuals or neighborhoods that possess one or more of these resiliency factors.

Lessening the impact of wealth on segregation and concentrated neighborhood poverty and the ensuing impact on health is possible through capitalizing on and increasing resiliency factors in low-income communities of color. In addition, understanding, illuminating, and addressing the social and economic policies that play a role in creating and reinforcing residential segregation in the United States is critical to designing solutions to eliminate health inequities.

Education and Health: Neglected Schools in Struggling Neighborhoods

An additional way wealth impacts health is through education. Wealth and segregation impact access to quality education, which in turns influences employment opportunities as well as access to benefits, income, and wealth accumulation. Public health practitioners have consistently illustrated the link between education and health across multiple pathways and for multiple health outcomes. Generally, improved educational outcomes are associated with improved health outcomes. However, the majority of state governments provide fewer dollars per student to their highest-poverty school districts than to their lowest-poverty school districts.[16] This educational funding disparity forms a consistent pattern across U.S. communities despite the clear evidence that high-poverty schools need *greater* resources to meet the same standards. This fact is even codified in the No Child Left Behind Act, wherein Congress established a standard that states should provide districts with *additional funding* per low-income student equal to an additional 40% of the average per student amount. Despite this awareness, funding gaps between wealthy and poor districts within states remain, and have even increased in some states.[16] In addition, most states also have a funding gap between schools with the most African American and Latino students and those with the fewest.[16] Finally, there is also evidence of substantial within-district funding disparities favoring wealthier white students at the expense of poorer African American and Latino students within the same school district.[16]

Nationally, only an estimated 68% of those who entered 9th grade graduated with a regular diploma in 12th grade. Comparatively, only 50% of all black students, 51% of Native American students, and 53% of all Hispanic students graduated from high school. Black, Native American, and Hispanic males fare even worse, with 43%, 47%, and 48% graduating, respectively.[17] Education correlates with health through multiple pathways. An important aspect is that adults need a high school diploma in order to be able to compete effectively for jobs that pay a living wage, which in turn provides people with the financial resources they need for healthy, productive lives. Neighborhoods in which many residents are high school dropouts are more likely to have higher unemployment, poorer quality housing, poorer schools, and possibly less stable families. This not only impacts individual health, but also impacts the health of the entire neighborhood. Middle and upper class families can point to low test scores and poor-quality schools as a basis for their decision to move away in favor of better schools in the suburbs, which further depletes the neighborhood of resources and a tax base. Thus, the abysmally poor graduation rates of poor African American and Latino children being tolerated in the United States are contributing greatly to maintaining a status quo of economically deprived, racially segregated, and generally under-resourced neighborhoods mired in severe social dysfunction. It is within this context that health inequities are created and perpetuated.

Why Place Matters: Social and Health Inequity in Alameda County

Place matters because it is through place that these critical determinants of health—wealth accumulation, neighborhood segregation and poverty, and access to high-quality education—concentrate and mutually reinforce each other. Like many U.S. cities and counties, Alameda County faces profound and persistent racial and class-based health inequities. Tracking health indicators by race provides important information about the disparate outcomes of people within various racial categories and suggests the powerful role that racism, both present and past, plays in determining health outcomes in this county. Understanding how race and racism may mediate the powerful influence of social and economic forces on health outcomes in Alameda County requires further exploration of the complex interplay of a variety of local, social, and economic factors and how their distribution across the county may be strongly influenced by race. Tracking social phenomena such as segregation can guide us in exploring the social inequities that lead to health inequities and offer hints at solutions. According to standard measures of residential segregation, Alameda County has among the highest levels of residential segregation for African Americans in the San Francisco Bay Area. Oakland, the county's largest city, ranks as the second most segregated city for African Americans in California.

While significant health inequities can be found for almost every racial and ethnic group, the magnitude of racial health inequities in Alameda County is most serious for African Americans, Latinos, Pacific Islanders, and Native Americans. In Alameda County, African Americans experience relative disadvantage in virtually all major health indicators including: coronary heart disease, diabetes, stroke, AIDS, cancer, asthma, infant mortality, low birth weight, and homicide. In fact, of the 19 key health indicators tracked longitudinally by the Alameda County Public Health Department, African Americans have the worst outcomes in 16 of them.

Local mortality data illustrate the result of concentrated disadvantage by place. Higher rates of mortality occur in certain geographic areas, as seen in Figure 20.1, which shows the spatial distribution of death from all causes by census tract. The highest rates of mortality (shown in black) are largely concentrated in the low-income communities West Berkeley, North Oakland, West Oakland, and East Oakland, as well as a few areas in Cherryland, Fairview, and Hayward. People living in these areas have mortality rates that are 1.4 times higher than the countywide rate of 704.3 per 100,000. The corresponding life expectancy in these high-mortality areas is up to 10 years less than other areas of the county (shown in light gray).

In Alameda County, higher rates of disease are also observed in low-income neighborhoods. Neighborhood of residence is linked to all-cause mortality, cause-specific mortality, coronary heart disease, low birth weight, perceived health status, and rates of violent crime. In Alameda County, the neighborhood in which people live serves as an all too accurate predictor of their mortality rate. Figures 20.2 and 20.3 demonstrate the strong association between the all-cause mortality rate and neighborhood poverty. Mortality steadily increases as the level of neighborhood poverty increases, so neighborhoods with the lowest proportion of poor households have better health than those neighborhoods in the middle, which, in turn, fare better than those in neighborhoods with the highest levels of poverty. This "social gradient" provides strongly suggestive evidence that the quality of the social environment itself plays an important role in determining health outcomes.

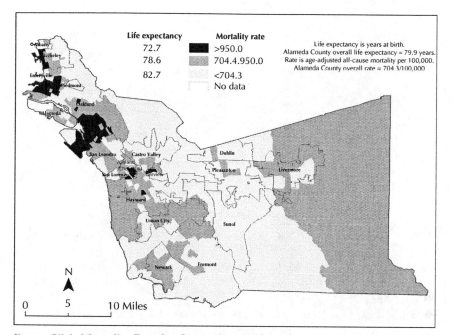

FIGURE 20.1 Mortality Rate by Census Tract, Alameda County.
SOURCE: Alameda County vital statistics files, 2001–2005.

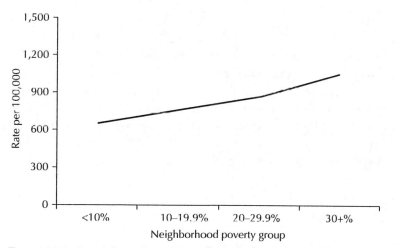

FIGURE 20.2 Age-Adjusted Mortality Rate by Neighborhood Poverty Level.
Alameda County, 2001–2005

The social gradient holds true across most racial/ethnic groups. African
Americans, Asians, and whites living in poorer neighborhoods die at higher
rates compared to their counterparts living in more affluent neighborhoods.
Whether living in poor or rich neighborhoods, African Americans experience the highest rates of death compared to other groups. Death rates rise

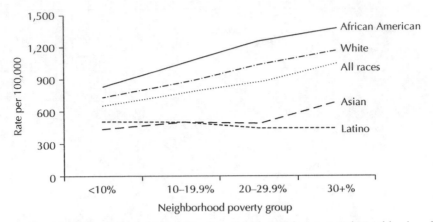

FIGURE 20.3 Age-Adjusted Mortality Rate by Race/Ethnicity[a] and Neighborhood Poverty Level. Alameda County, 2001–2005
SOURCE: C.J.L. Murray, S.C. Kulkarni, C. Michaud, et al., "Eight Americas: Investigating Mortality Disparities across Races, Counties, and Race-Counties in the United States," 3(9) e260 PLoS Medicine.
NOTES: Local data for Native Americans are not available but national data for this population indirectly show the same pattern of health outcomes by income.

substantially for Asians in the highest poverty neighborhoods. Latinos appear to be the exception, with about the same mortality observed regardless of poverty level. African Americans, followed by Latinos, are most likely to live in higher poverty neighborhoods (with over 20% of residents living in poverty). In 2003, nearly 41% of African Americans and 26% of Latinos resided in higher poverty neighborhoods, compared to 12% of Asians and 4% of Whites.

Several hypotheses might explain the apparent paradox reflected in the lack of a significant social gradient for Latinos in Alameda County, including the so-called "healthy-migrant theory" which posits that the immigration process itself may select for a healthier subpopulation. In addition, Latino immigrants may have health and social behaviors that are health protective, including healthier diets, greater inclination toward physical activity, and a greater cultural reliance on social and peer networks.[18,19] As immigrants acculturate, evidence suggests that they lose some of these protective health behaviors.[20] Public health interventions that attempt to strengthen and support these protective health and social behaviors while addressing the social inequities that contribute to health inequities will lead to improved health outcomes among all Alameda County residents.

Public Health as a Social Justice Enterprise

In Alameda County and elsewhere, to truly eliminate these health inequities, public health must be viewed as a social justice enterprise, recognizing and targeting root causes of social inequity. Injustice thrives where imbalances of power and privilege are found. The pervasive influence of persistent social, political, and economic forces that create and maintain striking patterns of inequitable wealth distribution, residential racial segregation, and educational disparities in the United States remain largely invisible to the general public. A close examination of how these rigid, apartheid-like patterns of societal organization are maintained, despite the successful elimination of legalized forms of racism following the civil rights movement, reveals that at its very roots the problem lies with a persistent inequity in the distribution of social, political, and economic power among racial groups in the United States. Therefore, the relevant question for public health practitioners becomes: how do we support and participate in movements that aim to build social, political and economic power for low-income communities of color?

In this society, privilege primarily flows along race, class, and gender lines, and to some extent, immigration status. Consequently, many social and economic policies favor whites, particularly wealthy white males. Examples of policies that have privileged whites while disadvantaging people of color include the GI Bill, redlining practices, welfare policy, urban renewal policies, education funding policies and practices, drug use and incarceration policies, housing policies, and health insurance policies. In essence, these policies and practices can be collectively described as affirmative action for whites. Cumulatively, they have created and continue to reinforce the United States' particular race and class social hierarchy. Any acute strain on society, whether it is economic recession, a predatory lending and foreclosure crisis, new drug epidemics such as crack cocaine, communicable disease epidemics such as influenza, or natural disasters such as Hurricane Katrina, will exact its greatest toll on low-income communities of color that are at the very bottom of the privilege and power hierarchy.

In addition to the presence of significant imbalances in power, injustice also thrives where truth is absent. Without both of these elements—truth and power—justice cannot exist. The public health "truth" is the powerful influence of the social determinants in the generation of health disparities. Innumerable detailed studies published in peer-reviewed journals describe the clear relationship between various "social determinants of health" and health outcomes. Entire journals are dedicated to these topics. Yet, despite the widespread distribution of evidence, we see relatively little progress in core health measures for our most socially, politically, and economically marginalized populations. This is because public health has still largely ignored the issue of power and its skewed distribution throughout society. Our work in communities tends to focus on individual-level behavioral change models, intensification of service delivery, and issue-specific community mobilization efforts. Rarely do public health agencies focus squarely on building upon indigenous social, political, and economic power in low-income communities of color.

Designing Public Health Practice to Achieve Health Equity

Expanding the Traditional Scope of Public Health Department Work

Alameda County Public Health Department (ACPHD) has adapted the Bay Area Regional Health Inequities Initiative's (BARHII) Framework for Health Equity (see Figure 20.4) to explain the comprehensive scope of work necessary to address stark differences in health outcomes by income, race/ethnicity and place. The framework is not meant to represent a comprehensive and explanatory logic model; rather, it is a simplified depiction of a spectrum of potential intervention points for a public health practice that is cognizant of and focused on the powerful structural causes of

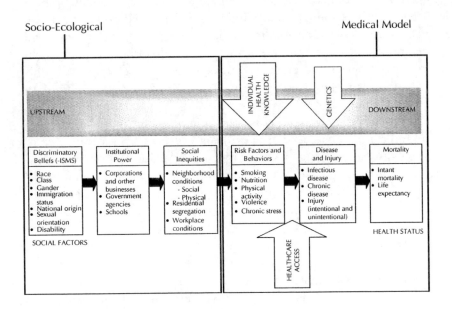

FIGURE 20.4 A Framework for Health Equity.
SOURCE: Adapted by ACPHD from the Bay Area Regional Health Inequities Initiative, Summer 2008.

health disparities in addition to the "downstream" consequences. Public health departments traditionally work on the right side of the figure—providing immunizations, diabetes education, smoking cessation, and other services to individuals in need. These public health strategies are essential because they affect risk behaviors and access to health care services, which we know influence health outcomes.

However, despite a general effort by our national health leadership to acknowledge the role of "social determinants" in influencing health outcomes, the federal government perspective on health inequities continues to focus predominantly on disease-specific remedial strategies.[21-23] Many federal public health organizations frequently frame the issue of racial health disparities primarily from a medical perspective. As a result, the solutions proposed tend to focus on the intensification of individual medical and case management services to the population most afflicted. In this way, "determinants of health" are often limited to those that are perceived as amenable to individual behavior modification approaches such as tobacco cessation and drug treatment, counseling against high-risk sexual behaviors, and education regarding the consequences of poor nutrition and physical inactivity. Efforts based on this "medical model" have demonstrated limited efficacy in addressing health inequities. In addition, such approaches are generally resource intensive and consequently unsustainable after the initial infusion of resources begins to dwindle.

One can see by moving "upstream" on the BARHII Framework that health inequities do not merely arise from individual variation in genes, medical care access, health knowledge, and risk behaviors/risk factors. The economic, social, and physical environments, as well as available services in neighborhoods all shape behavioral choices and disease risks. The policies and practices of powerful institutions strongly influence the environments where people live, work, and play. Finally, social structures can be instruments of oppression and discrimination by creating differential access to power, resources, life chances, and opportunities—all of which determine the distribution of health and disease within the population. To address the *root causes of health inequities*, ACPHD is bridging downstream and upstream public health activities highlighted in the BARHII framework.

In the process of bridging downstream and upstream approaches, ACPHD is also intentional about the ecological levels of its strategies. Local public health interventions are generally focused at one of four levels: (1) individual, (2) group, (3) neighborhood/community, and (4) the larger society/policy arena. Individual and group-focused interventions frequently are heavily characterized by specific clinical and preventive services such as risk factor screening, immunization, and targeted educational campaigns. Individual and group level interventions dominate local public health practice in the United States in large part due to the programmatic requirements embedded in most of the major federal and state public health funding streams, as well as years of socialization in the medical model as the only model for taking action.

Public health interventions that focus on conditions in neighborhoods or other "places" are rare despite the fact that many of the exposures to known social determinants of disease occur at the neighborhood level. It is particularly at the neighborhood level that the physical and social environments manifest their deleterious influence on low-income racial and ethnic communities in Alameda County and elsewhere. Some public health departments are working with community residents to build leadership skills and other capacity so that neighborhood residents can exercise more powerful roles in local planning and decision making. However, some researchers have critiqued public health approaches that focus *exclusively* on working within communities to build social capital. They argue that pure social capital building approaches present "a model of the social determinants of health that excludes any analysis of structural inequalities (e.g., class, gender, or racial/ethnic relations)."[24] Conversely, others are critical of approaches that focus primarily on legal efforts designed to dismantle specific policies and practices that have a racially discriminatory effect. Such approaches often fail to directly involve the affected community members and consequently do not lead to a sustained increase in community capacity.

This dichotomy can be oversimplified in the following question. Are health inequities due to something wrong within low-income minority neighborhoods, or are they due to something wrong with U.S. society that results in a concentration of health inequities in certain neighborhoods? Our contention is that this is not an either-or situation. Eliminating health inequities will require sophisticated public health interventions that simultaneously address both the internal neighborhood context (low social cohesion, neighborhood disorganization, and lack of leadership) and the structural context (discriminatory political, economic, and social policies), bridging strategies that focus on place and those that focus on policy.

The rarest of all local public health interventions are those directed to the larger society and policy arena. And yet it is in this arena where public health interventions hold their greatest potential. While public health leaders have supported social policies that have a direct and obvious impact on access to health services, such as universal health insurance, relatively little organized public health support exists for other policies that benefit health, such as universal preschool access, improved public school funding, living wage employment, affordable housing, land use planning reform, quality and affordable public transportation, immigration reform, criminal justice reform, and economic development.

What makes the fight for equity hopeful is that the social, political, and economic forces that produce health inequities in low-income communities are identifiable and actionable. They include long-standing and pervasive local, regional, state, and federal policies that reinforce rigid patterns of social and material disparities between racial and economic groups in this country, ultimately leading to persistent health inequities. Over time these forces have taken many forms including racially restrictive covenants on property, economic redlining in banking practices, school segregation, housing and urban renewal policies, disinvestment in public transportation, discriminatory zoning practices, law enforcement racial profiling, differential incarceration policies related to drug use and possession, and other deliberate governmental policies and practices. The cumulative impact of these discriminatory policies is a well-structured racial and class apartheid in Alameda County and elsewhere in the United States. While some of these policies and practices have been successfully challenged and reversed, others remain intact. The legacy of decades of these discriminatory policies is indelibly stamped in the health inequities that we are faced with in 2009.

A useful concept for understanding this legacy is that of "institutionalized racism" put forward by Dr. Camara Jones. Jones defines institutionalized racism as

> differential access to the goods, services, and opportunities of society by race. Institutionalized racism is normative, sometimes legalized, and often manifests as inherited disadvantage. It is structural, having been codified in our institutions of custom, practice, and law, so there need not be an identifiable perpetrator. Indeed, institutionalized racism is often evident as inaction in the face of need.[25]

Institutionalized racism *causes* unhealthy neighborhoods by systematically starving certain communities of access to key social goods, such as education, health care, adequate housing, recreational amenities, and other assets and opportunities, thereby directly creating adverse social and physical environments within these communities. ACPHD has strategically focused on addressing institutional racism because of the pervasive impact it can have on wealth, segregation, education, and other social determinants of health. In addition, residents, staff, partners, and health department leadership have all named racism as a key barrier to achieving health equity and healthy communities.

Countering these powerful social and environmental forces is unquestionably a daunting task. Nevertheless, it is only by eliminating these forces that health inequities can be eliminated. The question for local health departments is: what effective strategies can be employed to address these underlying structural forces that play such a powerful role in producing and perpetuating health disparities?

Alameda County's Working Principles and Three-Pronged Approach

Effective strategies to reduce and eventually eliminate health inequities must be multifaceted and long term. They must also involve institutions beyond the sectors of public health and medicine. In addition, they must address the power differentials that have contributed to the creation and maintenance of social and health inequities. ACPHD has recently identified ten *principles* that guide how and with whom we address the challenge of eliminating health inequities.[26]

1. Exploring the *historical forces* that have left a legacy of racism and segregation is critical to moving forward with the structural changes needed to provide living wages, affordable housing, excellent education, clean air, and other social conditions in neighborhoods that now experience disadvantage.

2. *Working across multiple sectors* of government and society is basic to making the structural changes necessary. Such work should be in partnership with community advocacy groups that continue to pursue a more equitable society.

3. *Measuring and monitoring the impact* of social policy on health to ensure gains in equity is essential. This will include instituting systems to track governmental spending by neighborhood and tracking changes in measures of health equity over time and place to help identify the impact of adverse policies and practices.

4. Groups that are the most affected by inequities must have a voice in identifying policies that will make a difference as well as in holding government accountable for implementing these policies. A high level of *public participation* is needed with attention to outreach, follow-through, language, inclusion, and cultural understanding. Government and private funding agencies should actively support resident capacity to engage.

5. Acknowledging the *cumulative impact of stressful experiences and environments* is crucial. For some families, poverty lasts a lifetime and is perpetuated throughout multiple generations, leaving family members with few opportunities to make healthful decisions.

6. The developmental needs and transitions of *all age groups* should be addressed. While infants, children, youth, adults, and elderly require age appropriate strategies, the largest investments should be in early life because important foundations of adult health are laid in early childhood.

7. Changing community conditions requires extensive *work on land use policy* to address the location of toxic sites, grocery and liquor stores, affordable housing and transportation, the primacy of the

automobile, access to opportunities for physical exercise and building social supports, and overall quality of life.

8. The *social fabric of neighborhoods* needs to be strengthened. Residents need to be connected and supported and believe that they hold power to improve the safety and well-being of their families. All residents need to have a sense of belonging, dignity, and hope. Neighborhood assets should be maximized to address this issue.

9. While low-income people and people of color face age-old survival issues, *new challenges* brought on by the global economy, climate change, U.S. foreign policy, and the need for immigration reform and energy alternatives are also relevant and should be addressed in the context of equity.

10. Because of the cumulative impact of multiple stressors, our overall approach should shift *toward changing community conditions* and away from blaming individuals or groups for their disadvantaged status. Eliminating inequities in Alameda County is a huge *opportunity to invest in community.* Inequity among us is no longer politically and morally acceptable and we all stand to gain by eliminating it.

ACPHD's efforts to address and eliminate health inequities have centered on three main strategies: (1) building the internal capacity of staff and creating an organizational culture that supports staff in addressing health inequities; (2) working closely with neighborhoods in community-capacity building efforts; and (3) addressing the root causes of health inequities through local policy work. These three areas are supported by innovative research and data analysis and in each area, connecting with programs and services is an important aspect. Each area is an essential part of a multifaceted approach to eliminating health inequities. While the three strategies provide a framework for action and day-to-day work, the 10 principles provide guidance for staff in how to approach this work from a social justice perspective.

1. Institutional change and internal capacity building

Institutional Change: As illustrated in the Framework for Health Equity, many local health departments, including ACPHD, have developed an infrastructure and organizational culture that is built around addressing the issues highlighted in the three boxes to the right in Figure 20.4, or those within the medical model. While ACPHD has demonstrated numerous successes in these areas, to truly address health inequities, programs and policies also need to act through the three boxes on the left, in the social-ecological area. This means that ACPHD has had to fundamentally rethink its infrastructure and organizational culture. This entails becoming an organization that can not only address the needs of individuals, but can also enact broader solutions, including community-capacity building efforts and policy change aimed at the fundamental processes of injustice.

An essential part of moving our organization forward has been undertaking a participatory strategic planning process, which occurred in 2006 and 2007. This process included: internal discussions on racism, gender discrimination, and class exploitation; seven community forums, including one for Spanish-speaking residents; dialogues with the Public Health Commission, ACPHD staff, and Alameda County youth about their vision for a healthy Alameda County; interviews with the Alameda County Board of Supervisors and other key stakeholders; an online survey to gather input from all ACPHD staff; and two planning retreats to finalize the plan. The plan will be incorporated into all divisional work plans and all of our efforts to address health inequities will be guided and supported by our strategic plan. For more information on the strategic plan, visit http://www.acphd.org/healthequity/strategic.

Box 20.2 Alameda County Public Health Department Strategic Plan 2008–2013

1. Transform our organizational culture and align our daily work to achieve health equity.
2. Enhance public health communications internally and externally.
3. Ensure organizational accountability through measurable outcomes and community involvement.
4. Support the development of a productive, creative, and accountable workforce.
5. Advocate for policies that address social conditions impacting health.
6. Cultivate and expand partnerships that are community driven and innovative.

Internal Capacity Building: A key issue that arose during the strategic planning process was the need for internal capacity building, which is exemplified in Strategic Directions 1 and 4. As staff must address increasingly complex issues, avenues and mechanisms must be in place to increase internal capacity. To change organizational culture and redefine practice, staff will need opportunities to learn and apply new skills. As organizational culture shifts, staff will need ongoing training and support in order to respond as the organization changes.

In the ACPHD experience, it has been essential to have staff from all levels who can examine and discuss social justice with diverse audiences; collect, analyze, and present data on health inequities in innovative ways; interpret the literature on social justice issues; facilitate difficult discussions around issues such as racism and move people toward action; understand, respect, and work with community residents; support youth interns from the community; and help other staff develop their skills. In addition to being logistically necessary, building staff capacity in these areas also creates a shared knowledge and language around social justice and increases solidarity and critical mass amongst staff. The staff continues to work with national, state, and local partners, universities, and others to increase our understanding of and ability to address these issues. We have created a five-module Public Health 101 training series for all staff that covers: (1) the history of public health; (2) cultural competency and cultural humility; (3) undoing racism; (4) social and health equity; and (5) community capacity building. Training on policy development is offered to staff members who are engaging in more focused policy work.

Numerous training opportunities and a wealth of literature on staff development, leadership, facilitation, management, and organizational culture can be adapted to focus on social justice and the needs of local health departments. By tying workforce development and organizational change to social justice, local health departments can strategically assess needs, create learning opportunities, and develop a staff that is capable and supported in tackling the difficult issues that arise when trying to address root causes of health inequities.

2. Building community capacity

Community capacity has been defined as "the characteristics of communities that affect their ability to identify, mobilize, and address social and public health problems."[27] Community capacity is considered to be a socially protective factor for community residents.[28] It is also a method for combating social inequities such as poverty, racial disparities, unemployment, and other social determinants of health. [28-30] Such assets may help explain why not all poor communities suffer disproportionately poor health outcomes. In Alameda County, the best example of this phenomenon is the so-called "Latino Health Paradox." As mentioned earlier, Alameda County's Latinos have lower overall age-adjusted mortality rates than Alameda County whites. While in the United States wealth and health are closely tied together, the existence of low-income subpopulations with better health outcomes supports the idea that health outcomes do not have to be inextricably tied to poverty levels. At a minimum it would seem that other less well understood factors, in addition to poverty, have the potential to substantially influence the health outcomes of communities. What are these factors, and how are they health protective? The Latino Health Paradox suggests that certain health protective factors in the culture and social milieu that can be identified and enhanced in a manner that would inure to the benefit of the broader community. These factors sometimes referred to as resiliency factors, may include strong social networks, meaningful employment opportunities, positive adult–youth relationships, and accessible venues for civic and political participation. Public health departments must become more adept at facilitating ongoing community-level processes that acknowledge cultural strengths and build upon the resiliency factors within each cultural group.

ACPHD has designed a community-centered, place-based, multicomponent intervention designed to build neighborhood-level community capacity. *The goal of the intervention is to build political, social, and economic power within low-income communities of color within Alameda County.* This approach borrows heavily from popular education principles expounded by Brazilian educator Paulo Freire and builds directly upon existing community assets and strengths. The approach focuses on identifying neighborhood assets, most specifically its leaders, and facilitating a coherent and supportive neighborhood social, economic, and political infrastructure that will allow these leaders to enhance the natural resiliency of their communities and thereby improve long-term health outcomes. Empowerment and community capacity building are vital for changing structural factors that perpetuate negative community conditions.[31–36] It is this "social action that promotes participation of people, organizations and communities toward the goals of increased individual and community control, political efficacy, improved quality of life and social justice" that is key strategy to achieving social and health equity.[37]

Overview of the City/County Neighborhood Initiative. In conjunction with partners from county, city, and community-based agencies, religious and neighborhood improvement organizations, ACPHD leads an intervention to build community capacity and social action in two Oakland neighborhoods in Alameda County: Sobrante Park and the Hoover Historic District. These communities were chosen because of their high rates of crime, violence, poverty, and health problems. In addition, these neighborhoods were known for their community assets (grassroots groups, community-based organizations, schools, and churches) and history of citizen civic participation.

The City/County Neighborhood Initiative (CCNI), a multiyear intervention, has four main goals on the pathway to reducing violence and health inequities:

1. Empower residents to speak and act effectively on their own behalf.
2. Build grassroots organizations that can leverage the power of the community.
3. Win concrete improvements in people's lives.
4. Alter the relations of power so institutions are accountable and responsive to the community.

To realize these goals, the CCNI has implemented a six-component intervention in each neighborhood, which is supported by a "Core Team" of representatives from local schools, churches, neighborhood associations, community-based associations, and city and county departments.

What follows is a description of the CCNI intervention components in Sobrante Park. For more information about CCNI activities in both neighborhoods, see the CCNI page of the ACPHD web site, http://www.acphd. org/healthequity/ccni.

Component 1: Community assessment and issue selection
In 2004, ACPHD reached out to community partners to implement surveys with adults and youth. These surveys had the dual purpose of: (1) identifying neighborhood assets, needs, and priorities; and (2) mobilizing adult and youth residents to gain awareness of neighborhood conditions that affect their health. Community building with residents in Sobrante Park continued by involving 60 residents in a series of interactive community trainings where they discussed survey results, identified priorities, and established action teams on the following topic areas:

1. Improving a local park, Tyrone Carney Park, and the surrounding streetscape;
2. Reducing drug use and dealing; and,
3. Increasing positive youth activities.

Component 2: Resident Action Council (RAC)
In early 2005, ACPHD organized RAC, which is the planning and decision-making body for residents to address neighborhood priorities. Currently, 20 adults and 20 youth serve on RAC and the council members receive facilitation, administrative and technical support from ACPHD. RAC is organized into subcommittees to mobilize residents around neighborhood priorities, and members report back on their progress at monthly RAC meetings.

One of the most active Sobrante Park RAC committees is focused on renovating Tyrone Carney Park and the surrounding streetscape. Their activities have included: conducting a neighborhood walk-through and several meetings with a local architect to help formulate draft designs and obtaining input from more than 150 on the final streetscape designs. A committee member wrote a successful grant for $30,000 to the City's Neighborhood Project Initiative requesting funds for the project.

Component 3: Leadership training
In 2005, ACPHD provided RAC members with 16 hours of initial leadership training to develop their practical skills in community organizing, neighborhood problem solving, and political advocacy. Since then, ACPHD has developed and begun implementing additional training modules, including: unlearning oppression and racism, action planning, public speaking, meeting facilitation, asset mapping, media advocacy, and fundraising. Trainings are offered in both English and Spanish.

Component 4: Community mini-grant program
To further support leadership development and social cohesion among residents, ACPHD developed a Mini-Grant Program to fund resident-initiated community improvement projects. The Mini-Grant Program is administered by a committee of 6 youth and adult RAC members who plan and implement the program, and make all funding decisions. In addition, they assist grantees in developing project ideas, writing proposals, and implementing activities.

Component 5: Time bank
In 2005, ACPHD collaborated with RAC and a local church to develop the Sobrante Park Time Bank (SPTB), modeled after the International Time Banking movement (http://www.timbanks.org). In the SPTB, members earn one Time Dollar for each hour of service they provide to another resident or organization, which they can spend to receive a service. The SPTB supports RAC by enhancing community relationships, and by providing incentives for residents to volunteer for RAC-sponsored activities. By 2007, the SPTB had grown to nearly 200 English- and Spanish-speaking individual and organizational members who have exchanged hundreds of service hours.

Component 6: Capacity building with youth
Using a framework of positive youth development, CCNI engages youth ages 12–24 years in programs to improve the social and physical conditions in their neighborhoods. Youth organizing in Sobrante Park began with a youth-led survey completed by 100 Sobrante Park youth. The survey identified two priorities: addressing the lack of healthy youth activities

and addressing youth violence. Several youth involved in RAC initially formed *It's on Y.O.U.* (Youth with One Understanding) to organize diverse youth, develop youth leadership, and produce an annual neighborhood event, "Keeping It Real." This day-long community fair, held in 2006 and 2007, has provided a youth-friendly venue for health education on violence prevention, nutrition, and physical activity.

It's on Y.O.U. is also part of the *Oakland Youth Movement* (OYM) that brings together youth from Sobrante Park and West Oakland to conduct participatory action research with their peers. In 2007, OYM youth administered surveys to 200 youth, which identified the following action issues: (1) high rates of violence, drug use and trafficking; (2) lack of youth activities; (3) limited youth employment opportunities; (4) litter and blight. OYM has presented the survey results to the Alameda County Board of Supervisors, the mayor of Oakland, the Oakland City Council, Oakland Police Department, ACPHD, and to neighborhood residents. As a result of OYM's presentations, momentum is building—more youth are signing on to work for a positive change.

Evidence of change in neighborhood capacity. Evidence of positive change supports the community-capacity building strategy.[38] Evaluation data show that the CCNI has met many of its short and intermediate-term goals. In interviews, residents reported that CCNI had helped them build relationships with other residents, particularly across ethnic and age groups. Residents further reported building their skills to identify and solve problems, and greater numbers are taking leadership roles at Resident Action Council meetings.

Residents have also worked with CCNI staff and local policy makers to meet their action priorities. For example, RAC successfully petitioned the City of Oakland to install new stop signs and other traffic safety improvements. Along with positive outcomes for residents, the CCNI has strengthened local partners and helped them obtain resources, such as funding, technical assistance and access to data. For example, a local church in Sobrante Park became the fiscal agent for the Time Bank program, providing new skills for those involved and strengthening the church as a resource to the community.

In Sobrante Park, notable community-level changes have been observed through the analysis of surveys. In 2007, 52% of those surveyed reported feeling that the neighborhood is a safe place to live, as compared with 44% in 2004. More people in 2007 reported being involved in neighborhood activities than in 2004. In 2007, there was less blight and more cleanliness: about one in two people surveyed reported that their neighborhood was cleaner than in 2004, and one in five reported the condition of their parks improved. In 2007, a greater percentage of residents reported that they were prepared for natural and man-made disasters.

ACPHD has examined a variety of local data to confirm residents' perceptions of change and to determine additional community outcomes. For example, ACPHD corroborated resident perceptions of increased cleanliness by examining City records, which showed that more than 200 blighted properties had been abated since September 2004. By mapping traffic injury deaths, ACPHD found a correlation between streetscape improvements made in 2006 and reduced traffic injuries and deaths at several dangerous intersections. ACPHD has also examined change over time for several measures of crime and violence; however, changes have not yet been found due to the challenges of conducting data analysis in small geographic areas. ACPHD is currently monitoring additional indicators of community health, including: truancy and suspensions from school; child abuse and neglect; enrollment in benefits programs (Medi-Cal, food stamps), overall mortality, and morbidity for asthma and diabetes. Over time, ACPHD plans to combine data over several years to yield more stable rates.

To have an impact on systemic problems such as crime, violence, and health inequities, ACPHD will need to continue to work with residents, community partners, and other government agencies to build community power to advocate for interventions that seek to impact upstream issues—such as policies that improve schools, increase the availability of jobs/job training, create and support reentry programs, and address environmental justice issues with regard to land use.

3. Public policy: Tackling society's inequities

Politics is the struggle over the allocation of resources in all aspects of social existence. Counteracting the forces that control the distribution of social goods and create the conditions in neighborhoods that lead to health inequities is a daunting task for local public health departments. This is particularly true when local public health departments are confronted with the neighborhood-level consequences of these broader societal and political forces. While many potent discriminatory forces have been struck down in law, their long-term legacy remains—for example, profound residential racial segregation exists today although some of the laws that overtly created segregation have been struck down. Evidence indicates that residential segregation is improving for some groups, but improvement is modest and gradual in pace. It is therefore difficult to observe progress in undoing social inequities in the timeframe of most typical public health interventions.

Examples abound of disease-specific public health interventions that target the broader social, economic, and political spheres such as tobacco control and automotive safety efforts (e.g., changes in laws relating to seatbelts, motorcycle helmets, and drunk driving). However, public health efforts that target the broader social determinants of health such as education, land use planning, wages, benefits and employment, transportation, and housing are rare. If one adopts the position that health inequities ultimately emanate from the fundamental power imbalances that are consciously maintained in our society, then one must conclude that efforts to build social, political and economic power within those communities that suffer most from health disparities is the only sustainable long-term solution. Local public health departments can support the righting of this power imbalance by highlighting the health implications of a variety of policy choices. Health agencies can legitimize grassroots community-led efforts through reviews of the research, data analysis, and "health impact assessments" to make tangible the impacts of certain policy choices.

For many years, ACPHD has asserted the public health interests of our low-income residents of color in various policy arenas. Most often, this is done in partnership with community-based organizations in order to leverage our credibility and legitimize their claims. However, the vast array of different venues for protecting these interests makes this approach very challenging. As a result, we have begun a systematic process for creating a policy agenda that will help us prioritize our policy activities while keeping them community centered.

Developing a Local Policy Agenda

Local public health departments should engage in systematic and ongoing policy change efforts for three reasons. First, the need for equity-based local policy is great. While the resources dedicated to such work remains extremely limited in most local public health departments, attention to the important role of public health in making healthy public policy is likely to increase and help garner the needed resources. With current low levels of available funds, the process for prioritizing policies must be especially well planned, politically strategic, and grounded in community participation. Second, the most tangible contribution of public health departments to policy change is our unique position as objective health experts. As such, it is important to maintain a consistent methodology that uses data to inform the work. Third and most importantly, we are faced with new and shifting opportunities based on changes in the political and economic environments. A mechanism for ensuring an equity and community focus will ground policy activities, keeping them community centered.

Box 20.3 Examples of Core Criteria

- Is the policy "upstream"? (See BARHII Framework)
- Does the policy play on our strengths as a public health department?
- Do we have preexisting strategic relationships with stakeholders involved with the issue or policy?
- Is there evidence that the policy will help meet our goals and further our adopted platform?
- Is there a related indicator available in order to measure the impact of the policy?
- Can we set an ambitious, coherent target for purposes of evaluating action?
- Do we have staff capacity to pursue the policy?
- Is the policy politically feasible and cost effective?
- Is the policy "community driven"?

For a more in-depth look at the criteria and how they are applied, visit http://www.acphd.org/healthequity/placematters.

Our department developed a set of questions—referred to as *Core Criteria*—to help us and our stakeholders build a local policy agenda to address social inequities in Alameda County (see Box 20.3). The questions help us assess internal capacity, as well as the relevance, viability and efficacy of proposed policies. While we have no way to guarantee a "community-driven" process and outcome, the process planned and followed to date involves community residents and community-based organizations in all phases of work. Without significant public input, we would run the risk of exacerbating conditions that are the legacy of historical exclusion of poor people and people of color from decision-making venues.

Our two-stage process for building a local policy agenda includes (1) needs assessment and (2) stakeholder engagement. The following section describes these stages of work and identifies the many ways we endeavor to keep the work community centered.

Needs assessment

We defined the goal of our local policy agenda as follows: ACPHD promotes health equity through a community-centered local policy agenda focused on criminal justice, economic development, education, housing, land use, and transportation. These six areas were identified as serious social issues in Alameda County with links to health inequities. We further limited the scope of our policy work by focusing on the County's geographic area with the most severe health inequities—the City of Oakland.

The actual needs assessment had three components: literature review, key informant interviews, and compilation of baseline indicators. Literature reviews explored connections between specific social conditions and health, as well as evidence-based policy interventions. Key informant interviews, held with representatives from local advocacy, community-based, membership-based, and government organizations, grounded the research in the local context, as well as the current policy environment. Baseline indicators of local health outcomes and social factors provided quantitative evidence of current local conditions. We will continue to use these indicators to monitor changes in social conditions over time. Each component of the needs assessment informed the others through an iterative process. For instance, both key informant interviews and literature reviews helped us identify baseline data that best illustrate current social conditions and inequities. We also used the data generated through key informant interviews and from the baseline indicators to hone our literature review.

The key informant interviews were critical to the process, serving two vital functions: first they grounded our reading of the literature and data collection in local community needs and current political environment and second, the interviews helped to establish relationships with various community stakeholders already involved in pursuing more equitable social and economic conditions. Building strong, trusting relationships with community stakeholders is essential because they are often the gatekeepers for successful involvement in policy change. Many of our current policy activities (some are described in the section "Examples of On-going Policy Activities") directly result from the relationships established through these interviews.

The information revealed in the needs assessment was helpful for establishing *policy-specific criteria* for each of the six policy areas. These criteria informed our analysis of whether proposed or existing policies are likely to promote health equity. For instance, the baseline indicator, "One Year (High School) Attrition Rates by Race/Ethnicity" revealed large differences between races, yet the literature reviews and key informant interviews revealed that certain policies intended to increase academic achievement have had an unintended negative consequence of encouraging attrition. We translated these "findings" into the criterion, "Does this policy decrease the likelihood of attrition among Oakland's *most vulnerable students*?" In so using the policy-specific criteria, we will not necessarily ignore or eliminate policies that do not meet every criterion, but instead, use the criteria to better weigh policy options against what could become an unmanageably large policy agenda. Specific policies that meet these criteria are incorporated into the policy agenda only if they are also aligned with the priorities of our stakeholders—priorities revealed in the second stage of our process: stakeholder engagement.

Stakeholder engagement

All policies we eventually pursue will be aligned with the priorities expressed by the three groups participating in this process: (1) community and government organizations; (2) residents; and (3) public health department staff. We will reach out to community and government stakeholders for in-depth discussions on the political and economic feasibility of specific policies given the current policy environment. We will ask them to consider potential strategies for affecting policy change, focusing on how the public health department can support current policy activities, spearhead new activities, and build multisector partnerships. The needs assessment and policy-specific criteria will frame and inform these discussions.

We will engage resident groups, such as neighborhood associations, as well as membership-based, issue-specific organizations. With the intent of ensuring the policy agenda's relevance to local resident needs, discussions will be organized around the broad issue areas (criminal justice, economic development, education, housing, land use, and transportation). Residents will be asked to prioritize the issues that "resonate" with their view of local society and conditions in their neighborhoods, as well as give feedback on strategies and policies that will most effectively address these issues.

Key staff from across the ACPHD will be asked to assume responsibility for finalizing and implementing the policy agenda. Using information collected from the other stakeholder groups in conjunction with the needs assessments, policy-specific criteria and overall criteria, issue-specific staff workgroups will vet all potential policies and determine which to incorporate in the "final" local policy agenda. A broad representation of ACPHD staff comprise these workgroups, and as a result, will keep this local policy agenda grounded in and integrated with the ongoing work of the entire health department, rather than creating a silo for policy work.

The relationship building function of this engagement process is central to effective change. Strong, trusting relationships with each of the stakeholder groups are essential for effectively implementing the local policy agenda. By inviting these groups to participate, we anticipate commitment to the partnership and support for the policies that make up the local agenda. This is especially important given that policy advocacy around the broader determinants of health is not yet widely seen as a core function of local public health departments. Ongoing partnerships are needed to sustain momentum.

Implementing the Local Policy Agenda

With the local policy agenda complete, ACPHD issue-specific workgroups will move forward with implementation. They will prioritize action steps and choose strategies such as Health Impact Assessments and giving testimonies to move the agenda forward. Much of their work will be coordinated with community stakeholder activities, whether they be residents, community organizations, advocacy groups, or other government agencies. An emphasis across all workgroups will be community capacity building, especially among residents impacted by health inequities. ACPHD and the partners we work with hold this as a priority not only because community capacity building promotes positive health outcomes and helps shift power imbalances, but also because voting constituents can put direct pressure on decision makers and build political will in ways that government agencies cannot.

The workgroups will have two additional functions. First, each issue-specific workgroup is responsible for tracking federal and state policies that will impact—either positively or negatively—our local policy efforts, and making recommendations to our ACPHD Legislative Council, which evaluates federal and state level policies relevant to public health. Connecting the local policy agenda work to state and federal efforts is essential for long-term success. In addition, workgroups will field requests from stakeholders for advocacy around policies not included in the local policy agenda. Responding to such requests is important for being accountable to our stakeholders, for building and maintaining strong relationships, and for maintaining flexibility around unexpected policy issues as they arise.

As we create the local policy agenda, we are simultaneously building political will for its implementation. In addition to knowing there is political will among constituents, public officials need information in order to make tough policy decisions. They need dependable and accurate local data. As such, we created the report, *Life and Death from Unnatural Causes: Health and Social Inequity in Alameda County.*[26] This report highlights the health inequities in Alameda County, reviews the historical forces that have contributed to these inequities, summarizes the evidence that ties them to social inequities, and identifies their policy implications (see Box 20.4). The report is targeted to decision makers and agency heads around the county and is intended to raise awareness and legitimize and mobilize policy work. Through briefings related to the report, decision makers are coming to understand the connections between policies in areas they have not traditionally seen as health related and the profound health inequities that are morally unconscionable and contradictory to the progressive values they espouse.

Box 20.4 Life and Death from Unnatural Causes: Health and Social Inequity in Alameda County

As indicated, ACPHD published a comprehensive report, *Life and Death From Unnatural Causes: Health and Social Inequity in Alameda County*, for use by local public officials and policy advocates. This report states:

It is the role of the Alameda County Public Health Department (ACPHD) to inform the public and public officials of what research and local data reveal about health inequities in Alameda County. While acknowledging that the political will for implementing some of the suggested policies is limited, it is important that the ACPHD offer our professional judgment about how to bring equal resources and opportunities to all communities. We are committed to working with stakeholders and decision makers across sectors to identify, prioritize, and advocate for policy solutions based on analysis of potential health and social equity impacts...The importance of, and our commitment to, working collaboratively across sectors and with various stakeholders—neighborhood residents, community-based organizations, advocacy groups, local planners, and government agencies—to influence policy change is underscored.

The report describes the nature and magnitude of health inequities in the county as they specifically relate to place, income, and race and goes further to examine inequities in key economic, social, physical, and service environments that contribute to the health inequities. These include: segregation, income and employment, education, housing, transportation, air quality, food access and liquor stores, physical activity and neighborhood conditions, criminal justice, access to health care, and social relationships and community capacity. In each of these 11 areas policy goals and strategies are offered for possible adoption and action. (http://www.acphd.org/healthequity/)

Additional Examples of Ongoing Policy Activities

1. *Supporting elderly Chinese American residents seeking rent stabilization.* A wealthy real estate developer and generous political contributor had interpreted a 10-year-old affordable housing agreement between his real estate company and the City of Oakland in a manner that permitted him to evict elderly long-term renters in order to convert his building to market rate condominiums. In response to a request from neighborhood activists, ACPHD weighed in on the part of the elderly renters noting the well documented public health literature that illustrates the deleterious impact

of disruptions to neighborhood social networks on the health outcomes of elderly communities of color. The evidence-based testimony served to bolster and legitimize the position of neighborhood advocates whose cause benefited from the credibility of the public health department in what otherwise might have been perceived simply as a parochial political struggle.

2. *Environmental justice partnership to hold port accountable.* ACPHD's partners with residents, community groups, and other government agencies to hold the Port of Oakland accountable for its impact on West Oakland residents. West Oakland residents—predominantly African American—have the lowest life expectancy in the county, 7.8 years lower than the county average. Residents have long attributed the high rates of asthma and other respiratory diseases to the practices of their largest and most powerful neighbor: the Port of Oakland. Science is catching up with residents' interpretations of their own experiences and has revealed that port operations, particularly diesel trucks, are contributing to a major local health inequity. In response to the outrage around this issue, the Port of Oakland engaged a diverse set of stakeholders, including ACPHD, representatives of elected officials, business, the Air District, residents, and community-based organizations, in a planning process for reducing the health risks associated with its operations. While working with the Port of Oakland in this public engagement process, we are continuing to strategize with our community partners on how to ensure that the port is responsive to community needs. Such activities include collaborating on briefs demonstrating how taxpayers subsidize unhealthy port policies, testifying as health experts at public meetings, and analyzing port policies with a health equity lens.

3. *Working with transportation advocates to close gaps in transit service.* Public health involvement in transportation decisions has grown in recent years as increasing biking and walking is seen as a necessary antidote to bad eating habits, sedentary lifestyles, and the attendant obesity and diabetes epidemics. Unfortunately, public health experts generally have not highlighted the link between health inequities and transportation inequities. For example, there is a large disparity in funding for transit services (usually bus service) used by low-income people compared to funding for transit services used wealthier commuters (usually rail). Through well-researched policy briefs and testimonies, outreach to decision makers, and partnerships with transit advocates, we are increasing awareness about the links between transportation and health inequities and have already seen increased equity in the distribution of regional transportation resources.

4. *Including community groups and residents in data collection, analysis, interpretation, and dissemination of results.* With such skills, community members themselves can better advocate and represent their interests in the policy arena. ACPHD supported a youth community group which

had advocated for a free and reduced-price student bus pass that was threatened with elimination by the transportation commission. The youth were interested in surveying their peers to document how the increase in the student bus pass prices would affect the lives of area youth and to examine the local experience of young bus riders. They requested and received assistance from ACPHD in developing a survey instrument and database, inputting results, and conducting simple statistical analysis. The youth group administered surveys to over 1000 middle and high school transit riders and their survey findings were used to mobilize the broader community to successfully advocate for the continuation of the discounted student bus pass.

5. *Assessing the health impact of housing displacement.* A membership-based, housing rights organization asked ACPHD to partner on a project to understand the health impacts of displacement due to rising housing costs and dilapidated public housing. Working together with their members who reside in the poorest areas of the county, we are looking for the pathways between displacement and poor health outcomes in those neighborhoods. In addition, using qualitative data of member experiences, we will attempt to contextualize and illustrate what is known from current literature on this topic. We will report the findings and make preliminary policy recommendations. The organization will use the results to develop a campaign for healthy housing and affordable housing policies.

Conclusion

In virtually every public health area, be it immunization, chronic disease, injury prevention, HIV/AIDS, sexually transmitted infections, obesity, or disaster preparedness, local public health departments and the people they serve must confront the consequences of structural poverty, institutional racism and other forms of systemic injustice. Disproportionate public health resources are expended in neighborhoods where unhealthy social and physical environments reflect the cumulative impact of profound and unjust social, political, and economic forces. By designing approaches that specifically identify existing assets and build social, political, and economic power among residents of afflicted neighborhoods, local public health departments can begin to sustainably reduce and move toward eliminating health inequities in low-income communities of color. In addition, local public health departments must simultaneously seek opportunities to strategically partner with advocates for affordable housing, labor rights, education equity, environmental justice, transportation equity, criminal justice reform, and other disciplines to change norms and apply pressure regarding the distribution of those critical social goods that have a powerful influence on health outcomes. Without such a commitment, local health departments will not be able to reduce and eliminate the health inequities that plague communities across the nation. The human cost of this lack of commitment to social justice is too great to justify. The opportunities for pursuing social justice that present themselves are too great to ignore: local public health departments have the ability and the opportunity to work with residents, advocates, other organizations, and governmental agencies to eliminate health inequities and ensure that all of those that we serve have the opportunity to live a healthy life.

Acknowledgments

Acknowledgments to Alameda County Public Health Department and City of Oakland staff, Sobrante Park and West Oakland Resident Action Council members, and our community partners for their program design contributions in community capacity building, internal capacity building, and policy development. These individuals include: Claudia Albano, Sara Bedford, Evette Brandon, LaToya Carroll, Amy DeReyes, Joe DeVries, Arly Flores-Medina, Deborah Fowler-Jones, Sandi Galvez, Jaron Isom, Tammy Lee, German Martinez, Korin Merle, Iris Merriouns, Councilmember Nancy Nadel, Gabriel Orozco, Arnold Perkins, Councilmember and Vice Mayor of Oakland Larry Reid, Anita Siegel, Valerie Street, Sheryl Walton, Kimi Watkins Tart, Africa Williams, and Pam Willow.

References

1. S.A. Huie, P.M. Krueger, R.G. Rogers, and R.A. Hummer, "Wealth, Race, and Mortality," 84(3) *Social Science Quarterly* (2003): 667–684.
2. A.T. Wenzlow, J. Mullahy, S.A. Robert, and B.L. Wolfe, *An Empirical Investigation of the Relationship Between Wealth and Health Using the Survey of Consumer Finances*. Draft-Russell Sage Foundation, 2003.
3. N.E. Adler, J. Stewart, S. Cohen, et al., *Reaching for a Healthier Life: Facts on Socioeconomic Status and Health in the U.S.* The John D. and Catherine T. MacArthur Foundation Research Network on Socioeconomic Status and Health, 2007: 43.
4. N. Krieger, D.H. Rehkopf, J.T. Chen, P.D. Waterman, E. Marcelli, and M. Kennedy, "The Fall and Rise of U.S. Inequities in Premature Mortality: 1960–2002," 5(2) *PLOS Medicine* (2008): e46.
5. N. Krieger, J.T. Chen, B.A. Coull, and J.V. Selby, "Lifetime Socioeconomic Position and Twins' Health: An Analysis of 308 Pairs of United States Women Twins," 2(7) *PLoS Medicine* (2005): e162.

6. J.W. Lynch, G.A. Kaplan, S.J. Shema, "Cumulative Impact of Sustained Economic Hardship on Physical, Cognitive, Psychological, and Social Functioning," 337(26) *New England Journal of Medicine* (1997): 1889–1895.

7. R.G. Wilkinson, "Income Distribution and Life Expectancy," 304(6820) *British Medical Journal* (1992): 165–168.

8. N.A. Ross, M.C. Wolfson, J.R. Dunn, J.M. Berthelot, G. Kaplan, and J. Lynch, "Relation Between Income Inequality and Mortality in Canada and in the United States: Cross Sectional Assessment Using Census Data and Vital Statistics," 320(7239) *British Medical Journal* (2000): 898–902.

9. R. Kochhar, "The Wealth of Hispanic Households: 1996 to 2002," Pew Hispanic Center Report, October 2004. Available at: www.pewhispanic.org.

10. National Institutes of Health (US), *NIH Strategic Research Plan to Reduce and Ultimately Eliminate Health Disparities* (2000 Oct. 6z). Available from http://www.nih.gov/about/hd/strategicplan.pdf.

11. M. Whitehead, *The Concepts and Principles of Equity and Health*, WHO, EURO Report. 1991.

12. P. Braveman and S. Gruskin, "Defining Equity in Health," 57 *Journal of Epidemiology and Community Health* (2003): 254–258.

13. I. Kawachi, S.V. Subramanian, and N. Almeido-Filho, "A Glossary for Health Inequalities," 56 *Journal of Epidemiology and Community Health* (2002): 647–652.

14. P.A. Jargowsky, *Stunning Progress, Hidden Problems: The Dramatic Decline of Concentrated Poverty in the 1990s* (Washington, DC: The Brookings Institution, May 2003).

15. A.T. Geronimus, "Understanding and Eliminating Racial Inequalities in Women's Health in the U.S.: The Role of the Weathering Conceptual Framework," 56 *Journal of the Medical Women's Association* (2001): 133–136.

16. *The Funding Gap 2004: Many States Still Shortchange Low-Income and Minority Students*. The Education Trust. Available at: http://www2.edtrust.org/EdTrust/Product+Catalog/searchpubs2.htm#ff

17. *Losing Our Future: How Minority Youth Are Being Left Behind by the Graduation Rate Crisis*. The Civil Rights Project at Harvard University, Urban Institute, Advocates for Children of New York, the Civil Society Institute. Available at: www.urban.org/Uploaded PDF/410936_LosingOurFuture.pdf

18. K.S. Makrides and J. Corell, "The Health of Hispanics in the Southwestern United States: An Epidemiological Paradox," 101(3) *Public Health Reports* (1986): 253–265.

19. W.A. Vega, H. Amaro, "Latino Outlook: Good Health, Uncertain Progress," 15 *Annual Review of Public Health* (2001): 39–67.

20. M.E. Weigers and M.S. Sherraden, "A Critical Examination of Acculturation: The Impact of Health Behaviors, Social Support and Economic Resources on Birth Weight Among Women of Mexican Descent," 35(3) *International Migration Review* (2001): 804–839.

21. CDC, Office of Minority Health, *Eliminating Racial & Ethnic Health Disparities*. http://www.cdc.gov/omh/AboutUs/disparities.htm

22. *National Heart, Lung, and Blood Institute Strategy for Addressing Health Disparities FY 2002–2006*. http://www.nhlbi.nih.gov/resources/docs/plandisp.htm#m

23. HRSA, Office of Minority Health, *Eliminating Health Disparities in the United States*. http://www.hrsa.gov/OMH/OMH/disparities/default.htm

24. C. Muntaner, J. Lynch, and G. Davey Smith, "Social Capital, Disorganized Communities, and the Third Way: Understanding the Retreat from Structural Inequalities in Epidemiology and Public Health," 31(2) *International Journal of Health Services* (2001) 213–237.

25. C.P. Jones, "Levels of Racism: A Theoretic Framework and a Gardener's Tale," 90 *American Journal of Public Health* (2000): 1212–1215.

26. M. Beyers, J. Brown, S. Cho, et al., *Life and Death from Unnatural Causes: Health and Social Inequity in Alameda County (Executive Summary)*. Community Assessment, Planning, Education, and Evaluation (CAPE) Unit, Alameda County Public Health Department. Oakland, CA, 2008. http://www.acphd.org/AXBYCZ/Admin/DataReports/unnatural_causes_exec_summ.pdf

27. R.M. Goodman, M.A. Speers, K. McLeroy, et al., "Identifying and Defining the Dimensions of Community Capacity to Provide a Basis for Measurement," 25 *Health Education and Behavior* (1998): 258–278.

28. E.C. Kieffer and J. Reischman, *Final Report: Contributions of Community Building to Achieving Improved Public Health Outcomes*. Report to the Aspen Institute Roundtable of Community Change (Ann Arbor: MI, August, 2004).

29. J.D. Bell, J. Bell, R. Colmenar, et al., *Reducing Health Disparities Through a Focus on Communities* (Oakland, CA: PolicyLink, 2002).

30. M. Minkler and N. Wallerstein, "Improving Health through Community Organization and Community Building: A Health Education Perspective," in *Community Organizing and Community Building for Health*, ed. M. Minkler (New Brunswick, NJ: Rutgers University Press, 2005).

31. P. Hawe, M. Noort, L. King, B. Lloyd, and C. Jordens, "Multiplying Health Gains: The Critical Role of Capacity-Building in Health Promotion," 39 *Health Policy* (1997): 29–42.

32. M. Minkler, "Community Organizing among the Elderly Poor in the United States: A Case Study," 22 *International Journal of Health Services* (1992): 303–316.

33. A.J. Scultz, B.A. Israel, A.B. Becker, and R.M. Hollis, "It's a 24-Hour Thing...A Living-For-Each-Other Concept: Identity, Networks, and Community in an Urban Village Health Worker Project," 24(4) *Health Education and Behavior* (1997): 465–480.

34. J.B. Mondros and S.M. Wilson, *Organizing for Power and Empowerment* (New York: Columbia University Press, 1994).

35. P. Hawe, "Making Sense of Context-Level Influences on Health" 13(4) *Health Education Research* (1998): i–iv.

36. I. Serrano-Garcia, "The Ethics of the Powerful and the Power of Ethics," 22 *American Journal of Community Psychology* (1994): 1–20.

37. N. Wallerstein, "Powerlessness, Empowerment and Health: Implications for Health Promotion Programs," 6 *American Journal of Health Promotion* (1992): 197–205.

38. L. Maker, T. Lee, M. Luluquisen, and K. Gilhuly, *Community Capacity-Building in Sobrante Park and West Oakland: An Evaluation Update 2004–2006* (Oakland, CA: Alameda County Public Health Department, CAPE Unit. August 14, 2008), http://www.acphd.org/healthequity/ccni/docs/evaluation/eval_report_2004_2006.pdf

21

Institutionalizing Health Equity and Social Justice in King County, Washington

NGOZI OLERU, MICHAEL GEDEON, AND MATÍAS VALENZUELA

In February 2008, Martin Luther King Jr. County in Washington State launched a bold and comprehensive new initiative with the goal of promoting fairness and opportunity for all. It was bold because it challenged county government to begin examining its operations and the impacts of programs and decisions in the lives of residents. It was comprehensive because it incorporated major sectors of government—including health and human services, transportation, the natural and built environment, and the criminal justice system—as well as community voices.

ML King County committed to making equity and social justice central to its work by engaging in three levels of action:

- Policy development and decision making: King County government would ensure that promoting equity is intentionally considered in the development and implementation of key policies and programs and in making funding decisions.
- Delivery of county services: By working with partners and the community, the county and its departments would identify and mitigate inequities; all executive departments began in 2008 to intentionally promote equity in new and existing activities.

- Community partnerships: ML King County would be a catalyst for mobilizing, educating, and meaningfully engaging communities. The main aim is to incorporate and empower community voice in county decision making.

Inequities: The Persistent Problem

In 1964, Dr. Martin Luther King Jr. proclaimed, "I have the audacity to believe that peoples everywhere can have three meals a day for their bodies, education and culture for their minds, and dignity, equality and freedom for their spirits." While more than four decades have passed, this nation is still burdened by vast disparities in wealth, health, and opportunities.

Dr. Martin Luther King Jr. County is not exempt from this grim picture. Consider the following facts:

- A child in south King County is more than twice as likely to drop out of high school as one in east King County.
- A worker making between $15,000 and $25,000 a year is almost 12 times less likely to have health insurance than one making $50,000 or more per year.
- A youth of color is six times more likely than a white youth to spend time in a state or county correctional facility.
- A southeast Seattle, Auburn or Federal Way resident is five times more likely to die from diabetes than a resident of Mercer Island.
- A Native American baby is four times more likely to die before his or her first birthday than a white baby.

Inequities that exist at all levels of society have persistent, profound, and long-lasting effects. And people with lower incomes, people of color, and those in disenfranchised communities are losing ground. They are more likely to begin their lives with inadequate infant care, to be not ready to learn when they get to school, to play in unsafe neighborhoods, to receive a low-quality education, to be less likely to find a good job that pays a livable wage, to be less healthy, to be prone to disease, and to die earlier.

The gulf between the rich and the poor is widening, a fact that can be seen in the great disparities in our neighborhoods around the county. While many of our communities thrive, some neighborhoods increasingly must confront the conditions that lead to poor health, underemployment, poor education, incarceration, loss of opportunity, and an unsafe living environment.

The stressors of racism and discrimination also contribute to poor health. A highly educated, professional African American woman is more than twice as likely to have a child with very low birth weight, compared to a white woman with a high school diploma or less.

Searching for and Creating Solutions

Improving a community's well-being requires the recognition that a person's condition is not just the product of individual characteristics—genetics, behavior, and lifestyle choices—but more importantly of underlying, root causes. These root causes, generally referred to as the social determinants of health, are powerful independent predictors of health outcomes. Key social determinants include, but are not limited to: income and other forms of wealth; affordable, quality housing; quality education; employment; safe neighborhoods and community recreation sites; social support; and transportation. Social determinants, collectively, form the fabric that clothes the health and well-being of the individual and families in the community.

Rates of illness and death increase as socioeconomic status decreases. Research shows that individual health is substantially influenced by the social and environmental context. Health and life expectancy increase with every step up the social hierarchy; meaning that wealthier people live longer, healthier lives.

Racism has played a substantial historical role in the distribution of these social determinants in the United States. A consequence of this legacy of racial discrimination is that people of color are disproportionately represented among the poor. As a result, people of color are more likely to have lower incomes, a lower quality education and fewer job opportunities than whites. The long-standing pattern of racial discrimination in the distribution of key social determinants has itself become an important determinant of health. Historical policies and practices that separate communities on the basis of income and race have resulted in the poor and people of color becoming concentrated in racially segregated neighborhoods. While neighborhood poverty, housing, and school segregation in King County may not reach the extreme levels experienced in some other U.S. metropolitan areas, the patterns in how they help create and sustain inequities are similar.

In King County, in addition to limiting socioeconomic opportunities, living in poor neighborhoods can have a direct negative impact on people's well-being. Poor neighborhoods are often close to freeways and other sources of environmental pollutants. Streets may be unsafe and housing run-down. The unhealthy neighborhood environment can become the social context that promotes unhealthy behaviors ranging from crime to poor nutrition. Poor neighborhoods have a low property tax base and less political power to implement the upkeep or restoration of parks and other recreational areas. The complex multitiered influences of social structures, power, income, education, and a myriad of other determinants combine in a powerful, systematic way to affect the quality of people's lives.

Correcting a History of Inequities

How can persistent inequities be overcome? Evidence is mounting that focusing on the determinants of health and well-being can improve the health and well-being of disadvantaged communities. Not surprisingly, these conditions are already present in thriving communities. Inequity, by its very definition, means that the benefits of progress are reaching some sectors of society, but not others. Hence, there are solutions that are working for some populations, but not others. Addressing inequities must therefore include expanding for all people what are known to be the contributors to well-being and a better quality of life that currently are enjoyed by only some.

Though it may be more challenging to craft how to foster these conditions in struggling neighborhoods and communities, every community has its strengths and assets, which should be the foundation of improvements. There are examples, locally, nationally, and internationally, where successes have been achieved, especially when comprehensive approaches are taken that combine policies with appropriate programs and services.

For example, over the past several decades, women across the globe have made extraordinary advances in achieving a more equitable standing in society and creating more fair systems. Globally not all societies have achieved the same level of progress, but in many societies women have made significant advances by gaining a voice, political representation, real economic power and more. In countries where women have achieved a more equal standing, the consequences have been astounding, ranging from higher literacy rates to reduced infant mortality, reduced population growth, and more rapid economic development.

For its part, asthma and housing quality is one of the best studied examples of how physical and social characteristics of the built environment are associated with health status. Public health efforts locally and nationally have focused on improving indoor environmental quality, and now they have moved into a broader effort to improve the built and social environment to promote health. This strategy includes addressing exposure to indoor asthma triggers and the underlying structural conditions which increase trigger exposure. Partnerships with public housing agencies and community-based organizations can incorporate healthy homes guidelines and principles of healthy community design into the physical redevelopment of public housing. In addition, resident-led community building activities promote social cohesion and interaction.

In King County, recent rates for childhood hospitalizations due to asthma have declined as local asthma control efforts, such as those described above, have intensified. Along these lines, the Seattle-King County Healthy Homes study, which included low-income children with poorly controlled asthma and targeted English, Spanish, and Vietnamese-speaking families, showed that a home visiting program was able to reduce asthma symptoms and produce improvements in the quality of life of the child's caregiver.

It is possible both to create new programs and to redesign existing programs to make a difference in addressing inequities. As part of King County's effort to correct a history of inequities, the goal is to expand the programs and activities that have achieved the desired effect, modify existing programs to incorporate pro-equity elements, and create new programs and policies that will explicitly address local inequities.

Community Empowerment

Equity and social justice are fundamentally about communities having an equal voice in shaping their future. A new park will have a much greater benefit to the surrounding community if its residents help design it. An underserved community is much more likely to have the bus service it needs if its members can influence the service delivery.

Yet, the historical disadvantages some communities face can be substantial barriers to having this voice. If residents move frequently in order to find affordable housing, cannot take time off work, do not know whom to call or where to go to voice their concerns, or simply lack faith that they will be heard, they will continue to be left out. A key ingredient to promoting equity and social justice is to engage communities and support them in developing their voice and shaping their future.

Clear and Constant Focus

Information about the economy and the population's income, health or education is usually reported as an average for the country or a particular region, which disguises the severe poverty, crime, preventable illnesses, and homelessness that persist in some communities. As a result, inequities are out of focus, or even worse, out of mind for many institutions, businesses, and privileged communities.

A key ingredient in formulating solutions is the need for intentional and systematic focus on inequities, including devoting resources to their measurement. As noted earlier, the facts alone are disturbing and compelling. However, to promote progress and prevent equity and social justice from returning to the back burner when the next crisis erupts, these issues and trends should be tracked and reported regularly.

Making progress requires King County and other local organizations to become more intentional and systematic about examining equity when developing policies, making funding decisions, and delivering services. Whether it is a zoning policy, a park improvement project, or a drug treatment program, the persons or groups making decisions should start by answering two questions: How does this policy, funding decision, or service affect underserved communities? How can it be used as an opportunity to work upstream and positively impact community conditions that support everyone?

National Momentum

Both nationally and in the Pacific Northwest, organizations are coming together to develop and share strategies for creating and promoting equity. These innovative strategies are important in order to maintain the focus on equity and to learn from each other.

At the national level, two initiatives, *Place Matters* and the Dellums Commission, are identifying root causes and proposing upstream approaches to creating and promoting equity. Both are initiatives of the Health Policy Institute of the Joint Center for Political and Economic Studies, whose mission is to ignite a "Fair Health" movement that gives people of color the inalienable right to equal opportunity for healthy lives. (For more information, see www.jointcenter.org).

A King County team examined the situation in this region for young men of color within the six domains in the national Dellums Commission Report (health, education, family support and child welfare, workforce and economic development, juvenile and criminal justice, and media), and highlighted possible next steps. Another King County team is one of over 20 teams participating in the national learning community called *Place Matters*. The King County *Place Matters* team is focusing its efforts on addressing the social conditions that lead to poor health. The work of both teams contributed to shaping and launching King County's Equity and Social Justice Initiative.

Five other important partners of King County's initiative include the Multnomah County (Oregon) Health Equity Initiative, the Alameda County (California) *Place Matters* Initiative, the Washington State Governor's Interagency Coordinating Council on Health Disparities, and the City of Seattle's Race and Social Justice Initiative.

Examples across the country show paths to achieving equity through social justice by creating or refocusing policies and practices rooted in the social determinants. Undoing decades of misguided policies, overt neglect, and the unintended consequences of past policies will take many years of persistent and steady effort.

Now Is the Time to Act

Government is better prepared than ever before to address inequities and injustices. Correcting inequities and promoting equal opportunity for all residents are the essence of what government should do. The goal must be to transform the privileges that some enjoy into basic rights for everyone.

Embracing the principles of equity and social justice can lead to a future where all residents of King County have real opportunities for quality education, livable wages, affordable housing, health care, and safe and vibrant neighborhoods. In this vision of the future, in stark contrast to the distressing indicators cited earlier, a much healthier and more prosperous picture of King County would emerge.

- If all King County residents had access to jobs paying a living wage, then 390,000 fewer individuals would be living in or near poverty and instead could better enjoy the high quality of life that this region has the potential to offer.
- If every school in King County were as excellent as the schools in the most privileged communities, then nearly 1,000 more youth of color would graduate from high school each year and would be prepared to take on the challenges of economic diversification and global change.
- If all people in King County lived in healthy environments, had the knowledge to make healthy lifestyle choices, and could access high quality and affordable health care, then preventable illnesses and chronic diseases would become rare occurrences in this region while long, healthier, and fuller lives would be the norm for all residents.

Promoting equity and social justice will benefit everybody. All residents of King County would benefit from a better-educated workforce, more businesses that provide livable wage jobs, safer communities, fewer residents without health insurance, and a shrinking demand for criminal justice and crisis services.

Guiding Principles for King County, Its Communities and Partners to Assure Equity

King County government is well positioned to be a catalyst for change in partnership with local communities and organizations. It has regional responsibilities for transportation, criminal justice, health, natural resources, parks, human services, and other critical services. It also is a municipal provider of services to hundreds of thousands of residents in unincorporated areas. Moving forward with an initiative focused on promoting equity and social justice presents many practical challenges and barriers. The following set of principles can help guide groups around these barriers.

- **Address the root causes of inequities.** The presence of inequities is a signal of inadequate economic, environmental, and other conditions that have existed for years. King County should use its collective expertise to identify these conditions and the opportunities to improve them.
- **Actively seek out and promote decisions and policies aimed at equity.** Many, if not most, decisions made in the public sector directly or indirectly impact conditions that influence the health and well-being of communities. While these decisions should not worsen the disparities in disadvantaged communities, the bar must be set higher. The decisions of King County government and its partners should promote equity through improving conditions that lead to a thriving community.
- **Empower communities.** The residents of the community are the best source of information on what is happening in their neighborhoods and what will or will not work. Their involvement combined with the expertise and technical know-how of King County and other institutional partners is a powerful model for positive and equitable change that will lead to more effective policies, decisions, and services.
- **Work across agencies and departments.** Too often, agencies work in "silos" when the best solution can come from an unexpected source and by working across disciplines. For example, a park can encourage physical activity for adults and provide after-school alternatives for youth. If agencies join together to creatively support the needs of a community, then they become co-producers of a community's health and well-being.
- **Recognize and honor cultural differences.** There is a need to understand, value, and work with the diversity and differences that exist in

the community. Tennis courts may be used constantly in one community and largely vacant in another community whose preferred activity is soccer. Home-based family services may be an effective program unless the social worker through a misunderstanding of cultural norms offends the clients and is unable to establish trust and confidence. If the programs and services are not designed and delivered in a culturally appropriate manner, they stand little chance of being effective.

· **Aim for long-term, permanent change.** While a new initiative can generate a burst of activity, real change will require long-term, sustainable strategies. Leveraging resources, regularly measuring progress, maintaining visibility, and embedding equity and social justice within an organizational culture are key components of a sustainable initiative. Policies and programs must be concrete and sustainable over time.

These directions represent a starting point for a way of thinking and doing that promotes fairness, equal opportunity, and community vitality for all residents of King County. It is a start on the long, but ultimately most rewarding, journey toward equity and social justice.

Steps and Actions

Starting in 2008, King County government began concrete steps to build momentum toward Dr. King's vision, focusing on three areas of action: policy development and decision making; delivery of county services, and engagement in community partnerships. These initial steps alone do not represent the full breadth of potential opportunities. They serve as catalysts for action and create the milieu for the kind of discussions and innovations that will lead to clear and ambitious pathways of equitable opportunities for all King County residents.[1]

Policy Development and Decision Making

King County has committed to ensuring that promoting equity is intentionally considered in the development and implementation of key policies and programs and in funding decisions.

2008 Highlight

By assessing equity impact, King County can determine whether policies and programs advance a shared agenda of fairness, spread burdens fairly, and help address historic patterns of institutional bias and discrimination. To this end, King County developed an Equity Impact Review Tool.

A training curriculum was created for the Equity Impact Review Tool, and county staff is being trained to use it. Several departments have used the tool. All departments described equity impacts of program reductions in their business plans.

Delivery of County Services

In 2008 all executive departments reviewed their work and committed to specific actions that promote equity and social justice. The following are the examples of those activities.

2008 Highlights

Adult and Juvenile Detention—Adult and Juvenile Detention along with the Department of Community and Human Services revised information and assistance provided to incarcerated women about available services. This revision to the program was in response to an observation that women of color were much less aware of the services that were offered, and were less likely to have attempted to access the services even when they knew about them.

Community and Human Services—With its partners Community and Human Services has been reviewing its prevention and early intervention services for the population birth to age three, crafting and implementing strategies to mitigate inequities in these early childhood services. Among its activities, the department developed culturally and linguistically appropriate outreach materials for Somali, Spanish, and Vietnamese families in response to data on utilization of birth to three prevention services for children with developmental disabilities.

Development and Environmental Services—Development and Environmental Services has begun the process of rewriting the zoning code. The goal is to allow for greater flexibility for developers and encourages more vibrant, mixed use neighborhoods in return for providing public benefit such as mixed income housing, walkability and sustainability. Public meetings were held in the two demonstration project neighborhoods in early 2009.

Executive Office—The Executive Office coordinated the launch of Opportunity Greenway in Summer 2008, offering court-involved young adult students the chance to learn about and train for high wage and high demand "green jobs." Approximately, 50 high school students were introduced to green jobs in three 6-week educational internships programs operated through YouthSource.

Executive Services—To determine if the new Healthy Incentives employee benefits program was having inequitable impacts on county employees, staff collected information on employee positions with lower participation rates in the health initiative's wellness assessment. The results showed lower participation rates among jobs lacking regular access to computers such as roads crews, carpenters, and maintenance workers. As a result, the benefits staff developed and implemented an outreach plan to those employees with lower participation with the goal of decreasing their health expenses and encouraging participation in interventions to improve health. Data show that the plan was successful in increasing participation in most cases.

Management and Budget—To promote engagement and leadership from under-represented groups in neighborhood revitalization activities, the Office of Management and Budget supported the design and facilitation of an inclusive public process to create a community vision for Skyway Park through the county's interdepartmental Community Enhancement Initiative. Encouraged by strong participation and the successful implementation of early action items in the park, this project has been expanded to produce a wider community agenda for neighborhood revitalization, addressing the root causes of long-standing and persistent inequities.

Natural Resources and Parks—Natural Resources and Parks conducted a GIS-based equity assessment which mapped benefits (e.g., proximity to a park or trail) and burdens (e.g., proximity to a wastewater regulator facility) related to demographic variables such as race, income, and language. This analysis helped to identify and promote action on potential areas of disproportionality in the department's facility locations and service delivery.

Public Health—To increase availability of health information for people with limited English proficiency, Public Health developed a translation policy and system. The policy includes processes for creating translations of consistently high quality and has innovative translation guidelines, resources, and best practices. Included are language maps for King County, priority language tiers with 20 languages, quality translation vendors chosen in a competitive process, and a translation worksheet to guide the translation process.

Transportation—Along with key partners, Transportation has been actively engaged with community organizations, schools, businesses, and residents to elicit their feedback about possible changes to bus routes in the southeast Seattle area and southwest King County in light of Link light rail service and RapidRide starting in 2009. Activities have included over a dozen sounding board meetings, mailings to over 92,000 addresses, a multilingual hotline, questionnaires, and other materials translated in seven languages, and numerous community discussions, public speaking engagements, and other intensive community outreach activities.

Internal Education and Communication

Hundreds of King County employees at all levels have participated in dialogues about equity and social justice. Discussions followed a screening of the ground-breaking PBS series *Unnatural Causes: Is Inequality Making Us Sick?* The dialogues served to educate employees about the root, underlying causes of inequities and to spark a dialogue among staff about how to best address inequities within their programs, divisions and departments.

Community Partnerships

King County has committed to supporting capacity building of local organizations and communities and to more effectively listen to and involve community members in creating solutions to inequities.

2008 Highlight

The Initiative's Community Engagement Team, comprised of King County staff and community partners, has been providing leadership to engage communities in dialogues and actions related to equity and social justice.

Over 100 people have been trained to facilitate dialogues involving screening of the PBS documentary *Unnatural Causes: Is Inequality Making Us Sick?* Throughout King County, discussion and dialogues have already taken place with over 100 groups. These groups cross many sectors of the community, including education, criminal justice, human services, public health, youth, and faith-based groups.

Hundreds of King County residents attended three Town Halls meetings in 2008—one led by King County Executive Ron Sims, a second hosted by the King County Council, and a third one focusing on neighborhoods and health.

Conclusion

Within state and local governments, all agencies have a role in contributing to a healthy community. Transportation, parks, education, health, justice, medical treatment, housing, and other service systems can break out of their traditional silos and work together to respond to the needs of communities. The historical response by most institutions has been to focus on the downstream crises of individuals and families. More prisons, social workers, homeless shelters, treatment beds, and emergency health care services are often the priorities. Yet, what is needed is a focus on all parts of the stream—upstream, midstream, and downstream.

The metaphor of a stream provides insights about the connection between the underlying conditions or social determinants in a community and the health and well-being of individuals and families. When the upstream foundational conditions of a community—environmental, social, economic, and political—are neglected, the implications are a much greater set of downstream problems experienced by individuals and families and significant costs incurred by everyone. The King County Equity and Social Justice Initiative places a focus on working upstream, thus finding solutions to problems before they develop, at a policy level and across sectors of society—communities, governments, and businesses.

It may take many years, but embedding equity in all the work of King County and its partners will produce the social change that will result in a steady reduction in the demand for crisis services and interventions and a commensurate increase in the ability to further support the conditions that promote thriving communities.

Notes

1. The Inter-Departmental Team of the King County Equity and Social Justice Initiative has been central in leading and coordinating these steps and actions.

22

Street Science: Local Knowledge and Environmental Justice

JASON CORBURN

Introduction

A dust cloud from the rubble of the former World Trade Center in lower Manhattan was swirling overhead when I entered a public meeting about local air quality on October 2001. Entering the meeting, I overheard a middle-aged woman who lives in nearby Battery Park City ask her anxious-looking friend: "How can two 100-story buildings disintegrate into thin air—given all the things in those buildings that were never meant to disappear into thin air—and that air be perfectly safe to breathe?" Almost on queue, Joel A. Miele Sr., the city's commissioner of the Department of Environmental Protection, came over the microphone and insisted that the air quality, while it might cause nagging discomfort, "is not a health problem. It is human nature," he continued, "to be worried and skeptical, but you can rest assured there is no danger from breathing the air."

This chapter is reprinted from Jason Corburn, *Street Science: Community Knowledge and Environmental Health Justice*, pp. 1–11, 35–45, 213–217, by permission of the MIT Press. Copyright 2005 Massachusetts Institute of Technology.

The woman next to me was not buying it: "I don't trust them for a minute. We feel physically sick when we stay there, sore throats, burning eyes, rashes." Mary Mears, a spokeswoman for the U.S. Environmental Protection Agency (EPA) got up to calm the uneasiness in the crowd: "You can see the dust, you can taste the dust, you can smell the smoke," she said. "I can understand why people are not convinced based on the evidence they see. By the time I get to work I feel like I was licking the sidewalk."

The EPA and the city's Department of Health had tested the air and tests revealed that only a few samples of heavy metals, asbestos, and other pollutants exceeded health safety levels; of 442 air samples the EPA analyzed for asbestos, only 27 exceeded safety levels.[1] "The chances of being exposed now are miniscule," noted commissioner Miele.

Walking out of the meeting, I caught up with the woman who had been sitting next to me. I asked whether the meeting had reassured her. She commented:

> What did they tell us? Essentially, that after they study the effects of the air on a variety of populations for the next few years they'd have lots of interesting data to report. They thoughtfully described their studies for us, although I noted the lack of research on immune system disorders, the type of problem I have. Their comments on stress and psychosomatic disorders alienated lots of people in the audience, and we let them know it. Since I didn't have high expectations for the meeting, I was not disappointed. The most important information for me came from an environmental advocacy group up Broadway from me—they did a Freedom of Information filing with the EPA, New York State, and New York City. Yesterday they got a huge file from the EPA that contains findings which appear to be wildly at variance with what they're putting out publicly. This group hasn't had time to go through the many inches of reports but it seems clear that there's lots of bad things going on down here—again no surprise, as is the fact the State denied them their records because it is a crime scene and NYC asked for 24 more days to respond. As expected, no one in the audience believed the experts—they believed in their noses, they believed in the fires. And they told the experts that they had to do better—which, being clueless academics, they won't be able to.

Almost a month later, on November 1, 2001, the New York City Council held another hearing, which ended in plans for yet another. The same story line seemed to be emerging: while the smoke plume continued to rise, locals were getting sick but the air, according to the experts, was safe. The locals were skeptical of the experts and the experts, while sympathetic, largely dismissed that the dust cloud was causing any serious illness. Policy makers were left in a quandary over what to do.

Community Knowledge and Environmental Health Controversies

Stories like these are not unique. Something unexpected happens, unexplained health problems arise, and residents want some assurance that they are not in danger. While residents share stories, scientists and technicians attempt to show, using techniques such as risk assessment that no strong causal connections exist between the dangers residents perceive and the health problems that worry them. Policy makers, administrators, and city planners are often left to decide who to believe and what course of action to take.

Should a community defer to professionals, trusting that their findings are accurate and that they are sharing all the information they have? Do professionals have an obligation to take account of community-generated information and to incorporate it, somehow, into their formal analyses? Should local accounts of health risk ever trump expert knowledge? Can we imagine a situation in which we should *not* put our lives and community well-being in the hands of technical experts? Or, would relying on community assessments of environmental health inevitably lead to inadequate protection because locals tend to ignore regional, national, and global factors that influence health?

This chapter addresses these questions by highlighting the ways in which community-generated information can, in fact, be used to improve environmental health decision making. Many communities, particularly disadvantaged groups seeking environmental justice, are increasingly rejecting the idea that professional scientists should be left alone to define, analyze, and prescribe solutions for the environmental health hazards they face. Instead, these groups are demanding meaningful participation in assessments and decisions, and pragmatic action to improve community health. I argue that residents' organized community knowledge can improve scientific inquiry and environmental health decision making. The framework for environmental health justice that joins local insights with professional techniques is a combination that I call "street science." "Street science" does not devalue science, but rather re-values forms of knowledge that professional science has excluded and democratizes the inquiry and decision-making processes.

I begin from the position that understanding the links between environmental pollution and public-health problems no longer can be viewed as purely technical problems to be left exclusively to professionals. Concerned lay publics, especially the most disadvantaged populations experiencing the greatest risks and health problems, are demanding a greater role in researching, describing, and prescribing solutions for the hazards they face. When local experience conflicts with the conclusions of experts, residents often question how professionals create, define, and prioritize "problems" and which problems warrant attention. Communities are demanding to "speak for themselves." By drawing on their first hand experience—here called local knowledge—they are engaging in their own brand of science. This new science puts pressure on environmental and public health decision makers to find new ways of fusing the expertise of professional practitioners and scientists with the "contextual intelligence" that only local residents possess. As such, street science can contribute to the general knowledge base of policy making and highlights the ways local knowledge differs from professional knowledge. In this chapter I describe how street science operates in practice, and offer a practical framework for fusing local and professional knowledge with the aim of achieving environmental health justice.

Typically, research into environmental health decision making asks how science *influences* policy. Science is seen as "speaking truth" to controversial environmental and human-health-risk decision making. In this view, politics is seen as a separate entity that is informed by science. Scientific knowledge is thus presumed to be shaped outside institutional, cultural, and historical contexts—not something integral to and evolving with political decision making. I challenge this idea and instead suggest that scientific knowledge is always "co-produced;" science and politics are interdependent, each drawing from the other in a dynamic iterative process. Before further defining the "co-production" of scientific expertise, this chapter highlights why community knowledge should become an integral part of environmental health problem solving.

Why Local Knowledge and Environmental Health Justice?

Several issues remain largely unaddressed in the environmental policy and public health literatures. First, increasing evidence suggests that local knowledge has contributed positively to the formulation of more sustainable resource-management practices and development decisions, especially in the developing world.[2] Yet, little work has examined how this type of knowledge might improve environmental decisions in Western contexts. In developing countries, Andean potato farmers, Indian foresters, and Haitian community-health workers have revealed how their "indigenous knowledge" improved the local environment, development, and human health conditions.[3] Even the World Bank and other international agencies have acknowledged that local people have their own scientific knowledge and practices, and that to assist them professionals must understand something about that knowledge. For example, the 1999 *World Development Report* noted that local knowledge, on par with additional capital, is the key to sustainable social and economic development, reducing poverty, and improving health.[4] Surprisingly, little work has explored whether and how local knowledge can be applied in U.S. urban settings where the populations are largely the poor, immigrants, and people of color.

Second, a growing body of literature suggests that inequalities in environmental health, morbidity, and mortality result from a combination of poverty, discrimination, political disenfranchisement, environmental exposures, *and* biologic agents.[5] The implication of this renewed interest in *social epidemiology* is that disease is less and less believed to be caused by a specific identifiable biological agent and instead that a host of social, economic, political, and biological conditions contribute to well-being.[6] Much of this work has recognized that "health" is not just the absence of disease, but the conditions and capabilities—material, physical, social, and biological—that enable populations to make healthy lifestyles choices, avoid disease, and prolong life.[7]

In order to identify these conditions and capabilities, social epidemiologists have turned to the populations suffering the most—such as African Americans, immigrants, and farm workers—to understand how their daily experiences influence morbidity, mortality, and access to health-promoting resources more generally. The tendency of social epidemiologists has been to turn the "social determinants" of health into covariates in a regression model.[8] This quantification of social experience often misses the social contexts, networks and subjective understandings that tell the complex story of what it means to live with environmental exposure and disease burdens.[9] Attention to the meanings people attach to their experiences living in polluted neighborhoods and with persistent disease burdens, and how this experience shapes social action, could further our understanding of inequalities in environmental health burdens. To extend the work of social epidemiology, this chapter explores how the local knowledge of disadvantaged populations can influence both the research and decision-making agendas attempting to reverse the health inequalities afflicting residents of urban America.

Third, public health has a rich history of studying how *place*—the geographic areas where we live, learn, work, and play—structures population health. From the work of nineteenth-century Europeans such as Edwin Chadwick, Rudolf Virchow, and Fredrick Engels, to the efforts of early American reformers such as Alice Hamilton and Florence Kelley, there was a recognition that the condition of one's neighborhood, housing, and workplace helped explain differences in life expectancy and morbidity among different class, racial, and ethnic groups.[10] The recent revival of "place-focused" public health emphasizes how, for example, neighborhoods and the "built environment" structure health status, not act merely as background to other lifestyle or risk factors.[11] Place is central to the study of health inequalities because place is increasingly understood as the primary site where the impact of macro-social structures are played out in everyday life.[12] Local knowledge is a crucial resource for under standing how neighborhoods structure both physical and social exposures, and how it can assist epidemiologists and policy makers in structuring effective place-based interventions.

Fourth, while environmental justice activists, some agency staff, and many intergovernmental institutions around the world have "rediscovered" the importance of local knowledge in environmental health decision making, along with this recognition has come a tendency to romanticize local knowledge as always in harmony with natural and human systems and as superior to other ways of knowing.[13] Compelling evidence shows that local knowledge can sometimes lead to naive or even detrimental environmental, public health, and development decisions.[14] In addition, some commentators suggest that the "rediscovery" of local knowledge is a way to shift the burden of proof to resource-starved residents and exonerate the state's responsibility to protect the least well-off.[15] Others claim that focusing on localism can serve as a smoke screen for political control by private interests. While conflating local knowledge with private interests is without merit, particularly in community-based environmental health controversies, local knowledge in environmental health problem solving is both valuable and limited.

Fifth, one difficulty that local knowledge presents is that its insights are often very contextual, while policy making tends to make general rules. Much of the work on local knowledge is ethnographic and deeply contextual, and few general patterns or lessons are offered. Advocates of local knowledge have been understandably hesitant to "scale up" or generalize their findings and insights—largely out of fear of inaccurate decontextualizations, oversimplifications, and unjustified generalizations.[16] One result is that professional decision makers have not found ways to incorporate the important understandings from studies of local knowledge into the more generalized practice of policy making. Scaling up knowledge from local settings to more general policy is a necessary task in environmental health because of the extreme heterogeneity in ecosystems and human-environment linkages. But local knowledge can be used to improve environmental health decisions while maintaining a heightened sensitivity to the contextually specific qualities of this knowledge.

Finally, the fields of urban planning and public health have increasingly embraced the importance of "local," "public," and bottom-up, as opposed to top-down, approaches to research and decision making.[17] This view is reflected in practices such as community-based participatory research (CBPR) and community planning.[18] One aim of these approaches is to enhance the democratic character of decisions by challenging the technocratic model of public decision making. Advocates of these approaches reject the "deficit" model of citizen participation, which assumes that the public is largely ignorant and in need of education regarding environmental and scientific problem solving, and instead embrace a "complementary" model.[19] The complementary view assumes that citizens have political rather than technical insight, so citizens are asked to offer values while experts retain autonomy over technical issues. This misses what practitioners and analysts of local knowledge have come to understand, namely that technical expertise is "co-produced."[20] I borrow the term *co-production* from the field of science and technology studies and use it here to suggest that scientific knowledge and political order are interdependent and evolve jointly. Yet, how the fusing of different kinds of knowledge occurs in the co-production process rarely has been examined in community-based environmental health controversies.

Street Science and Participatory Action Research

While street science is a practice of knowledge production that embraces the co-production framework, it is also a process that builds on existing participatory models of knowing and doing. Street science ought to be conceptualized as a process that encompasses many of the key principles of the broad set of participatory research methods increasingly called participatory action research (PAR) and community-based participatory research (CBPR). However, street science differs from these techniques by not taking as a priori truths the meanings and definitions of issues framed by professionals. Many participatory-research processes aim to make the *methods* of inquiry more legitimate by opening up participation to lay persons and giving community members an opportunity to prioritize issues. They also tend to create processes for building public consensus around research results and interpretations, and involve these same publics in action to improve their situation. Rarely are problem definitions, meanings, and purposes open for negotiation or reframing by lay people in these processes. Street science, by embracing the co-production model of expertise, is a process that emphasizes the need to open up both problem framing and subsequent methods of inquiry to local knowledge and community participation. Street science raises the contentious political questions that professional "techno-science" tries to silence by often claiming that an issue is "purely technical." Importantly, street science should be thought of as an overarching process that embraces many of the ideals from action research, community-based participatory research, popular epidemiology, and joint fact-finding, but differs from each of these in significant ways. The driving concept in action research is that information gathering and knowledge production ought to start by engaging in and changing practice.[21] The idea might be described as turning the traditional research paradigm of "ready-aim-fire" (i.e., hypothesis, tests, new theory) on its head; "fire-aim-ready" (action, methods, theory). Street science embraces the action research idea of starting with practice, but rejects this model for failing to explicitly challenge the deficit model.

Participatory action research (PAR) attempts to make action research more democratic by emphasizing that the individuals and groups impacted by an action must be involved in practice.[22] PAR also recognizes that actions often are more effectively implemented and more likely to meet the needs of a population if these same people are involved in problem solving. This process does not specify how to manage potential conflicts between professional knowledge and that of other participants, particularly lay people. While the "practitioners" in PAR are often professionals and lay people—often the poor and people of color—how to engage a specific group of lay people is generally not specified. This model differs from street science because it tends to embrace the complementary, not the co-production, model.

Community-based participatory research (CBPR) embraces the action paradigm of PAR and specifies that community members, particularly from underserved groups and/or geographic areas, are crucial participants and that action ought to be oriented toward community improvement.[23] In addition, CBPR emphasizes "capacity building" of community members (i.e., participants are better-off after the process), improving relationships between community members and "outsiders" (i.e., government agencies, academics, other professionals), and incorporating local knowledge into the research process. CBPR models tend to adhere to the overarching objectives of the sponsoring organization (such as academics operating under a research grant) and structure community participation to address these predetermined objectives.

These definitions reflect the prevailing tendencies for each practice, and little agreement exists even among practitioners of these methods. For example, the National Institute of Environmental Health Sciences (NIEHS) and the W.K. Kellogg Foundation have both emphasized the importance of CBPR for reshaping environmental health research and addressing health disparities.[24] While the NIEHS definition of CBPR emphasizes "information sharing," Kellogg's stresses the creation of "learning communities." For some practitioners, the NIEHS CBPR framework might imply one-way information exchange while Kellogg's paradigm demands dynamic two-way communication that includes long-term relationship building.

Popular epidemiology is another form of CBPR that closely resembles street science.[25] Brown defines *popular epidemiology* as the process where lay people "gather scientific data and other information and also direct and marshal the knowledge and resources of experts in order to understand the epidemiology of disease."[26] While street science embraces many of the ideas and methods of popular epidemiology, it is a process that is not limited to epidemiological investigations or methods. Street scientists can question the appropriate research and action frameworks for the questions they decide are important to study. Street science also encompasses a wider spectrum of questions and methods than popular epidemiology, and street scientists often question whether "epidemiology" and "risk" are the right frames around which to structure research and intervention strategies. Street science also embraces a wider range of legitimate knowledge-making and communication techniques than popular epidemiology. For example, street scientists might use street murals, hand-drawn maps, and other images to understand and communicate what they know.

Finally, street science builds from a collaborative method of resolving public scientific disputes called *joint fact-finding*.[27] Most often used when technical issues are in dispute, joint fact-finding is a process that makes explicit that science-intensive controversies involve value judgments, that a range of stakeholder interests must be involved in data gathering and analysis, and that environmental dispute resolution techniques, including neutral mediation, should be used to assist stakeholders in resolving controversies. Professional analysts from a range of disciplines usually are selected by the mediator and other stakeholders to represent interests from the private sector, government, academia, and nongovernmental organizations (NGOs). While joint fact-finding does not have an explicit community action orientation, nor does it necessarily include participants from disadvantaged communities, the collaborative method provides a framework for how professional and lay knowledge might be fused in environmental health problem solving. However, for joint fact-finding to embody the ideals of street science, the process must explicitly embrace the social justice components of some of the other collaborative methods mentioned above.

Professionals must learn how to view their practice in a more open-ended way, managing uncertainty by acknowledging the limits to their expertise and meaningfully valuing other kinds of knowledge. Such open-ended engagement requires a special kind of interaction with community members, especially those bearing the brunt of society's ills. As public administrators, especially urban planners, are increasingly forced to play a mediating role between scientists, policy makers, and various publics, they will need to learn new ways of taking account of the local knowledge embedded in the communities within which they work. Street science offers a way for environmental health decisions to draw from the best science has to offer while also upholding the democratic ideals of participation and justice. But how has it been used in practice?

The Movement for Environmental Health Justice and Street Science

The environmental health justice movement combines citizen activism and environmental health problem solving with demands for civil and human rights.[28] Many communities around the world seeking environmental health justice are engaging in street science, often forging research and action partnerships with outsiders, to address the problems they face. Here are a few brief examples, all of which are part of the larger movement for environmental health justice across the United States.

In Los Angeles, Communities for a Better Environment (CBE) has organized poor Latinos to monitor air toxics and address children's health. Partnering with researchers from the University of California, CBE activists formed a "bucket brigade" to take street-level air samples, to analyze these data according to local conditions, and to use these data to address respiratory-health issues facing local Latino children. These bucket brigades are groups of local activists that use a low-tech method for taking air samples "on the street," or where one breathes. CBE has used young people and other community members to take samples of toxic emissions from oil refineries in Contra Costa County. The brigades rely on local knowledge, such as reports of fouls odors, seeing or hearing a release from the plant, and reports of nausea, eye and throat irritation, or other health symptoms, in order to determine when and where to take samples.

In Boston another environmental justice organization, Alternatives for Community and Environment (ACE), is collaborating with professional scientists, including some from the Harvard School of Public Health, to address asthma and air pollution in the Roxbury section of Boston.[29] ACE organized students to map neighborhood land uses and found 15 diesel bus and truck garages within one-half mile of an elementary school. The organization then tapped the knowledge of high-school students to count truck traffic at a neighborhood intersection and identified over 150 diesel vehicles passing through neighborhood streets every hour. Combing the knowledge of young people, their maps, and traffic surveys, ACE partnered with Harvard and the Northeast States for Coordinated Air Use Management to take particulate samples of their own, further documenting the air-pollution problem in their neighborhood. The street science of ACE activists has lead to a state-funded but locally operated comprehensive air-monitoring system, which provides hour-to-hour data on particulate matter pollution over the Web and via telephone.

In San Francisco, the People Organizing to Demand Environmental and Economic Rights or PODER, have organized low-income residents within the Mission District of San Francisco to address environmental, public health, and redevelopment concerns and to help build a land-use agenda within the larger environmental justice movement. As part of their involvement in the Mission Anti-Displacement Coalition, PODER and its members helped develop a grassroots, comprehensive plan for the Mission that was presented to the San Francisco Planning Commission, Planning Department, and Board of Supervisors in July 2003. PODER also has developed a model for EJ groups to partner with one another, and they helped coordinate a report entitled "Building Healthy Communities from the Ground Up: Environmental Justice in California" in coalition with Communities for a Better Environment and the Environmental Health Coalition, another EJ group located in San Diego. In Albuquerque, New Mexico, the South West Organizing Project (SWOP) and the Southwest Network for Environmental and Economic Justice (SNEEJ), have collaborated with one another to organize residents in Veguita, New Mexico, to address water contamination issues. The organizations trained residents to test their drinking-water wells and perform a community survey of water and illegal-dumping concerns in the South Valley of Albuquerque. This work eventually convinced the U.S. Environmental Protection Agency (EPA) to issue a half-million-dollar grant to the local community and water district to plan, build, and maintain a water-distribution and sanitary-sewer system. SWOP also organized residents to perform air monitoring around the Intel Corporation's Rio Rancho facility as a way to pressure the company to address environmental health issues for workers and communities along the U.S.–Mexico border. SWOP is a unique EJ group because their partnerships span multiple issues (water and air quality, workers rights, globalization) and multiple constituencies (low income, Latino/as, youth and elderly, immigrants).

The work of all these groups aims to combine environmental justice organizing with issues of population health. Each group has forged a collaborative research partnership with one or a host of outside professionals to help them combine community knowledge and experience with professional methods of researching and documenting inequitable environmental health burdens. When community organizations such as these engage in the science of environmental health, they grapple not only with understanding complex environment–human health interactions, but also with how to create more democratic partnerships with scientific and political elites that have traditionally ignored their concerns.

Democracy, Science, and Local Knowledge

A fundamental aspect of environmental health justice is the creation of more democratic partnerships between professionals and the public. This ongoing challenge was perhaps best articulated by John Dewey, in his 1954 work *The Public and Its Problems,* where he highlighted the struggle or "problem" of engaging a citizenry in political processes increasingly dominated by technically elite professionals. Dewey's response was a division of labor; experts would analytically identify problems and citizens would set a democratic agenda for addressing them. The central challenge for Dewey was to devise methods and conditions of public debate, discussion, and persuasion where experts and citizens could integrate their knowledge and understandings. He called for participatory processes to increase the democratic character of decisions, where experts were not asked to judge the efficacy of particular policies, but to act as "interpreters and teachers" to help citizens debate in a way that would reflect the "public interest."[30]

While Dewey's analysis remains important for understanding the democratic challenge presented by street science, his analysis did not fully anticipate the influence of the specialized analyst, operating largely removed from any public discourse, on public policy. Nor did Dewey find the information and knowledge that experts (or lay people for that matter) have problematic; science and expertise for Dewey offered a body of facts and methods that only entered the rhythms and influences of politics at a later stage. Finally, Dewey focused on the optimal procedural conditions for reciprocal dialogue among scientists and lay people, but he did not fully anticipate that the content of the scientist-lay conversation might be problematic; scientists may be unable to translate their information into the ordinary language of everyday practice and publics may be unable to translate their knowledge into the specialized language of science. Thus, the rise of the professional analysts, or technocrat, and an uncritical faith in science as facts and truths, are key components for understanding why professionals tend to ignore community knowledge in environmental health decision making. Theda Skocpol, in her book *Civic Engagement in American Democracy,* notes that "today's professionals see themselves as experts who can best contribute to national well being by working with other specialists to tackle complex technical and social problems."[31] Skocpol continues that these privileged professionals no longer see their role as "working closely with and for non-professional fellow citizens" or helping to lead "locally rooted" associations for problem solving. The view that public problems ought to be analyzed by a group of autonomous, highly trained and specialized professionals, who offer their dispassionate findings to decision makers, is partially rooted in the belief that facts and values can be separated easily. The positivist view of neutral fact-finding as informing value-laden politics remains a powerful decision-making model in environmental politics.[32]

Perhaps most influential in this view is that one form of rationality has come to dominate environmental politics—where science is the only legitimate form of expertise. Technocrats argue that experience in a given area and training in the specialized collection and systematic analysis of information allow them as professionals to tackle issues with neutrality and dispassionate objectivity.[33] Yet political scientists have regularly challenged the technocratic model. For example, Charles Lindblom and David Cohen, in their polemic 1979 book *Usable Knowledge: Social Science and Social Problem Solving*, argue not only that has social policy making relied too heavily on professionals, but that professional knowledge has not contributed any more than ordinary knowledge to social problem solving. In their strong claim, Lindblom and Cohen[34] argue for *useable knowledge*, as opposed to the professional knowledge that dominates modern policy making. The problem with professional knowledge is that it has not delivered on its promise of making better, more efficient, cheaper, more fair or more just social decisions. Nor have the policy sciences contributed a great deal, they argue, to solving some of our most pressing social problems. Lindblom and Cohen[35] argue for a reintegration of "ordinary knowledge" into policy making in order to make it more responsive to the needs of the public and to remove the barriers between professional policy makers and citizens.

According to policy analysts like Linblom and Cohen, professionals should not be entrusted to speak for lay publics, especially concerning complex environmental health controversies. Richard Sclove echoes these concerns in his 1995 book *Democracy and Technology*. Sclove claims that professionals are ill-suited to ensure that science and technology serve democracy because experts normally are more preoccupied with the mechanisms of science and not its structural bearing on society.

Sclove also notes that since "experts enjoy a privileged position within today's inegalitarian political and economic structures, they tend to share with other elites an unstated, and usually quite unconscious, interest in suppressing general awareness of technologies' public, structural face."[36] Additionally, since scientists often have similar backgrounds, professionally socialize, and tend to acquire specialized competence at the expense of integrative knowledge and experience, they are unrepresentative of the "public" and should not be expected to understand or communicate the everyday knowledge of lay people. Clearly, scientific and technical professionals hold important contributions for environmental health problem solving, but they alone cannot be expected to ensure science and its results serve the larger society, particularly the least well-off. Lay people often are in a better position than professionals to make judgments over the democratic character of science because they experience how science impacts their everyday lives, from the repetitive mechanical tasks on the factory floor, to navigating inadequate mass-transit systems, to substandard housing and inferior medical care. Thus, to be scientifically and technologically "literate" is to have knowledge and experience not only about a technology's internal principles of operation, but also about how it influences democracy and social justice within the context where it is deployed.[37] Lay people are not only well-situated for this task, they are often more knowledgeable than professionals and therefore ought to be considered local experts in their own right.

The Co-Production of Environmental Health Expertise

Since both professionals and lay people have "expert" contributions to make to environmental health decisions, we might think about expertise as being "co-produced." Jasanoff and Wynne[38] refer to "co-production" to describe the interdependence of scientific knowledge and political order. As mentioned above, in the co-production model, scientific knowledge and social order evolve jointly; science is understood as dependent on the natural world, as well as on historical events, social practices, material resources, and institutions that contribute to the construction, dissemination, and use of scientific knowledge. Political decision making, in the co-production framework, does not take "scientific knowledge" as a given, but seeks to reveal how science is conducted, communicated, and used. The co-production model problematizes knowledge and notions of expertise, challenging hard distinctions between expert and lay ways of knowing. Finally, the co-production model emphasizes that when science is highly uncertain, as in many environmental health controversies, decisions are inherently "trans-science"—involving questions raised by science but unanswerable by science alone.[39]

Decision making in the co-production model requires a negotiation among the always partial and plural positions of professionals and lay people.[40] The co-production model also destabilizes the dominant view in science policy making that science can be uncritically accepted as "fact" and "truth." The destabilizing stories and emphasis on the need for "negotiating expertise" suggest that a deliberative politics is necessary for the co-production of expertise.

In an attempt to articulate how science might be co-produced, Funtowicz and Ravetz call for an "extended peer community" where professionals and publics collaboratively review evidence aimed at improving scientific knowledge:

> When problems lack neat solutions, when environmental and ethical aspects of the issues are prominent, when the phenomena themselves are ambiguous, and when all research techniques are open to methodological

criticism, then the debates on quality are not enhanced by the exclusion of all but the specialist researchers and official experts. The extension of the peer community is then not merely an ethical or political act; it can possibly *enrich the process of scientific investigation.*[41] (emphasis added)

The explicit recognition of both professional information and local knowledge—and that neither ultimately can put to rest the uncertainty of environmental health problems—can encourage decision makers to acknowledge the necessity of renewal, flexibility, and adjustment as key elements of decision-making success. Instead of portraying themselves as the "source of certainty," professional decision makers can highlight the necessity for contingent decisions that must be open to renegotiation as new information becomes available. This means that the professional's role must be reconceptualized from "guarantor of safety" to "guarantor of recognition"—of new knowledge, new voices, new ideas, new possibilities, and new directions for interventions.

Robert Reich gives an eloquent account of how this practice of public deliberation can spur civic discovery. He suggests that professionals seize the opportunity for the public to deliberate over what it wants by:

convening of various forums ... where citizens are to discuss whether there is a problem and, if so, what it is and what should be done about it. The public manager does not specifically define the problem or set an objective at the start ... Nor does he take formal control of the discussions or determine who should speak for whom...In short, he wants the community to use this as an occasion to debate its future.

Several different kinds of civic discovery may ensue ... The problem and its solutions may be redefined ...Voluntary action may be generated ... Preferences may be legitimized...Individual preferences may be influenced by considerations of what is good for society ... Deeper conflicts may be discovered ... Deliberation does not automatically generate these public ideas, of course, it simply allows them to arise. Policy making based on interest group intermediation or net benefit maximization, by contrast, offers no such opportunity.[42]

Both Reich's vision and the process articulated by Funtowicz and Ravetz help frame what the co-production process might look in practice. However, if co-production requires a negotiation between experts and local people, communities should be weary and enter with caution. As Arnstein's[43] classic essay on the "ladder of citizen participation" highlighted, public participation can often backfire when the professionals controlling such processes do little to understand the residents of disenfranchised, low-income communities and do even less to meaningfully listen to and include them in decisions. Arnstein wrote that "there is a critical difference between going through the empty ritual of participation and having the real power needed to affect the outcome of the process."[44]

According to Judith Innes, a professor of urban planning at the University of California, Berkeley, urban planners are attentive to the power dynamics that occur in public dialogues and increasingly "depict planners as embedded in the fabric of community, politics, and public decision-making."[45] Drawing from critical theory and communicative ethics, this view of planning attempts to ensure, much like Dewey's original problem, that public processes are structured to allow the least powerful, politically disenfranchised to meaningfully participate. In order to accomplish this, a distribution of extra resources, assistance, and guidance to disenfranchised groups by planners may be necessary in order for meaningful and fair public deliberations.[46] The communicative view of planning is employed most often when finding an acceptable policy solution depends on appealing to and mobilizing citizens' knowledge of local or regional conditions, when policy issues have a strong ethical component, and when experts are strongly divided over an issue.[47] As planning practitioners are increasingly asked to mediate between professionals and disenfranchised communities in local environmental health decision making, understanding the benefits and limits of communicative practice becomes a necessary component of the co-production process.

Yet, deliberative forums, especially those involving environmental decisions, rarely have found a way to avoid granting science and technical expertise a privileged position in the discourse.[48] Even some of the most collaborative processes advanced by advocates of consensus building, such as joint fact-finding, have been unable to place science and technical expertise on par with lay knowledge, and these advocates instead recommend not pursuing joint fact-finding when "significant power imbalances among the parties" in a policy dispute exist.[49] Technical language remains a prerequisite for most deliberative forums, often creating an intimidating and "disciplining" barrier for lay citizens seeking to express their disagreements in the language of everyday life.[50] Speaking the language of science, as well as the jargon of a particular policy community, remains an essential, but often tacit, credential for participation in environmental health decision making—even in the new deliberative forums. The process of street science offers a model for interconnecting and coordinating the different but inherently interdependent discourses of citizens and professionals through the co-production process.

Street Science as Deliberative Practice

While traditional policy making focuses on "problems" and "decisions," deliberative policy science has emphasized *practices* as its unit of analysis.[51] Practice is admittedly a difficult concept. The concept of practice is an attempt to develop a unified account of knowing and doing.[52] Practice emphasizes that knowledge, knowledge application, and knowledge creation cannot be separated from action; knowing and doing are intimately related.[53]

Street science is a practice; a practice of science, political inquiry, and action. Street science is not merely a synonym for action. Street science integrates the actor, her resources, and her external environment in one "activity system," in which social, individual, and material aspects are interdependent.[54] The focus in such activity systems is on the way the different elements *relate* to each other rather than just on the elements themselves. As Keller and Keller put it:

> An individual's knowledge is simultaneously to be regarded as representational and emergent, prepatterned and aimed at coming to terms with actions and products that go beyond the already known. Action has an emergent quality, which results from the continual feedback from external events to internal representations and from the internal representations back to enactment.[55]

Street science in this view acknowledges that the world in which we operate is always to a large extent provisional and improvisational. Action never is controlled completely by the actor, but is influenced by the contingencies of the physical and social world.[56] An important aspect of street science is its social character. Street science originates and evolves in a community—whether community is defined geographically, culturally, or socially. Street science also distances itself from mentalistic and subjectivistic views of judging, assessing, and knowing.[57] Street science is a public process that originates and has meaning within a particular community. People learn about the world in shared public processes in which they test what they have learned, often through public discourse.

Central to the communicative dimension of street science are stories. Stories are central to the generative, emergent quality of action in context. Actors negotiate reality by telling *stories* about their own and other people's actions within the various elements of their community. Stories, however, are not merely representations of actions and consequences; stories are generative. As a form of discourse, by telling stories actors simultaneously shape, grasp, and legitimate both their actions and the situation that gave rise to their actions.[58] While the co-production model and deliberative practice offer frameworks for how street science might happen, they hardly help with understanding its content.

Street Science and Environmental Health Practice

This chapter has suggested that when professionals fail to acknowledge the value street science brings to environmental health decision making, their work misses important information, is less effective, and is less democratic. Yet, local knowledge is not something that professionals likely will be able to acquire on their own, even those who may be committed to fusing street science with their professional work. Street science is not merely a set of methods and techniques that anyone can learn with enough attention and practice. Rather, it is as much a process as it is particular information. Even if professionals understood the local knowledge in a particular place or community and how to gather it, they could not necessarily export this insight to another "place" or community without going through the processes associated with street science. The processes communities use to mobilize knowledge, including organizing coalitions, gathering and sharing information, assessing options for action, and building partnerships with professionals, all suggest that street science is something that never can be ignored by professionals concerned with both using the best available science and achieving democratic decision making.

Street science also can speak to professional concerns, particularly those of urban planners and spatial epidemiologists, about how the qualities of places and the "built environment" are linked to the health of populations. For professionals the dominant models for intervention remain policy sectors (e.g., transportation, housing, environment, public health, etc.), largely constructed from economic and social policy objectives. Distinct functions have been privileged in regulation over the interconnection of multiple activities in regions, communities, and neighborhoods. The insights from street scientists have revealed the importance of local context and that the dominant regulatory modes are providing inadequate protection for disadvantaged populations. For example, the current regulatory framework presumes that environmental laws are geographically neutral; they should apply equally everywhere, within the relevant jurisdiction, and therefore advances in protecting the environment should benefit everyone equally. Yet, the inattention to geographic place may limit the current environmental management system from addressing the community-based hazards raised here. Current environmental regulations focus primarily on three methods of hazard management. The first approach is to control the activity causing the pollution (e.g., energy production, agriculture, transportation), and, the EPA regulates by industrial sector. A second approach is to target an agent or specific pollutant (e.g., lead, asbestos, radon), a scenario usually only used to control perceived immediate threats to human health. The third and most widely used approach targets the medium or, less frequently, the route of exposure (e.g., drinking water, ambient air, pesticides on food). Yet, when professionals begin to consider street science, they will need to understand better the characteristics of a place and learn from locals how to tailor interventions that most effectively address the needs of a place and the diverse populations in urban neighborhoods.

Street Science as the "Jazz of Practice"

I have suggested that professionals ought to stop seeing themselves as static purveyors of a technical rationality (or any specific rationality for that matter) and instead engage critically with the tensions and contradictions that are inherent to their own decision making and in the thinking of the publics they are supposed to serve. In short, professionals ought to become, borrowing from Donald Schon, "reflexive practitioners."[59] The case studies have shown that professionals must make new commitments in their work in order to understand the insights of populations suffering from disproportionate environmental exposure and disease burdens and to enable, not stymie, the work of street scientists. This type of practice will likely be unfamiliar terrain for most professionals. Therefore, a metaphor of something familiar—jazz—can best describe this new ideal professional practice. Jazz music is about improvisation, creativity, and building a group sound. The jazz musician builds on and responds to the actions and tones of other musicians in the group. While the musician reacts in the moment, she does not enter the "jam session" unprepared or without a repertoire of responses. Jazz musicians have a keen sense of history—the origins of the music, those who came before them, and the riffs and arrangements that define the genre. In the *jazz of practice*, professionals will bring their conventional "tool kit" but be rewarded for improvising and being creative. They also will be encouraged to forge new partnerships and to be open to new interpretations of seemingly routine situations.

While jazz is largely about improvisation, accepted rules of procedure exist—when to solo, how to yield to another musician, when to break with tone and how to "bring back the rhythm." It is untrue that anything goes. In the *jazz of practice*, professionals still will bring their disciplinary methods, but they also must learn and respect the rules and norms—the everyday rhythms—of the cultures and communities with whom they work.

Finally, jazz music emerged out of the struggle by African Americans for recognition and equality. To be a jazz musician is to embody and continue the struggle for justice, racial equality, and an end to all discrimination. In the *jazz of practice*, professionals are expected to situate themselves in this struggle and make this a centerpiece of their work. By being playful, improvisational, and open to new "players," the *jazz of practice* encourages professionals to reinvent and remake existing models of environmental health decision making.

Toward Environmental Health Justice

Street science is no panacea. Yet, when street science identifies hazards, highlights previously ignored questions, provides hard-to-gather data, involves difficult-to-reach populations, and expands the possibilities for intervention alternatives, science and democracy are improved. When street science is meaningfully considered by professionals, they are more likely to understand the claims made by the publics they are supposed to serve—and these same publics are more likely to, in turn, trust the professionals. Improved trust is likely to ease the work of professionals and allay community fears that interventions are not addressing their priorities. Fundamentally, street science is about the pursuit of environmental health justice. Mobilizing local knowledge helps disadvantaged communities organize and educate themselves, as well as increases control over the decisions that impact their lives. Communities also benefit from the mobilization of street science, by shifting the environmental discourse from protest and refusal to engagement with problem solving. Community groups can use street science to complement other actions they may be involved in, such as lawsuits. Finally, street science pursues environmental health justice by explicitly valuing the different rituals of learning that communities use to understand, analyze, and act upon the problems they face. Table 22.1 summarizes some of the ways street science contributes to the professional and community pursuit of environmental health justice.

The main goal of this chapter was to contribute to a better descriptive, analytic, and prescriptive understanding of local environmental health knowledge. Like the jazz funeral that mourns death in its first line and celebrates life in its second, encourages both the repulsion of dominant modes of professional rationality while optimistically attempting to restructure professional–local interactions toward more democratic environmental health decision making. The case for street science is strong; improved scientific information, a method for community organizing, and a way to

TABLE 22.1. How *Street Science* Pursues Environmental Health Justice

Helping professionals:

- Identifies hazards: reveal some problems that professionals may have missed and raise new questions about hazards that matter most to those most impacted by hazard exposures.
- Provides good data: some information is inaccessible to outsiders; professional data is always partial and sketchy.
- Improves access to difficult-to-reach informants/clients: local knowledge can make reluctant community members, such as immigrants and non-English speakers, participate and can overcome disincentives to participation, such as poverty.
- Expands scope of implementation alternatives: "expands the pie" of considerations for interventions.
- Improves implementation success: by recognizing various actors, perspectives, practices and traditions that influence the effectiveness of local policy.
- Increases understanding of community claims: in order to work well with communities, professionals need to understand what residents think, what they do, and what they want, and street science is one way to organize this information.
- Increases trust and credibility: with skeptical publics.
- Recognizes the fallibility of local knowledge: incorporating local knowledge into public debate, opens it up to scrutiny, criticism and testing.

Helping communities:

- Organizing: build community coalitions through production and sharing of information, practices, and images.
- Empowerment: educate, raise awareness, and develop self-help strategies through mobilization of knowledge and action strategies.
- Recognition: residents have important information, can be trusted, are not ignorant, and are not dependent on professionals for problem solving.
- Improves intra-community decision making: provides new information for local groups to help themselves, define priority issues and learn what is important to constituents.
- Enhance community control: local knowledge mobilization, organizing and local decision-making are all attempts by disadvantaged groups to enhance control over their own lives.
- Shifts environmental discourse: from protest and refusal to positive demands and engagement in problem solving.
- Supplements other actions: street science can contribute to other problem-solving strategies such as lawsuits.
- Rituals of learning: street science mobilization legitimizes alternative ways of learning about problems, such as through story-telling, visual images, theatrical performance, and community tours.

ensure interventions are contextually relevant. As the health and well-being of disenfranchised urban residents and their neighborhoods hangs in the balance, street scientists are proving that environmental health decisions can be more democratic, more just, and more protective for everyone.

Notes

1. S. Saulny and A.C. Revkin, "E.P.A. Says Air is Safe, But Public is Doubtful," *New York Times*, sec. B, col. 1, metropolitan desk (October, 2001): 9.
2. S. Brush, "Potato Taxonomies in Andean Agriculture," in *Indigenous Knowledge Systems and Development*, ed. D. Brokensha, D. Warren, and O. Werner (Lanham, MD: University Press of American, 1980): 37–47; R. Chambers, *Whose Reality Counts? Putting the Last First* (London: ITDG, 1997); J.C. Scott, *Seeing Like A State: How Certain Schemes to Improve the Human Condition Have Failed* (New Haven, CT: Yale University Press, 1998).
3. J.D. VanderPloeg, "Potatoes and Knowledge," in *An Anthropological Critique of Development: The Growth of Ignorance*, ed. M. Hobart (London: Routledge, 1993), 209–227; P. deGuchteneireetal, I. Krukkert, and G. von Liebenstein, *Best Practices on Indigenous Knowledge, UNESCO's Management of Social Transformation Programme (MOST) and the Centre for International Research and Advisory Networks (CIRAN)* (The Hague: Netherlands Organization for International Cooperation in Higher Education, 1999); P. Farmer, *Infections and Inequalities* (Cambridge, MA: Harvard University Press, 1999).
4. World Bank, *World Development Report 1998/1999: Knowledge for Development*, 1999. Available at http://econ.worldbank.org/wdr/ (accessed April 25, 2009).
5. R.G. Evans, M.L. Barer, and T.R. Marmot, eds., *Why Are Some People Healthy and Others Are Not? Determinants of Health of Populations* (New York: Aldine de Gruyer, 1994).
6. L. Berkman and I. Kawachi, *Social Epidemiology* (London: Oxford University Press, 2000).
7. The World Health Organization defines "health" as "a state of complete physical, mental, and social well-being and not merely the absence of disease or infirmity." www.who.int/aboutwho/en/definition.html.
8. Ana Diez-Roux, "Bringing Context Back Into Epidemiology: Variables and Fallacies in Multilevel Analysis," 88(2) *American Journal of Public Health* (1998): 216–222.
9. S. Steingraber, *Living Downstream: A Scientist's Personal Investigation of Cancer and the Environment* (New York: Vintage Books, 1998).
10. Nancy Krieger, "Theories for Social Epidemiology in the 21st Century: An Ecosocial Perspective," 30 *International Journal of Epidemiology* (2001): 668–677; S. MacIntyre, S. MacIver, and A. Sooman, "Area, Class, and Health: Should We Be Focusing on People or Places," 22 *Journal of Social Policy* (1993): 213–234.
11. S. MacIntyre, A. Ellaway, and S. Cummins, "Place Effects on Health How Can We Conceptualize, Operationalize, and Measure Them?" 55(1) *Social Science and Medicine* (2002): 125–139.
12. Kevin Fitzpatrick and Mark LaGory, *Unhealthy Places: The Ecology of Risk in the Urban Landscape* (New York: Routledge, 2000); M. Fullilove, *Root Shock: How Tearing Up City Neighborhoods Hurts America, and What We Can Do About It* (New York: Ballantine Press, 2004).
13. A. Agarwal, "Dismantling the Divide Between Indigenous and Scientific Knowledge," 26(3) Development and Change (1995): 413–439; D.M. Warren, G.W. von Liebenstein, and L. Slikkerveer, "Networking for Indigenous

Knowledge," 1(1) *Indigenous Knowledge and Development Monitor* (1993): 2–4.

14. D. Buege, "The Ecologically Noble Savage Revisited," 18(1) *Environmental Ethics* (1996): 71–88; K. Milton, *Environmentalism and Cultural Theory: Exploring the Role of Anthropology in Environmental Discourse* (London: Routledge, 1996).

15. L. Gibbs, "Risk Assessment from a Community Perspective," 14(5/6) *Environmental Impact Assessment Review* (1994): 327–335; S. Krimsky, "Epistemic Considerations on the Values of Folk-wisdom in Science and Technology," 3(2) *Policy Studies Review* (1984): 246–264.

16. I borrow the idea of "scaling up" from the work of M. Dethrick, *Dilemmas of Scale in America's Federal Democracy* (Cambridge: Cambridge University Press, 1999).

17. P. Healey, *Collaborative Planning: Shaping Places in a Fragmented Society* (London: Macmillan, 1997); M. Minkler, ed., *Community Organizing and Community Building for Health* (New Brunswick, NJ: Rutgers University Press, 1997); B.A. Israel, A.J. Schulz, E. A. Parker, and A.B. Becker, "Review of Community-based Research: Assessing Partnership Apporaches to Improve Public Health," 19 *Annual Review of Public Health* (1998): 173–202.

18. M. Minkler and N. Wallerstein, eds., *Community-based Participatory Research for Health* (San Francisco, CA: Jossey-Bass, 2003); J. Forester, *The Deliberative Practitioner* (Cambridge, MA: The MIT Press, 1999).

19. B. Wynne, "Knowledge in Context," 16 *Science, Technology, and Human Values* (1991): 111–121.

20. S. Jasanoff and B. Wynne, "Science and Decision Making," in *Human Choice and Climate Change,* ed. S. Rayner and E. Malone (Columbus: Battelle Press, 1998): 1–87; L. Susskind and M. Elliot, *Paternalism, Conflict, and Co-Production* (New York: Plenum, 1983).

21. J. Dewey, *Democracy and Education: An Introduction to the Philosophy of Education* (New York: The Free Press, 1944); M. Horton, *The Long Haul: An Autobiography* (New York: Teachers College Press, 1998); L.D. Brown and R. Tandon, "Ideology and Political Economy in Inquiry: Action Research and Participatory Research," 19 *Journal of Applied Behavioral Science* (1983): 277–294.

22. R. Chambers, *Whose Reality Counts? Putting the First Last* (London: ITDG, 1997); Paulo Freire, *Education for Critical Consciousness* (New York: Continuum Books, 1974); W.F. Whyte, *Street Corner Society* (Chicago: University of Chicago Press, 1943); O. Fals Borda and M.A. Rahman, eds., *Action and Knowledge: Breaking the Monopoly with Participatory Action Research* (New York: Apex Press, 1991).

23. Israel et al. (1998), Note 17; Minkler and Wallerstein (2003), Note 18.

24. W.K. Kellogg Foundation,: Community Partnerships Toolkits (2003). Available at http://www.wkkf.org/Pubs/CustomPubs/CPtoolkit/CPtoolkit/, (accessed June 20, 2009); L.R. O'Fallon and A. Dearry, "Community-based Participatory Research as a Tool to Advance Environmental Health Sciences," 110(Suppl. 2) *Environmental Health Perspectives* (2002): 155–159; L.R. O'Fallon, G.M. Wolfe, D. Brown, A. Dearry, and K. Olden, "Strategies for Setting a National Research Agenda that is Responsive to Community Needs," 111 *Environmental Health Perspectives* (2003): 1855–1860.

25. P. Brown and E.J. Mikkelsen, *No Safe Place: Toxic Waste, Leukemia, and Community Action* (Berkeley, CA: University of California Press, 1990).
26. P. Brown, "Popular Epidemiology and Toxic Waste Contamination: Lay and Professional Ways of Knowing," 33 *Journal of Health and Social Behavior* (1992): 269.
27. J.R. Ehrmann and B.L. Stinson, "Joint Fact-finding and the Use of Technical Experts," in *The Consensus Building Handbook*, ed. L. Susskind, S. McKearnen, and J. Thomas-Lamar (Thousand Oaks, CA: Sage, 1999) 375–399; C. Ozawa, *Recasting Science: Consensual Procedures in Public Policy Making* (Boulder, CO: Westview Press, 1991).
28. R. Bullard, *Dumping in Dixie: Race, Class, and Environmental Quality* (Boulder, CO: Westview Press, 1990); G. Di Chiro, "Environmental Justice From the Grassroots," in *The Struggle for Ecological Democracy*, ed. Daniel Faber (New York: Guilford Press, 1998),104–136; L. Cole and S. Foster, *From the Ground Up: Environmental Racism and the Rise of the Environmental Justice Movement* (New York: NYU Press, 2000).
29. P. Loh and J. Sugerman-Brozan, "Environmental Justice Organizing for Environmental Health: Case Study on Asthma and Diesel Exhaust in Roxbury Massachusetts," 584 *Annals of the American Academy of Political and Social Science* (2002): 110–124.
30. J. Dewey, *The Public and Its Problems* (Chicago: Gateway Books, 1954).
31. Theda Skocpol, "Advocates Without Members: The Recent Transformation of American Civic Life," in *Civic Engagement in American Democracy*, ed. T. Skocpol and M.P. Fiorina (Washington, DC: The Brookings, 1999): 495.
32. F. Fischer, *Citizens, Experts, and the Environment: The Politics of Local Knowledge* (Durham, NC: Duke University Press, 2000); J. Habermas, "Technology and Science as 'Ideology'," in *Toward A Rational Society: Student Protest, Science, and Politics*, ed. J. Habermas (Boston: Beacon Press, 1970), 81–122.
33. G. Benveniste, *The Politics of Expertise* (Berkeley, CA: Glendessary Press, 1972).
34. C.E. Lindbloom and D.K. Cohen, *Usable Knowledge: Social Science and Social Problem Solving* (New Haven, CT: Yale University Press, 1979).
35. Ibid.
36. R. Sclove, *Democracy and Technology* (New York: Guilford Press, 1995): 50–51.
37. D. Nelkin, "Science and Technology Policy and the Democratic Process," in *Citizen Participation in Science Policy*, Peterson, ed. (Amherst, MA: University of Massachusetts Press, 1984): 18–39.
38. Jasonoff and Wynne (1998), Note 20.
39. A.M. Weinberg, "Science and Trans-science," 10 *Minerva* (1972): 209–222; S. Jasonoff, *The Fifth Branch: Science Advisors as Policy Makers* (Cambridge, MA: Harvard University Press, 1990).
40. D.J. Haraway, "Situated Knowledges: The Science Question in Feminism and the Privilege of Partial Perspective," in *Simians, Cyborgs, and Women: The Reinvention of Nature*, D.J. Haraway, ed. (New York: Routledge, 1991), 183–202; S.G. Harding, *Whose Science? Whose Knowledge?: Thinking from Women's Lives* (Ithaca, NY: Cornell University Press, 1991).

41. S. Funtowicz and J. Ravetz, "Post-normal Science: An Insight Now Maturing," 25(7) *Futures* (1993): 752–753.
42. R.B. Reich, "Policymaking in a Democracy," in *The Power of Public Ideas*, ed. R.B. Reich (Cambridge, MA: Harvard University Press, 1988): 144–146.
43. S.R. Arnstein, "A Ladder of Participation," 35 *Journal of the American Institute of Planners* (1969): 216–224.
44. Ibid., 216.
45. J.E. Innes, "Planning Theory's Emerging Paradigm: Communicative Action and Interactive Practice," 14(3) *Journal of Planning Education and Research* (1995):183.
46. J. Habermas, *The Theory of Communicative Action, Vol. 1* (Cambridge: Polity Press, 1984); J. Forrester, *Planning in the Face of Power* (Berkeley, CA: University of California Press, 1989.
47. S. Yearley, "Computer Models and the Public's Understanding of Science: A Case-Study Analysis," 29 *Social Studies of Science* (1999): 845–866.
48. C.P. Ozawa and L.E. Susskind, "Mediating Science-intensive Public Policy Disputes," 5(1) *Journal of Policy Analysis and Management* (1985): 23–39; D.J. Amy, *The Politics of Environmental Mediation* (New York: Columbia University Press, 1987).
49. Ehrmann and Stinson (1999), Note 27.
50. M. Foucault, *Discipline and Punish: The Birth of the Prison* (New York: Vintage Books, 1977).
51. F. Fischer and J. Forrester, *The Argumentative Turn in Policy Analysis and Planning* (Durham, NC: Duke University Press, 1993).
52. Dewey (1994), Note 21.
53. H. Putnam, *Pragmatism: An Open Question* (Cambridge, MA: Blackwell, 1995).
54. M. Callon, "Some Elements of a Sociology of Translation: Domestication of the Scallops and Fishermen of St. Brieuc Bay," in *Power, Action, and Belief: A New Sociology of Knowledge?*, ed. J. Law (London: Routledge, 1986): 196–232; B. Latour, *We Have Never Been Modern* (Cambridge, MA: Harvard University Press, 1993).
55. P. Keller and M. Keller, *Visual Cues: Practical Data Visualization* (Los Alamitos, CA: IEEE Computer Society Press, 1993): 127.
56. Putnam (1995), Note 53.
57. Ibid.
58. J.A. Throgmorton, *Planning as Persuasive Storytelling: The Rhetorical Construction of Chicago's Electric Future* (Chicago: University of Chicago Press, 1996).
59. D. Schon, *The Reflective Practitioner* (New York: Basic Books, 1983).

23

Measuring Social Determinants of Health Inequities: The CADH Health Equity Index

BAKER SALSBURY, ELAINE O'KEEFE, AND JENNIFER KERTANIS

Introduction

In 2000, testifying before Congress, then Surgeon General Dr. David Satcher made the bold pronouncement that we must eliminate, not merely reduce, health disparities in the United States. His leadership set the stage for a more vigorous response to our long-standing and growing national shame. More recently, the emphasis on disparities—unwarranted differentials in health status in population groups—obscures the twin issues of etiology and causality, and deflects our attention from the root causes of these disparities, that is, inequities.

There is considerable irony in observing the public health discipline, promoter and guardian of *primary prevention*, seduced into the popular mantra of decrying individual health behaviors and the feverish seeking of

The resource materials that Connecticut Association of Directors of Health (CADH) developed for Health Equity Index (HEI) users provides added detail and instruction on topics such as data gathering and analysis, incorporating community-based participatory research principles, forming alliances with communities, building capacity within the local health department (LHD), partner agencies and communities, influencing the policy process, tracking social determinants and correlations with population health trends over time, and other practical information. The reader can access these materials at www.cadh.org.

national health insurance coverage. While a society-wide solution to health inequities must certainly encompass both downstream and upstream issues, the irrefutable logic of prevention teaches us that only by reversing the tide of social and economic inequities will we actually eliminate health inequities. Attacking inequities is truly the bedrock of primary prevention and the foundation of major public health accomplishments in past centuries.

The Connecticut Initiative

The Connecticut Association of Directors of Health, Inc. (CADH), a state affiliate of the National Association of City and County Health Officials (NACCHO), began to address the issue of health inequities by first surveying local health directors regarding their perceived role in addressing health inequities. This survey revealed a widespread belief that local health departments (LHDs) should act more decisively on the social determinants of health as a fundamental part of their mandate for primary prevention. Equally widespread was the perception that local health directors were, for the most part, ill-equipped to meet the special challenges of eliminating health inequities. Among concerns raised were lack of specialized training, limited resources, only rudimentary knowledge of social epidemiology, and uncertain political/public support.

Fueled by these findings, CADH established a coalition of stakeholders united by a shared commitment to alter the underlying conditions that give rise to these inequities. Known as the Health Equity Action Team or HEAT, this coalition includes representation from diverse local, regional, and state-wide organizations as well as several national groups. As its overarching goal, the HEAT coalition aims to persuade Connecticut to adopt a public health agenda focusing on conditions, not symptoms, and to adopt structural, statutory, and policy changes emphasizing prevention, not treatment.

Underlying the HEAT initiative are three premises:

- Health inequities are morally reprehensible, originating in deeply ingrained inequities that particularly impact the poor and those of color.
- These inequities are discernable and measurable, thus they can be eliminated through organized design and action.
- Change will be prompted and driven by people in their communities, along with the nation's three thousand health departments as the appropriate vehicle to convene and facilitate this movement.

This chapter describes the HEAT effort to confront the root causes of health inequities through the creation and application of a unique measurement tool and an equally important process of community engagement and advocacy.

The CADH Health Equity Index

Since 2006, CADH has focused on creating a tool to measure the social and economic determinants of health called the Health Equity Index (HEI). This novel tool will assist local communities to identify and advance policy agendas that will achieve equitable social and economic conditions. Funding for the development and piloting of the HEI derives from multiple sources including the Connecticut Universal Health Care Foundation, the Connecticut Health Foundation, the Joint Center for Political and Economic Studies in Washington DC and the W.K. Kellogg Foundation.

Several important assumptions underlie the construction of the Index. Foremost is the premise that social conditions are major determinants of health. These conditions, such as income, residence, education, and occupation, help determine risk behaviors, environmental exposures, and access to resources that promote health. Larger institutional forces affect these determinants, forces that include social injustice based on race, class, gender, and age; segregation; lack of political control and access to decision-making structures; and public and corporate policies that affect labor markets, trade, taxes, wages, and land use regulations.

The HEI is designed to locate, quantify, and measure the social determinants that prompt health inequities between different population groups, not as a tool to measure health outcome data commonly examined in community health assessments. The HEI measures the essential conditions associated with inequities in health: employment, adequacy of housing, poverty rates, and other contextual circumstances and examines correlations with critical health outcomes such as excessive morbidity and premature mortality.

Constructing the HEI

To design a credible instrument, CADH and its consultants reviewed existing indices, "health gauges," and similar instruments used in the United States and other countries. They stressed design fundamentals, methodologies, and utility at the community and/or neighborhood level. The latter consideration is of particular relevance to Connecticut where health departments often serve relatively small jurisdictions without formal county geopolitical structure.

The final HEI instrument consists of two elements, described in detail below:

- A *Core Index*, quantitative in nature, yielding both scores (for comparisons) and correlations, to assess the strength and significance of relationships among variables.
- A *Complementary Indicator* framework, qualitative in nature, for direct field application "on the ground" by those community groups and institutions desiring a more penetrating analysis of factors particularly relevant to their geography or populations.

The Core Index

The purpose of the Core Index is to conduct finely scaled measurements of social, economic, and environmental conditions in a particular community and then assess the impact of these conditions on population health status by testing the strength of their relationships to demographics and health outcomes, both also measured at that same community level.

Social determinants: The domains of interest. After considerable research and deliberation, we concluded that the most important conditions impacting health status could be captured in nine domains, a framework we termed the "Social Determinants of Health Inequities":

1. Economic security and financial resources
2. Livelihood security and employment opportunity
3. School readiness and educational attainment
4. Environmental quality
5. Availability and utilization of quality medical care
6. Adequate, affordable, and safe housing
7. Community safety and security
8. Civic involvement
9. Transportation

Components: The subcategories. Within each Social Determinant, *Components* specify broad subcategories of interest. For example, the Determinant "Adequate, Affordable and Safe Housing" includes these components: Affordability, Ownership, Value, and Condition.

Indicators: The actual measures. Within each Component, *Indicators* measure the specific characteristic or condition of interest. For example, housing affordability contains the following indicators:

- Rental vacancy rate
- Percentage of households paying more than 30% of income for rent
- Percentage of households paying more than 30% of income for mortgage
- Percentage of median household income needed to afford two-bedroom rental
- Estimated percentage of households unable to afford two bedroom, fair market rent

Selecting the indicators. While existing community health assessments and indices have generated hundreds of measures of interest, identifying and adhering to strict criteria for inclusion in the HEI was necessary to assure that every community was measuring the same phenomena, and that measures and scales did not deviate over time. Thus, HEI Indicators were chosen following these criteria:

- Availability—accessible and affordable
- Numerator and denominator—all data expressed in rates
- Reliable—consistently collected and compiled data, recognized sources
- Valid—measures what it purports to measure
- Sensitive—monitor changes over set periods
- May be disaggregated into target groups of interest
- Compelling—resonates with public and policy makers

Scores

All Indicator data, originally captured at the continuous or interval level, are categorized in a six-point ordinal scale, ranging from low to high, that is, the more favorable a specific condition is in a census tract or zip code, the higher the score. Scores may be calculated at the Indicator, Component, and/or Determinant levels, as well as deriving a *summative* score for the total Core Index Index (see Figure 23.1). Any community, therefore, may compare its "score" at any level of measurement with any other community that has used the HEI.

Correlations

The most powerful function of the Core Index is to locate and measure the impact of specific community "conditions" on population health status. The Indicators described above are statistically analyzed for the strength of their relationship to two additional data sets, drawn from the same community-level populations: (1) Demographic variables that include age, gender, educational attainment, race/ethnicity, median household income, place of residence, female-headed households, and households with children under 18; and (2) Health Outcome data that includes 49 variables

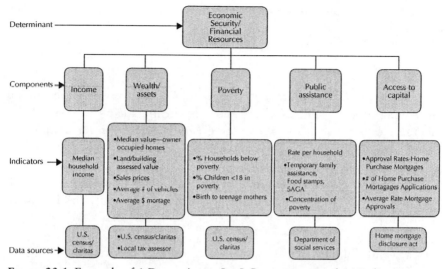

FIGURE 23.1 Example of 1 Determinant, Its 5 Components, and 14 Indicators.

drawn from the following categories: communicable diseases, maternal and child health, mental health treatment and outcomes, prenatal care, age-adjusted mortality rates, years of potential life lost, intentional and unintentional injuries. The variables in these two data sets had to meet the same strict criteria for inclusion as the Indicators. Using statistical software, Pearson Product Moment correlations are run to test significance levels and strength of relationships between and among these three data sets.

Complementary indicators

To supplement and provide community context to the data produced by the Core Index, the HEI incorporates a second measurement schema termed Complementary Indicators. As contrasted with the tightly scaled Core Index, Complementary Indicators are qualitative in design, intended to assist communities in exposing the "lived experience" of their neighborhoods, exploring and documenting their perceived environment.

Gathering Complementary Indicator data will entail questionnaires, surveys, key interviews, and focus groups. As an example, if the Core Index reveals starkly low scores in the Housing Determinant and correspondingly high rates of childhood lead poisoning and emergency room admissions for asthma, the community may choose to investigate the quality of housing stock, safety of neighborhoods, environmental conditions of abandoned lots, number of parks and open space in the area for exercise, and a host of other relevant local factors that may contribute to the elevated lead poisoning rates and asthma visits experienced by residents.

HEI and GIS Mapping

Mapping is another facet of the HEI construct and a powerful means of identifying and explaining where and why health inequities exist. Said the ancient, *"Tell me where a man lives; I will foretell you the manner of his passing."* In the twenty-first century, we learn again the importance of place, as we marry epidemiology, environmental health, and social justice through the instrumentalities of Geographical Information System (GIS) Mapping. Through mapping, communities that apply the HEI will be able to

- locate and illuminate the physical relationships between people, health outcomes, and the built environment;
- flag the specific neighborhoods where residents experience negative (and positive) health outcomes; and
- illustrate for policy makers the tangible relationships linking land use, economics, urban planning and public health.

Testing the Instrument

The HEI's Core Index was pretested using data collected in two contiguous but highly diverse municipalities, Hartford and West Hartford, Connecticut. The pretest served to answer several questions: Are the data available and collectable at the local (i.e., neighborhood) level? Are the data collection and analysis processes achievable at reasonable costs and time frames? Most important, do the data reveal meaningful relationships between social determinants, place, demographics, and measurable health outcomes?

The answers to all these questions appear to be yes. In mid-2007, CADH completed an introductory analysis of the first level of data, the total Core Index score for each neighborhood and its relationship to demographics and health outcomes. As predicted from the literature, low Core Index scores were strongly associated with higher levels of chronic disease, injuries, emergency room admissions, premature mortality from multiple factors. Certain results seem especially striking; premature *mortality* from multiple forms of cancer was strongly correlated with low Core Index scores, while cancer *incidence* was strongly related to high-scoring neighborhoods, presumably highlighting the value of comprehensive health insurance and preventive screening.

Similarly, findings revealed correlations between demographic data and total Core Index scores for each neighborhood. Scores correlated significantly with certain attributes of race, ethnicity, age, income, and education. Specifically, low Core Index scores were found to correlate with a higher percentage of

- Hispanic racial/ethnic groups
- Black/Hispanic racial/ethnic groups
- Female-headed households with children under 18
- Residents with less than 12th grade education
- Residents with less than 9th grade education

Conversely, the higher the Core Index score, the higher the percentage of:

- White racial/ethnic groups
- Higher median household income levels
- Bachelors degrees
- Advanced degrees
- Older residents

Thus, the first test of the Core Index demonstrated that interactions between demographic and health outcome variables and total Core Index scores were predictable. Testing and analysis is being conducted at the next level, the Components, and subsequently at the Indicator level, where examination of correlations will allow us to illuminate the specific "conditions" that impact community health.

Applying the HEI: From Tool to Action

The HEI is both a measurement instrument and an inherently political tool. It represents a major departure from our preoccupation with urging people to improve their health behaviors, in favor of a paradigm in which public health joins with other disciplines and local communities to alter those social and economic circumstances that allow health inequities to thrive. This is truly primary prevention and a fitting response to the Institute of Medicine's famous dictum that the purpose of public health is to "assure the conditions in which people may be healthy."

The success of the HEI will depend entirely on engaging local communities to provoke institutional and structural policy changes. This calls for a political strategy that includes building broad-based coalitions with genuine community roots. Communities choosing to employ the HEI will necessarily operate in a political arena involving allocation of public and private resources, zoning and land use, economic development, regulatory processes, and the like. To be effective in this highly charged arena calls for strategic planning and action on the part of LHDs in partnership with their communities, and political/governance structures, as described in the following narrative.

Local Health

Local health departments embracing the challenge will play a large role in the HEI process. In Connecticut, the HEAT defined this role to include that of convener, facilitator, technical expert, social epidemiologist, and advocate. While LHDs are generally familiar with these functions, employing the HEI calls for a reorientation and even transformation of contemporary local public health practice. The essential elements of this paradigm shift include organizational analysis and capacity building, acculturation of the public health workforce, and strategic planning that embodies a social justice perspective whereby:

- The organizational vision and values of the LHD clearly reflect a commitment to the principles of health equity and social justice.
- The stated mission and scope of practice of the health department incorporates social determinants and a commitment to redress inequities.
- The concept of health embraced by the LHD has a heightened focus on the social and economic injustices that shape health outcome and less on the individual, behavioral, and medical dimension of health.

Workforce development and acculturation is essential to the evolution of practice that must occur in LHD's that utilize the HEI. The staff within these LHDs will want to explore the origins of health inequity, the social processes that generate these inequities, and ways to link their work with a social justice agenda. Their attitudes, beliefs, and practices will largely determine the LHD's ability to support and sustain the HEI process. The experience of Ingham County Health Department, MI provides a useful example. Ingham County used structured dialogue to raise awareness of the social determinants of health and to instill "a new responsiveness to the root causes of health inequity" in the daily practice of their health department. They also created a preliminary assessment tool to enable LHDs to evaluate their practice through a social justice lens (see Chapter 14). This tool will help LHDs to reframe and strengthen the internal capacity of their organizations as they prepare to apply the HEI.

Community Collaboration

Working *with* communities is the only way to apply the HEI. Most local public health practitioners will concede the difficulties of such collaboration, even when the cause concerns a single, pressing issue like infant mortality or AIDS. This is not the case with the HEI, where the issue is primary prevention and the purpose may at first appear intangible and ambiguous.

Truly engaging communities in the HEI process demands an approach to building partnerships, one that transcends conventional community health assessment and participatory planning efforts. In order for the HEI process to emerge as a truly collaborative venture, the participants will need a common vision and stated mission, and a process that is both perceived and actually managed democratically. Community engagement, a precursor to community mobilization, requires that all partners share in the definition of the "community," the values and democratic principles anchoring the project, and the implementation of the total HEI initiative.

As local communities engage and begin to mobilize, LHDs will develop supportive relationships with those groups experiencing health inequities. Ultimately, the greatest change will occur from building social, political and economic power among residents of impacted areas at the neighborhood level. The process of identifying and prioritizing the conditions that contribute to health inequities and effecting change must be driven and owned by local communities.

LHDs and other institutional/agency partners can work collaboratively with local communities to build capacity in the following ways:

- Identify and support existing neighborhood coalitions to advance the health equity agenda.
- Provide training in areas such as leadership, policy development, community mobilization, and advocacy.
- Offer grants to community groups mobilizing for change.
- Provide technical assistance on data collection, analysis, and community health improvement planning.
- Help to identify local regulations, laws, and policies that bear on social, political and economic conditions/inequities and draft changes or create newly proposed regulations/policies with community input.

To avoid the imbalance of power that often impedes the effectiveness of community health collaborations, the process must be agile and will necessarily change as actual communities become involved in applying the HEI tool and in determining what issues and outcomes are of most importance to their particular circumstances and health concerns. While no single method or approach will ensure the realization of effective community collaboration and investment, we present some key elements of this process as a basic frame on which to build a locally nuanced community engagement experience.

Phase one—laying the foundation

It will be most advantageous for LHDs to convene a *core health equity team* very early to steer the process and serve as the springboard for subsequent levels of community involvement. The composition of this group will vary but should include balanced representation of those closely linked to and/or derive from communities that bear the brunt of health inequities. Representation of existing coalitions whose work and purpose includes health equity as a goal and public and private sector organizations whose missions have direct bearing on the social determinants of health should also be represented. This initial outreach to engage residents is critical to establish a credible foundation for professional-community collaboration.

Like LHDs, the core health equity team will need orientation to the issues of health inequity and social justice and the purpose of the HEI initiative. Once that foundation is established, the core team will be better positioned to create a vision embraced by the group and to refine their mission and roles. Likely roles would include the following:

- Providing input during the core index data collection phase and troubleshooting issues that arise
- Participating in media, institutional, and other community education to begin shifting the local/regional dialogue on health from an individual/personal focus to social and economic conditions and social responsibility
- Shaping and orchestrating the process for dissemination of core index results
- Designing an inclusive process to use the core index findings to identify problems that may be turned into community issues for further inquiry
- Articulating ways to integrate complimentary indicator research and/or other Community-Based Participatory Research (CBPR) approaches to supplement and "contextualize" the data from the core index
- Identifying, recruiting, and nurturing the involvement of others who must be engaged in the process
- Identifying ways that the LHD and other agencies can most effectively work to support and build capacity of communities to engage in change efforts
- Developing a framework for identifying local policy and structural change targets and for advancing actions for change

- Developing a community strategic planning process that identifies priorities and is assimilated into the LHD strategic plan and plans of other organizations/institutions that have a direct bearing on redressing health inequities.

Phase two—community capacity building and priority setting

Once the core index is compiled, results can be shared and vetted in community forums, neighborhood group discussions, civic dialogue, key informant interviews, and other venues, with core health equity team members actively participating in presentations of data and follow-up actions. Mapping is a particularly effective way to communicate local data to residents and policymakers, and is one of the methods that might be used to share findings in communities that employ the HEI.

At this juncture, it will be important to develop a larger health equity coalition with dominant representation from the most affected communities. This broader coalition can identify issues for further investigation based on the core index results and analysis, and other local priorities and situational factors that influence health experience as identified by the community. The coalition should inform and drive additional local research on complementary indicators, including identifying the topics/issues to be explored and the methods of investigation.

Once the extended community investigation of complementary indicators has yielded satisfactory findings, the next logical move is to construct a plan to focus change efforts on the issues of highest importance. Many ways exist to orchestrate a community-driven process that aims to identify critical issues and set priorities for action. The voice of those experiencing health inequities must remain audible and imprinted on whatever strategic plan emerges from the HEI data analysis and discourse around the findings. Maintaining a two-way, flexible relationship between authentic community members and professionals is also paramount to the longevity and success of the effort. Developing a democratic process and framework for identifying local policy and structural change targets is thus another critical function of the health equity coalition.

Phase three—effecting policy change

At some point, the HEI process should yield specific local policy and structural change objectives, strategies for advancing change through sustained and collaborative efforts, and actions to produce desired change in impacted communities. This local policy and structural change agenda should be solidified in the plans and priorities of the LHD, and other organizations with a vested interest in advancing health equity, as well as in the platforms of political institutions and leadership.

The need for continued collaboration and support of communities striving to change inequities is particularly acute at this stage of the process. LHDs and others involved in public health surveillance must continue monitoring health inequities in local populations and measure changes over time. The ultimate test of the impact of the utility of the HEI will be the extent to which it can ameliorate adverse social and economic conditions in ways that translate to health status improvements.

In summary, the community engagement process envisioned is founded on the tenets of community-based participatory research including the following:

- Building on community strengths, resources and relationships
- Assuring equitable participation in the interpretation and application of local data to address local priorities
- Using data to produce positive change of direct benefit to communities
- Promoting reciprocity in exchange of knowledge and resources among professional agencies and communities
- Committing to a sustained effort to promote health equity

Political/Governance Structures

In all primary prevention—from fluoridation of water to national child immunization policy—public health is engaged in complex political processes involving the allocation of scarce public resources to achieve positive health outcomes. Eliminating health disparities, our nation's stated primary health-related goal, will require focused efforts to identify and act on the specific conditions giving rise to health inequities, as these conditions are ordinarily the result of decades of policies and regulations that result from an imbalance of wealth and power. The HEI process must be strategic in enlisting decision makers early in the cause, whether mayor, town council, county commissioner, or governor. With decision makers engaged, gates open to the municipal offices critical to HEI implementation such as housing, education, zoning, and public safety. In turn, HEI will provide these local agencies and authorities with detailed determinants and correlations central to their missions.

In summary, applying the HEI is a multifaceted and political process that requires a decided and sustained commitment to the public health mission of primary prevention. The index provides LHDs with an effective tool to quantify and measure the social determinants of health inequities, but it is only a starting point. The data alone will have limited if any impact on community health outcomes. Rather, it will take the collaboration and coordination of multiple sectors, including community organizations, government entities, residents, and policy makers, to apply the data in ways that change the circumstances that foster health inequities.

Evaluation

Applying a conventional public health evaluation model to this multidiscipline, multisector venture would be challenging and perhaps unreasonable. Yet the public urgently requires knowledge about the efficacy of primary prevention interventions that aim to change the root causes of disproportionate injury and illness. While the ultimate impact of HEI application is the elimination of health inequities, it is equally critical for all involved to learn about the process, the assumptions, the milestones, and to distinguish effectiveness from effort. To that end, CADH devised this introductory framework:

Process indicators—health departments

- Proportion of LHD staff embracing social justice tenets
- Proportion of LHD staff trained in HEI principles and methodologies
- Degree to which LHD strategic plans incorporate health inequities identification and amelioration

Process indicators—collaborations

- Degree to which Health Equity Team represents the actual constituencies of the community
- Degree to which Health Equity Team meaningfully involve the multiple organizations and institutions focusing on community engagement and improvements
- Proportion and relevance of complementary indicators derived from community collaborators
- Number, frequency, and depth of media placements publicizing the progress of the Team

Process indicators—politics/governance (using a city as an example)
- Written, public statement from chief elected official (CEO), committing support and resources for proposed term of the project
- Joint statement from CEO and legislative body agreeing to the principles, purposes, goals, and allocation of resources for the term of the project
- Written directive to all municipal agencies and commissions regarding positive involvement and true assistance over term of project

Outcomes—Short and Medium-term

While the true impact of community HEI implementation will be measured over many years, there are discernible outcomes that can be observed almost immediately, and remain in place.

Outcome indicators—health departments

- Production and use of comprehensive strategic plan should be based on measurable multiyear objectives for removing health inequities.
- Epidemiology programs identify, collect, measure, analyze, and publish status of conditions related to population health (e.g., annually refresh HEI data and outputs).
- Staffing reflects the community populations it serves.
- Health Department programs work in close collaboration with other city departments and jointly publish periodic assessments tracking reductions in health inequities.

Outcome indicators—collaborations

- Health Equity Team matures, grows, constitutes a permanent Community Health Council; staffing and resources contributed through the LHD, and multiple city agencies.
- Community Health Council establishes measurable objectives and timetable for reduction or removal of conditions impacting population as identified in HEI.
- Council, jointly with LHD Epidemiology program, publishes a biannual progress report on meeting published objectives and consequent improved population health.

Outcome indicators—governance

- Establishment of permanent Commission on Health Equity
- Legislative enactment requiring public participation in new regulatory mechanism: For example, "Health Impact Assessment" for all economic development projects using tax dollars
- Review and restatement of city ordinances and regulations to ensure "conditions" impacting population health are exposed and measured

These indicators are intended as a practical *starting point*. Evaluation of the HEI experience should ultimately require an inclusive process that generates information of true value to all collaborators. This means providing opportunities for partner agencies/institutions and community residents to participate in the creation of the evaluation purpose, design, and methods as well as in analyzing and disseminating the findings. HEI sites may well choose to develop their own particular evaluation questions and methods.

Conclusion

We are at the proverbial crossroad in public health practice. Attacking and eliminating the root causes of excessive morbidity and premature mortality calls for the public health workforce and our collaborators to work together for *primary prevention* to an unprecedented degree in our history. If we truly seek a nation of equal health opportunity, where alterable health inequities cease to exist, public health practice must return to its roots. Our forebears offer inspiration for the journey. Their legacy of advocating social change that led to true improvements in the health status of the most disenfranchised populations can be ours, if we dare to turn our gaze to the underlying causes of health inequities.

Our future success rests in large part on the extent to which we broaden our focus to include social determinants as the rightful domain of public health practice. Perhaps this is what the Institute of Medicine (IOM) meant by "assuring the conditions in which people may be healthy." To suggest such fundamental change and realignment in social, environmental, and economic policy and practices places public health squarely in the turbulent political arena, no longer a bystander or technical expert, but now a player. This critical transformation will require intelligence, patience and courage. The stakes are high, for to veer from the course is to accept the failure of public health to fulfill its core mission.

The Connecticut HEI is based on three premises: that social inequities giving rise to health inequities are morally reprehensible; that social, economic and environmental inequities can be discerned, measured, and changed; and that the nation's nearly 3,000 health departments are an appropriate and likely catalyst of community-driven efforts to eliminate inequities. Hopefully, the Index will stimulate a reinvention of local public health practice and a firestorm of community and political activism. The times call for no less than a revolution in thought and action on the solution to our national disgrace of health inequities, and we are on the cusp of that historic movement.

24

Place Matters: Building Partnerships among Communities and Local Public Health Departments

GAIL C. CHRISTOPHER, VINCENT LAFRONZA, AND NATALIE BURKE

Communities across America continue their struggle with increasing health inequities and increasingly tighter budgets, and chronic diseases have become the drivers of morbidity and mortality. Without a healthy population, no country can survive well and continue to improve the quality of life for each consecutive generation. Achieving sustained population health improvements necessitates addressing the root causes of poor health outcomes. This chapter presents lessons learned from the experiences of community partnerships participating in the national initiative, entitled, *Place Matters*. It argues for increased focus on addressing the social determinants of health and explores implications for the vital role of local health departments (LHDs) in eliminating health inequities.

Background

In 2002, the W.K. Kellogg Foundation awarded the Joint Center for Political and Economic Studies a $7 million grant to establish a Health Policy Institute that would contribute to improving the health of underserved and diverse people by informing policy and sharing promising practices. Designed to improve the health of participating communities, the

Place Matters demonstration program supports multidisciplinary teams to address social factors that lead to poor health. As of fall 2008, the national learning community of 16 teams or partnerships is responsible for designing and implementing strategies that address the social determinants of health affecting residents in 21 counties and three cities.

Place Matters: Leveraging a Transdisciplinary Approach

A growing body of research clearly indicates that interventions targeting the social determinants of health can indeed modify patterns of health, illness, and health inequities. Addressing fundamental causes of health inequity (e.g., employment, education, poverty, housing, etc.) through action and policy development and measuring the indicators associated with social determinants of health are at the heart of *Place Matters*. Legal liability and fragmented funding streams have encouraged local public health departments, other governmental agencies, and community-based organizations to function primarily in isolation. The competitive funding environment restricts opportunities for data/information sharing, the leveraging of resources, or sustained, meaningful collaboration that could protect and improve heath status. The *Place Matters* initiative provides a framework for multisector/transdisciplinary teams to engage in place-based collaboration and strategies to produce long-term change at a community level. Participating teams target improvements directed at social determinants of health through policy innovation, community engagement, advocacy, and activism. Teams reflect a diversity of partners, populations, priorities, leadership, resources, experience, ideologies, and spheres of influence. As a result of that diversity, *Place Matters* sites are well positioned to leverage their capacities to affect policy change.

A multisector/transdisciplinary approach allows teams to develop strategies, priorities, and goals that can best meet the needs of the communities they represent and serve. The teams work together to inform policy agendas at the local and state levels. Collaborations such as the *Place Matters* teams seek community support for their efforts by relying on organizations and leadership well known, trusted, and vetted. At the same time, they are able to welcome emerging organizations and leadership to their partnerships, ensuring increased opportunities for sustainability and success in achieving their policy objectives. Ultimately, their efforts across sectors and organizations will ensure sustainable change rooted in effective policies that shape and frame the social factors that produce or inhibit health at the local level. These approaches aimed at fundamental causes seek to create the best possible conditions in which people can be healthy. The participating county and city teams are listed below:

- Alameda County, CA
- Baltimore, MD
- Bernalillo County, NM
- Boston, MA
- Cook County, IL
- Cuyahoga County, OH
- Jefferson County, AL
- King County, WA
- Marlboro County, SC
- Mid-Mississippi Delta Counties: Coahoma, Washington, and Sunflower, MS
- Orleans Parish, LA
- Prince George's County, MD
- San Joaquin Valley Counties: Fresno, Kern, Kings, Merced, Madera, and Tulare, CA
- Sharkey-Issaquena Counties, MS
- Wayne County, MI
- Washington, DC

Similar to other national efforts, participation in this national community provides an important venue for state and local public officials/administrators and community leaders to engage in innovative initiatives designed to reduce health inequities and to benchmark their activities in a coordinated effort. Working with county officials and community leaders and informed by the relevant literature, *Place Matters* will assist participants to establish performance indicators specific to each county or jurisdiction and designed to identify and monitor progress toward health inequities reduction/elimination.

Building Capacity to Address Social Determinants of Health

The national public health community is increasingly aware of the growing inequities in health and well-being as measured at the county level. These alarming data depict increasing racial segregation and an overall widening of inequities in health, life expectancy, education, income, and a myriad of other measures of social progress.

Social determinants of health refer to conditions of society such as quality and affordability of housing, level of employment and job security, standard of living, availability of mass transportation, quality of education, forms of clean economic development, poverty, distribution of goods and services, chronic stress, and workplace conditions that reflect *root causes* of community and individual health and well-being.[1] Such causes are racism, class exploitation, and sexism. We also know that developing strategies that effectively address health determinants is a challenging work. Participation in regional and national communities such as *Place Matters* provides a safe place to assist counties (1) test approaches for identifying important social determinants and health, (2) develop/measure interventions that involve multisector partners, (3) identify which interventions are associated with the desired outcomes, and (4) determine which social determinants that have the greatest potential to reduce inequities.

During our work over the past several years, participating community and institutional leaders have endorsed the need to convene as a national learning community to provide peer support, critique, and to explore opportunities for knowledge sharing and movement building with colleagues

In a 2006 landmark article, Murray, et al.,[2] identified eight Americas, or population groups. Specifically, they identified the following groups:

1. Asian, population 10.4 million, average income $21,566, 80% high school graduates, living in counties where Pacific Islanders make up less than 40% of the Asian population.
2. Northland low-income rural white, population 3.6 million, average income $17,758, 83% high school graduates. These are whites living in the northern plains and Dakotas with 1990 county-level per capita income below $11,775 and population density less than 100 persons/km².
3. Middle America, population 214 million, average income $24,640, 84% completed high school. This group includes all whites not included in the Northland low-income America or in the poor living in Appalachia or Mississippi, as well as Asians not included in America 1 and Native Americans not included in America 5.
4. Low-income whites in Appalachia and the Mississippi Valley include 16.5 million people with an average per capita income of $16,390 and a high school graduation rate of 72%.
5. Western Native American, population one million, average income $10,029, 69% high school graduates. These Native Americans live in the mountain and plains areas, usually on reservations.
6. Black middle America, population 23.4 million, average income of $15,412, 75% of them have completed high school.

7. Southern rural low-income black, population 5.8 million, average income $10,463, 61% high school graduation rate.
8. High-risk urban black, population 7.5 million, average income $14,800, high school completion rate of 72%.

Place Matters teams represent communities that fall within six of these eight Americas designations. Despite the increasing evidence base, many public/community health practitioners struggle with the notion that their programs should address social issues. How could individual programs tackle deep-rooted injustices related to racial and class discrimination, socioeconomic disadvantage, poor housing stock, and a myriad of other social forces that drive population health status? Shouldn't public health practitioners just focus on their mission to provide everyday public health services such as preventing the spread of West Nile Virus, inspecting restaurants, family planning programs, immunizations, and communicable disease surveillance? Can access to services for all community residents reduce inequities in health?

These questions are understandable as this work presents unique challenges for public health practitioners. History has shown that indeed one agency simply cannot respond to these issues, nor should one agency attempt to do so.

Public health practitioners are searching for effective practice models. It is challenging to develop one fully inclusive model that tackles all relevant forces driving the social determinants of health with *Place Matters* communities. As a first attempt, Figure 24.1 presents a phenomenological snapshot of the forces (some of which are social determinants) identified by participating *Place Matters* teams. This draft model depicts those forces that *Place Matters* teams seek to influence. The "community health and well-being" (the shaded box on top) reflects the target goal or endpoint. The remaining boxes reflect the mid-level factors that influence and largely determine health outcomes, including the small dark grey boxes on the left that reflect critical social determinants of teams have identified. The directional arrows indicate the interrelationships among social determinants of health and community structures available as potential assets to achieve health equity.

Place Matters challenges participants working in health care settings to develop strategies that convene groups outside of the traditional health arena to expand their collective spheres of influence. Teams must intentionally design such strategic expansion to impact the social determinants of health in action within a given community. As of fall 2008, our model remains a work in progress. We will refine it based on input and lessons learned from the national learning community.

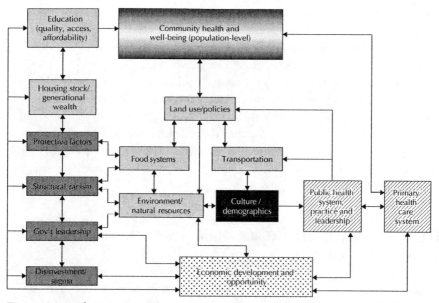

Figure 24.1 *Place Matters* Phenomenological Social Determinants of Health Model.

Notes:

1. The Shaded Box: Community health status (outcome measures of disease, health, and well-being).
2. The Doted Box: Economic foundation needed to provide employment opportunities for sustainable communities.
3. The Striped Boxes: Traditional primary care and public health capacity.
4. The Light Gray Boxes: Mission-specific disciplines supported by organized community structures typically operating outside of the health arena.
5. The Black Box: Critical social determinants of health related to culture and demographics often not well supported by organized community structures.
6. The Dark Gray Boxes: Critical social determinants of health often overlooked in public health and health care service delivery systems.

While the construct and reality of "place" are critically important and place-based strategies have proved to be effective, we also know first-hand from the *Place Matters* learning community that broader social and political forces influence the social determinants of health in each locale. These forces, for example, include the significant disinvestment that we see in both rural and inner-city environs and the long-term deterioration of communities driven by such disinvestment. Perhaps most striking is the absence of generational wealth that exists among residents living in *Place Matters* communities. While we find similarities in the forces influencing the social determinants of health in each locale, great variability exists in the interrelationships among the determinants and strength in which these determinants impact health. Addressing social determinants of health in each community, therefore, requires developing and testing approaches that will work in the unique circumstances within participating locales.

The results of this work demonstrate that "place" per se is not what determines and drives this phenomenon, but larger social forces and injustices within American society, which result in an accumulation of negative conditions in certain communities. For example, the federal policies governing reservation-based tribal lands caused the absence of generational wealth among American Indian/Alaska Native communities remains a primary cause of long-term poverty cycles. Though the policy antecedents differ, we believe many of the *Place Matters* communities are in similar positions.

The Power of Multisector Collaborative Work—Three *Place Matters* Case Examples

To illustrate the diversity of approaches undertaken to address health inequities, we include in the following section three *Place Matters* case examples. Specifically, these examples illustrate the relevance of structural racism and gender discrimination as fundamental causes of inequality in health outcomes. The case examples also highlight the importance of collaborative action to address racism and gender discrimination as no one community-based entity has adequate influence on these determinants of health.

Baltimore City *Place Matters* Team

The Baltimore *Place Matters* Collaborative for Health Equity includes representatives from Baltimore City Council, Associated Black Charities, the Baltimore City Health Department, Mid-Atlantic Association of Community Health Centers, Cradle to College Pipeline, the Maryland Health Care Coalition, and a Maryland State Delegate/Legislative Health Disparities Champion, and so forth.

Targeted change

The Baltimore City team will facilitate changes in housing and education conditions that contribute to the poor health of children, youth, and families— thus producing better health outcomes for Baltimore City residents. Through their work, they plan to influence leadership and leverage relationships to develop policies and institutional transformation necessary to eliminate the systemic racism, its historic impacts, and the resulting inequities in housing and education in Baltimore.

The Baltimore *Place Matters* team is committed to a collaborative approach toward health equity that recognizes and complements the work on health inequities well underway in Maryland. Through collaboration with policy makers, public and private organizations, and local citizens, they seek to engender a new paradigm of thought that promotes the reduction of health disparities using the framework of the social determinants of health. With a focus on education, mobilization, and advocacy, the team seeks to utilize data and national best practices to inform the development of public policies that have a measurable impact on reducing health disparities affecting children, youth, and families in Baltimore.

Anticipated results and outcomes

The Baltimore team will support the development of well-educated advocates including parents, policy makers, and influential civic and business leaders who understand the correlation between historical and structural racism and the health inequities that exist in Baltimore. Achieving that level of understanding along with supporting data, political pressure, community engagement, and effective strategies, will produce an improved framework for policy making and funding decisions. The barrier of structural racism will be diminished and eliminated over time through equitable policy decisions related to housing and education while producing improved health outcomes related to obesity, CVD, diabetes, substance abuse/tobacco/alcohol/drugs, and premature births/low birth weight.

Wayne County *Place Matters* Team

The Wayne County *Place Matters* team plans to reduce infant mortality and in particular disparities in infant mortality by *valuing womanhood*. The team will achieve this by addressing the fundamental social determinants of health such as social isolation, social perception of women, and racism.

Michigan currently ranks among the worst five states with regard to racial and ethnic disparities in infant mortality rates (IMR). In Wayne County, infant mortality is more than twice as prevalent in African American population as compared to whites (16/1,000 of live births versus 5.3/1,000 live births respectively). While this disparity is largely due to higher low birth weights in the African Americans as compared to Caucasians (14.4% versus 6.6% of live births) other factors such as health behaviors, socioeconomic factors, environmental conditions, access to health care, availability of services where most needed, and mental health issues also contribute to the disparity.

Collaborative partners

The Wayne County team includes representatives from Wayne County Health and Human Services, Wayne County Department of Public Health, Detroit-Wayne County Community Mental Health Agency, Detroit-Wayne County Health Authority, Michigan Department of Community Health, Oakland University School, Oakwood Health System, Michigan Chronicle, representatives from targeted communities, elected officials, youth groups, parenting groups, law enforcement, faith-based institutions, and so forth.

Targeted actions

The team will employ a multipronged approach to address the value of women in the county, by seeking to improve policies that support women while providing direct public health services related to preconception and interconception care. The Wayne County team is developing a curriculum targeted at self-esteem in girls. In addition to the curriculum, the team will produce a white paper to analyze key policies in the county that shape the social determinants of health and assess whether those policies actively value and support women or hinder and burden them. In an effort to develop an ongoing awareness and dialogue related to valuing womanhood within the county, the team will develop a monthly column in The Chronicle newspaper that would speak to the importance of self-worth, self-reliance, and self-mastery in women. It will also explore the best ways for women to leverage structural supports already in place to lead to better education, employment, and housing.

Anticipated results and outcomes

The team plans to raise awareness regarding poor birth outcomes for women in the county and to clarify the connections between those outcomes and factors such as a social isolation, livable wage, education, and racism. In doing so, they plan to persuade policy makers to consider nonhealth-related legislation through the lens of the social determinants of health, leading to a policy agenda that supports women and improved birth outcomes, particularly for women of color.

Place Matters in King County

King County's *Place Matters* effort is organized into three tiers. A King County *Place Matters* team functions as a small planning group and includes eight representatives of Public Health—Seattle and King County and the King County Executive's Office. A larger Community Planning Group consists of individuals who are interested in this work, and representing 20 community-based organizations, social service and public health agencies, and the University of Washington. The broad inclusion of multisector agencies and professionals ensures the inclusion of all the social determinant factors that fully represent the issues that impact health outcomes. A third group of community members paired with agency representatives will be trained to facilitate community dialog sessions to provide input to various parts of the King County *Place Matters* initiative.

In King County, there are racial disparities in well-being that are influenced by such factors as income and access to living wage jobs, educational attainment and access to resource-rich schools, neighborhoods, and access to safe, affordable housing, criminal justice involvement, and institutionalized racism. These disparities in income, educational attainment, housing, and criminal justice involvement result in health inequities.

Social inequalities of race, gender, and class interacts with inequalities of institutional power to create neighborhood conditions, both physical and social environments that contribute to individual risky behaviors. These neighborhood conditions and risky behaviors, directly and indirectly through chronically elevated stress, result in unequal distribution of disease and mortality.

Inequities exist in almost every social issue of concern to the residents of King County. Young black men are disproportionately represented in King County's juvenile justice system. Minority youth are 5.6 times more likely to be in jail or prison. Children of color are disproportionately represented in the child welfare system. African American youth are over 4 times more likely to be placed in foster care in King County. Rates of college education among people of color are much lower than their white counterparts. Twenty-three percent of African American males have a Bachelor's degree compared with 50% of white males in King County. Children and adults of color are more likely to be living in poverty than whites. The median income of white households is almost twice that of African American households. The unemployment rate for white males ages 16–24 is 13%, compared to African American males at 26% and Native American males at 27%. African American babies are three times as likely and Native American babies are four times more likely to die before their first birthdays than white, Latino, and Asian babies. African Americans die as a result of diabetes at 3.3 times the rate and Native Americans at 2.3 times the rate of whites in King County.

In addition to the basic tenet of social justice that everyone should have equal opportunity for health and well-being, the burden of poor health is borne by the whole community. The economy is impacted by health inequity through reduced productivity, increased health care costs, and the shift of health care costs from the uninsured to the insured, resulting in a greater burden on business, which bears the costs of health care for the insured. Communities and countries with large gaps between rich and poor have worse health outcomes for both groups than communities and countries where the gap is smaller. Health inequities are both influenced by and contribute to economic disparities, so they impact the health of the whole community, not just those populations with disparate health outcomes.

King County's initiative will impact health inequity in two ways. King County's program investments and policy decision-making processes can impact the root causes of inequity by consciously evaluating new and current programs and policies through the lens of their impact on people of color and people in poverty. In addition, the King County *Place Matters* team, understanding that racism is a result of unequal distributions of power and privilege, seeks to change the process to give communities more voice in King County programs and policy decisions (see Chapter 21).

Targeted actions

The King County team proposes to accomplish the following:

1. Increase the capacity of King County departments to identify actions that will increase health and well-being and decrease health inequities by developing a health equity impact assessment (HEIA) process by which new and existing King County programs, initiatives and policies will be assessed by King County departments for their impact on health equity.
   a. A draft tool for HEIA will be developed by the *Place Matters* team/and introduced to the Community Planning Group in order to gather community input into its development.
   b. The draft tool will be presented for Executive Review and application of a pilot process to test it among selected King County departments.
   c. The tool will be piloted with staff from selected King County departments, to be used in their planning decisions for developing the 2009 Budget.
2. Enhance the voice of communities in decision making, to increase their power and reduce power inequity within the county by conducting community dialogs facilitated by community members paired with King County staff, to provide community members with a forum in which to give input on proposed programs and policies and to represent their communities on issues of concern to them.

   a. A core group of community members and King County staff will be trained in Technology of Participation (ToP), a facilitation method that encourages participation by all members of a dialog group and that results in identification of priorities truly reflective of the group.

    b. Using the ToP facilitation method, community dialogs will be conducted throughout the county, among targeted communities, for the purpose of raising community awareness about the social determinants of health and beginning an input process for policy development and implementation and for obtaining community input on the piloted HEIA.

Anticipated results and outcomes

Community dialogs function as an intervention on social inequalities by educating people and giving them a voice, often leading to effective engagement and mobilization. A HEIA tool will support an intervention to gain institutional power. The combination of these two strategies will result in improved neighborhood conditions and reduced risky behaviors, which will improve health outcomes. Once the process has been piloted, it will move to full implementation. The HEIA process will be adopted in an Executive Order and all King County Departments will use the tool for assessing new and current programs and policies. This will begin a culture change that becomes self-sustaining as this process becomes the normal way of doing business for King County departments.

Challenges to Advancing Health Equity

While the *Place Matters* demonstration sites are making progress, this work presents challenges. Through our collective experience from the efforts of this national learning community, the following nine challenges emerge.

1. *Politics*—Public health practice remains strongly tied to political ideology. While public health practice comprises both public and private sector infrastructure, in the public sector, elected officials appoint a majority of public health officials at every level of government. Because newly elected officials and the public often lack knowledge of public health practice, misconceptions about the scope of practice persist, particularly with respect to government action to address social issues. Designing intervention strategies that attempt to influence social determinants of health is often viewed as a high risk activity with the propensity for criticism by some constituents as supporting a liberal agenda. We do not know of any scientific evidence that would support the validity of this fear. In truth,

addressing social issues that drive population health status will benefit society as a whole. Obvious social and financial costs accompany the increasing inequalities in health status. Chronic disease takes more lives prematurely than infectious disease. We believe that the increase in chronic disease presents unique opportunities for public health practitioners and our partners to clarify connections between chronic disease and social determinants. Prime examples of these connections relate to the obesity epidemic. The food desert in many of our inner cities, inadequate policies that govern our children's school environments, the lack of safe and affordable housing, and increasing unemployment and underemployment are familiar to the public. *Place Matters* demonstration sites are experimenting with approaches that leverage these opportunities to demonstrate how acting on these negative social factors benefits the public's health.

2. *Structural racism*—Advancing health equity in the United States requires public health practitioners to acknowledge the importance of structural racism and to develop strategies that unravel the systemic inequities in all levels of public and private sector policy making. According to the Aspen Institute, structural racism refers to "...a system in which public policies, institutional practices, cultural representations, and other norms work in various, often reinforcing ways to perpetuate racial group inequity. It identifies dimensions of our history and culture that have allowed privileges associated with "whiteness" and disadvantages associated with "color" to endure and adapt over time.[3]" (See Chapter 7.) Leaders from several *Place Matters* communities have identified arenas of policy reform that will reduce the institutional practices that sustain disadvantage. Such experimentation holds great promise for long-term improvement in the health status of entire populations.

3. *Framing social determinants of health*—Demonstration sites all struggle with how to frame and communicate about health inequity and their efforts to eliminate it. Health equity is challenging to explain to those unfamiliar with the concept of equity. We often rely on organizations within social movements to help frame the constructs used. This may not be the most effective strategy to build support and momentum from the public. The credit and overall economic crises may provide ideal opportunities to make the case for legitimizing this work. How do we best leverage rising unemployment and the housing crisis to mobilize action that results in equitable outcomes for all communities? What new partners will public health practitioners need to be effective? What groups are already engaged in these issues that public health practitioners can support?

4. *Leadership*—How do health officials and other community leaders leverage their positions of influence to address health equity and legitimize government's role in such action? What is the balance between supporting

advances in equity versus risking termination by a mayor or governor? We believe a majority of health officials want to advance health equity but do not necessarily believe they have either the support or the knowledge to take action.

5. *Workforce*—Sixty percent of the public health workforce will retire in 2020.[4] Local governments fill a majority of positions with professionals that lack formal training in public health. Often, compensation packages are not sufficiently competitive to attract well-qualified candidates. Based on evaluation data, the national learning community created by *Place Matters* provides great value to participants to share ideas and test new approaches to addressing social determinants of health.

6. *Resources*—Governments and many philanthropic entities fund action dedicated to specific diseases and individual services or programs. *Place Matters* teams struggle to find creative ways to coordinate a variety of funding streams that will expand their capacity to implement their plans. Improving health outcomes in the U.S. requires significant public and private sector investments that specifically address health determinants, not diseases.

7. *Approaches*—Several demonstration sites are designing plans to address the obesity epidemic. While personal responsibility is certainly part of the solution, individuals living in unsafe neighborhoods that lack grocery stores and a built environment that provides safe recreational outlets simply cannot be expected to beat the odds. In addition, as long as the purchasing processed and fast foods high in trans fats remains the most economical option, families with limited means living on the edge of financial catastrophe will continue to purchase low-cost calories.

8. *Building evidence*—Participating teams struggle with measuring progress. While county jurisdictions have massive amounts of data available, the teams have not been able to establish cause–effect relationships between specific action on social determinants of health and actual health outcomes. Perhaps this is an unrealistic expectation. Various government agencies maintain data reflective of social determinants of health (e.g., affordable housing, employment conditions). These data systems were not designed to interface across agencies responsible for each discipline. Creating a data systems architecture that permits linked analyses is costly. As county government budgets continue to shrink, finding dedicated resources becomes unlikely. In addition, agency leadership in nonhealth related disciplines may not see the utility of investing in efforts to monitor social determinants of health.

9. *Public health workforce development and succession planning*—A 2002 national survey estimated a rapidly aging public health workforce and predicted retirement rates as high as 45% through 2007.[4] Few doubt

that many workers postponed their retirement plans in the wake of current poor economic conditions, but increases in civil service position openings in state and local governments are still expected. Anticipated workforce shortages present opportunities for workforce development strategies that focus on recruiting and training operatives that facilitate leadership development in transdisciplinary approaches to agency management supportive of social determinants of health practice models.

Leveraging National and Regional Learning Communities to Propel Movement Building

The power of collaboration truly enables a community to achieve goals and realize visions that transcend achievements within the reach of an individual organization. Partnerships reflective of a given community can play a critical role in health protection and improvement in rural areas where it is not always fiscally prudent to establish a fully functioning governmental local public health agency. These partnerships can collaborate effectively with state or other regional public health entities that may be responsible for an entire territory but may not have any meaningful understanding of community life in the service delivery areas. Demonstration programs such as *Place Matters* also suggest that public health practice in the United States is much more than mere service delivery; it is a social enterprise that weaves art and science, and requires leadership, commitment, flexibility, and perseverance.

Partnerships Can Advance the Health Equity Movement

Health equity partnerships provide a unique catalyst function to promote change needed to produce a healthier society, which requires moving beyond services that address disease to taking action that measures and produces health. Partnerships can play an intermediary role for issues that may present challenging political situations for state or local governments. Partnerships may also bring credibility to policy agendas and may garner additional, critical support beyond the traditional purview of community health programming.

Partnerships focused on advancing health equity can provide critical linkages to community residents and larger service delivery systems that influence individual and population health outcomes. These are not necessarily mutually exclusive foci but a partnership must spend time together planning how individual entities can best contribute to a larger vision that a collaborative effort is bound to create. This challenging work requires investments in leadership, financial resources, and commitment. The 2003 IOM report strongly encourages multisector, collaborative approaches that involve all public health system actors in order to improve the public's health and well-being. *Place Matters* also teaches us that in the current definitions of organizational arrangements, partnerships are not substitutes for public health agencies nor are public health agencies by themselves sufficient components of a public health infrastructure. As Murrey et al. note,

> Disparities in mortality across the eight Americas, each consisting of millions or tens of millions of Americans, are enormous by all international standards. The observed disparities in life expectancy cannot be explained by race, income, or basic health-care access and utilization alone. Because policies aimed at reducing fundamental socioeconomic inequalities are currently practically absent in the U.S., health disparities will have to be at least partly addressed through public health strategies that reduce risk factors for chronic diseases and injuries.

The past century has brought great advancements in health. In 1900, no county public health agencies existed. In the early phases they were fairly successful at controlling infectious disease. Now, with chronic disease as our most significant threat, we require new organizational structures, paradigms, and skills. Moreover, government's role in combating infectious disease has evolved into a fairly standard practice. But this is clearly not the case for chronic disease, as the extent of government influence over the conditions in which chronic disease has increased remains quite limited. Public health agencies are struggling to organize comprehensive action to reduce chronic disease, as a new voluntary accreditation program begins for local public health practice. Now is the time to ask: How might we structure an arrangement of public and private organizations to advance health equity? What types of agencies are needed? European communities are experimenting with investment strategies that produce population health while the United States has shifted its national attention to anticipate bioterrorism events and war, and more recently, natural disasters. "Historically, our public health culture championed a scientific approach to emerging threats and supported the principals of social justice and improved health and health care for all. That culture has shifted in a post-September 11, 2001, world."[5] Meanwhile, U.S. life expectancy rates are slipping behind other nations, and the most significant threats to health remain outside the direct purview of medicine and public health practice. But partnership approaches can make enormous differences in communities despite these challenges.

Our collective learning from equity programming clearly shows the need to build broader systems to address health and that doing so is both challenging and valuable. Over time, we believe that it will be possible to measure our collective success through positive changes reflected in social indicators. In this light, demonstration programs like *Place Matters* and other similar initiatives will help organized efforts move from data to action that will address social determinants of health. We look forward to continuing a collaborative learning journey that holds great promise.

Notes

1. Dennis Raphael, ed., *Social Determinants of Health* (Toronto: Canadian Scholars Press, 2004): 1.
2. Murray, C.J.L., Kulkarni, S.C, Michaud C., Tomijima, N., and Bulzacchelli, M.T. "Eight Americas: Investigating Mortality Disparities across Races, Counties, and Race-Counties in the United States," 3(9) *PLoS Medicine* (September 2006): 1513–1524.
3. The Aspen Institute Roundtable on Community Change, (June 2004): 11.
4. Association of State and Territorial Health Officials, State Public Health Employee Worker Shortage Report: A Civil Service Recruitment and Retention Crisis (2004).
5. B. Berkowitz, R. Nicola, V. Lafronza, and B. Beckemeier, "Turning Point's Legacy," 11(2) *Journal of Public Health Management and Practice* (2005): 97–100.

PART IV

Shifting Consciousness and Paradigms

25

Unnatural Causes: Using Media to Build a Constituency for Health Equity

LARRY ADELMAN

By now the evidence is overwhelming that the social and economic conditions that surround us drive population health outcomes even more than behaviors, genes, or health care. But the *story* of how society shapes our health has been all but absent from the mainstream media.

This is particularly troublesome since the majority of Americans gets most of its health information from the media, according to a 2005 Kaiser Family Foundation poll.[1] They are more likely to read an article about a new cholesterol drug or "10 Foods That Will Let You Live to Be 100" than one about how living wage laws, universal preschool or quality affordable housing can improve our health by improving living standards and the quality of life.

The conventional story locks us into an individual, biomedical model which equates health with health care, sees prevention as little more than trying to change health behaviors, and views technological advances and genetic research as the key to future health improvements. It removes individuals from their social context, ignoring how forces outside the body—the jobs people do, the money they make, the neighborhoods they inhabit, the resources people can access—can get under our skin and pattern health outcomes as surely as germs and viruses.

California Newsreel's documentary series *Unnatural Cause: Is Inequality Making Us Sick?* ruptures the prevailing "right choices" discourse and opens up a space for a broader way of thinking about health, for a different story that connects population health not just to behaviors, meds and genes but to the socioeconomic structures and policies that generate unequal access to the resources people need to gain control over the conditions of their lives.

But one film series does not transform consciousness or shift paradigms by itself. In that spirit, *Unnatural Causes* was conceived as part of a broad-based, multitiered communications and public engagement campaign that would use the series' PBS broadcast and DVD release to inject these ideas about health equity into a broader public dialogue. The campaign was intended to help reframe the national discourse about health and what society can and should do to tackle health inequities. More than 10,000 events involving *Unnatural Causes* exploring how institutions and public policies produce patterns of health and illness have taken place across the country within the first five months of the series' release.

While it is premature to gauge the project's impact and success,[2] this chapter describes the goals of the series, the strategies behind the engagement campaign, some of the campaign elements, tools, and companion activities undertaken, and draws some inferences about prospects and obstacles to building a transformative health equity movement.

Background to Production: A Paucity of Popular Tools

When California Newsreel first began researching a documentary exploring the root causes of health inequities in the wake of our earlier series, *Race—The Power of an Illusion,*[3] we were struck by the hundreds of academic journal articles on the social determinants of health and health inequities (usually called "disparities" at the time). The research suggested a new and potentially transformative way of addressing population health, a path rooted in collective action to improve access for all to the social conditions for health.

But we were also astonished that except for a couple of books and an occasional magazine article, virtually no popular media—not print, TV, nor web—had disseminated these findings to the general public.[4] What we termed the "Big Three"—medical care (particularly health insurance and drugs), behaviors, and genes—still monopolized the health discussion. Popular media—and public policy—remained locked in the old individual, biomedical discourse where health is equated with health care, prevention is mostly limited to individual behavioral change, and the future of health is tied to technological advances, especially genetic research.

These medical technology and so-called right choices stories had in fact become so dominant that they were the default "commonsense" prism, or metaframe, through which much of the public filters, interprets, and gives meaning to information on population health.[5]

But the right choices, or behavioral, frame removes individuals from their daily context and ignores social factors, while reinforcing the divide between "them" (those who make the "bad" choices) and "us." As a result, even when the media do run an occasional story spotlighting differences in population health outcomes, the reader or viewer is more often likely to blame the victims for making the wrong choices than make the connections to underlying injustices. "Unfortunate, but not necessarily unfair," is a common refrain; hierarchies are part of life; the poor and minorities get sick because they have unlucky genes or lack the fortitude and self-discipline to eat right, exercise and abstain from drugs and alcohol. In other words, this individualist "right choices" and "lifestyle" frame inhibits organized political action.

Yet the research (much of which is cited elsewhere in this book) suggested that not only are the choices that people make constrained by the choices they have, but many health outcomes have nothing to do with individual choice. They result from circumstances outside people's control. Government and business decisions over which individuals have little say can expose people to health threats or health promoters: the location of toxic dumps and oil refineries, the quality of schools, factory closings and the shifting of jobs overseas, locations of parks, freeways and public transit, the wages and benefits jobs pay, regulation of the mortgage market and foreclosures, and even fiscal policy.

As we learned more about health equity, we realized that a documentary which brought the data to life and translated the research into a form popular and compelling would fill a huge void. Further, a film that explored the root causes of health inequities could reveal how a more just and equitable society that works for everyone is not just politically correct rhetoric but has life and blood consequences. Conversely, the lens of health equity could bring into view how the often hidden structures of class and racism operate to shape opportunity in the United States.

Social determinants also had an "Aha!" factor going for it. While the dynamic, cumulative and mutually constitutive pathways by which the economic and social environment become embodied and structure patterns of health and disease might be extraordinarily complicated, the basic concept—that greater economic equality, racial justice, and caring communities are issues as critical to the public's health as diet, tobacco, and exercise – is simple and easy to grasp once a light has been shined on it. The continuous wealth-health gradient gives even the white middle class a stake in the issue.

The timing for such a film also seemed propitious. The health insurance crisis, ever-rising medical costs, lost productivity due to chronic illness, and the inability of current programs to reverse the obesity and diabetes epidemics had opened a window of receptivity to new ideas about why people get sick in the first place.

Most important, a growing number of organizations and individuals were working on health equity, yet were stymied and frustrated by the lack of media resources that could help them communicate and advance the new social determinants of healthy equity framework among their constituents, the general public and policy makers.[6] While these network was fragmented and disconnected, with organizations often isolated from others, especially from those working in nonhealth arenas such as labor, racial justice, or housing, we found them to be committed and eager to build a larger movement for health and social justice.

We asked ourselves: Might it be possible to produce a documentary film series that could help change the conventional health story by rendering visible the forces which are beyond an individual's control that shape health? Could we tell a compelling tale that centers social justice, empowerment and collective action as fundamental to achieving health and well-being? Most of all, could we produce a good film series as well as one that was useful—one that would be used widely?

A vision for what would eventually become *Unnatural Causes: Is Inequality Making Us Sick?* began to take shape. The series would not consist of two-minute YouTube clips (though clips are posted on YouTube). Rather it would run a demanding four hours all together, broken into seven modules, an essay that respected the complexity of its subject matter and the intelligence of its audience while translating the data into powerful and compelling stories of real people and real communities struggling for better health. We also wanted to deconstruct and question viewers' own taken-for-granted understandings about health rather than just grandly presenting a new idea. Most of all, the series needed to demonstrate that health inequalities are not natural, not accidental, and not inevitable. As David Williams of Harvard University's School of Harvard's School of Public Health says in the series, "These are not acts of God, and they don't happen by chance." They result largely from policy decisions that Americans as a body politic have made, and can certainly make differently if we had the political will.

Producing such a film series was a daunting but compelling challenge. At California Newsreel we have always made the distinction between a good film and a useful film. Not all good films are useful, though all useful films must be good. If a film on health equity were to be successful, it would have to respond to and advance the needs of the field—the educators, practitioners, organizers, and advocates—so that it would be widely used and not just watched. We didn't want to preach to the choir but rather saw our role as providing the choir resources that could help them better sing their song.

This goal implied that we would also have to produce companion materials that could help users integrate the film screenings into a larger organizational strategy, set objectives, assess capacity, optimize the viewing experience and serve as a prelude to further action. That meant the production of Community Action Toolkits, Discussion Guides, Policy Guides, Backgrounders, Quizzes, Handouts, and other resources. But most of all, we would have to engage in an ongoing discussion with prospective users right from the start and build a community around the film and its objectives.

Distribution Precedes Production: Building a User Network

Rather than produce a film and then distribute it to an audience, we began by identifying the needs of potential users. We involved and built relationships with interested organizations even before a frame of film was shot. Not only did their input enhance our chances of producing a useful film series, their having a voice in the work also gave them a stake in ensuring its successful dissemination.

First, we circulated a background paper outlining our thinking and proposing the concepts the series might address to selected health equity scholars and advocates. In Winter 2005, we attended a small meeting of Washington, DC-based health equity advocates where these ideas were discussed. We received invaluable feedback and most importantly, enough enthusiasm and commitments for assistance that we decided to go ahead with the project.[7]

We recruited two sets of advisors. The first, our Scientific Advisors, helped ensure that we understood the basic concepts, brought our attention to key studies, experiments and research, and got our facts right. They provided consultation, reviewed film treatments, and critiqued rough cuts.[8]

We also established an Outreach Advisory Board, a small brain trust of advocates and leaders which helped ensure that the series best served the needs of the field by working with us on messaging, outreach and communications, and otherwise held us accountable. They helped develop the public engagement campaign that would use the series and ancillary tools to educate, organize, and advocate for health equity.[9]

We also brought McKinney & Associates on-board as our media relations and publicity consultant to begin shaping communications strategies rather than wait until completion and release of the series.

In consultation with our advisors, we set the following goals for the project:

- Increase media, public, and policy makers' attention to the extent of health inequities, their root causes, and that they are an issue of urgent national concern.
- Reveal that health inequities are not "natural" but avoidable and preventable, in many ways a consequence of decisions we as a society have made—and can make differently.
- Help introduce the importance of social and economic policies (jobs, labor, housing, racial justice, land use, etc.) into discussions of health.
- Inject consideration of health consequences into debates over social and economic policies.
- Demonstrate that tackling health inequities is not a special interest issue but is in the common public interest.
- Direct media and policy maker attention to hopeful, innovative, and community-based initiatives for health equity.

We finally initiated production in the winter of 2006 with an orientation workshop for our entire production team in Boston at the offices of our production partners, Vital Pictures, that grounded everyone in the core concepts of health equity.[10,11]

Moving Forward: A Public Engagement Strategy Takes Shape

The *Unnatural Causes* public engagement campaign would be run not by one central intelligence but rather more as a neural network, with each partner communicating with and contributing to the whole. We understood as well that no documentary film series could—or would—lead a social movement. But if we could provide the rich but fragmented network of organizations, programs and initiatives working on health inequities and social justice a compelling film series, and accompanying support tools they would use them, each in their own way. They would use them to deepen the conversation, build interdisciplinary links to new partners, generate solidarity among peoples, organizations and regions struggling for better health, and help set the groundwork for a health equity movement.

In June 2006, the Health Policy Institute of the Joint Center for Political and Economic Studies and California Newsreel convened a strategic planning kick-off meeting in Washington, DC. The meeting brought together 50 leading health equity advocates and other stakeholders from around the country to view early film clips and brainstorm how best to take advantage of the series to advance public awareness, engage electoral officials and concerned organizations, and mobilize political will. We discussed the campaign's message framework and partnership building. We also set up an Outreach Steering Committee of a dozen members who would continue to serve as a sounding board, review messages and materials, and help to recruit additional outreach partners.

We drafted an *Unnatural Causes* public engagement strategy document that would dovetail with health equity initiatives led by the Joint Center of Political and Economic Studies, the National Association of County and City Health Officials, the Praxis Project, the American Public Health Association, PolicyLink, and others. The Strategy was built around four complementary and overlapping objectives:

1. Reframing the Health Conversation: Press and Publicity

We would capitalize on the PBS broadcast and release of *Unnatural Causes* to reach beyond TV critics and galvanize press attention to the key messages of the series, while giving a platform to some central characters and spokespeople in print, radio, and the Web. Off-the-critics pages press outreach would focus on feature writers, columnists, and producers who cover social and economic issues in major daily news media (e.g., Washington Post, USA Today, NPR), popular media (e.g., The Today Show), ethnic media (e.g., La Opinion, Native American Calling), constituency media (e.g., AFL-CIO, AARP), talk radio (e.g., The Thom Hartmann Show), and the placement of opinion pieces. We would also reach out to web sites and bloggers, and present the series and its findings at the conventions of appropriate professional associations, including journalists.

Viral marketing would also play a role in publicity. Video clips and "power punch" graphics would be posted on popular Web, video, and social networking portals for easy download and e-forwarding.

The campaign's general message was straightforward: Our health and well-being depends on more than our meds, our behaviors and our genes. Society matters. Improving the conditions in which we are born, live, work and play are as vital to our health as diet, smoking and exercise.

2. Engaging the Neural Network: Targeted Outreach

What was most exciting to us—and ultimately more effective than a film confined to a TV broadcast or theatrical release—was the prospect of recruiting organizations already working in public health and/or social justice to organize their own screenings and discussions of *Unnatural Causes* across the country. We would build a network of several hundred Outreach Partners eager to organize launch events, convene internal trainings, community dialogues, policy forums, town-hall meetings, and other events. Each of these efforts would in turn also stimulate other events, in an ever widening circle. We directed our outreach efforts toward four distinct groups of potential Outreach Partners:

Public health organizations: Building the new consensus

Public and community health agencies, organizations and alliances would serve as the leads in the public engagement campaign since many already were committed to tackling health inequities, at least in name. They would use the series as an internal training tool to strengthen the capacity of staff and leadership, as well as externally to organize alliances and partnerships with other stakeholder groups, and to educate the public and government officials.

Nonhealth organizations: Broadening the coalition

Not surprisingly, we made housing, community development, business, racial justice, child advocates, education, religious, labor, and other non-medical organizations a top priority. After all, the central theme of the series is that greater equity and justice in nonhealth arenas—neighborhoods, jobs, schools, and so forth—is critical to improving population health. The engagement of nonpublic health organizations would also be needed to drive public policy change.

At the same time, when nonhealth groups examine and communicate the health consequences of economic and social policies, they can more effectively leverage their own social and economic justice reform proposals whose impacts on health traditionally have not been taken into account in the policy and decision-making process. The more these groups integrate the health consequences of social policy into their own advocacy work, the more the movement for equity in all arenas, including health, will advance.

Elected officials and the policy community: Change from within

We also wanted to encourage policy forums and briefings for federal, state, and local officials. These would occur within legislative committees and caucuses (such as the Congressional Black Caucus Health Braintrust) and executive agencies as well as through the relevant professional associations of government officials such as the National Conference of Mayors and the National Association of State Legislators.

Highlighting community-based equity efforts: Pressure from below

The health equity stories spotlighted in *Unnatural Causes* should especially strengthen those grassroots organizations advocating greater empowerment and social justice in their own communities. They could use the series to raise the local profile of their own work and integrate it with health concerns. Community-based organizations are widespread. But few have until now seen, let alone communicated their work, through the lens of health equity.

3. DVD Distribution

California Newsreel, a leading distributor of social issue documentaries (www.newsreel.org), would release the series on DVD as a core audio visual text for use in college and university course work, professional schools, community-based education, for professional and staff development and continuing education. We decided not to release the series in home video. The additional music and archival footage license fees for the home video market would increase the costs while the home video market for the series would be negligible. The goal was organizational use not individual viewing.

4. The Online Action Center: Campaign Support Tools

Building outreach partnerships was just a first step. But how could Partners actually use *Unnatural Causes*? How could organizations integrate the series into their work? Who were their natural allies? What next steps could they advocate? How could we help organizations plan effective screenings that would serve not as onetime events but as momentum-building steps toward further involvement?

As indicated earlier, watching a film and using a film are different. Most people, including our Outreach Partners, are conditioned by the viewing experience of Hollywood films—sitting in a darkened theater, attention fixed and absorbed by the action on the screen. But the real subject of a film about social justice is not that depicted on the screen but rather the audience, or more precisely, the (often unarticulated or even subconscious) attitudes and beliefs the audience holds about that subject.

We created an Online Action Center to help prospective *Unnatural Causes* users. It is housed on the series companion web site at www. unnaturalcauses.org and contains planning and discussion guides, backgrounders, handouts, and other tools that prompt new questions, spark conversations, and organize new alliances between everyone who needs to be involved in the effort to make us healthier: health workers, government officials, educators, labor unions, city planners, church leaders, and other groups.

The tools in the Action Center help Partners and others organize screenings, build interest in the issue, reach out to the press, and optimize the impact of their screenings. They were designed to serve several different screening contexts:

- **Trainings** that build skills, competencies, support, and commitment among both staff and leadership.
- **Community dialogues** that engage community voices and identify major concerns, assess readiness, and generate action ideas.
- **Cross-sectoral screenings and forums** that bring nonhealth stakeholders (housing, planning, racial justice, labor, business) into the health equity conversation, build alliances and partnerships among different sectors, and construct a broader base of support for wide-reaching equity initiatives.
- **Town-hall meetings** that explore root causes of health and illness, challenge government or corporate decisions that adversely affect health, and identify and advocate for innovative initiatives and policies that can make a difference.
- **Policy forums and briefings** that bring a perspective based upon the social determinants of health equity, government officials, and staff in different departments.
- **Media outreach** that encourages reporters to focus more broadly on social conditions, historical context, corporate actions and government policies, rather than just how individuals can change behaviors or protect themselves.

We started developing Action Center tools while editing the series:

- The Action Toolkit, developed with the Praxis Project, presents organizations with a step-by-step planning process to assess their capacity, set clear goals and objectives, and identify the types of screenings—internal trainings, briefings for government officials, policy forums for agencies and staff, community dialogues, and/or town-hall meetings—that can best advance their work. The Toolkit also helps organizations determine the most appropriate episodes to screen.

- The Discussion Guide enriches the screening itself by providing previewing activities, comprehension questions, reflection, and suggestions for identifying activities and next steps for each of the episodes.
- The Policy Guide helps organizations connect their growing interest with specific social and economic policies that can promote health equity.
- Backgrounders include position papers and articles that describe core concepts as well as talking points.
- Handouts and Power-Points such as "Ten Things to Know About Health," "The Health Olympics" and "The Health Literacy Quiz" help to illustrate key concepts, raise questions, chart health trends and data, and develop strategies.
- "For the Press" includes press releases, publicity tips and other materials groups can use to work with local journalists and win better press coverage of their work.
- A "Connect-Up!" data base allows individuals to get involved by connecting to health equity organizations working in their locale or on a topic of their interest.

These plus other tools are all posted on the www.unnaturalcauses.org companion web site, along with interactivities, an "Ask the Experts" online forum, lesson plans, "mythbuster" video clips, podcasts, and more. The *Unnatural Causes* Web site serves as a unique entry point and online gathering place not only for Outreach Partners but also for the public, health equity advocates, students, teachers, the press and others.

Building the Network: The Public Engagement Campaign Takes Off

We knew that the success of the engagement campaign would depend upon recruiting and communicating regularly with outreach partners during production. We met and consulted with many organizations personally, but also reached out to potential partners in other ways.[12]

Perhaps most critically, we conducted more than 30 work-in-progress screenings at meetings and conferences ranging from the American Public Health Association to Black Women's Agenda. These screenings provided invaluable feedback and the final films were better as a result. But the screenings also gave groups a stake and sense of ownership in the series, and became more committed to using and promoting it as a result. Several national organizations consulted closely with us as they planned to use the series.

Our Scientific and Outreach Advisors also presented clips from *Unnatural Causes* and discussed the campaign at the many conferences where they presented.

A temporary web site (posted while we designed the much more ambitious *Unnatural Causes* companion site) served as a communications hub for Outreach Partners. The site described the project and included a video clip, posted news, and updates, as well as health equity tools and handouts (e.g., "Ten Things to Know about Health") as they were developed. The web site also included a page where organizations could sign up to be included as Outreach Partners.

We published an e-newsletter that included regular updates and reports along with news of companion tools as they were developed and posted on the temporary web site. By the time of the series' release, more that 4,200 subscribers were receiving the newsletter.

Meanwhile, listservs such as the Spirit of 1848 (a caucus of APHA) and SDOH (York University, Toronto) discussed and built excitement about the series and its companion tools among health equity scholars and advocates.

As a result, when *Unnatural Causes* was finally broadcast by PBS and released on DVD by California Newsreel in the Spring of 2008, hundreds of organizations already had plans in place for promoting and using the series.

Our partnership with the *National Association of County and City Health Officials* (NACCHO) offers one illustration of how the campaign operated. A NACCHO senior staff member served on both our scientific and outreach advisory boards. Early on, he arranged for us to make a presentation to the NACCHO Health Equity and Social Justice Strategic Direction Team. NACCHO supported and began to recruit local public health departments to organize a "town-hall meetings" campaign using the series, funded in part by the California Endowment. The campaign was introduced in a plenary session at the NACCHO 2007 annual conference where clips from *Unnatural Causes* were also screened and the participation of local public health departments solicited. In February 2008, we conducted two six-hour workshops on using the series and its companion tools for California health departments.

By the time of the Spring 2008 PBS broadcast, 112 county and city public health departments (plus four state departments) were planning screenings of *Unnatural Causes* as part of efforts to move the health discussion toward root causes and tackling inequities. Local public health departments began conducting internal trainings, interagency policy forums, and community dialogues (commonly built around issues of housing, land use, and racism), often in partnerships with other government agencies and community-based groups. Some highlights are as follows:

- Several health departments partnered with local organizations to sponsor local public premieres and kick-off health equity initiatives. The Boston opening at the Kennedy Library, for example, was introduced by Boston Mayor Thomas Menino, featured Massachusetts Secretary of Health and Human Services, Dr. Judyann Bigby, and was attended by a standing room only crowd of 750.
- Chicago and Cook County Public Health Departments trained 80 discussion leaders.
- Four companion health equity reports were written and released to date (e.g., Alameda County's (CA) "Life and Death from Unnatural Causes") which attracted additional press coverage and the attention of local officials.
- PBS stations in six cities—Chicago, Pittsburgh, Columbus, Kansas City, Santa Rosa (CA) and Louisville—produced and broadcast their own companion programs in cooperation with local public health departments.
- King County (Seattle) executive Ron Sims announced a new "Equity and Social Justice" initiative that will evaluate all county social policy through an equity lens. They are using *Unnatural Causes* to build understanding and support among various county groups.

NACCHO is just one among more than 250 other Outreach Partners who are undertaking campaigns using *Unnatural Causes*. A few examples of other campaign activities are as follows:

- The ISAIAH/Gamaliel Interfaith Network of 90 congregations, community groups, unions, and public health officials in Central Minnesota is building a transformative health campaign around *Unnatural Causes* forums to drive state health policy beyond the narrow debate over health insurance.
- Black Women's Agenda, a coalition of 16 national African American women's organizations, is using the series to mobilize members around preterm births using a racial and economic justice framework.
- The Service Employees International Union (SEIU) is using the series in their "Community Strength" campaign to advocate for social policies that improve community well-being.
- The 16 *Place Matters* county-level teams, a project of the Joint Center's Health Policy Institute, is using the series to win support for their respective health equity initiatives from other county organizations.

- The California Pan Ethnic Health Network (CPEHN) is hosting convenings throughout the state to develop place-based policy approaches to health equity, using clips from the series as the conversation starter, followed by a panel of local leaders sharing their advocacy experiences in land use and planning.
- The Health Trust of Silicon Valley offered mini-grants up to $1,500 supporting 32 community organizations convening screenings and dialogues. Grantees have been blogging about their experiences and will come together in 2009 to develop a regional health equity strategy. The Blue Cross/Blue Shield Foundation of Minnesota produced television and online spots as well as opinion pieces to drive viewers to the broadcast, hosted screenings with health and nonhealth partners throughout the state, and is distributing 250 DVDs to encourage grantees to hold screenings, while hosting a web-based calendar and blog for organizations to network and share lessons-learned and next steps.
- Health professionals can earn Continuing Education Credits in an online course built around *Unnatural Causes* and offered by San Francisco State University with the American Public Health Association, while the Boston Public Health Commission is developing units for high school "Health" courses.
- The Centers for Disease Control (CDC) and other government agencies are featuring *Unnatural Causes* in workshops and conferences, as they begin to focus increasingly on population health.
- Policy Forums have been convened on Capitol Hill, several state legislatures and for local and state agency heads to begin injecting health considerations into discussions of economic and social policy.

Challenges and Opportunities

As of August 2008 (5 months after the series' release) more than 10,000 events had already taken place across the country, many more than we ever anticipated. The campaign is ongoing and growing, with more organizations using *Unnatural Causes* every week (most groups using *Unnatural Causes* are *not* official outreach partners but operate independently).[13] They are using the series, or parts of it, repeatedly and in different settings, both internally and externally, reaching out to government agencies, students, nonprofits, community organizations, policy makers and the general public. Like particles of dust in the upper atmosphere around which hailstones coalesce, it is almost as if organizations had been waiting for a film to appear so they could finally bring the message of how social institutions and policies produce health inequities to a broader public.

Unnatural Causes users find that screenings offer both advantages and challenges different than more targeted educational, training, and organizing tools. *Unnatural Causes* touches viewers on several levels. It tells human stories that make abstract concepts real and personal while providing an emotional connection to the viewer that can motivate and encourage. The series is not prescriptive but rather helps people come to their own insights and stimulates rich dialogues. Because *Unnatural Causes* ties the patterning of health outcomes to social and institutional structures (what Michael Marmot calls "the cause of the causes"), it enables a broader discussion of society, its power arrangements, politics, values, and possibilities for change.

But users also need to undertake a thorough planning process to optimize the impact of *Unnatural Causes* since most have little experience integrating documentaries effectively into their work. Many organizations ask us what they should do, what next steps they should advocate. We resist answering this question for several reasons. One, we do not know. But even if we did, we believe organizations will be more successful if they perform their own assessment to determine what kind of event is most desirable and realistic given their own capacity, allies, and local situation. Instead, we suggest that people use the Action Tool kit on the *Unnatural Causes* Web site that walks them through an event planning process, from self-assessment and objective setting all the way to next steps.

We have noticed one or more of the following missteps are common to screenings that fall short of their promise. First, many organizations began using *Unnatural Causes* externally before they have transformed their own practice and developed the expertise and commitment to health equity among both leadership and staff.

Second, they do not articulate one or two simple and clear objectives for the screening event, let alone integrate it into a larger organizational health equity strategy; instead, they too often try to accomplish too many things at once, precluding deeper, more directed conversations directed toward a specific end.

Third, government agencies sometimes invite communities and the general public to attend events but do not involve them or their representatives in the planning or as panel participants. Or if they do, they do not yet have an understanding of health grounded in social determinants.

And fourth, organizations fail to identify action opportunities that can inspire participants, resonate with their interests and capacity, and offer specific ways for the audience to get involved. It is important to gather and communicate possibilities and solutions, both short and long term, not just health threats. At the end of every screening, the big issue is always: what can we do? Without event organizers thinking through and suggesting specific follow-up "asks" or next steps ahead of time, audiences can easily feel overwhelmed by the scale of the problem. The screening then becomes a onetime event rather than a step toward further involvement and momentum is lost.

On the other hand, many groups are impatient. They want to take action that can "fix" health inequities now. But tackling health inequities is not a matter of a new program or service. It is deeply implicated in the class and racial structures that disempower communities and generate inequalities, especially the deregulation and corruption of the democratic process that disproportionately channel resources, power, and wealth to corporate interests at the expense of working people and the poor.

Building a movement able to advocate effectively for the social changes needed to achieve health equity is a long-term struggle. Media like *Unnatural Causes* are no substitute for that movement. But media can help prepare the groundwork for such a movement by telling a new story that reframes the way health is perceived and discussed.

Used properly, *Unnatural Causes* can help build a corps of committed organizations who ask not just what individuals can do to be healthy, but how they can build the foundations for health communities. It can help engage thousands of people in the challenge of organizing communities and building alliances to create neighborhoods, schools, workplaces and economies that promote good health. It can help people understand that tackling health inequities is not just about healthy behaviors but unavoidably a public matter of politics, of people working with their neighbors and coworkers and engaging in struggles over how government allocates resources, regulates corporate power and implements the principles of democracy. Most of all, *Unnatural Causes* can help people spread that message and inspire action.

We each are responsible for making healthy choices, of course. But the social dimension and responsibility for the health of our communities is a story long hidden from view. But if the movement that is building around the country is any indication, it will not be for long.

Notes

1. *Kaiser Family Foundation Health Poll Report Survey*, conducted June 2–5, 2005, published July 18, 2005 (http://www.kff.org/kaiserpolls/pomr071805oth.cfm).
2. As of this writing, California Newsreel is developing a survey instrument and evaluation of the impact of Unnatural Causes. The results will be posted on www.unnaturalcauses.org

3. *Race-The Power of an Illusion,* 3 x by 56 minutes, DVD, California Newsreel: 2003 (www.pbs.org/Race).
4. Michael Marmot's book *The Status Syndrome* (New York: Henry Holt, 2004) had just been published but received little press or promotion in the United States. Some attention was being paid to *racial* disparities in health, thanks to the Institute of Medicine's 2002 report *Unequal Treatment: Confronting Racial and Ethnic Disparities in Health Care,* books by Thomas LeVeist and others, and the U.S. Department of Health and Human Services *Healthy People 2010* objectives. But much of the work remained focused on issues of access and treatment in health care rather than the production of health and illness in the first place.
5. See especially Axel Aubrun, Andrew Brown, and Joseph Grady, "External Factors vs. Right Choices: Findings from Cognitive Elicitations and Media Analysis on Health Disparities and Inequities in Louisville, Kentucky," *Cultural Logic* (May, 2007); Lori Dorfman, Lawrence Wallack, and Katie Woodruff, "More Than a Message: Framing Public Health Advocacy," in *Prevention is Primary,* ed. Larry Cohen, Vivian Chavez, and Sana Chehimi (San Francisco, CA: John Wiley & Sons, 2007) 121–138; Joseph Grady and Axel Aubrun, "Provoking Thought, Changing Talk: Discussing Inequality," and Lori Dorfman and Lawrence Wallack, "Provoking Thought, Changing Talk: Putting it into Practice," in *You Can Get There from Here,* The Social Equity and Opportunity Forum of The College of Urban and Public Affairs, Portland State University, April 2007 (*www.bmsg.org/documents/TalkingInequality-1.pdf*).
6. The Health Policy Institute of the Joint Center for Political and Economic Studies (www.jointcenter.org) was launching a seven-pronged Fair Health movement with social determinants at its core, including a national "Place Matters" initiative. The National Association of County and City Health Officials (NACCHO; www.naccho.org) already had commissioned a health equity and social justice advisory group, developed a social justice framework for public health practice, and had just published the first edition of this book. The Praxis Project (www.thepraxisproject.org) was training community-based organizations to advocate effectively for health equity. PolicyLink (www. policylink.org) had just initiated a health and place project, complementing the work of the Prevention Institute (www.preventioninstitute.org). The MacArthur Network on Socio-Economic Status and Health (*www.macses.ucsf. edu/*) was beginning work on a handbook summing up the research on the social determinants of health (published in 2007 as *Reaching for a Healthier Life*). Paula Braveman, director of the Center on Social Disparities on Health at the University of California, San Francisco (familymedicine.medschool. ucsf.edu/csdh/), had been lobbying for a decade to win support for a national commission that would sum up the research on health equity and make national policy recommendations, not unlike the Black and Acheson reports in the United Kingdom. And Michael Marmot had just convened the WHO Commission on the Social Determinants of Health. The Spirit of 1848 listserv shared health justice news and information among scholars and practitioners around the country, while York University, Canada's SDOH listserv had many American subscribers. Several universities and public health departments were increasingly focusing on the social determinants of health inequities while the W.K. Kellogg Foundation had been funding fellows in health disparities.

7. The meeting with coexecutive producer Llew Smith and the author was hosted by Brian Smedley, then policy director of Opportunity Agenda, and Barbara Krimgold of the Center for the Advancement of Health, and also attended by Richard Hofrichter, senior policy analyst, NACCHO; Makani Themba-Nixon, executive director, The Praxis Project; Gwen McKinney, president, McKinney & Associates; and Dora Hughes, then the legislative health aide to Senator Edward Kennedy. Later we also met with Gail Christopher, DN, then director of the Health Policy Institute of the Joint Center for Political and Economic Studies.

8. Scholarly Advisors: Dolores Acevedo-Garcia, Harvard University School of Public Health; Nancy Adler, Chair, MacArthur Network on Socio-Economic Status and Health and Director, Center for Health and Community, University of California, San Francisco; Paula Braveman, MD, Director, Center on Social Disparities in Health, University of California, San Francisco; Gail Christopher, DN, then Director, Health Policy Institute, Joint Center for Political and Economic Studies; Troy Duster, Professor Sociology, New York University and former President, American Sociological Association; Camara Jones, MD, Research Director, Social Determinants of Health, Centers for Disease Control (CDC); Ichiro Kawachi, MD, Harvard School of Public Health; Nancy Krieger; Harvard School of Public Health; Brian Smedley, then Project Director, Opportunity Agenda; S. Leonard Syme, Professor of Epidemiology (Emeritus), School of Public Health, University of California-Berkeley; Makani Themba-Nixon, Executive Director, The Praxis Project; David Williams, Norman Professor of Public Health, Harvard School of Public Health. The members of the MacArthur Network on Socio-Economic Status and Health were also wonderfully generous with their time and counsel.

9. Outreach Advisors: Georges Benjamin, MD, Executive Director, American Public Health Association; Gail Christopher, then Director, Health Policy Institute of the Joint Center for Political and Economic Studies; Makani Themba-Nixon, Executive Director, The Praxis Project, and Richard Hofrichter, senior analyst, health equity, NACCHO. It is no exaggeration to say that without the help of our scholarly and outreach advisors, this project would never have gotten off the ground. We cannot thank them enough.

10. Llew Smith served as coexecutive producer and series producer and helped develop the project with the author. Christine Herbes-Sommers served as series senior producer. For a complete list of production credits, go to www.unnaturalcauses.org.

11. Production funding was generously provided by the Ford Foundation; National Minority Consortia of Public Television; John D. and Catherine T. MacArthur Foundation; W.K. Kellogg Foundation; the California Endowment; Joint Center for Political and Economic Studies Health Policy Institute; Kaiser Permanente; Nathan Cummings Foundation; Annie E. Casey Foundation; Akonadi Foundation, the Falk Fund, and the Wallace A. Gerbode Foundation. Additional public engagement and outreach funding was provided by the Robert Wood Johnson Foundation, the W.K. Kellogg Foundation, the California Endowment, the Open Society Fund, and the Akonadi Foundation.

12. Rachel Poulain, MPH, served as Director of Outreach and led this effort.

13. More than 6,000 DVDs had been distributed to organizations by California Newsreel as of August 25, 2008.

26

Talking about Public Health: Developing America's "Second Language"

LAWRENCE WALLACK AND REGINA G. LAWRENCE

In their classic analysis of American culture, *Habits of the Heart*, Robert Bellah and his colleagues[1] argued that the first "language" of American life is individualism. This is a language centered on the values of freedom, self-determination, self-discipline, personal responsibility, and limited government. The language of individualism is easy for most Americans to use, because it taps into values reinforced by dominant societal myths endlessly repeated in the popular culture. But although it may be this country's first language, individualism is not a sufficient language for advancing public health. Bellah and his colleagues also identified a second language in US culture—a language of interconnectedness. This is a language of egalitarian and humanitarian values, of interdependence and community. We have drawn on literature from the fields of sociology and political science as well as from public health to suggest how that second language could be more clearly articulated in order to talk more effectively to the general public, journalists, and policymakers about public health. By *public health* we refer in a broad sense to the question of how a society balances considerations of personal responsibility and social accountability in public

This chapter is reprinted with permission from *American Journal of Public Health* 95(2005): 567–70. Copyright 2005 American Public Health Association.

policies that impact health. *Public health* focuses on the *health of popula-tions*. But despite wide agreement among public health professionals on that general approach, what it *means* to focus on the health of popula-tions is not necessarily well defined.

A substantial body of theoretical and empirical work shows that the state of the public's health unavoidably reflects systemic forces as well as individual behaviors. Indeed, "a key class of determinants of health is the full set of macrosocio-economic and cultural factors that operate at the societal level,"[2] necessitating interventions that span the many levels of the society in which any given health problem exists.[3,4] Ironically, many professionals in the field of public health believe in the importance of social determinants of health yet routinely rely on strategies that largely ignore social determinants in favor of individual, behavioral approaches to improving health. Although this disconnect between public health theory and practice has several sources, including the structural and philosophi-cal limitations of conventional public health,[5] a significant cause is the fact that a language to properly express the unique public health approach has not been adequately developed.

The lack of a well-developed language for talking about public health has serious consequences that extend beyond how public health profes-sionals spend their working hours. Public policies that reflect the disciplin-ary theory of public health remain difficult to enact in the United States. Egalitarianism, humanitarianism, and social responsibility—values that lie at the core of a social justice orientation to public health[6,7]—often seem inadequate to respond effectively to the moral resonance of individualism. Yet in a culture preoccupied with personal responsibility and suspicious of governmental power, it is imperative for the public health profession to tap into these countervailing values in order to become more effec-tive advocates for the public health approach to the nation's many health challenges.

Values and Public Health in the United States

Although it is useful to analyze cultures in terms of their dominant beliefs, cultures of developed societies typically exhibit multiple value systems, with various subgroups weighting those values differently.[8] Despite the well-documented prominence of individualism in US culture,[9-11] equality, compassion, community, and social responsibility have, throughout US his-tory, motivated people, particularly marginalized groups, to act collectively to address social problems.[12,13] Although support for egalitarian values is more limited in the United States than in many other Western democracies, and the term *welfare* is highly unpopular,[14] many Americans nevertheless believe that government and society have a responsibility to ensure that the opportunities to build a successful life be enjoyed roughly equally by all—beliefs that, research shows, are rooted in humanitarian values.[15-17]

Empirical research also suggests, however, that most Americans do not articulate these values nearly as easily as they use the language of individualism. For example, when researchers asked members of the public to explain their support for or opposition to social welfare policies, they found that those who opposed such policies did so in terms of abstract principles like personal responsibility and limited government. But the abstract principles of equality, fairness, and compassion that underlie social welfare policies were not readily articulated even by supporters of those policies.[18] In other words, these people knew that they supported these policies, but they couldn't easily explain why.

And therein lies the rub: these values of equality, fairness, and compassion are closely associated with public health. One of the most visible definitions of public health is "the process of assuring the conditions in which people can be healthy."[19] In the context of public health, each element of that definition—process, assuring, conditions—evokes values beyond individualism. Yet the predominance of the first language of individualism makes the mission of public health often seem somewhat alien to the general public, as well as policymakers, journalists, and other elites. For example, public health focuses on "conditions" that make *populations* more or less healthy, which shifts both the causal explanation of public health problems and their potential solutions away from a sole focus on individual choice. These are relatively complicated explanations compared with the simple ones generated by the more reductionist language of individualism.

Take the example of obesity: it is much simpler to believe that people are obese because they eat too much and don't exercise enough. News coverage has framed the issue predominantly in terms of personal responsibility, the frame also favored by those who oppose policy changes such as eliminating junk food from schools and requiring better food labeling. Although the balance of public discourse now seems to be shifting, until recently most news coverage did not convey the idea that people are also obese because our society is organized in a way that encourages overconsumption of fat-laden, high-calorie food (through advertising, marketing, and an economic system requiring 2 wage earners) and limits outlets for physical activity (for example, by elimination of physical education in schools and heavy reliance on automobiles).[20] In the first language, the point that people need more self-discipline simply needs to be asserted and its assumptions (e.g., personal responsibility) are intuitively grasped and expected conclusions reached. In the second language, the point that society needs to be organized in a healthier way must be explained, because the assumptions (e.g., social accountability, shared responsibility) are not easily grasped and the conclusion needs to be argued. As cognitive linguist George Lakoff has revealed, the metaphors underlying the language of individualism form a coherent and compelling package rooted in widely accepted moral values.[21] The political virtues of limited government and personal responsibility correspond, at a subconscious level, with many Americans' mental model of personal morality in which self-reliance is a moral obligation. Government policies that interfere with the mechanisms of personal responsibility and self-discipline are therefore seen, in a sense, as immoral. Thus, a predominant belief is that "people should accept the consequences of their own irresponsibility or lack of self-discipline, since they will never become responsible and self-disciplined if they don't have to face those consequences."[21] When seen through this lens, many social welfare and public health policies look like wrongheaded efforts to "protect people from themselves," thus (immorally) undermining self-discipline.

Consequently, the language of public health seems foreign ("Sounds like central planning— didn't they fail at that in the old Soviet Union?"), and its paternalistic objectives and methods for protecting the health of populations (government as national nanny) can be difficult to support. Even the public health data amassed over the years that demonstrate empirically the relation between social inequality and health inequality[22-25] can be hard for the public to understand, in part because the predominant moral framework makes it easier for people to imagine what one person might or might not do to be healthy compared with what society might collectively do to ensure health for the population. Thus, individualism, as the "dominant orientation in the United States…profoundly restricts the content of public health programs."[5]

Developing the Language of Interconnection

As Dan Beauchamp,[6] Ann Robertson,[7] and others have noted, the moral framework underlying the public health approach differs from the predominant moral framework of individualism. Robertson argued that health promotion "represents a moral/ethical enterprise" and that the language of public health is essentially "a moral discourse that links health promotion to the pursuit of the *common* good" (emphasis added).[7] Focusing on the health of populations inevitably raises questions about the health effects of how society is organized—questions difficult to raise in a public discourse suffused with individualism.

Perhaps intuitively recognizing this difficulty, many public health advocates tend to fall back on a language of service provision and behavior change—clear, concrete, easily understandable approaches. But that strategy reinforces the first language of individualism by emphasizing a risk factor approach that leads to a discourse about behavioral strategies and treatments for existing conditions.[5]

Discussion of social, political, and economic context is often only cursory. When these contextual issues—the more complicated story of public health—are not discussed, their importance is implicitly diminished and efforts to improve the health of populations are weakened. To advance public health with the necessary comprehension and urgency requires articulating an overarching value that we call *interconnection*. Interconnection is not a new idea. It invokes long-held ideals associated with the words *public, social,* and *community.* Indeed, as Dan Beauchamp argued nearly 20 years ago, the practice of public health is premised on a "group principle" that "has tended to be subordinated to the language of individual rights." But "public health as a second language," he wrote, "reminds us that we are not only individuals, we are also a community and a body politic, and that we have shared commitments to one another and promises to keep."[26] Echoing Beauchamp, Robertson[7] called for the development of a "moral economy of interdependence" in which beliefs about justice and need are informed by a sense of mutual obligation that "acknowledges our fundamental interdependence."[7] Various contemporary thinkers have also begun to develop this language of interconnection.

Lakoff,[21] for example, envisioned a language of "cultivated interdependence" in which those who have been nurtured accept a corresponding responsibility to nurture others. Political theorist Mary Ann Glendon[27] argued for challenging the notion of the "self-determining, unencumbered individual, a being connected to others only by choice."[27] And political theorist Joan Tronto[28] argued for developing an "ethic of care" that would recognize that "humans are not fully autonomous, but must always be understood in a condition of interdependence."[28] She argued, "The moral question an ethic of care takes as central is not—What, if anything, do I (we) owe to others? But rather—How can I (we) best meet my (our) caring responsibilities?"[29] Underlying all these visions is the belief that human existence is as much social as individual and that individual well-being depends to a significant degree on caring and equitable social relationships. Recognizing human interconnection broadens the moral focus of individual responsibility for one's self and family to include shared responsibility for societal conditions.

Without the glue of interconnection, in fact, egalitarian and humanitarian ideals can lack moral heft. Robertson,[7] for example, based her proposed language of public health on the recognition of need. But to be effective in advancing public health, the notion of need must (as Robertson also suggested) be couched in terms of *shared* needs and reciprocity. It is less compelling to argue that autonomous individuals "should" help one another than to argue that our individual well-being is inescapably a product of the quality of our social relationships.[28]

There are instances in which public health professionals have effectively articulated this language of community to enhance population health. One example is the "reframing" of violence from being seen primarily as a criminal justice issue to being seen as a public health issue. For instance, over a 10-year period in California, the Violence Prevention Initiative engaged in a comprehensive, $70 million campaign to reduce the toll of handgun violence on youths. By highlighting the fact that handguns were the number 1 killer of young people in the state, emphasizing the role of social conditions in violence against youths, advancing specific public policies to reduce gun availability and increase violence prevention, and mobilizing citizen involvement to change "What's Killing Our Kids," the Violence Prevention Initiative helped to pass more than 300 local ordinances in 100 cities and counties and a dozen statewide laws limiting gun availability—and to secure an unprecedented increase in state-funded violence prevention efforts.[30,31] A significant factor in the campaign's success was the resonance of its underlying *moral* messages: gun violence is not just the fault of young people's behavior, but of social arrangements created by adults, and adults have a shared obligation to improve these arrangements for the benefit of all. When young people are killing young people, the campaign argued, it's everyone's problem, and the appropriate response stems from compassion for young people rather than the fear-based, punitive approach of tougher criminal penalties.

There are also signs that Americans' understanding of interconnection is evolving in other policy areas in ways that may be of help to public health advocates. For example, many Americans use a cultural model of interdependency[31] to think and talk about the environment, a belief that species within ecosystems are interrelated and mutually dependent such that disturbances to one species will likely affect others. This model, which is now "widespread and thoroughly integrated into American culture," draws on "core American values" that include a sense of obligation to our descendants.[32] It may provide resources for thinking about human interdependence as well. Globalization may also be forcing Americans to come to grips with the reality of human interconnectedness. From the increased recognition that our inexpensive consumer goods may be produced by children working in foreign sweat shops to the new reality of diseases such as severe acute respiratory syndrome (SARS) that travel quickly around the globe, Americans may be less inclined to see

their country as an island. Yet recognizing the pragmatic reality of interconnection does not necessarily lead to accepting the normative value of interconnection, a fact also exemplified in the public panic surrounding SARS
and other communicable diseases. A challenge for public health advocates is
to capitalize on increasing understanding of the interconnectedness of global
health without simply fanning xenophobizc fears.

Conclusion

Developing the language of interconnection is crucial because once the
moral focus is broadened, the definition of and response to public health
problems can expand. As a moral and conceptual lens on the world, individualism restricts the range of public understanding, oversimplifying
complex and multifaceted problems, boiling them down to their individual
roots while leaving social responsibility and collective action largely out of
the picture. Although personal responsibility is undeniably a key to health,
so are a range of social conditions that are shaped not just by our individual choices, but by our collective choices manifest in public policy.

Accepting C. Wright Mill's challenge to "continually...translate personal
troubles into public issues,"[33] public health advocates can help the public
to see the causal connections between their own well-being and that of others. All humans have needs that others must help them to meet, especially
in the complex social, economic, and political systems of today. A society
that accepts the reality of human interconnection and effectively structures
itself so that egalitarian and humanitarian values are more fully reflected
in public policy will be a society that better understands the meaning of
public health and responds more appropriately to its challenges. It will be
a society that not only talks about community but translates its values into
caring—and more effective—public policy.

Work on this article was partly supported by a Robert Wood Johnson
Foundation Innovator's Award to Lawrence Wallack. Also, the authors
express their appreciation to Dan Beauchamp and to Richard Hofrichter,
who reviewed an early version of this article and provided important guidance, and to the anonymous reviewers.

Notes

1. R.N. Bellah, R. Madsen, W.M. Sullivan, A. Swidler, and S.M. Tipton, *Habits of
the Heart*. 2nd ed. (Berkeley, CA: University of California Press, 1996).
2. J.W. Frank, "The Determinants of Health: a New Synthesis," 1 *Current Issues
in Public Health* (1995): 233.

3. Institute of Medicine, *Promoting Health* (Washington, DC: National Academy Press, 2000).
4. J.B. McKinlay, "The Promotion of Health through Planned Sociopolitical Change: Challenges for Research and Policy," 36 *Social Science & Medicine* (1993): 109–117.
5. J.B. McKinlay and L. Marceau, "To Boldly Go," 90 *Am J Public Health* (2000): 25.
6. D.E. Beauchamp, "Public Health as Social Justice," 12 *Inquiry* (1976): 3–14.
7. A. Robertson, "Health Promotion and the Common Good: Theoretical Considerations," 9(2) *Critical Public Health* (1999): 124.
8. T. Michael, R. Ellis, and A. Wildavsky, *Cultural Theory* (Boulder, CO: Westview Press, 1990).
9. J.W. Kingdon, *America the Unusual* (Boston, MA: Worth Publishers, 1999).
10. S.M. Lipset, *Continental Divide* (New York: Routledge, 1991).
11. S. Feldman, "Structure and Consistency in Public Opinion: the Role of Core Beliefs and Values." 32 *American Journal of Political Science* (1988): 416–440.
12. G. Wood, *The Radicalism of the American Revolution* (New York: Alfred A. Knopf, 1992).
13. V. Sapiro, "The Gender Basis of American Social Policy," 101(2) *Political Science Quarterly* (1986): 221–238.
14. R.K. Weaver, R.Y. Shapiro, and L.R. Jacobs, "The Polls—Trends: Welfare," 59 *Public Opinion* (1995): 606–627.
15. *Fighting Poverty in America: A Study of American Public Attitudes* (Washington, DC: Center for the Study of Policy Attitudes, 1994).
16. *The Values We Live By: What Americans Want From Welfare Reform* (New York: Public Agenda, 1996).
17. S. Feldman and M.R. Steenburgen, "The Humanitarian Foundation of Public Support for Social Welfare," 45 *American Journal of Political Science* (2001): 658–677.
18. S. Feldman and J. Zaller, "The Political Culture of Ambivalence: Ideological Responses to the Welfare State," 36 *American Journal of Political Sciencei* (1992): 268–307.
19. Institute of Medicine, *The Future of Public Health* (Washington, DC: National Academy Press; 1988).
20. R.G. Lawrence, "Framing Obesity: the Evolution of Public Discourse on a Public Health Issue," 9(3) *Harvard International Journal of Press Politics* (2004): 56–75.
21. G. Lakoff, *Moral Politics: What Conservatives Know that Liberals Don't* (Chicago, IL: University of Chicago Press, 1996): 97.
22. M. Marmot and R.G. Wilkinson, *Social Determinants of Health* (Oxford: Oxford University Press, 1999).
23. I. Kawachi, B.P. Kennedy, and R.G. Wilkinson, *The Society and Population Health Reader: Income Inequality and Health*, Vol. 1 (New York: The New Press, 1999).
24. R. Wilkinson, *Unhealthy Societies: The Afflictions of Inequality* (New York: Routledge, 1996).
25. J.A. Auerbach and B.K. Krimgold, eds., *Income, Socioeconomic Status, and Health: Exploring the Relationships* (Washington, DC: National Policy Association, Academy for Health Services Research and Health Policy, 2001).

26. D. Beauchamp, "Community: the Neglected Tradition of Public Health," *The Hastings Center Report* (December 1985): 34.
27. M.A. Glendon, *Rights Talk: The Impoverishment of Public Discourse* (New York: Free Press, 1991): 12.
28. J. Tronto, *Moral Boundaries: A Political Argument for an Ethic of Care* (New York: Routledge, 1993): 162.
29. J. Tronto, *Moral Boundaries: A Political Argument for an Ethic of Care* (New York: Routledge, 1993): 137.
30. L. Wallack, "The California Violence Prevention Initiative: Advancing Policy to Ban Saturday Night Specials," 26 *Health Education & Behavior* (1999): 841–857.
31. L. Wallack, A. Lee, and L. Winett, "A Decade of Effort, a World of Difference: the Policy and Public Education Program of the California Youth Violence Prevention Initiative," *Report to The California Wellness Foundation* (Woodland Hills, CA: California Wellness Foundation, 2003).
32. W. Kempton, J.S. Boster, and J. Hartley, *Environmental Values in American Culture* (Cambridge, MA: MIT Press, 1999): 61.
33. C.W. Mills, *The Sociological Imagination* (New York: Oxford University Press, 1959): 187.

27

Helping Public Health Matter: Strategies for Building Public Awareness

MAKANI THEMBA-NIXON

Public health. Sounds benign enough. Two good words brought together to describe how government and nonprofit agencies work together to ensure our safety and well-being. And, polling data show that, once people understand what services live behind the term, public health enjoys strong public support.

A 2004 poll by Research!America and the American Public Health Association revealed that nearly three-quarters of respondents believe that their communities benefit from public health services and more than half knew someone who works in the public health field. Those numbers shot up even higher when respondents were asked if they benefited from specific services, such as child immunization programs, restaurant inspections, or sexual assault hotlines.

Yet, when asked to rank public health related research among other national priorities, including homeland security, education, and job creation, the ranking drops much lower to the bottom half of respondents. In polling overall, even fewer people express support for raising the public revenues required to sustain these services.

Given the political realities of shrinking resources and competing budgets, public health workers can no longer ignore the fact that we need to communicate with our public about what we do, why it matters, and why it deserves serious investment.

Beyond Scare Tactics

Two primary misconceptions operate in public health communications. *Misconception 1: Most people don't know nearly as much as we do.* Effective communication begins with a clear understanding of how much the people we are talking to know and the many nontraditional ways they know it. An effective message speaks to people in their own idiom, their most familiar, even intimate way of speaking. It requires a healthy respect and understanding of the incredible experience our "audience" brings to bear. Knowing this requires that we listen at least twice as often as we speak.

Misconception 2: We must communicate more information on "the problem." The more they see how bad it is, the more likely they are to act. People are rarely scared into action. Most of us are fairly jaded by now and have already assumed the worst. So it is no surprise that the media effects research confirms that it is practical information on what they can do about an issue versus the severity of a problem that moves us. Not that we do not need to communicate that our issue is a serious one—we do. We must make sure that we do not leave it at that. Besides, oftentimes our audience already knows that the problem is serious before we begin.

Bottom-line. *Talking about the problem is much less important than offering understandable solutions.* Or put another way, concrete action is more important than education though both are necessary.

Good messages are affective (they touch us emotionally), effective (they convey what we need to understand), and connect with shared dreams and beliefs. They cause to surface, what James Scott called in his seminal book *Domination and the Arts of Resistance,* the **hidden transcript**. This hidden transcript constitutes the private conversations most of us have about the injustice, the unfairness of those in power; about the "right thing" we ought to do but feel too difficult to undertake on our own; and even that which we fear. People are more willing to act in circumstances when that hidden transcript is unearthed and they can see that it is widely shared, that they constitute the majority; that they are not alone. It is like someone else saying out loud what you were thinking all along. Of course, this shared recognition requires that a message—a galvanizing one—be grounded in the language and idiom and even the dreams of our target audience. So how do we begin? With good listening skills and lots of planning.

Effective Media Planning

Developing a communications plan requires attention to strategic planning. Although it is clear that time is tight and there is so much to do, staff and management input into this process—beyond the person tasked with day-to-day communications—is important. Staff investment in the process up front helps create clarity and confidence down the line.

Set clear goals. What are you trying to accomplish? What outlets are you trying to reach? This is the most important step in preparing for media advocacy because it will define what you communicate about and to whom you will be communicating. Identifying goals require an honest assessment of your program's strengths and weaknesses, the political climate, and thorough research of the available options.

Know who you are talking to. Most media advocacy is focused on policymakers because it is often policymakers who have the power to enact the desired change. In some cases, groups use media advocacy to mobilize supporters as a preliminary step in targeting policymakers. It is important to note that although media can support efforts to build a base of support, one cannot build a broad base of support for their issue using media alone. That is why most groups shape their media strategy to target policymakers and support their base building goals and incorporate community organizing strategies (i.e., canvassing, phoning, coalition building, etc.) into their overall plan.

Spend time researching how your "targets" get their information. Most elected officials and other gatekeepers read the editorial pages of local newspapers to gauge community concerns. Television news and radio talk shows also help set the public agenda and affect the "public conversation" on a particular issue. In any case, knowing the target will help you shape a more effective and efficient strategy.

Know what you're saying. Now you are ready to take the final step in preparation: developing a message. A message is not a soundbite or a slogan (although it can help shape them). It is the overarching theme that neatly frames your initiative for your target audience. Messages should be relatively short, easy to understand, emotive, and visual. The message should reflect the hard work and research that went into developing the initiative and should be supportive of the overall strategy.

It is best to *test messages on friends and coworkers*—especially those who are not familiar with your issue. Colleagues who work on similar issues are another good resource. Listen carefully to feedback: Did the message convey the importance of your issue? Did they "get" it? Keeping your target in mind, use the input to help shape and refine your message.

Facing the Budget Monster

Perhaps the toughest communication task is selling the public on funding—especially when our programs are on the chopping block. We begin by translating the issue from abstract cuts into human *stories*. What are the compelling stories behind the budget negotiations? Here are some places to start looking (see Table 27.1).

TABLE 27.1. Questions for Budget Story Themes

POTENTIAL BUDGET STORY THEMES	WHERE TO BEGIN
Raising new revenues	How long has it been since new revenues were raised? How much do these revenues really amount to when you control for inflation? What are some of the good proposals? Any recent tax cuts causing problems?
Pulling open the budget curtain	What is the real process? Who has influence?
Health and health care threats and losses	What is at stake? Who will be hurt? What cuts have broad impact if only the public knew?
Cessation and treatment makes a difference	A grandma who was finally able to quit smoking. A cancer survivor receiving program support. In what ways is our work making a difference?
Youth programs and interventions that changed lives	Are young people learning important lessons of democracy and activism? Better indicators for youth health and well-being? Let the public know.
Losing community resources	Are there losses and threats beyond health? Jobs? Buildings? Parks? Tally it up and tell the stories.
Who is on the frontlines	Who is hit the hardest by the cuts? Who is protected? If your state is like most, children, women, people of color, and seniors will be hurt the most. Look for disparate impact, bias, and unfairness in losses and benefits.
Making the case for developing public and nonprofit sectors as a vital part of the economy	Cutting public and nonprofit jobs hurts the economy even more than losing private sector (especially service) jobs. With budget cuts, you lose important higher wage jobs with benefits and local spending power. *What's the percentage of public and nonprofit jobs in your state, city or county?* In many states, about one in five jobs is created in the public or nonprofit sector. In some states, it's closer to one in four. Reporters need to understand that these jobs and programs are not mere fiscal "pork, but important engines of the state economy.

Developing Media Infrastructure

Translate all of the great data into even more compelling stories. Start by identifying and compiling a list of the right spokespeople. Who is the best person to deliver the message to which audience? Consider the breadth and diversity of communities affected. What are your opponents saying? Devise strong counter images and messages.

Identify a broad range of outlets through which to tell your stories, including media in languages other than English. Be sure to have spokespeople who can communicate in other languages as appropriate. These audiences are key potential supporters.

Make time to practice delivering messages so that everyone is comfortable and stays "on message," and that no one gets offtrack or says anything to contradict what you are trying to communicate. Role-play interviews and tough questions. Practice responding with your message without getting distracted. Remember when reviewing that you are communicating *with your target audiences*. The reporter is a conduit. Speak accordingly.

Avoid holding press conferences unless you are sure to attract press. When possible, look for other newsworthy events on which you can piggyback. Instead, work to cultivate reporters who are already covering your issues through one-on-one meetings and phone calls, and sending well-packaged, concise information with contact information for spokespeople. When packaging information, think of the data, spokespeople, and other information that reporters will need to do a good job covering the issue.

Public health professionals have great stories and even greater motivation to tell them because our success depends upon an informed public. With some attention to planning, story development, and audience, we can develop the media outreach mechanisms necessary to build greater awareness and support for this vitally important work.

28

The Ethics of the Medical Model in Addressing the Root Causes of Health Disparities in Local Public Health Practice

ANTHONY B. ITON

The Challenge of Eliminating Health Disparities

The second goal of Healthy People 2010 is to "eliminate health disparities among segments of the population, including differences that occur by gender, race or ethnicity, education or income, disability, geographic location, or sexual orientation."[1] Although eliminating health disparities is not listed as one of HHS Secretary Mike Leavitt's current HHS priorities, Secretary Leavitt has said that eliminating health disparities as they affect racial, ethnic, and underserved populations is a "critical goal" of HHS.[2] US Centers for Disease Control and Prevention Director, Dr Julie Gerberding, looks forward to the day that eliminating health disparities will become "part of the backbone and the culture of CDC" rather than a separate activity.[3]

Despite the apparently high priority that the elimination of health disparities receives in the public pronouncements of our nation's federal public health leaders, the public health strategies and practices that would operate to eliminate health disparities appear to be lacking. Quantitative research indicates that an estimated 83,570 excess deaths *each year* could be prevented in the United States if the black–white mortality gap could be eliminated.[4] However, HHS's Healthy People 2010 midcourse review indicates that there has been no overall progress in the nation regarding the second goal of eliminating health disparities.[5] Bottom line, health disparities are worsening. So there appears to be a large gulf between the stated goals of our national public health institutions and the presence of successful public health policies, strategies, and practices to eliminate health disparities.

The failure to develop an appropriate and responsive *public health practice* is the focus of this chapter. It is not an effort to reassert the scientific link between the physical and social environment and population health outcomes, and specifically the contribution of social, political, and economic policies to persistent and large health disparities. The evidentiary support for this linkage has been resoundingly demonstrated in decades of epidemiological, health services, and social science research, as well as in the recently released PBS documentary *Unnatural Causes*. Instead, I argue that public health practitioners (federal, state, and local) have failed to develop a focused, consistent, and comprehensive *public health practice* that is informed by and incorporates the abundant research evidence of the profound contribution of the social, economic, and physical environments to population health outcomes and health disparities. Given the clear tenets of the Public Health Code of Ethics, and the nation's stated commitment to eliminate health disparities, the commentary raises the question of whether current US public health practice is in fact ethical.

Public Health Code of Ethics

Public Health has a code of ethics. There are several principles of the Public Health Code of Ethics that directly inform public health practice strategies for the elimination of health disparities. The public health code of ethics says that

- public health should address principally the fundamental causes of disease and requirements for health, aiming to prevent adverse health outcomes (principle 1);
- public health should advocate and work for the empowerment of disenfranchised community members, aiming to ensure that the basic resources and conditions necessary for health are accessible to all (principle 4); and
- public health programs and policies should be implemented in a manner that most enhances the physical and social environment (principle 9).

How Does Our Public Health Practice Conform to the Dictates of This Challenge?

The backbone of US public health system is that of a governmental enterprise with federal, state, and local components. While one can easily define the public health system in the United States as consisting of a much broader array of nongovernmental entities, both nonprofit and for profit in addition to the federal-state-local governmental enterprise, it should at least follow logically that if the federal government sets a goal such as those laid out in Healthy People 2010, the public health governmental enterprise must be expected to work toward achieving that goal.

Definitions of public health practice are few and, in general, quite nonspecific. One useful definition of public health practice is: "the strategic, organized, and interdisciplinary application of knowledge, skills, and competencies necessary to perform essential public health services and other activities to improve the population's health."[6] (p 8) To understand what constitutes US public health practice, one would presumably look for federal, state, and local governmental public health activities that are widespread across states and territories, have realistic per-capita funding, and commonly accepted as effective, or ideally, evidence based. The practice of governmental public health in the United States is varied by virtue of the organizational and jurisdictional heterogeneity associated with what is constitutionally a state-led and driven function.

Nevertheless, when the federal government establishes a health priority through a combination of funding incentives and mandates, it can greatly influence and direct governmental public health practice in all of the 50 states and 3000 or so local health departments at the county, city, and district levels throughout the country.

In general, federal public health practice priorities can be categorized into four broad groupings: (1) specific communicable diseases (e.g., sexually transmitted diseases, tuberculosis, and HIV/AIDS), (2) vulnerable populations (i.e., maternal, child, and adolescent health), (3) critical healthcare services (e.g., childhood and adult immunizations, healthcare for the homeless), and (4) issues of national security (e.g., bioterrorism preparedness, pandemic influenza). Consequently, most state and local public health departments have developed corresponding practices in these areas.

One of the common characteristics of these core public health practice areas is that they are generally disease-specific and "categorical" in that they are not structured in a way that facilitates an examination of root causes that may be shared by several diseases.

The Medical Model

A disturbingly high proportion of state and federal grant-funded public health programs, including those designed to eliminate health disparities, are deeply rooted in the so-called medical model. Simply stated, the medical model posits that differential rates of disease and death between groups are primarily explained by differences in clinical risk factors, and risk behaviors, including healthcare seeking behaviors, among different population groups. The medical model focuses most heavily on certain proximate causes of morbidity and mortality, including genetics, healthcare access and quality, and individual behavior change strategies and health knowledge. As the medical model is focused primarily on individual behaviors and risks, it is most easily applicable to situations in which health disparities are narrowly defined as the differential incidence of certain specific diseases. Consequently, many federal health disparity elimination initiatives quickly devolve into a discussion of disease-specific strategies that largely ignore the socioecological context of those diseases. The medical model solutions proposed tend to involve the intensification of clinical services to specific populations and numerous variations on the theme of increasing patient–professional interactions among populations already afflicted with disease. Common disease roots in the socioecological context are often ignored. Examples of this narrow disease-specific focus abound.

For example, HHS's Initiative to Eliminate Racial and Ethnic Disparities in Health immediately devolves into a set of disease-specific initiatives focused on six diseases, infant mortality, cancer screening and management, cardiovascular disease, diabetes, HIV/AIDS, and immunizations. The "promising strategies" highlighted under each of these enumerated diseases are disproportionately clinically focused initiatives that are designed to improve individual health behaviors, increase early detection, and improve the clinical treatment of the diseases in question.[7] In short, the over-whelming emphasis of this HHS Initiative to Eliminate Racial and Ethnic Disparities in Health is the medical model. NIH's Strategic Research Plan to Reduce and Ultimately Eliminate Health Disparities acknowledges that health disparities are "the result of the complex interaction among biological factors, the environment, and specific health behaviors," and that "(i)nequalities in income and education also appear to underlie many health disparities in the United States."[8] (p 2) The plan envisions directing resources to better understand "the role of the environment and socioeconomic status in health disparities."[9] Despite these important insights into the social determinants of disease, the NIH plan places only limited emphasis on funding research or activities that seek to understand the role of the physical or social environment, economic and social policy, racial discrimination, or any of the major social determinants that the plan itself acknowledges underlie the very health disparities that NIH is trying to strategically reduce and ultimately eliminate.

The Socioecological Context of Health Disparities

While the medical model is undoubtedly important in ameliorating health disparities, particularly those related to the failures of our fragmented healthcare delivery system, the medical model *alone* can never success-fully eliminate racial and ethnic disparities that are largely driven by social inequalities that are *structural* in nature and inextricably intertwined with profound racial and ethnic disparities in income, education, housing, employment, and other important indicators of social power and opportu-nity. The ethical practice of public health must acknowledge the profound influence of the socioecological context of health disparities and seek to define effective new strategies that are truly intended to *eliminate* these disparities. Such strategies must understand the relevance of the immediate social and physical environment to the development of risk behaviors, such as smoking, physical inactivity, and low consumption of healthy foods.

These new strategies must also analyze and assess the health impacts of social policies related to land use planning, education, employment, housing, and wages, to name a few. Ultimately these new public health strategies must serve to build social, political, and economic power in low-income communities where health disparities are concentrated and exact an appalling human toll.

Place Matters

The *spatial* concentration of poverty and race, the remnants of an American system of de facto apartheid, remains a persistent problem in many parts of the United States. There is some evidence of improvement in this basic American demographic pattern[10]; however, the rate of this improvement is neither fast nor consistent. Consequently, the relevance of neighborhood, or *place*, to the geographical distribution of health dis-parities remains profound. Neighborhood remains an important context where in individual decisions about health behaviors may be constrained by limited access to opportunities and amenities, and negative social mes-sages that reinforce unhealthy individual behaviors. The performance and accountability of institutions within neighborhoods, including local gov-ernment, schools, businesses, and employers, also contribute to creating

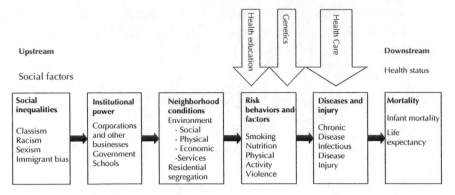

FIGURE 28.1 Health Disparities Logic Diagram.

conditions at the neighborhood level that is not conducive to healthy behaviors among residents of certain neighborhoods. Consequently, place matters. Successful public health strategies to eliminate health disparities must address the context of place in order to increase the likelihood that groups disproportionately affected by disparities will have greater opportunity to adopt healthy behaviors.

Figure 28.1 is an oversimplified framework for better understanding the context of health disparities in the United States.[11] The framework incorporates and legitimizes the medical model as an important part of the pathway leading to differential rates of disease and death between various population groups. However, the framework expands "upstream" and illuminates the socioecological model that recognizes that social inequalities in power drive biased institutional decision-making that creates adverse physical and social environmental conditions in low-income communities of color throughout the United States.

Public Health as a Social Justice Enterprise

Today social justice lives as more than an ideal; social justice serves as the underlying principle of many efforts to define and create a civilized society. It involves partnership among those affected by social justice issues and those who make policy to create change. Social justice policies address disparities between people and are designed to establish and improve equal treatment under the law, equal access to opportunity, and fair and equitable distribution of resources. Social justice policies often call for social change

—The Minneapolis Foundation,
A Framework for Social Change.[12]

Public health practitioners who purport to be committed to "eliminating health disparities" cannot labor in ignorance of the persistent social, political, and economic forces that create and reinforce such striking patterns of residential racial segregation, educational disparities, and profound wealth gaps. Ultimately, when forced to examine how these enduring, structural patterns of societal organization are maintained, despite the successful elimination of legalized forms of racism following the civil rights movement, one cannot but conclude that at its very roots, the problem lies with a persistent inequity in the distribution of social, political, and economic power among racial groups in the United States. If one accepts this conclusion, then the relevant and ethical question for public health practitioners is how to build social, political, and economic power for low-income communities of color.

Public health practice as a social justice enterprise is a concept of public health that recognizes and targets roots causes of social inequity. Social justice is a dynamic concept that takes on many different forms in different settings. Fundamentally though, the need for social justice efforts arises wherever significant power imbalances are found. In settings in which justice is in short supply, power will tend to concentrate according to lines of privilege. In this society, privilege primarily flows according to race, class, gender, and, to some extent, immigration status. Consequently, many social, political, and economic policies tend to favor whites, particularly wealthy White men. There are numerous specific examples of this including the GI Bill, redlining practices, welfare policy, urban renewal policies, education funding policies and practices, drug use and incarceration policies, federal housing subsidization policies, and health insurance policies. One can easily describe these policies and practices collectively as affirmative action for whites. Cumulatively, these policies and practices have created and continue to reinforce America's unique form of apartheid. Any general strain on society whether it be economic recession, new drug epidemics such as crack cocaine, communicable disease epidemic such as influenza, or natural disaster such as Hurricane Katrina, will exact its greatest toll on low-income communities of color that are at the very bottom of the American privilege and power totem pole.

Justice has two key ingredients: truth and power. Without either one of these ingredients, there cannot be justice. Public health practitioners are experts at identifying truth. We have innumerable detailed studies published in peer-reviewed journals describing the clear relationship between various "social determinants of health" and health outcomes. In fact, we have entire journals dedicated to these topics. Yet despite the truth being out there, we see relatively little evidence of steady progress in core health measures for our most socially, politically, and economically marginalized populations. This is because public health practice has still largely ignored the issue of power and its skewed distribution throughout our society. Our work in communities tends to focus on individual-level behavioral change models, intensification of service delivery, and issue-specific community mobilization efforts, namely, the medical model. Rarely do public health agencies focus squarely on building upon indigenous social, political, and economic power in low-income communities of color. Given the ethical precepts outlines in the Public Health Code of Ethics, that public health should address principally the fundamental causes of disease and requirements for health, aiming to prevent adverse health outcomes; that public health should advocate and work for the empowerment of disenfranchised community members, aiming to ensure that the basic resources and conditions necessary for health are accessible to all; and that public health programs and policies should be implemented in a manner that most enhances the physical and social environment, can we honestly say that our current American public health practice is ethical?

Notes

1. U.S. Department of Health and Human Services, *Healthy People 2010*. 2nd ed. *With Understanding and Improving Health and Objectives for Improving Health*. 2 vols. (Washington, DC: US Government Printing Office, 2000): 11.
2. HHS press release, January 9,2006. http://ncmhd.nih. gov/SawardsM.html (accessed May 7, 2008).
3. J.L. Gerberding, "Plenary session 4: improving health, eliminating disparities: visions for the 21st century," 15(Suppl. 2) *Ethnicity & Disease* (Spring 2005): S2–S78.
4. D. Satcher, G.E. Fryer, Jr, J. McCann, A. Troutman, S.H. Woolf, and G. Rust, "What If We Were Equal:?A Comparison of the Black-White Mortality Gap in 1960 and 2000," 24(2) *Health Affairs* (2005): 459–464.
5. HHSHP, "Executive Summary, Summary and Future Directions," *Midcourse Review* (2010):30. http://www.healthypeople.gov/Data/midcourse/ (Accessed May 7, 2008).
6. Association of Schools of Public Health, *Demonstrating Excellence in Academic Public Health Practice* (Washington, DC: Association of Schools of Public Health, June 1999).
7. Centers for Disease Control and Prevention Office of Minority Health, *Eliminating Racial and Ethnic Health Disparities*, http://www.cdc.gov/omhd/About/disparities.htm (accessed May 7, 2008).
8. NIH Strategic, *Research Plan to Reduce and Ultimately Eliminate Health Disparities*, FY 2002–2006: 2–3. Executive Summary.
9. Ibid.
10. G.T. Kingsley and K.L.S. Pettit, *Concentrated Poverty: Dynamics of Change Neighborhood Change in America*, Series No.5. Urban Institute (August 2007).
11. Bay Area Health Inequities Initiative, *Health Equity Conceptual Framework*, www.barhii.org. (accessed May 7, 2008).
12. N. Nagler, *Social Justice in Minnesota: a Framework for Social Change. The Minneapolis Foundation*, www. mplsfoundation.org/publications/PolicyPaper Social justice.pdf (accessed February 19, 2008).

29

Teaching Social Inequalities in Health: Barriers and Opportunities

CARLES MUNTANER AND HAEJOO CHUNG

The teacher of social inequalities in health (SIH) faces difficulties of both social technologies (aiming at changing society through education on SIH) and basic sciences (in order to educate she needs to understand SIH). We can identify two kinds of barriers to the effective tasks of teaching SIH: those internal to academia and those external, originating outside the academic world. In this chapter, we outline a series of internal and external barriers (see Table 29.1) and propose a number of mechanisms to explain them. More applied educational research is needed to determine the accuracy our conjectures. Next, we present a number of strategies that might help overcome the aforementioned barriers in teaching SIH (see Table 29.2). Because our academic experience including teaching social inequalities in health has occurred mostly in the Organization for Economic Cooperation and Development (OECD) countries (with the exception of Venezuela), we limit our analysis to wealthy capitalist countries.

Dedicated to the memory of Juan Carlos Garcia-Borron and Manuel Sacristan who suffered the consequences of teaching egalitarian values during Francisco Franco's fascist dictatorship in Spain.

TABLE 29.1. Internal and External Barriers to the Effective Tasks of Teaching SIH

	INTERNAL	EXTERNAL
Cultural and ideological	Medicalization or biological reductionism Scientism Empiricism	The dominant culture of most contemporary societies Individualism Nihilism Libertarianism Neoliberalism Many varieties of subjectivism and idealism
Political	Exploitation of undergraduate and PhD students and nontenured faculties Antiegalitarian behavior of SIH teachers that compromise their credibility	Direct censorship (e.g., fascist regimes) Self-censorship as a consequence of antiegalitarian political climate
Economic	"Soft money" employment contracts Emergence of powerful private donors Teachers' own class position in academia	A system dominated by private interest Privatization of public education and lack of investment in public universities

TABLE 29.2. Strategies That Might Help Overcome Barriers in Teaching SIH

IN AND AROUND CLASSROOMS	AT THE GOVERNMENT LEVEL
Teachers' affiliation with working-class unions and participation in collective bargaining Teachers' engagement with oppressed communities via community-based participatory action research Student community projects during SIH course work	Increased public funding for universities Limiting the role of corporate agendas in research and teaching Implementation of egalitarian policies that reduce the elitism in academia Alleviating class inequalities in university credentials

Barriers Internal to Academia

We distinguish between cultural (including ideological), political (power related), and economic barriers that hinder the teaching of SIH within contemporary academia.

Cultural and Ideological

A first barrier to teach SIH to health personnel is "medicalization" or "biological reductionism," the tendency to see public health problems exclusively in terms of biology and medicine (e.g., "race inequalities in health are due to inherited traits").[1] As these views reflect a strong curricular emphasis in biological sciences and a neglect of social sciences, a likely solution would be to increase the presence of social sciences among health care professionals (nurses, MDs, social workers, pharmacists, dentists, etc.). It is not surprising that the lack of enthusiasm toward integrating SIH in the population health agenda has often been advanced by leaders with training in those disciplines.[2]

Scientism, or the belief that science endows scientists with superior knowledge, can be a barrier as it tends to produce contempt for the views of deprived populations. It is not uncommon to see SIH researchers who entertain the notion that they know what is better for the "poor" and "minorities." For example, a team of public health researchers might be engaged in research on infant mortality in segregated poor communities while its members consider lack of jobs their first health related priority.[3]

Elitism, closely related to scientism manifests itself in academia with the belief in the superiority of the "educated" in particular those with credential from "top" institutions. Elitist attitudes may represent a serious threat to teaching SIH as the elitist teacher denounces social inequalities and at the same time reproduces and endorses them with regard to academia and educational credentials. Thus, in elitist environments, a working-class background can be held against students and be a cause for subtle or not so subtle discrimination.[4]

Empiricism (a term distinct from empirical) is the epistemology that neglects hypothetico-deductive systems (theories) with the pretence that all a scientist needs to do is to "let the data speak." When the common wisdom of a society includes engrained theories that perpetuate inequalities "race as biology, individualism" empirical research would tend to confirm that world view. For example, researchers can survey a community as a sum of individuals with indicators such as "race" and "education" and conclude that nonwhites have poor health because they do not study and they are to be held responsible for their situation. Alternatively, scientists can ask questions about geographical racial segregation, lack of political power, and economic disinvestment by governments (e.g., devolution in the United States) to obtain a very different explanation.[5] Thus, gradients in health in groups stratified by race or education are understood with appeal to "common sense" that is reifying that causes of health inequalities with some property of race or ethnicity (e.g., irresponsible blacks, fatalistic Latinos);[6] or of "vulnerable" and "disadvantaged" communities, what has been referred to as "blaming the community."[7]

The Weberian ethos of empirical social science has been particularly responsible for thwarting SIH teaching and research.[8] Thus, researchers are supposed to be neutral with regard to their scientific work under threat of not being objective, the result being self-censorship with regards to models that are portrayed as "value-driven" such as SIH. Yet public health and epidemiology (a technology and an applied science) need to declare their values. When a physician tries to resuscitate a dying patient, the deed reflects his values of life at the individual level. Similarly, the field of population health inherits a certain value at the aggregate level.

Political/Power

The use of power in academic organizations to extract labor from undergraduate and PhD students and nontenured faculty members can easily lead to situations of exploitation. When these practices are indulged by teachers of SIH, the contradictions between what is taught in the classroom and the behavior outside can become so shocking that they can alienate those who are victimized from SIH. Common mechanisms of exploitation are not giving credit for work performed (no coauthorship offered); stealing hypotheses, models or ideas or technical innovations; forcing students to conduct research against their interests, or which are not adequate for their goals or job descriptions, expecting overtime, showing disrespect and authoritarianism in scientific activities; using academic status to "appropriate" oneself from scientific ideas generated by persons in "lesser" institutions; and forcing subordinates to bow to authority rather than scientific truth. Other activities that can have a negative impact on the credibility of teachers of SIH are hoarding knowledge from students and faculty; tolerating inequities in academia itself for personal gain; posing or pretending to have special forms of knowledge; and subcontracting faculty to avoid working and as a result creating a precarious academic labor force.

The work organization of academic work itself interacts with the personality of teachers to promote a certain type of behaviors or personalities that are antiegalitarian. Among them we find extreme, "cut-throat" competition; individualism, lack of empathy, and solidarity; narcissism including grandiose sense of self-importance, expectations of being admired, sense of entitlement, interpersonal exploitation, or arrogant attitudes.

Economic

The modern university is controlled by capital and state elites, also known as the ruling class.[9] They serve class interests at home and abroad, for example, by providing the knowledge foundation to justify imperialism.[10] Its function is essential to promote the development of technology[11] and guarantee that upper middle classes spouse the values of the ruling class.[12] Therefore, the attitudes and production of academics is of extreme importance in maintaining the dominant political, economic, and cultural systems of most cotemporary societies.

The most powerful means of controlling the behavior (including attitudes) of scientists are soft money employment contracts. Under this employment relation, wages and job security are contingent on obtaining grants. This development, widely disseminated in the 1980s in U.S. major universities, ensures compliance with both business and government priorities and perspectives. Researchers write proposals with research questions that are appealing to funders (e.g., SES rather than class exploitation effects). Intellectual autonomy including the freedom to pursue research on SIH might be limited or seriously compromised (e.g., health disparities become a search for the genetics of ethnicity or the pharmacology of race). These compromises in which teachers of SIH engage not only can redirect research and interests (as attitudes are affected by behavior) but also generate incoherence between classroom and research output. For example, professors who teach social class might produce articles on SES; those who lecture on the health effects of sexism include only a "sex variable" in their papers.

A contemporary example of the influence of academia on SIH comes with the entrance of powerful private donors (Bill Gates and Warren Buffet, the two wealthiest individuals on the planet). The Bill and Melinda Gates foundation (ironically accountable only to a person who dropped out of college) has been able to influence global health research with a technocratic[13] and private market philosophy (e.g., microfinance, for profit "creative" capitalism;[14]) in direct competition with the WHO, which, at least in principle, has the potential to represent billions of citizens from its constituent countries. It is thus unlikely that researchers hired or financed by Gates will be independent and will promote private approaches to reducing health inequities even when evidence is missing (e.g., microcredits) or insufficient and controversial (Mexico's health reform).[15]

Some committed researchers are able to challenge the corporate interests of academia such as university investments, donor's or state's economic interests such as investments or real estate ownership, (e.g., hog industry in North Carolina[16]). Most researchers may unfortunately fall in line into bland, safe, and conventional scholarship[17] for fear of the very real economic and professional consequences of "red hunting."[18]

Unfortunately, unless teachers of SIH try to collectively overcome the contradictions that their class position in academia subjects them to, their efforts at teaching SIH lose legitimacy and effectiveness.

Barriers External to Academia

Cultural, political, and economic barriers to teaching SIH can also be external to academia. As larger social institutions (governments, private sector, citizens) tend to control the organization of academia, these are of utmost importance.

Cultural and Ideological

Egalitarian values in SIH (everyone has the same rights to health, according to their needs) run against the core of the dominant culture of most contemporary societies. Some of these cultural barriers (from which students and teachers are not immune) are individualism (i.e., all values are individual, only individual rights matter, self interest should be placed above any other consideration); nihilism (rejection of values and norms), libertarianism (individuals should be free to do what they want no matter how this affects the needs and wants of others), neoliberalism (e.g., private markets are optimal and self-regulated structures), and many varieties of subjectivism and idealism (e.g., postmodernism, religion, spiritualism).

Political

Many political regimes censor the teaching and publishing of egalitarian ideas.[19] First among them we find fascism[20] followed by various forms of authoritarianism that subject egalitarian scholars to various penalties such as labor market discrimination.[21] For example, dictatorships such as Francisco Franco's fascist regime in Spain (1936–1977) was merciless in jailing and torturing university professors who taught egalitarian philosophies.[22] One consequence of a climate where egalitarian views are ridiculed or shunned[23] is self-censorship, which can manifest itself in multiple ways: changing topics, watering down the content of what is taught in the classroom (class becomes SES; racism becomes race; and patriarchy becomes sex), compromising the content of courses (certain topics, authors or publications are considered "off limits"), or teaching only bland ("social capital," "social cohesion," "neighborhood disorganization"), or non-threatening, comfortable topics; (it is easier for a Canadian professor to teach about the public health effects of war using Iraq as an example than using Afghanistan, a war in which Canada is involved).[24]

Economic

Academic institutions are affected by the political economy of their home countries.[25] A system dominated by private interests is less likely to allow teaching of disciplines that criticize it as cause of inequalities. Privatization of public education and lack of investment in public universities should therefore be a major barrier to teaching SIH in market economies.

Solidarity, Realist Criticism, and Scientific Utopia: A Way Out toward Teaching Social Inequalities in Health

Teaching SIH requires both critical scientific realism and a dose of scientific "utopia" as teachers need to produce models and plan for societies without health inequalities that do not exist. These ingredients are hardly possible under the circumstances described earlier.

Individual barriers internal to academia can be overcome with different forms of collective action. Teachers' affiliation with working-class unions and participation in collective bargaining, as in several Scandinavian countries, will limit the elitism of teachers. Engagement with oppressed communities via community-based participatory action research can also prevent teachers of SIH from falling in some of the cultural, power, and economic barriers afflicting teachers of SIH. For example, a resident from the Johns Hopkins School of Medicine in Baltimore developed a joint SIH course with the participation of students from an African-American college adjacent to Johns Hopkins. Both teachers and students from the elite institution learned from the views on SIH of local Baltimore students. This engagement with exploited and oppressed communities can also be achieved via student community projects during SIH course work.[26] Community outreach and community engagement is a part of the recent anti neoliberal and globalization education strategies.[27] These innovations should be adopted or incorporated in courses of SIH.

At the government level, economic measures such as sufficient funding of public universities and limiting the role of corporate agendas in research and teaching (e.g., via wealthy charities a la Gates Foundation);[28] will remove barriers to teaching SIH. Governments can also implement egalitarian policies that reduce the elitism in academia. By reducing class inequalities in university credentials, governments can promote nonclassist views among teachers of SIH. For example, the Bolivarian revolution has changed the class composition of its MDs. While MDs used to originate almost exclusively from urban upper middle classes and refused the practice of medicine in poor areas, the new medical education under the program Barrio Adentro enrolls students from poor areas who are committed to serve their own communities after graduating. This program not only will change the class composition of the medical profession but also its classist and antiegalitarian attitudes.

In summary, although there are numerous barriers to teaching SIH, as the discipline runs against the ideological grain of most countries there are also opportunities to transform its content and educational practices that are cause for optimism.

Notes

1. R.C. Lewontin, S. Rose, and L. Kamin, *Biology, Ideology and Human Nature: Not In Our Genes* (London: Penguin, 1984).
2. K.J. Rothman, H.O. Adami, and D. Trichopoulos, "Should The Mission Of Epidemiology Include The Eradication Of Poverty?" 352(9130) *The Lancet* (1998): 810–813.
3. R.E. Aronson, K. Lovelace, J.W. Hatch, and T.L. Whitehead, "Strengthening Communities and the Role of Individuals in Community Life," in *Social Justice and Public Health,* ed. B. Levy and V. Sidel (Oxford: Oxford University Press, 2005): 433–449.
4. M.M. Tokarczyk and E.A. Fay, *Working Class Women in the Academy: Laborers in the Knowledge Factory* (Amherst, MA: The University of Massachusetts Press, 1993); R. Sennett and J. Cobb, *The Hidden Injuries of Class* (New York: Vintage, 1972).
5. M. Gomez and C. Muntaner, "Urban redevelopment and health in East Baltimore, Maryland: The Role of Communitarian and institutional social capital," 15(2) *Critical Public Health* (2005): 83–102.
6. C.E. Ross, J. Mirowsky, and W.C. Cockerham, "Social Class, Mexican Culture, and Fatalism: Their Effects on Psychological Distress," 11 *American Journal of Community Psychology* (1983): 383–399.
7. C. Muntaner and J. Lynch, "Income Inequality, Social Cohesion, and Class Relations: A Critique of Wilkinson's Neo-Durkheimian Research Program," 29(1) *International Journal of Health Services* (1999): 59–81.
8. A. Sadri, *Max Weber's Sociology of Intellectuals* (New York: Oxford University Press, 1992).
9. D.N. Smith, *Who Rules The University? An Essay in Class Analysis* (New York: Monthly Review Press, 1974).
10. D. Dickson, *The New Politics of Science* (Chicago: Chicago University Press, 1988).
11. D.F. Noble, *America By Design. Science Technology and The Rise of Corporate Capitalism* (New York: Oxford University Press, 1977).
12. N. Chomsky, *The Chomsky Reader* (New York: Pantheon Books, 1987).
13. A.E. Birn, "Gates's Grandest Challenge: Transcending Technology as Public Health Ideology," 366(9484) *The Lancet* (August 6–12, 2005): 514–519.
14. B. Gates, "How To Fix Capitalism," *TIME* (July 31, 2008): 26–33; N. Krieger, "Proximal, Distal, and the Politics of Causation: What's Level Got To Do With It," 98(2) *American Journal of Public Health* (February, 2008): 221–230.
15. J. Frenk, E. González-Pier, O. Gómez-Dantés, M.A. Lezana, and F.M. Knaul, "Comprehensive Reform to Improve Health System Performance in Mexico," 49(Suppl.1) *Salud Publica Mexicana* (2007): S23–S36; also in J. Frenk, et al., *The Lancet,* vol. 368(9546) (Oct 28, 2006):1524–34; A.C. Laurell, "Health

System Reform in Mexico: A Critical Review," 37(3) *International Journal of Health Services* (2007): 515–537.

16. S. Wing, R.A. Horton, N. Muhammad, G.R. Grant, M Tajik, and K. Thu, "Integrating Epidemiology, Education and Organizing for Environmental Justice: Community Health Effects of Industrial Hog Operations," 98(8) *American Journal of Public Health* (August, 2008): 1390–1397.

17. R. Jacoby, *The Last Intellectuals: American Culture in the Age of Academe* (New York: Noonday, 1987).

18. J. Kovel, *Hunting in the Promised Land: Anticommunism and the Making of America* (London: Cassell, 1997); C. Muntaner and M.B. Gomez, "Anti-Egalitarian, Legitimizing Myths, Racism, and 'Neo-McCarthyism' in Social Epidemiology and Public Health: A Review of Sally Satel's PC, MD," 32(1) *International Journal of Health Services* (2002): 1–17.

19. L.A. Coser, *Men of Ideas* (New York: The Free Press, 1997).

20. J.F. Marsal, *Pensar Bajo El Franquismo: Intelectuales y Política en la Generación de los Años Cincuenta* (Madrid: Peninsula, 1979).

21. Kovel, 1997, Note 18.

22. Marsal, 1979, Note 20.

23. Muntaner and Gomez, 2002, Note 18.

24. Chomsky, 1987, Note 12.

25. Noble, 1977, Note 11; Smith 1974, Note 9; Dickson, 1988, Note 10.

26. M. Cote, R.J.F. Day, and G. De Peuter, *Utopian Pedagogy : Radical Experiments Against Neoliberal Globalization* (Toronto : UTP, 2007).

27. Cote, et al., 2007, ibid.; P. McLaren and R. Farahmandpur, *Teaching Against Global Capitalism and The New Imperialism: A Critical Pedagogy* (Oxford: Rowan and Littlefield, 2005).

28. Cote, et al., 2007, Note 26.

APPENDIX A

Selected References

Acheson, Donald, *Independent Inquiry into Inequalities in Health* (London: The Stationery Office, 1998).

Aday Lu Ann, ed., *Reinventing Public Health: Policies and Practices for a Healthy Nation* (San Francisco, CA: Jossey-Bass, 2005).

Adler, Nancy E., Michael Marmot, Bruce S. McEwen, and Judith Stewart eds., *Socioeconomic Status and Health in Industrial Nations: Social, Psychological, and Biological Pathways* (New York: New York Academy of Sciences, 1999).

Agren, Gunnar, *Sweden's New Public Health Policy: National Public Health Objectives for Sweden* (Stockholm: Swedish National Institute of Public Health, 2003).

Anand, Sudhir, Fabienne Peter, and Amartya Sen, eds., *Public Health, Ethics, and Equity* (Oxford: Oxford University Press, 2004).

Arizona Public Health Association, *Living and Dying in Arizona: A Profile of Arizona's People and Their Health Needs*, An Arizona Public Health Association Health Status Report for Arizona, (Phoenix, AZ: Arizona Public Health Association, 1999).

Armstrong, H., P. Armstrong, and David Coburn, eds., *Unhealthy Times: The Political Economy of Health and Health Care in Canada* (Oxford: Oxford University Press, 2001).

Arno, Peter S., and Janis Barry Figueroa, "The social and economic determinants of health," in *Unconventional Wisdom: Alternative Perspectives on the New Economy*, ed. Jeff Madrick (New York: The Century Foundation Press, 2000): 93–104.

Asada, Yukiko and Thomas Hedemann, "A problem with the individual approach in the WHO health inequality measurement," 1: 2 *International Journal for Equity in Health* (2002) doi:10.1186/1475-9276-1-2

Asada, Yukiko, *Health Inequality: Morality and Measurement* (Toronto: University of Toronto Press, 2007).

Asthana, Sheena, and Joyce Halliday, *What Works in Tackling Health Inequalities Pathways, Policies and Practice Through the Lifecourse* (Bristol: Policy Press, 2006).

Bambas Nolen, Lexi, Paula Braveman , Norberto W. Dachs, et al., "Strengthening health information systems to address equity challenges," 83(8) *Bulletin of the World Health Organization* (August, 2005): 597–602.

Bambra, C., D. Fox, and A Scott-Samuel, "A politics of health glossary," 61 *Journal of Epidemiology and Community Health* (2007): 571–574.

Barfield, W.D., P.H. Wise, F.P. Rust, K.J. Rust, J.B. Gould, and S.L. Gortmaker, "Racial disparities in outcomes of military and civilian births in California," 150 *Archives of Pediatric and Adolescent Medicine* (October, 1996): 1062–1067.

Bashir, Samiya A., "Home is where the harm is: inadequate housing as a public health crisis," 92(5) *American Journal of Public Health* (May, 2002): 733–738.

Baum, F., "Health, equity, justice and globalization: some lessons from the people's health assembly," 55(9) *Journal of Epidemiology and Community Health* (2001): 613–616.

Bay Area Regional Health Inequities Initiative, *Health Inequities in the Bay Area* (Oakland, CA: Public Health Institute, 2008).

Beaglehole, Robert and Ruth Bonita, *Public Health at the Crossroads: Achievements and Prospects* (Cambridge: Cambridge University Press, 1997).

Beaglehole, Robert ed., *Global Public Health: A New Era* (Oxford: Oxford University Press, 2003).

Beaglehole, Robert, Ruth Bonita, Richard Horton, Orvill Adams, and Martin McKee,. "Public health in the new era: improving health through collective action," 363 *The Lancet* (June 19, 2004): 2084–2086.

Beauchamp, Dan E., "Public health as social justice," 8 *Inquiry* (1976): 3–14.

Beckfield, Jason and Nancy Krieger, "Epi + Demos + Cracy: Linking Political Systems and Priorities to the Magnitude of Health Inequities—Evidence, Gaps, and A Research Agenda," *Epidemiologic Reviews* (May 27, 2009). Advance access published online by the Johns Hopkins Bloomberg School of Public Health, Oxford Journals. doi: 10.1093/epirev/mxp002v2.

Bezruchka, Stephen, Tsukasa Namekata, and Maria Gilson Sistrom, "Is Our Society Making You Sick?" *Newsweek* (February 26, 2001): 14.

Bezruchka, Stephen, "Improving Economic Equality and Health: The Case of Postwar Japan," 98(4) *American Journal of Public Health* (April, 2008): 1–6.

Birn, Anne-Emanuelle, "Gate's Grandest Challenge: Transcending Technology as Public Health Ideology," http://image.thelancet.com/extras/04art6429web.pdf (accessed March 11, 2005).

Black, Douglas, J.N. Morris, C. Smith, and Margaret Whitehead, *Inequalities in Health* (Harmondsworth: Penguin, 1992).

Blane, David, Eric Brunner, and Richard Wilkinson, *Health and Social Organization: Towards a Health Policy for the 21st Century* (London: Routledge, 1996).

Bolaria, B. Singh and Rosemary Bolaria, *Racial Minorities, Medicine and Health* (Halifax, Nova Scotia: Fernwood, 1994).

Boufford, Jo Ivey and Phillip R. Lee, *Health Policies for the 21st Century: Challenges and Recommendations for the U.S. Department of Health and Human Services* (New York: Milbank Memorial Fund, September, 2001).

Boutain, D., "Social Justice as a Framework for Professional Nursing," 44(9) *Journal of Nursing Education* (2005): 404–408.

Braveman, Paula and Eleuther Tarimo, "Social Inequalities in Health Within Countries: Not Only an Issue for Affluent Nations," 54(11) *Social Science & Medicine* (June, 2002): 1621–1635.

Braveman, Paula and Sofia Gruskin, "Poverty, Equity, Health and Human Rights," 81(7) *Bulletin of the World Health Organization* (2003): 539–545.

Braveman, Paula, Barbara Starfield, and Jack Geiger, "World Health Report 2000: How it Removes Equity from the Agenda for Public Health Monitoring and Policy," 323 *British Medical Journal* (September 22, 2001): 678–681.

Braveman, Paula, Nancy Krieger, and James Lynch, "Health Inequalities and Social Inequalities in Health," 78(2) *Bulletin of the World Health Organization* (2000): 232–234.

Braveman, Paula. "Monitoring Equity in Health and Healthcare: A Conceptual Framework," 21(3) *Journal of Health, Population, and Nutrition* (September, 2003): 181–192.

Brink, Satya and Allen Zeesman, *Measuring Social Well-Being: An Index of Social Health for Canada*, R-97–9E. Hull, Quebec, Canada: Applied Research Branch, Strategic Policy, Human Resources Development Canada (June, 1997).

Burd-Sharps, Sarah, Kristen Lewis, and Eduardo Borges Martins eds., *The Measure of America: American Human Development Report 2008–2009* (New York: Columbia University Press, 2008).

Byrd, Michael and L.A. Clayton, *An American Health Dilemma. Volume 1. A Medical History of African Americans and the Problem of Race: Beginnings to 1900* (New York: Routledge, 2000).

Byrd, Michael and L.A. Clayton, *An American Health Dilemma. Volume 2. Race, Medicine, and Health Care in the United States: From 1900 to the Dawn of the New Millennium* (New York: Routledge, 2002).

Callinicos, Alex, *Equality* (London: Polity Press, 2000).

Calman, K.C., "Equity, Poverty, and Health for All," 314 *British Medical Journal* (1997): 1187–1191.

Carlisle, Sandra, "Health Promotion, Advocacy and Health Inequalities: A Conceptual Framework," 15(4) *Health Promotion International* (2000): 369–376.

Carroll, G., "Mundane Extreme Environmental Stress and African American Families: A Case For Recognizing Different Realities," 29 *Journal of Comparative Family Studies* (1998): 271–284.

Carter-Pokras, Olivia and Claudia Baquet, "What Is a 'Health Disparity,' " 117 *Public Health Reports* (September–October, 2002): 426–434.

Chang, W-C., "The Meaning and Goals of Equity in Health," 56 *Journal of Epidemiology and Community Health* (2002): 488–491.

Chen, Jarvis T., David H. Rehkopf, Pamela D. Waterman, et al., "Mapping and Measuring Social Disparities in Premature Mortality: The Impact of Census Tract Poverty Within and Across Boston Neighborhoods, 1999–2001," 83(6) *Journal of Urban Health: Bulletin of the New York Academy of Medicine* (2006): 1063–1084.

Chernomas, Robert, *The Social and Economic Causes of Disease* (Manitoba: Canadian Centre for Policy Alternatives, March, 1999).

Chung, Haejoo and Carles Muntaner, "Political and Welfare State Determinants of Infant and Child Health Indicators: An Analysis of Wealthy Countries," 63 *Social Science & Medicine* (2006): 829–842.

Chung, Haejoo and Carles Muntaner, "Welfare State Types and Global Health: An Emerging Challenge," 62 *Journal of Epidemiology and Community Health* (2008): 282–283.

Coburn, David, "Beyond the Income Inequality Hypothesis: Class, Neo-liberalism, and Health Inequalities," 58 *Social Science & Medicine* (2004): 41–56.

Coburn, David, "Income Inequality, Social Cohesion, and the Health Status of Populations: The Role of Neo-Liberalism," 51 *Social Science & Medicine* (2000): 135–146.

Cohen, Hillel W. and Mary E, Northridge, "Getting Political: Racism and Urban Health," 90(6) *American Journal of Public Health* (June, 2000): 841–843.

Collins, James, Jr., Richard J. David, Arden Handler, Stephen Wall, and Teven Andes, "Very Low Birthweight in African-American Infants: The Role of Maternal Exposure to Interpersonal Racial Discrimination" 14(9) *Poverty & Race* (September/October, 2005): 9–11.

Commission on Social Determinants of Health, *Closing the Gap in a Generation: Health Equity through Action on the Social Determinants of Health*, Final Report of the CSDH (Geneva: World Health Organization, 2008).

Comstock, R. Dawn, Edward M. Castillo, and Suzanne P. Lindsay, "Four-Year Review of the Use of Race and Ethnicity in Epidemiologic and Public Health Research," 159 *American Journal of Epidemiology* (2004): 611–619.

Cooper, Richard, Joan F. Kennelly, Ramon Rurzo-Arvizu, Hyun-Joo Oh, George Kaplan, and John Lynch, "Relationship Between Premature Mortality and Socioeconomic Factors in Black and White Populations of U.S. Metropolitan Areas," 116 *Public Health Reports* (September-October, 2001): 464–473.

Corburn, Jason, *Street Science: Community Knowledge and Environmental Health Justice* (Cambridge, MA: MIT Press, 2005).

Corburn, Jason, *Toward the Healthy City: People, Places, and the Politics of Urban Planning* (Cambridge, MA: MIT Press, 2010, forthcoming.)

Craig, Gary, Tania Burchardt, and David Gordon eds., *Social Justice and Public Policy: Seeking Fairness in Diverse Societies* (Bristol: The Policy Press, 2008).

Cummins, Steven, Sarah Curtis, Ana V. Diez-Roux, and Sally Macintyre, "Understanding and Representing 'Place' in Health Research: A Relational Approach," 65 *Social Science & Medicine* (2007): 1825–1838.

Cwikel, Julie G., *Social Epidemiology: Strategies for Public Health Activism* (New York: Columbia University Press, 2006).

Daniels, Norman, Bruce Kennedy, and Ichiro Kawachi, *Is Inequality Bad for Our Health?* (Boston: Beacon Press, 2000).

Davey Smith, G., C. Hart, G. Watt, D. Hole, and V. Hawthorne, "Individual Social Class, Area- Based Deprivation, Cardiovascular Disease Risk Factors and Mortality: The Renfrew and Paisley Study," 52 *Journal of Epidemiology and Community Health* (1998): 399–405.

Davey Smith, George, C. Hart, D. Blane, C. Gillis, and V. Hawthorne, "Lifetime Socioeconomic Position and Mortality: Prospective Observational Study," 314 *British Medical Journal* (1997): 547–552.

Davey Smith, George, Daniel Dorling, and Mary Shaw eds., *Poverty, Inequality and Health in Britain: 1800–2000, A Reader* (Bristol: Policy Press, 2001).

Davey Smith, George ed., *Health Inequalities: Lifecourse Approaches* (London: The Policy Press, 2003).

Davey Smith, George, "Income Inequality and Mortality: Why Are They Related?" 312 *British Medical Journal* (April 20, 1996): 987–988.

Davey Smith, George, "Learning to Live with Complexity: Ethnicity, Socioeconomic Position, and Health in Britain and the United States," 90(11) *American Journal of Public Health* (November, 2000): 1694–1698.

Diderichsen, F. and J. Hallqvist, "Social Inequalities in Health: Some Methodological Considerations for the Study of Social Position and Social Context," in *Inequality in Health: A Swedish Perspective*, ed. B. Arve-Pares (Stockholm: Swedish Council for Social Research, 1998): 25–39.

Diderichsen, Finn, Timothy Evans, and Margaret Whitehead, "The Social Basis of Disparities in Health," in *Challenging Inequities in Health: From Ethics to Action*, ed. Timothy Evans, Margaret Whitehead, Finn Diderichsen, Abbas Bhuia, and Meg Wirth (New York: Oxford University Press, 2001): 13–23.

Diez Roux, Ana, Sharon Stein Merkin, Donna Arnett, et al., "Neighborhood of Residence and Incidence of Coronary Heart Disease," 345 *New England Journal of Medicine* (July 12, 2001): 99–106.

Diez-Roux, Ana, "Bringing Context Back Into Epidemiology: Variables and Fallacies in Multilevel Analysis," 88(2) *American Journal of Public Health* (1998): 216–222.

Doyal, Leslie, *What Makes Women Sick: Gender and the Political Economy of Health* (New Brunswick, NJ: Rutgers University Press, 1995).

Drexler, Madeline, *Health Disparities and the Body Politic. A series of international symposia organized by the Working Group on Health Disparities at the Harvard School of Public Health* (Boston: Harvard School of Public Health, 2005).

Duleep, H.O., "Mortality and Income Inequality," 58 *Social Security Bulletin* (1995): 34–50.

Epstein, Helen, "Enough to Make You Sick?" *New York Times Magazine* (October 12, 2003).

Evans, R.G., M.L. Barer, and T.R. Marmot, eds., *Why Are Some People Healthy and Others Are Not? Determinants of Health of Populations* (New York: Aldine de Gruyter, 1994).

Evans, Timothy, Margaret Whitehead, Finn Diderichsen, Abbas Bhuiya, and Meg Wirth eds., *Challenging Inequities in Health: From Ethics to Action* (New York: Oxford University Press, 2001).

Ezzati, Majid, Ari B. Friedman, Sandeep C. Kulkarni, and Christopher Murray, "The Reversal of Fortunes: Trends in County Mortality and Cross-Country Mortality Disparities in the United States," 5(4) *PLoS Medicine* (April 2008): e66.

Fahrenwald, N., "Teaching Social Justice," 28(5) *Nurse Educator* (2005): 222–226.

Farmer, Paul, "Social Inequalities and Emerging Infectious Diseases," 2(4) *Emerging Infectious Diseases* (October–December, 1996): 259–269.

Farmer, Paul, *Infections and Inequalities: The Modern Plagues* (Berkeley: University of California Press, 1999).

Farmer, Paul, *Pathologies of Power: Health, Human Rights, and the New War on the Poor* (San Francisco: University of California Press, 2004).

Fee, Elizabeth and Nancy Krieger eds., *Women's Health, Politics, and Power: Essays on Sex/Gender, Medicine and Public Health* (Amityville, NY: Baywood, 1994).

Fein, Oliver, "The Influence of Social Class on Health Status: American and British Research on Health Inequalities," 10 *Journal of General Internal Medicine* (1995): 577–586.

Fitzpatrick, Kevin and Mark LaGory, *Unhealthy Places: The Ecology of Risk in the Urban Landscape* (New York: Routledge, 2000).

Forbes, I. ed., *Health Inequalities: Poverty and Policy* (London: Academy for Learned Societies for the Social Sciences, 2001).

Fort, Meredith, Mary Anne Mercer, and Oscar Gish, *Sickness and Wealth: The Corporate Assault on Global Health* (Boston: South End Press, 2004).

Freudenberg, Nicholas, "Time for a National Agenda to Improve the Health of Urban Populations," 90(6) *American Journal of Public Health* (June 2000): 837–840.

Freudenberg, Nicolas, Sandro Galea, and David Vlahov, *Cities and the Health of the Public* (Nashville, TN: Vanderbilt University Press, 2006).

Frohlich, Katherine L. and Louise Potvin, "The Inequality Paradox: The Population Approach and Vulnerable Populations," 98(2) *American Journal of Public Health* (February, 2008): 216–221.

Fullilove, Mindy Thompson, Lesley Green, and Robert E. Fullilove III, "Building Momentum: An Ethnographic Study of Inner-City Redevelopment," 89(6) *American Journal of Public Health* (June, 1999): 840–844.

Fullilove, Mindy Thompson, "Psychiatric Implications of Displacement: Contributions From the Psychology of Place," 153 *American Journal of Psychiatry* (1996): 1516–1523.

Fullilove, Mindy, *Root Shock: How Tearing up City Neighborhoods Hurts America, and What We Can Do about It* (Prescott, AZ: One World Press, 2005).

Galea, Sandro ed., *Macrosocial Determinants of Population Health* (Secaucus, NJ: Springer, 2007).

Gault, Barbara, Heidi Hartmann, Avis Jones-DeWeever, Misha Werschkul, and Erica Williams, *The Women of New Orleans and the Gulf Coast: Multiple Disadvantages and Key Assets for Recovery, Part I. Poverty, Race, Gender and Class.* Briefing Paper #D464 (Washington, DC: Institute for Women's Policy Research, October, 2005).

Geronimus, Arline T., "To Mitigate, Resist, or Undo: Addressing Structural Influences on the Health of Urban Populations," 90 *American Journal of Public Health* (2000): 867–872.

Geronimus, Arline T., "Understanding and Eliminating Racial Inequalities in Women's Health in the US: The Role of the Weathering Conceptual Framework," 56 *Journal of the Medical Women's Association* (2001): 133–136.

Geronimus, Arline T., and J. Phillip Thompson, "To Denigrate, Ignore, or Disrupt: Racial Inequality in Health and the Impact of a Policy-Induced Breakdown of African American Communities," 1 *Du Bois Review* (2004): 247–279.

Gilson, Lucy, "In Defence and Pursuit of Equity," 47 *Social Science and Medicine* (1998): 1891–1896.

Gilson, Lucy, "Re-addressing Equity: The Importance of Ethical Processes," in *Reforming Health Sectors*, ed. A. Mills (London: Kegan Paul, 2001).

Glyn, A. and D. Miliband, *Paying for Inequality: The Economic Costs of Social Injustice* (London UK: IPPR/Rivers Press, 1994).

Gostin, Lawrence O., "What Does Social Justice Require for the Public's Health? Public Health Ethics and Policy Imperatives," 25(4) *Health Affairs* (2006): 1053–1060).

Gostin, Lawrence O., Jo Ivey Boufford, and Rose Marie Martinez, "The Future of the Public's Health: Vision, Values, and Strategies," 23(4) *Health Affairs* (July/ August, 2004): 97–107.

Graham, Hilary and Michael P. Kelly, "Health Inequalities: Concepts, Frameworks and Policy," National Health Service, Health Development Agency. Briefing paper, 2005.

Graham, Hilary ed., *Understanding Health Inequalities* (Buckingham: Open University Press, 2000).

Graham, Hilary, "Social Determinants and Their Unequal Distribution: Clarifying Policy Understandings," 82(1) *The Milbank Quarterly* (2004): 101–124.

Graham, Hilary, *Unequal Lives: Health and Socioeconomic Inequalities*, (Berkshire, UK: Open University Press, 2007).

Green, Judith and Ronald Labonte eds., *Critical Perspectives in Public Health* (New York: Routledge, 2007).

Griffith, Derek M., Mondi Mason, Michael Yonas, et al., "Dismantling Institutional Racism: Theory and Action," 39 *American Journal of Community Psychology* (2007): 381–392.

Gwatkin, D.R., "Health Inequalities and the Health of the Poor: What Do We Know? What Can We Do?" 78(1) *Bulletin of the World Health Organization* (2000): 3–18

Hahn, R.A., E. D. Eaker, N.D. Barker, S.M. Teutsch, W.A. Sosniak, and N. Krieger, "Poverty and Death in the United States," 26(4) *International Journal of Health Services* (1996): 673–690.

Hamlin, Christopher, *Public Health and Social Justice in the Age of Chadwick. Britain 1800–1854* (London: Cambridge University Press, 1998).

Hartman, Chester and Gregory D. Squires, *There Is No Such Thing As A Natural Disaster: Race, Class, and Hurricane Katrina* (New York: Routledge, 2006).

Hayward, Karen and Ronald Colman, *The Tides of Change: Addressing Inequity and Chronic Disease in Atlantic Canada—A Discussion Paper*, Prepared for the Population and Public Health Branch, Atlantic Regional Office, Health Canada (July, 2003).

Health Canada, Health Promotion and Programs Branch, *Taking Action on Population Health*, A position paper for Health Promotion and Programs Branch staff. (Ottawa, Ontario: Health, Canada, 1998).

Healton, Cheryl and Kathleen Nelson, "Reversal of Misfortune: Viewing Tobacco as a Social Justice Issue," 94 *American Journal of Public Health* (2004): 186–191.

Heymann, Jody, Clyde Hertzman, Morris L. Barer, and Robert G. Evans eds. *Healthier Societies: From Analysis to Action* (New York: Oxford University Press, 2006).

Hillemeier, Marianne M., John Lynch, Sam Harper, and Michele Casper, "Measurement Issues in Social Determinants: Measuring Contextual Characteristics for Community Health," 38(6), Part II *HSR: Health Services Research* (December, 2003): 1645–1718.

Hodge, James G. and Lawrence O. Gostin, *Public Health Practice vs. Research: A Report for Public Health Practitioners Including Cases and Guidance for*

Making Distinctions (Council of State and Territorial epidemiologists, May 4, 2004).

Hofrichter, Richard ed., *Health and Social Justice: Politics, Ideology, and Inequity in the Distribution of Disease* (San Francisco, CA: Jossey-Bass/John Wiley, 2003).

Holland, P., L. Berney, D. Blane, G. Davey Smith, D.J. Gunnell, and S.M. Montgomery, "Life Course Accumulation of Disadvantage: Childhood Health and Hazard Exposure During Adulthood," 50 *Social Science & Medicine* (2000): 1285–1295.

House, James S. and David R. Williams, "Understanding and Reducing Socioeconomic and Racial/Ethnic Disparities in Health," in *Promoting Health: Intervention Strategies from Social and Behavioral Research*, ed. Brian D. Smedley and Leonard S. Syme (Washington, DC: National Academy Press, 2000): 81–115.

International Society for Equity in Health/Global Equity Gauge Alliance, *The Equity Gauge: Concepts, Principles, and Guidelines*, Global Equity Gauge Alliance and Health Systems Trust, 2003, http://www.gega.org.za/ (accessed July 31, 2009).

Irwin, A., N. Valentine, C. Brown, et al., "The Commission on Social Determinants of Health: Tackling the Social Roots of Health Inequities," 3(6) e106 *PLoS Med* (2006): 1–3.

Isaacs, Stephen L. and Steven A. Schroeder, "Class—The Ignored Determinant of the Nation's Health," 351(11) *New England Journal of Medicine* (2004): 1137–1142.

Isreal, Barbara, Barry Checkoway, Amy Schulz and Marc Zimmerman, "Health Education and Community Empowerment: Conceptualizing and Measuring Perceptions of Individual, Organizational, and Community Control," 21(2) *Health Education Quarterly* (Summer, 1994): 149–170.

Isreal, Barbara, Eugenia Eng, Amy J. Schulz, and Edith A. Parker eds., *Methods in Community Community-Based Participatory Research for Health* (San Francisco: Jossey-Bass, 2005).

Jackson, Sharon A., Roger T. Anderson, Norman J. Johnson, and Paul D. Sorlie, "The Relation of Residential Segregation to All-Cause Mortality: A Study in Black and White," 90(4) *American Journal of Public Health* (April, 2000): 615–617.

Jennings, Tim and Gert Scheerder, *Tackling Social Inequalities in Health: The Role of Health Promotion* (Brussels: Flemish Institute for Health Promotion/European Network of Health Promotion Agencies, 2002).

Jones, Camara Phyllis, "Race, Racism, and Epidemiological Practice," 154(4) *American Journal of Epidemiology* (August 15, 2001): 299–304.

Jones, Camara Phyllis, "Levels of Racism: A Theoretic Framework and a Gardner's Tale" 90(8) *American Journal of Public Health* (August, 2000): 1212–1215.

Jones, Loring, "The Health Consequences of Economic Recessions," in *Health and Poverty*, ed. Michael J. Holosko and Marvin D. Feit (New York: The Haworth Press, 1997): 50–64.

Judge, Ken, Stephen Platt, Caroline Costongs, and Kasia Jurczak, *Health Inequalities: A Challenge for Europe*, An independent report commissioned by, and published under the auspices of, the UK Presidency of the EU (October, 2005).

Kaplan, G.A., E. Pamuk, J.W. Lynch, J.W. Cohen, and J.L. Balfour, "Income Inequality and Mortality in the United States: Analysis of Mortality and Potential Pathways," 312 *British Medical Journal* (1996): 999–1003.

Kaplan, George A., "Health Inequalities and the Welfare state: Perspectives from Social Epidemiology," 17(1) *Norwegian Journal of Epidemiology* (2007): 9–20.

Kaplan, George and John W. Lynch "Is Economic Policy Health Policy?" [Editorial] 91(3) *American Journal of Public Health"* (2001): 351–352.

Karlsen, Saffron and James Y. Nazroo, "Relation between Racial Discrimination, Social Class, and Health Among Ethnic Minority Groups," 92(4) *American Journal of Public Health* (April, 2002): 624–631.

Karpati, Adam, B. Kerker, F. Mostashari, et al., *Health Disparities in New York City* (New York: New York City Department of Health and Mental Hygiene, 2004).

Karpati, Adam, Sandro Galea, Tamara Awerbuch, and Richard Levins, "Variability and Vulnerability at the Ecological Level: Implications for Understanding the Social Determinants of Health," 92(11) *American Journal of Public Health* (November, 2002): 1768–1772.

Kaufman, Jay S. and R.S. Cooper, "Seeking Causal Explanations in Social Epidemiology," 150(2) *American Journal of Epidemiology* (1999): 113–120.

Kawachi, Ichiro and Lisa Berkman eds., *Neighborhoods and Health* (New York: Oxford University Press, 2003).

Kawachi, Ichiro and Sarah P. Wamala eds., *Globalization and Health* (New York: Oxford University Press, 2008).

Kawachi, Ichiro, B. Kennedy, V. Gupta, and D. Prothrow-Stith, "Women's Status and the Health of Men and Women: A View from the States," 48 *Social Science & Medicine* (1999): 21–32.

Kawachi, Ichiro, Bruce P. Kennedy, and Richard G. Wilkinson eds., *The Society and Population Health Reader: Income Inequality and Health* (New York: The New Press, 1999).

Keleher, Helen and Berni Murphy, *Understanding Health: A Determinants Approach* (London: Oxford University Press, 2004).

Kennedy, Bruce, Ichiro Kawachi, Kimberly Lochner, Camara P. Jones, and Deborah Prothrow-Stith, "(Dis)respect and Black Mortality," in *The Society and Population Health Reader: Income Inequality and Health*, ed. Ichiro Kawachi, B. Kennedy, and R. G. Wilkinson (New York: New Press, 1999) 465–473.

Kim, Jim Yong, Joyce V. Millen, Alec Irwin, and John Gershman eds., *Dying for Growth: Global Inequality and the Health of the Poor* (Monroe, ME: Common Courage Press, 2000).

Kington, R. and H. Nickens, "The Health of African Americans: Recent Trends, Current Patterns, Future Directions," in *America Becoming: Racial Trends and Their Consequences*, Vol. 2. (Washington, DC: National Academy Press, 2001).

Krieger, James and Donna L. Higgins, "Housing and Health: Time Again for Public Health Action," 92(5) *American Journal of Public Health* (May, 2002): 758–768.

Krieger, Nancy and Anne-Emannuelle Birn, "A Vision of Social Justice as the Foundation of Public Health: Commemorating 150 Years of the Spirit of 1848," 88(11) *American Journal of Public Health* (November, 1998): 1603–1606.

Krieger, Nancy and S. Zierler, "What Explains the Public's Health?: A Call for Epidemiologic Theory," 7 *Epidemiology* (1996): 107–109.

Krieger, Nancy and Sofia Gruskin "Frameworks Matter: Ecosocial and Health and Human Rights Perspectives on Disparities in Women's Health—The Case of Tuberculosis," 56(4) *Journal of the American Medical Women's Association* (Fall 2001): 137–142.

Krieger, Nancy ed., *Embodying Inequality: Epidemiologic Perspectives* (Amityville, NY: Baywood, 2004).

Krieger, Nancy, D.H. Rehkopf, J.T. Chen, et al., "The Fall and Rise of U.S. Inequities in Premature Mortality 1960–2002," 5(2) *PLoS Medicine* (2008): e46.

Krieger, Nancy, D.L. Rowley, A. Herman, B. Avery, and M.T. Phillips, "Racism, Sexism, and Social Class: Implications for Studies of Health, Disease, and Well-Being," 9(Suppl. 6) *American Journal of Preventive Medicine* (1993): 82–122.

Krieger, Nancy, David R. Williams, and Nancy E. Moss, "Measuring Social Class in US Public Health Research: Concepts, Methodologies, and Guidelines," 18 *Annual Reviews of Public Health* (1997): 341–378.

Krieger, Nancy, J.T. Chen, and G. Ebel, "Can We Monitor Socioeconomic Inequalities in Health? A Survey of U.S. Health Departments' Data Collection and Reporting Practices," 112 *Public Health Reports* (1997): 481–494.

Krieger, Nancy, Kevin Smith, Deepa Naishadham, Cathy Hartman, and Elizabeth M. Barbeau, "Experiences of Discrimination: Validity and Reliability of a Self-Report Measure for Population Health Research on Racism and Health," 61 *Social Science & Medicine* (2005): 1576–1596.

Krieger, Nancy, Pamela D. Waterman, David H. Rehkopf, and S.V. Subramanian, "Race/Ethnicity, Gender and Monitoring Socioeconomic Gradients in Health: A Comparison of Area-Based Socioeconomic Measures—The Public Health Disparities Geocoding Project," 93(10) *American Journal of Public Health* (2003): 1655–1671.

Krieger, Nancy, "A Glossary for Social Epidemiology," 55 *Journal of Epidemiology and Community Health* (2001): 693–700.

Krieger, Nancy, "Discrimination and Health," in *Social Epidemiology*, ed. Lisa Berkman and Ichiro Kawachi (New York: Oxford University Press, 2000), 36–75.

Krieger, Nancy, "Does Racism Harm Health? Did Child Abuse Exist Before 1962? On Explicit Questions, Critical Science, and Current Controversies: An Ecosocial Perspective," 93(2) *American Journal of Public Health* (February, 2003): 194–199.

Krieger, Nancy, "Embodying Inequality: A Review of Concepts, Measures, and Methods for Studying Health Consequences of Discrimination," 29(2) *International Journal of Health Services* (1999): 295–352.

Krieger, Nancy, "Epidemiology and Social Sciences: Towards A Critical Reengagement in the 21st Century" 22 *Epidemiologic Reviews* (2000): 155–163.

Krieger, Nancy, "Epidemiology and the Web of Causation: Has Anyone Seen the Spider," 39 *Social Science & Medicine* (1994): 887–903.

Krieger, Nancy, "Genders, Sexes, and Health: What Are the Connections—and Why Does It Matter?" 32 *International Journal of Epidemiology* (2003): 652–657.

Krieger, Nancy, "Historical Roots of Social Epidemiology: Socioeconomic Gradients in Health and Contextual Analysis," 30 *International Journal of Epidemiology* (2001): 899–903.

Krieger, Nancy, "Ladders, Pyramids and Champagne: The Iconography of Health Inequities," 62 *Journal of Epidemiology and Community Health* (2008): 1098–1104.

Krieger, Nancy, "Proximal, Distal, and the Politics of Causation: What's Level Got To Do With It," 98(2) *American Journal of Public Health* (February, 2008): 221–230.

Krieger, Nancy, "Questioning Epidemiology: Objectivity, Advocacy, and Socially Responsible Science." 89(8) *American Journal of Public Health* (August, 1999): 1151–1153.

Krieger, Nancy, "Researching Critical Questions on Social Justice and Public Health: An Ecosocial Perspective," in *Social Injustice and Public Health*, ed. Barry S. Levy and Victor W. Sidel (New York: Oxford University Press, 2006), 460–479.

Krieger, Nancy, "Stormy Weather: Race, Gene Expression, and the Science of Health Disparities," 95(12) *American Journal of Public Health* (December, 2005): 2155–2160.

Krieger, Nancy, "The Health of Black Folk: Disease, Class and Ideology in Science," in *The Racial Economy of Health*, ed. Sandra Harding (Bloomington, IN: Indiana University Press, 1993): 161–169.

Krieger, Nancy, "The Ostrich, The Albatross and Public Health: An Ecosocial Perspective—Or Why an Explicit Focus on Health Consequences of Discrimination and Deprivation Is Vital for Good Science and Public Health Practice," 116(5) *Public Health Reports* (2001): 419–423.

Krieger, Nancy, "Theories for Social Epidemiology in the 21st Century: An Ecosocial Perspective," 30 *International Journal of Epidemiology* (2001): 668–677.

Krieger, Nancy, "Why Epidemiologists Cannot Afford to Ignore Poverty," 18(6) *Epidemiology* (November, 2007): 658–663.

Kruger, Jennifer Prah, "Health and Social Justice," 364 *The Lancet* (2004): 1075–1080.

Kuh, D. and Y. Ben-Shlomo eds., *A Lifecourse Approach to Chronic Disease Epidemiology* (Oxford: Oxford University Press, 1997).

Kuh, Diana, Rebecca Hardy, Claudia Langneberg, Marcus Richards, and Michael E.J. Wordsworth, "Mortality in Adults Aged 26–54 Years Related to Socioeconomic Conditions in Childhood and Adulthood: Post War Birth Cohort Study," 325 *British Medical Journal* (November 9, 2002): 1076–1080.

Labonte, Ronald and Matthew Sanger, "Glossary of the World Trade Organization and Public Health: Part I," 60 *Journal of Epidemiology and Community Health* (2006): 655–661.

Labonte, Ronald and Ted Schrecker, *Globalization and Social Determinants of Health: Analytic and Strategic Review Paper*, (Ottawa: University of Ottawa, March 11, 2006).

Labonte, Ronald, "Healthy Public Policy and the World Trade Organization: A Proposal for an International Health Presence in Future World Trade/Investment Talks," 13 *Health Promotion International* (1998): 245–256.

Labonte, Ronald, "International Governance and World Trade Organization (WTO) Reform," 12(1) *Critical Public Health* (2002): 65–86.

Labonte, Ronald, "Social Inclusion/Exclusion and Health: Dancing the Dialectic," in *The Social Determinants of Health: Canadian Perspectives*, ed. Dennis Raphael (Toronto: Canadian Scholars Press, 2004), 253–266.

Langone, John, "Trying to Bridge the 'Death Gap' Confronting Minority Groups," *The New York Times* (December 19, 2000): D7.

Lantz, P.M., J.S. House, J.M. Lepkowski, D.R. Williams, R.P. Mero, and J. Chen, "Socioeconomic Factors, Health Behaviors, and Mortality," 279 *Journal of the American Medical Association* (1998): 1703–1708.

LaVeist, T.A., "Why We Should Continue to Study Race But Do a Better Job: An Essay on Race, Racism, and Health," 6(1–2) *Ethnicity and Disease* (1996): 21–29

LaVeist, T.A. ed., *Race, Ethnicity and Health: A Public Health Reader* (San Francisco, CA: Jossey-Bass/John Wiley, 2002).

LaVeist, T.A., *Minority Populations and Health: An Introduction to Health Disparities in the United States* (San Francisco, CA: Jossey-Bass, 2005).

Leavitt, Judith, *The Healthiest City* (Madison, WI: University of Wisconsin Press, 1995).

Leon, David and Gill Walt eds., *Poverty, Inequality and Health: An International Perspective* (Oxford: Oxford University Press, 2001).

Levins, Richard and Cynthia Lopez, "Toward An Ecosocial View of Health," 29(2) *International Journal of Health Services* (1999): 261).

Levy, Barry S. and Victor W. Sidel eds., *Social Injustice and Public Health* (New York: Oxford University Press, 2005).

Li, Jianghong, Anne McMurray, and Fiona Stanley, "Modernity's Paradox and the Structural Determinants of Child Health and Well-Being," 17 *Health Sociology Review* (2008): 64–77.

Lilley, Susan, *An Annotated Bibliography on Indicators for the Determinants of Health*, (Manitoba: Health Promotion and Program Branch, Atlantic Regional Office, Health Canada, 2000), www.hc-sc.gc.ca/hppb/phdd/determinants_deter_biblio.html (accessed July 31, 2009).

Link, B.G. and J. Phelan, "Social Conditions as Fundamental Causes of Disease," 36 *Journal of Health and Social Behavior* (1995): 80–94.

Link, B.G. and J. Phelan, "McKeown and the Idea That Social Conditions Are Fundamental Causes of Disease," 92(5) *American Journal of Public Health* (May, 2002): 730–732.

Lloyd, Cathy E., Stephen Handsley, Jenny Douglas, Sarah Earle, and Sue Spurr eds., *Policy and Practice in Promoting Health* (London: The Open University, 2007).

Lockner, Kim, Elsie Pamuk, Diane Makuc, Bruce Kennedy, and Ichiro Kawachi, "State-Level Income Inequality and Individual Mortality Risk: A Prospective, Multilevel Study," 91(3) *American Journal of Public Health* (2001): 385–391.

Luna, Marcos, The Limited Role of Environmental Health for Social Justice, Paper presented at the 131st Annual Meeting of the American Public Health Association (San Francisco, CA: November 17, 2003).

Lutfey, Karen and Jeremy Freese, "Toward Some Fundamentals of Fundamental Causality: Socioecoomic Status and Health in the Routine Clinic Visit for Diabetes," 110(5) *American Journal of Sociology* (March, 2005): 1326–1372.

Lynch, John W., George A. Kaplan, and Elsie R. Pamuk, "Income Inequality and Mortality in Metropolitan Areas of the United States," 88(7) *American Journal of Public Health* (July, 1998): 1074–1080.

Lynch, John W., George Davey Smith, George A. Kaplan, and James S. House, "Income Inequality and Mortality: Importance to Health of Individual Income, Psychosocial Environment, or Material Conditions," 320 *British Medical Journal* (April 29, 2000) 1200–1204.

Lynch, John, "Income Inequality and Health: Expanding the Debate," 51 *Social Science & Medicine* (2001): 1001–1005.

Lynch, John, George Davey Smith, Sam Harper, et al., "Is Income Inequality a Determinant of Population Health? Part 1. A Systematic Review," 82(1) *The Milbank Quarterly* (2004): 5–99.

Maantay, Juliana, "Mapping Environmental Injustices: Pitfalls and Potential of Geographic Information Systems in Assessing Environmental Health Equity," 110(Suppl. 2) *Environmental Health Perspectives* (April, 2002): 161–171.

Maantay, Juliana, "Zoning, Equity and Public Health," 91(7) *American Journal of Public Health* (July, 2001): 1033–1041.

Macintyre, Sally, "Prevention and the Reduction of Health Inequalities," 320 *British Medical Journal* (2000): 1399–1400.

Macintyre, Sally, "Social Inequalities and Health in the Contemporary World: Comparative Overview," in *Human Biology and Social Inequality* 39th Symposium Volume of the Society for the Study of Human Biology, ed. S.S. Strickland and P.S. Shetty (Cambridge: Cambridge University Press, 1998): 20–33.

Mackenbach, J.P., *Health Inequalities: Europe in Profile*, UK Presidency of the EU, London (2005).

Marmot, M. and R. Bell, "Action on Health Disparities in the United States: Commission on Social Determinants of Health," 301(11) *Journal of the American Medical Association* (2009): 1169–1171.

Marmot, M. and S. Friel, "Global Health Equity: Evidence for Action on the Social Determinants of Health," 62 *Journal of Epidemiology & Community Health* (2008): 1095–1097.

McCoy, David, Lexi Bambas, David Acurio, et al., "Global Equity Gauge Alliance: Reflections on Early Experiences," 21(3) *Journal of Health, Population, and Nutrition* (September, 2003): 273–287.

McDonough, P., G.J. Duncan, D. Williams, and J. House, "Income Dynamics and Adult Mortality in the United States, 1972–1989," 87(9) *American Journal of Public Health* (1997): 1476–1483.

McGinnis, J.M. and William H. Foege, "Actual Causes of Death in the United States," 270 *Journal of the American Medical Association* (1993): 2207–2212.

McKinley, John, "The Case for Refocussing Upstream: The Political Economy of Illness," in *The Sociology of Health and Illness: Critical Perspectives*, ed. Peter Conrad, 8th ed., (New York: St. Martins Press, 2008) 578–591.

McKinley, John and Lisa D. Marceau, "To Boldly Go…," 90(1) *American Journal of Public Health* (January, 2000): 25–33.

Minkler, Meredith, Esme Fuller-Thomson, and Jack M. Guralnik, "Gradient of Disability Across the Socioeconomic Spectrum in the United States," 355(7) *The New England Journal of Medicine* (August 17, 2006): 695–703.

Minnesota Department of Public Health. *A Call to Action: Advancing Health for All Through Social and Economic Change* (St. Paul, MN: Minnesota Department of Health, 2001).

Miringoff, Marc and Marque-Luisa Miringoff, *The Social Health of the Nation: How America Is Really Doing* (New York: Oxford University Press, 1999).

Mitchell, Richard, Mary Shaw, and Danny Dorling, *Inequalities in Life and Death: What If Britain Were More Equal?* (London: The Policy Press, 2000).

Montague, Peter, "Wealth and Health," *Rachel's Environment & Health Weekly* 654 (June 10, 1999).

Morone, James A. and Lawrence R. Jacobs eds., *Healthy, Wealthy, and Fair: Health Care and the Good Society* (New York: Oxford University Press, 2005).

Moss, Nancy, "Socioeconomic Disparities in Health in the US: An Agenda for Action," 15(11) *Social Science & Medicine* (2000): 1627–1638.

Muntaner, Carles and John Lynch, "Income Inequality, Social Cohesion, and Class Relations: A Critique of Wilkinson's Neo-Durkheimian Research Program," 29(1) *International Journal of Health Services* (1999): 59–81.

Muntaner, Carles, Carme Borrell, Joan Benach, M. Isabel Pasarin, and Esteve Fernandez, "The Associations of Social Class and Social Stratification with Patterns of General and Mental Health in a Spanish Population," 32 *International Journal of Epidemiology* (2003): 950–958.

Muntaner, Carles, John Lynch, and George Davey Smith, "Social Capital and the Third Way in Public Health," 10(2) *Critical Public Health* (2000): 108–124.

Muntaner, Carles, John Lynch, and Gary L. Oates, "The Social Class Determinants of Inequality and Social Cohesion," 29(4) *International Journal of Health Services* (1999): 699–732.

Muntaner, Carles, William W. Eaton, and Chamberlain C. Diala, "Social Inequalities in Mental Health: A Review of Concepts and Underlying Assumptions," 4(1) *Health* (2000): 89–113.

Muntaner, Carles, "Commentary: Social Capital, Social Class, and the Slow Progress of Psychosocial Epidemiology," 33 *International Journal of Epidemiology* (2004): 1–7.

Muntaner, Carles, "Invited Commentary: Social Mechanisms, Race, and Social Epidemiology," 150(2) *American Journal of Epidemiology* (1999): 121–126.

Muntaner, Carles, "Teaching Social Inequalities in Health: Barriers and Opportunities," 27 *Journal of Public Health* (1999): 161–165.

Muntanter, Carles and Haejoo Chung, "Commentary: Macrosocial Determinants, Epidemiology, and Health Policy: Should Politics and Economics be Banned From Social Determinants of Health Research?" 29 *Journal of Public Health Policy* (2008): 299–306.

Myer, Ilan H. and Sharon Schwartz, "Social Issues as Public Health: Promise and Peril," 90(8) *American Journal of Public Health* (August, 2000): 1189–1191.

Nairn, R. F. Pega, T. McCreanor, J. Rankine, and A. Barnes, "Media, Racism, and Public Health Psychology," 11(2) *Public Health Psychology* (2006): 183–196.

National Research Council, *Eliminating Health Disparities: Measurement and Data Needs*, Panel on DHHS Collection of Race and Ethnicity Data, ed. Michele Ver Ploeg and Edward Perrin, Committee on National Statistics, Division of Social and Behavioral Sciences and Education (Washington, DC: National Academies Press, 2004).

Navarro, Vicente ed., *Neoliberalism, Globalization and Inequalities: Consequences for Health and the Quality of Life* (Amityville, NY: Baywood Press, 2007).

Navarro, Vicente, Carles Muntaner, Carme Borrell, et al., "Politics and Health Outcomes," 368 *The Lancet* (September 16, 2006): 1033–1037.

Navarro, Vicente, "The Politics of Health Inequalities Research in the United States," 34(1) *International Journal of Health Services* (2004): 87–99.

Navarro, Vincente ed., *The Political Economy of Social Inequalities: Consequences for Health and Quality of Life*, Vol. 1. (Amityville, NY: Baywood Press, 2000).

Navarro, Vincente and Carles Muntaner eds., *Political and Economic Determinants of Population Health and Well-Being: Controversies and Developments*, Vol. 2. (Amityville, NY: Baywood Press, 2004).

Navarro, Vincente and Leiyu Shi, "The Political Context of Social Inequalities and Health," 31(1) *International Journal of Health Services* (2001): 1–21.

Navarro, Vincente, "Assessment of the World Health Report 2000," 356 *The Lancet* (2000): 1598–1601.

Navarro, Vincente, "Health and Equity in the World in the Era of 'Globalization,'" 29(2) *International Journal of Health Services* (1999): 215–226.

Nazroo, James Y., "Genetic, Cultural, or Socio-economic Vulnerability? Explaining Ethnic Inequalities in Health," in *The Sociology of Health Inequalities*, ed. Mel Bartley, David Blane and George Davey Smith (Oxford: Blackwell, 1998), 151–170.

Nazroo, James Y., "The Structuring of Ethnic Inequalities: Economic Position, Racial Discrimination, and Racism," 93(2) *American Journal of Public Health* (February, 2003): 277–284.

Newman, Kathy, "Older, Healthier, and Wealthier: Study Finds Big Racial Disparities in Seniors' Growing Well-Being," *The Washington Post* (August 10, 2000).

Northridge, Mary and Peggy Shepard, "Environmental Racism and Public Health," 87 *American Journal of Public Health* (1997): 730–732.

Northridge, Mary, Gabriel N. Stover, Joyce E. Rosenthal, and Donna Sherard, "Environmental Equity and Health: Understanding Complexity and Moving Forward," 93(2) *American Journal of Public Health* (February, 2003): 209–214.

Nuru-Jeter, Amani, Tyan Parker Dominguez, Wizdom Powell Hammond, et al., "'It's the Skin You're In': African-American Women Talk About Their Experiences of Racism. An Exploratory Study to Develop Measures of Racism for Birth Outcome Studies," 13(1) *Maternal & Child Health Journal* (January, 2009): 29–39).

Oakes, J. Michael and Jay S. Kaufman eds., *Methods in Social Epidemiology* (San Francisco, CA: Jossey-Bass, 2006).

Olafsdottir, S, "Fundamental Causes of Health Disparities: Stratification, the Welfare State and Health in the United States and Iceland," 48(3) *Journal of Health & Social Behavior* (2007): 239–253.

Oliver, Adam, *Why Care About Health Inequality?* (London: Office of Health Economics, 2001).

Oliver, M. Norman and Carles Muntaner, "Researching Health Inequities Among African Americans: The Imperative to Understand Social Class," 35(3) *International Journal of Health Services* (2005): 485–498.

Ostlin, Piroska, Asha George, and Gita Sen, "Gender, Health and Equity: The Intersections," in *Challenging Inequities in Health: From Ethics to Action,* ed. T. Evans, M. Whitehead, F. Diderichsen, A. Bhuiya, and M. Wirth (New York: Oxford University Press, 2001), 175–189.

Pappas, Greg, S. Queen, W. Hadden, and G. Fisher, "The Increasing Disparity in Mortality between Socioeconomic Groups in the United States, 1960 and 1986," 329(2) *New England Journal of Medicine* (1993): 103–109.

Paradies, Yin, "A Systematic Review of Empirical Research on Self-Reported Racism and Health," 35 *International Journal of Epidemiology* (2006): 888–901.

Parker, Edith, Lewis H. Margolis, Eugenia Eng, and Carlos Henriquez-Roldan, "Assessing the Capacity of Health Departments to Engage in Community-Based Participatory Public Health," 93(3) *American Journal of Public Health* (March, 2003): 472–476.

Pearce, Neil and George Davey Smith, "Is Social Capital the Key to Inequalities in Health?" 93(1) *American Journal of Public Health* (January, 2003): 122–129.

Phelan, Jo C., Bruce G. Link, Ana Diez-Roux, Ichiro Kawachi, and Bruce Levin, "'Fundamental Causes' of Social Inequalities in Mortality: A Test of the Theory," 45 *Journal of Health and Social Behavior* (September, 2004): 265–285.

Poland, B., D. Coburn, A. Robertson, and J. Eakin, "Wealth, Equality, and Health Care: A Critique of a 'Population Health' Perspective on the Determinants of Health," 46(7) *Social Science and Medicine* (1998): 785–798.

Politics of Health Group, *UK Health Watch 2005: The Experience of Health in an Unequal Society*. London, 2005.

Porter, Dorothy, *Health, Civilization and the State* (New York: Routledge, 1999).

Potvin, Louise, Sylvie Gendron, Angele Bilodeau, and Patrick Chabot, "Integrating Social Theory Into Public Health Practice," 95(4) *American Journal of Public Health* (April, 2005): 591–595.

Power, C. and S. Matthews, "Origins of Health Inequalities in a National Population Sample," 350 *The Lancet* (1997): 1584–1585.

Powers, Madison and Ruth Faden, *Social Justice: The Moral Foundations of Public Health and Health Policy* (Oxford: Oxford University Press, 2006).

Prescott-Allen, Robert, *The Wellbeing of Nations: A Country-by-Country Index of Quality of Life and the Environment* (Washington, DC: Island Press, 2001).

Public Health Agency of Canada, *The Chief Public Health Officer's Report on the State of Public Health in Canada, 2008*. Ottawa, Ontario, 2008.

Pulido, Laura, "Rethinking Environmental Racism: White Privilege and Urban Development in Southern California," 90(1) *Annals of the Association of American Geographers* (March, 2000): 12–40.

Putnam, Sarah and Sandro Galea, "Epidemiology and the Macrosocial Determinants of Health," 29 *Journal of Public Health Policy* (2008): 275–289.

Raphael, Dennis ed., *Social Determinants of Health: Canadian Perspectives*, 2nd ed. (Toronto: Canadian Scholars' Press, 2008).

Raphael, Dennis, "Public Health Units and Poverty in Ontario: Part of the Solution or Part of the Problem?" Material in this paper was presented at the All-Members Meeting of the Association of Local Health Authorities, Toronto, Canada (February 1, 2002).

Raphael, Dennis, "Addressing the Social Determinants of Health in Canada: Bridging the Gap Between Research Findings and Public Policy," 24(3) *Policy Options* (March, 2003): 35–40.

Raphael, Dennis, "Barriers to Addressing the Societal Determinants of Health: Public Health Units and Poverty in Ontario, Canada," 18(4) *Health Promotion International* (2003): 415–423.

Raphael, Dennis, "Getting Serious About the Social Determinants of Health: New Directions for Public Health Workers," 15(3) *Promotion and Education* (June, 2008): 15–20.

Raphael, Dennis, "Health Effects of Economic Inequality," A paper based on a presentation made as part of the University of Toronto's School of Continuing Studies Lecture Series, the Economic Fabric (January 29, 1999).

Raphael, Dennis, "Health Inequalities in Canada: Current Discourses and Implications for Public Health Action," 10(2) *Critical Public Health* (2000): 193–216.

Raphael, Dennis, "Public Health Responses to Health Inequalities," 89(6) *Canadian Journal of Public Health* (November/December, 1998): 380–381.

Raphael, Dennis, "The Limitations of Population Health as a Model for a New Public Health," 17(2) *Health Promotion International* (2002): 189–199.

Raphael, Dennis, "The Question of Evidence in Health Promotion," 15 *Health Promotion International* (2000): 355–367.

Raphael, Dennis, *Social Justice is Good for Our Hearts: Why Societal Factors—Not Lifestyles—are Major Causes of Heart Disease in Canada and Elsewhere* (Toronto: CSJ Foundation for Research and Education, 2002).

Rawh, Viriginia A., Ginger Chew, and Robin S. Garfinkel, "Deteriorated Housing Contributes to High Cockroach Allergen Levels in Inner-City Households," 110(Suppl. 2) *Environmental Health Perspectives* (April, 2002): 323–327.

Ridde, Valery, "Reducing Social Inequalities in Health: Public Health, Community Health, or Health Promotion," 14(2) *Promotion and Education* (2007): 63–67.

Ridde, Valery, "Reducing Social Inequalities in Health: Public Health, Community Health, or Health Promotion?" 14(2) *Promotion and Education* (2007): 63–67.

Robertson, Ann, "Critical Reflections on the Politics of Need: Implications for Public Health," 47(10) *Social Science and Medicine* (1998): 1419–1430.

Robertson, Ann, "Health Promotion and the Common Good: Theoretical Considerations," 9(2) *Critical Public Health* (1999): 117–133.

Ronzio, C.R., E. Pamuk and G.D. Squires, "The Politics of Preventable Deaths: Local Spending, Income Inequality, and Premature Mortality in U.S. Cities," 58 *Journal of Epidemiology and Community Health* (2004): 175–179.

Rose, G., *The Strategy of Preventive Medicine* (Oxford: Oxford University Press, 1992).

Rosen, Lawrence and Deirdre Imus, "Environmental Injustice: Children's Health Disparities and the Role of the Environment," 3(5) *Pediatrics* (September/October, 2007): 524–528.

Ross, N.A., M.C. Wolfson, J.R. Dunn, J-M. Berthelot, G.A. Kaplan, and J.W. Lynch, "Relation Between Income Inequality and Mortality in Canada and the United States: Cross-Sectional Assessment Using Census Data and Vital Statistics," 320 *British Medical Journal* (2000): 898–902.

Rubin, I. Leslie, Janice T. Nodvin, Robert J. Geller, W. Gerald Teague, Brian L. Holtzclaw, and Eric I. Felner, "Environmental Health Disparities: Environmental and Social Impact of Industrial Pollution in a Community—the Model of Anniston, AL," 54 *Pediatric Clinics of North America* (2007): 375–398.

Scambler, Graham and Paul Higgs, "Stratification, Class and Health: Class Relations and Health Inequalities in High Modernity," 33(2) *Sociology* (1999): 275–296.

Scambler, Graham, *Health and Social Change: A Critical Theory* (Buckingham: Open University Press, 2002).

Schalick, L.M., W.C. Hadden, E. Pamuk, V. Navarro, and G. Pappas , "The Widening Gap in Death Rates Among Income Groups in the US: 1967–86," 30 *International Journal of Health Services* (2000): 13–26.

Schulz, Amy and Mary Northridge, "Social Determinants of Health: Implications for Environmental Health Problems," 31(45) *Health Education & Behavior* (2004): 1–17.

Schulz, Amy J. and Leith Mullings eds., *Gender, Race, Class and Health: Intersectional Approaches* (San Francisco, CA: Jossey-Bass 2005).

Schulz, Amy J. and Leith Mullings eds., *Gender, Race, Class, and Health: Intersectional Approaches* (San FranciscoCA: Jossey-Bass, 2005): Chapter 1.

Schulz, Amy, David R. Williams, Barbara A. Isreal, and Lora Bex Lempert, "Racial and Spatial Relations as Fundamental Determinants of Health in Detroit," 80(4) *The Milbank Quarterly* (2002): 677–707.

Schulz, Amy, Edith Parker, Barbara Isreal, and Tomiko Fisher, "Social Context, Stressors and Disparities in Women's Health," 56 *Journal of the Medical Women's Association* (2001): 143–149.

Scott-Samuel, A., "Health Impact Assessment—Theory Into Practice," 52 *Journal of Epidemiology and Community Health* (1998): 704–705.

Scott-Samuel, Alex and Eileen O'Keefe, "Health Impact Assessment for Healthy Public Policy: The Way Ahead," Contributing Papers, the 3rd HIA International Workshop on Global and Regional Challenges for Healthy Society, Nakhon Pathom, Thailand (July 19–21, 2006).

Scriven, Angela and Sebastian Garman eds., *Public Health: Social Context and Action* (London: Open University Press, 2007).

Sen, Amartya, "Economic Progress and Health," in *Poverty, Inequality, and Health: An International Perspective*, ed. David Leon and Gill Walt (Oxford: Oxford University Press, 2001) 333–345.

Sen, Amartya, "Elements of a Theory of Human Rights," 32(4) *Philosophy and Public Affairs* (October, 2004): 315–356.

Sen, Amartya, "Mortality as an Indicator of Economic Success and Failure," 108 *The Economic Journal* (January 1998): 1–25.

Sen, Gita, A. George, and P. Ostlin, "Engendering Health Equity: A Review of Research and Policy," in *Engendering International Health: The Challenge of Equity*, ed. Gita Sen, A. George, and P. Ostlin (Cambridge, MA: MIT Press, 2002).

Shavers, Vicki and Brenda S. Shavers, "Racism and Health Inequity Among Americans," 98(3) *Journal of the National Medical Association* (March, 2006): 386–396.

Shaw, Mary, Danny Dorling, and George Davey Smith, "Poverty, Social Exclusion and Minorities," in *Social Determinants of Health,* ed. Michael Marmot and Richard Wilkinson (New York: Oxford University Press, 1999).

Siegrist, Johannes and Michael Marmot eds., *Social Inequalities in Health: New Evidence and Implications* (Oxford: Oxford University Press, 2006).

Singh, Gopal K. and Robert William Blum, "Morbidity and Mortality Among US Adolescents," 86(4) *American Journal of Public Health* (April, 1996): 505–512.

Smedley, Brian D. and S. Leonard Syme eds., *Promoting Health: Intervention Strategies from Social and Behavioral Research* (Washington, DC: National Academy Press, 2000).

Smith, David Barton, *A House Divided: Race and Healing A Nation* (Ann Arbor, MI: University of Michigan Press, 1999).

Sofaer, Shoshanna, *Performance Indicators: A Commentary from the Perspective of an Expanded View of Public Health* (Washington, DC: Center for the Advancement of Health and the Western Consortium for Public Health, March, 1995).

Soobader, M., C. Cubbin, G.C. Gee, A. Rosenbaum, and J. Laurenson, "Levels of Analysis for the Study of Environmental Health Disparities," 102 *Environmental Research* (2006): 172–180.

Sorlie, Paul D., Eric Backlund, and Jacob B. Keller, "US Mortality by Economic, Demographic, and Social Characteristics: The National Longitudinal Mortality Study," 85(7) *American Journal of Public Health* (1995): 949–956.

Spitzer, Denise, "Engendering Health Disparities," 96(Suppl. 2) *Canadian Journal of Public Health* (March–April, 2005): 578–596.

Standing, H., "Gender and Equity in Health Sector Reform Programmes: A Review," 12(1) *Health Policy and Planning* (1997): 1–18.

Starfield, B., J. Hyde, J. Gervas, and I. Heath, "The Concept of Prevention: A Good Idea Gone Astray?" 62 *Journal of Epidemiology and Community Health* (2008): 580–583.

Stephens, C., "The Policy Implications of Health Inequalities in Developing Countries," in *Human Biology and Social Inequality*, 39th Symposium Volume of the Society for the Study of Human Biology, ed. S.S. Strickland and P.S. Shetty (Cambridge: Cambridge University Press, 1998): 288–307.

Subramanian, S.V. and Ichiro Kawachi, "Income Inequality and Health: What Have We Learned So Far?" 26 *Epidemiologic Reviews* (2004): 78–91.

Szreter, Simon, "Rethinking McKeown: The Relationship Between Public Health and Social Change," 92(5) *American Journal of Public Health* (May, 2002): 722–725.

Tesh, Sylvia, *Hidden Arguments: Political Ideology and Disease Prevention Policy* (New Brunswick, NJ: Rutgers University Press, 1988).

Alvin Tarlov and Robert F. St. Peter eds., *The Society and Population Health Reader, Volume II, A State and Community Perspective* (New York: The New Press, 2000), 230–252.

Thiele, Bret, "The Human Right to Adequate Housing: A Tool for Promoting and Protecting Individual and Community Health," 92(5) *American Journal of Public Health* (May 2002): 712–715.

Thomas, Stephen B., "The Color Line: Race Matters in the Elimination of Health Disparities," 91(7) *American Journal of Public Health* (July, 2001): 1046–1048.

Townson, Monica, *Health and Wealth: How Social and Economic Factors Affect Our Well Being* (Ontario: Canadian Centre for Policy Alternatives, 1999).

van de Mheen, D., *Inequalities in Health: To be Continued? A Lifecourse Perspective on Socio economic Inequalities in Health* (Rotterdam: Erasmus University, Rotterdam, 1998).

Vega, Jeanette and Alec Irwin, "Tackling Health Inequalities: New Approaches in Public Policy," 82(7) *Bulletin of the World Health Organization* (July, 2004): 482–483.

Waitzman, N.J. and K.R. Smith, "Separate but Lethal: the Effects of Economic Segregation on Mortality in Metropolitan America," 76 *The Millbank Memorial Fund Quarterly* (1998): 341–373.

Wallace, Barbara C. ed., *Toward Equity in Health: A New Global Approach to Health Disparities* (New York: Springer, 2008).

Wallace, Roderick and Deborah Wallace, "Structured Psychosocial Stress and Therapeutic Failure," 12(3) *Journal of Biological Systems* (2004): 335–369.

Wallace, Roderick, Deborah Wallace, and Robert Wallace, "Coronary Heart Disease, Chronic Inflammation, and Pathogenic Social Hierarchy: A Biological Limit to Possible Reductions in Morbidity and Mortality," 96(5) *Journal of the National Medical Association* (2004): 609–619.

Wallack, Lawrence, "The Role of Mass Media in Creating Social Capital: A New Direction for Public Health," in *Promoting Health: Intervention Strategies from Social and Behavioral Research*, ed. Brian D. Smedley and Leonard S. Syme (Washington, DC: National Academy Press, 2000), 339–367.

Wallerstein, Nina and Bonnie Duran, "Using Community-Based Participatory Research to Address Health Disparities," 7(3) *Health Promotion Practice* (July, 2006): 312–323.

Weber, Lynn, "Reconstructing the Landscape of Health Disparities Research: Promoting Dialogue and Collaboration between Feminist Intersectional and Biomedical Paradigms," in *Gender, Race, Class, and Health: Intersectional Approaches*, ed. Amy J. Schulz and Leith Mullings (San Francisco, CA: Jossey-Bass, 2006), 21–59.

White, P., "Urban Life and Social Stress," in *The New Europe: Economy, Society, and Environment*, ed. D. Pinder (Chichester: Wiley, 1998).

Whitehead, M., "The Concepts and Principles of Equity and Health," 22(3) *International Journal of Health Services* (1992): 429–445.

Whitehead, M. and F. Diderichsen, "International Evidence on Social Inequalities in Health," in *Health Inequalities—Decennial Supplement*, ed. F. Drever and M. Whitehead, DS Series No. 15, Office for National Statistics (London: The Stationery Office, 1997): 45–69.

Whitehead, Margaret, "Health Policies, Health Inequalities, and Poverty Alleviation: Experiences from Outside Latin America and the Caribbean," in *Investment in Health: Social and Economic Returns* (Washington, DC: Pan American Health Organization, 2001).

Wiilst, William H., "Public Health and the Anticorporate Movement: Rationale and Recommendations," 96(8) *American Journal of Public Health* (August, 2006): 1370–1375.

Wilkinson, Richard and Michael Marmot eds., *Social Determinants of Health: The Solid Facts*. World Health Organization, 1998.

Wilkinson, Richard, *The Impact of Inequality: How to Make Sick Societies Healthier* (New York: The New Press, 2005).

Wilkinson, Richard, *Unhealthy Societies: The Afflictions of Inequality* (New York: Routledge, 1996).

Williams, A. and R. Cookson, "Equity in Health," in *Handbook of Health Economics*, ed. J.P. Newhouse and A.J. Culyer (North Holland, The Netherlands: Elsevier, 1999: 1863–1908).

Williams, David and C. Collins, "U.S. Socioeconomic and Racial Differences in Health: Patterns and Explanations," 21 *Annual Review of Sociology* (1998): 349–386.

Williams, David R., "Race and Health: Basic Questions, Emerging Directions," 7 *Annals of Epidemiology* (1997): 322–333.

Williams, David R., "African-American Health: The Role of the Social Environment," 75(2) *Journal of Urban Health: Bulletin of the New York Academy of Medicine* (June 1998): 301–321.

Williams, David R., "Race and Health Issues in Kansas: Data, Issues, and Directions," in *The Society and Population Reader: A State and Community Perspective*, ed. A.R. Tarlov and Robert F. St. Peter (New York: The New Press, 2000) 236–258.

Williams, David R., "Race and Health: Trends and Policy Implications," in *Income, Socioeconomic Status and Health: Exploring the Relationships*, ed. J.A. Auerbach and B.K. Krimgold (Washington, DC: National Policy Association, 2001) 67–85.

Williams, David R., "Racial/Ethnic Variations in Women's Health: The Social Embeddedness of Health," 92(4) *American Journal of Public Health* (April, 2002): 588–597.

Williams, David R., "The Health of Men: Structured Inequalities and Opportunities," 93(5) *American Journal of Public Health* (2003): 724–731.

Williams, David R. Harold W. Neighbors, and J.S. Jackson, "Racial/Ethnic Discrimination and Health: Findings from Community Studies," 98(Suppl. 1) *American Journal of Public Health* (2008): S29–S37.

Williams, David R. and Chiquita Collins, "Racial Residential Segregation: A Fundamental Cause of Racial Disparities in Health," 16(5) *Public Health Reports* (September/October, 2001): 404–416.

Williamson, D.L., "The Role of the Health Sector in Addressing Poverty," 92 *Canadian Journal of Public Health* (2001): 178–183.

Wing, Steven, "The Limits of Epidemiology," in *Illness and the Environment: A Reader in Contested Medicine*, ed. Steve Kroll-Smith, Phil Brown, and Valerie J. Gunter (New York: New York University Press, 2000).

Wolff, Edward N., "Racial Wealth Disparities: Is the Gap Closing?" Policy Brief No. 66. (New York: Levy Institute, 2001).

Wolff, Edward N., "Recent Trends in Living Standards in the United States," The Levy Economics Institute Working Paper No. 502 (New York: The Jerome Levy Economics Institute, May, 2001).

Wolff, Edward N. *Top Heavy: A Study of the Increasing Inequality of Wealth in America*, 2nd ed., (New York: The Twentieth Century Fund, 2001).

Wolfson, M.C., G Kaplan, and J. Lynch, "The Relationship between Income Inequality and Mortality is not a Statistical Artefact: An Empirical Assessment," 319 *British Medical Journal* (1999): 953–957.

Woodward, A. and I. Kawachi, "Why Reduce Health Inequalities," 54(12) *Journal of Epidemiology and Community Health* (2000): 923–929.

Woolf, Steven H., "Future Health Consequences of the Current Decline in U.S. Household Income," 298(16) *Journal of the American Medical Association* (October 24/31, 2007): 1931–1933.

Woolf, Steven H., "Social Policy as Health Policy" 301(11) *Journal of the American Medical Association* (2009): 1166–1169.

Woolf, Steven H., Robert E. Johnson, and Jack Geiger, "The Rising Prevalence of Severe Poverty in America: A Growing Threat to Public Health," 31(4) *American Journal of Preventive Medicine* (2006): 332–341.

World Health Organization, *25 Questions & Answers on Health and Human Rights*, Health & Human Rights Publication Series Issue No. 1, (Geneva: WHO, July, 2002).

World Health Organization, Commission on Social Determinants of Health, "Achieving Health Equity: From Root Causes to Fair Outcomes," Interim Statement (Geneva: WHO, 2007).

World Health Organization, Secretariat of the Commission on Social Determinants of Health. "Action on the Social Determinants of Health: Learning From Previous Experiences," A background paper prepared for the Commission on Social Determinants of Health (Geneva: WHO, March, 2005).

Wright, Erik Olin, "The Logics of Class," in *Social Class: How Does It Work?*, ed. Annette Lareau and Dalton Conley (New York: Russell Sage Foundation, 2008) 329–349.

Yalnizyan, A., *The Growing Gap: A Report on Growing Inequality Between Rich and Poor in Canada* (Toronto: Center for Social Justice, 1998).

Yen, I.H. and G.A. Kaplan, "Neighborhood Social Environment and Risk of Death: Multilevel Evidence from the Alameda County Study," 149(10) *American Journal of Epidemiology* (1999): 898–907.

Yen, I.H. and S. L. Syme, "The Social Environment and Health: A Discussion of the Epidemiologic Literature," 20 *Annual Review of Public Health* (1999): 287–308.

Young, Iris Marion, "Structural Injustice and the Politics of Difference," in *Social Justice and Public Policy: Seeking Fairness in Diverse Societies*, ed. Gary Craig, Tania Burchardt and David Gordon (Bristol: The Policy Press, 2008).

APPENDIX B

Guidelines for Achieving Health Equity in Public Health Practice

Based on the Modification of the Essential Services of Public Health 1–5, 8, 10

The purpose of the Guidelines for Health Equity is, at a minimum, to identify the needs of local health departments (LHDs) and their constituents and to ensure that they have a means to evaluate the effectiveness of their practice in achieving health equity. These guidelines are meant to serve as advice, not performance standards. In addition, they are designed to increase awareness of and draw attention to health inequity, provide a method for evaluating accountability, and enable LHDs to gain a portrait of their capacity to address it. Finally, their intent is to equip LHDs to set priorities, compare themselves to other agencies, and educate elected officials and other institutions that influence health about what they can accomplish.

The three essential criteria for these guidelines are as follows: (1) they maintain a focus on root causes of health inequity; (2) they are feasible; and (3) they inspire alternative ways of thinking more comprehensively about organizing public health practice.

The phenomenon of health inequity requires that we move from an improvisational approach to a more comprehensive one, returning to a larger social context that defined the origins of public health. In devising guidelines, our assumptions are that (1) building internal capacity and capability, and shifting the philosophy and culture regarding how the work of public health is done; (2) developing strong relationships with community organizations within a Community-Based Participatory Research Model; and (3) generating strategy for reforming public health policy to enable action and remove constraints.

1. Monitor Health Status and Track the Conditions That Influence Health Issues Facing the Community

- Obtain and maintain data that reveal inequities in the distribution of disease. Focus on information that characterizes the social conditions under which people live that influence health.
- Lead or participate in health impact assessments of policies, programs, or plans relevant to living conditions that affect health.
- Compile comprehensive data on health resources and health threats (e.g., on schools, parks, housing, transportation, economic well-being, and environmental quality) through relationships or partnerships with relevant state and local agencies.
- Identify specific population subgroups or specific geographic areas characterized by (1) either an excess burden of adverse health or socioeconomic outcomes; (2) an excess burden of environmental health threats; and (3) inadequacies in human resources that affect human health (e.g., quality parks and schools).
- Support research that explores the social processes and decisions through which inequalities of race, class, and gender generate and maintain health inequities.

2. Protect People from Health Problems and Health Hazards

- Prevent the further growth of environmental inequities and social conditions that lead to inequities in the distribution of disease, premature death, and illness.
- Play a leadership role in reducing or mitigating existing social and economic inequities and conditions that lead to inequities in the distribution of disease, premature death, and illness.

3. Give People Information They Need to Act Collectively to Improve Their Health

- Make available to residents data on health status and conditions that influence health status by race, ethnicity, language, and income.

- Conduct and disseminate research that supports and legitimizes community actions to address the fundamental environmental, social, and economic causes of health inequities.
- Develop or support mass media educational efforts that uncover the fundamental social, economic, and environmental causes of health inequities.

4. Engage with the Community to Identify and Eliminate Health Inequities

- Enhance residents' capacity to conduct their own research and share departmental information, based on the principles of Community-Based Participatory Research and the National Environmental Justice Advisory Council's community collaboration principles.
- Learn about the values, needs, major concerns, and resources of the community. Respect local, community knowledge; scrutinize and test it.
- Promote the community's analysis of, and advocacy for, policies and activities that will lead to the elimination of health inequities.
- Promote and support healthy communities and families through progressive practices in existing service delivery and programs, based on principles of social justice.
- Support, implement, and evaluate strategies that tackle the root causes of health inequities, in strategic, lasting partnerships with public and private organizations and social movements.
- Engage in dialogue with residents, governing bodies, and elected officials about governmental policies responsible for health inequities, improvements being made in those policies, planning initiatives, and priority health issues related to conditions not yet being adequately addressed.
- Routinely invite and involve community members and representatives from community-based organizations in strategic planning processes and promotion of health.
- Provide clear mechanisms and invitations for community contributions to LHD planning, procedures, and policies.
- Assist in building leadership among affected residents and respect their existing leadership, thereby honoring their capacity.
- Provide technical assistance to communities with respect to analyzing data, setting priorities, identify levers of power, and develop strategies.
- Engage with the public health system and related institutions in comprehensive planning.
- Use grant funding to support community-based programs and policies.
- Connect with relevant social movement organizations.

5. Develop Public Health Policies and Plans

- Advocate for comprehensive policies that improve physical, environmental, social, and economic conditions in the community that affect the public's health, recognizing that health policy is social policy.
- Enable residents to sustain their advocacy activity and support their capacity to become involved in regulatory activity.
- Support revisions of statutes that govern LHDs and other regulations and codes to ensure nondiscrimination in the distribution of public health benefits and interventions.
- Promote public investments in community infrastructure, for example, education, childhood development, mass transit, employment, healthy design in the built environment, and neighborhood grocery stores that sustain and improve community health.
- Focus on policies related to primary prevention and improving social and economic conditions, not just remediation of conditions.
- Monitor relevant issues under discussion by governing and legislative bodies

8. Maintain a Competent Public Health Workforce

- Develop an ongoing educational program and structured dialogue process for all staff across departments and divisions that (1) explores the evidence of health inequity and its sources; (2) explains the nature of the root causes of health inequities and the ways in which practice may be changed to address those root causes; (3) examines the values and needs of the community, and (4) assists in providing core competencies and skills to do what is necessary to achieve health equity.
- Make sensitivities to, and understanding of, root causes of health inequities part of hiring, including willingness to learn, cultural humility, creativity, listening skills.
- Develop an assessment of and training to improve staff knowledge and capabilities about health inequity.
- Conduct an internal assessment more generally of a department's overall capacity to act on the root causes of health inequities, including its organizational structure and culture.
- Recruit the public health workforce from those disproportionately affected and also those with education, training, and experience in addressing inequitable social and environmental conditions.
- Hire staff with skills, knowledge and abilities in community organizing, negotiation, power dynamics, and the ability to mobilize people, particularly from communities served.

- Recruit staff with more culturally and academically diverse backgrounds, with knowledge of the population they serve in relation to racial, ethnic, class, and gender characteristics, as well as social and economic conditions in the jurisdiction.
- Mentor and inspire staff to address health inequities in their local jurisdiction.
- Establish greater flexibility in job classifications to tackle the root cause of health inequity.
- Develop relations with high schools and colleges to ensure that diverse groups of youth will seek to join the public health workforce.
- Develop antiracism training as part of building a competent workforce.

10. Contribute to and Apply the Evidence Base of Public Health and Relevant Fields

- Develop public health measures of neighborhood conditions, institutional power, and social inequalities that lead to prevention strategies focused on the social and environmental determinants of health.
- Include knowledge based on social and economic context, subjective understandings, history, and social experience, beyond quantifiable data from epidemiological investigation, in informing decision making and action.
- Stay current with the literature on health equity, synthesize research, and disseminate as applicable to staff and community.
- Evaluate and disseminate knowledge of findings and efforts related to health equity.

APPENDIX C

How Social Justice Becomes Embodied in Differential Disease and Mortality Rates

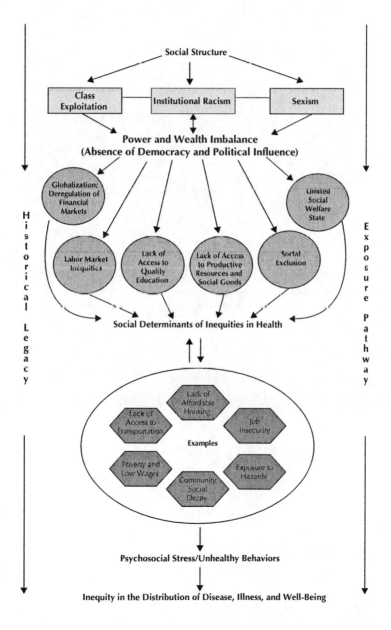

APPENDIX D

Eliminating Health Inequity: The Role of Local Public Health and Community Organizing

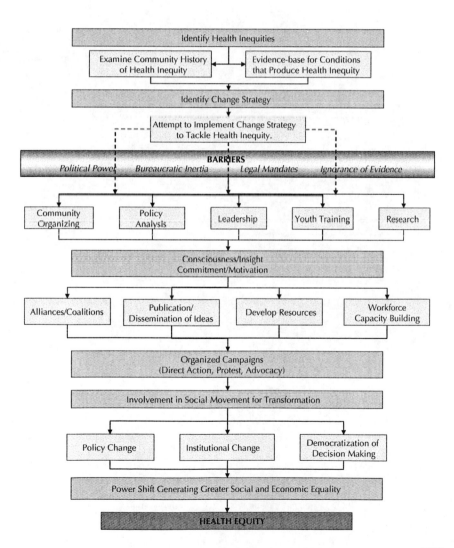

APPENDIX E

People's Charter for Health

People's Health Movement

Preamble

Health is a social, economic and political issue and above all a fundamental human right. Inequality, poverty, exploitation, violence and injustice are at the root of ill-health and the deaths of poor and marginalised people. Health for all means that powerful interests have to be challenged, that globalisation has to be opposed, and that political and economic priorities have to be drastically changed.

This Charter builds on perspectives of people whose voices have rarely been heard before, if at all. It encourages people to develop their own solutions and to hold accountable local authorities, national governments, international organisations and corporations.

Vision

Equity, ecologically-sustainable development and peace are at the heart of our vision of a better world - a world in which a healthy life for all is a reality; a world that respects, appreciates and celebrates all life and diversity; a world that enables the flowering of people's talents and abilities to

559

enrich each other; a world in which people's voices guide the decisions that shape our lives.

There are more than enough resources to achieve this vision.

The Health Crisis

"Illness and death every day anger us. Not because there are people who get sick or because there are people who die. We are angry because many illnesses and deaths have their roots in the economic and social policies that are imposed on us."

(A voice from Central America)

In recent decades, economic changes world-wide have profoundly affected people's health and their access to health care and other social services.

Despite unprecedented levels of wealth in the world, poverty and hunger are increasing. The gap between rich and poor nations has widened, as have inequalities within countries, between social classes, between men and women and between young and old.

A large proportion of the world's population still lacks access to food, education, safe drinking water, sanitation, shelter, land and its resources, employment and health care services. Discrimination continues to prevail. It affects both the occurrence of disease and access to health care.

The planet's natural resources are being depleted at an alarming rate. The resulting degradation of the environment threatens everyone's health, especially the health of the poor. There has been an upsurge of new conflicts while weapons of mass destruction still pose a grave threat.

The world's resources are increasingly concentrated in the hands of a few who strive to maximise their private profit. Neoliberal political and economic policies are made by a small group of powerful governments, and by international institutions such as the World Bank, the International Monetary Fund and the World Trade Organisation. These policies, together with the unregulated activities of transnational corporations, have had severe effects on the lives and livelihoods, health and well-being of people in both North and South.

Public services are not fulfilling people's needs, not least because they have deteriorated as a result of cuts in governments' social budgets. Health services have become less accessible, more unevenly distributed and more inappropriate.

Privatisation threatens to undermine access to health care still further and to compromise the essential principle of equity. The persistence of preventable ill health, the resurgence of diseases such as tuberculosis and malaria, and the emergence and spread of new diseases such as HIV/AIDS are a stark reminder of our world's lack of commitment to principles of equity and justice.

Principles of the People's Charter for Health

4. The attainment of the highest possible level of health and well-being is a fundamental human right, regardless of a person's colour, ethnic background, religion, gender, age, abilities, sexual orientation or class.
5. The principles of universal, comprehensive Primary Health Care (PHC), envisioned in the 1978 Alma Ata Declaration, should be the basis for formulating policies related to health. Now more than ever an equitable, participatory and intersectoral approach to health and health care is needed.
6. Governments have a fundamental responsibility to ensure universal access to quality health care, education and other social services according to people's needs, not according to their ability to pay.
7. The participation of people and people's organisations is essential to the formulation, implementation and evaluation of all health and social policies and programmes.
8. Health is primarily determined by the political, economic, social and physical environment and should, along with equity and sustainable development, be a top priority in local, national and international policy-making.

A Call for Action

To combat the global health crisis, we need to take action at all levels - individual, community, national, regional and global - and in all sectors. The demands presented below provide a basis for action.

Health as a Human Right

Health is a reflection of a society's commitment to equity and justice. Health and human rights should prevail over economic and political concerns.

This Charter calls on people of the world to:
1. Support all attempts to implement the right to health.
2. Demand that governments and international organisations reformulate, implement and enforce policies and practices which respect the right to health.
3. Build broad-based popular movements to pressure governments to incorporate health and human rights into national constitutions and legislation.
4. Fight the exploitation of people's health needs for purposes of profit.

Tackling the Broader Determinants of Health

Economic Challenges

The economy has a profound influence on people's health. Economic policies that prioritise equity, health and social well-being can improve the health of the people as well as the economy.

Political, financial, agricultural and industrial policies which respond primarily to capitalist needs, imposed by national governments and international organisations, alienate people from their lives and livelihoods. The processes of economic globalisation and liberalisation have increased inequalities between and within nations.

Many countries of the world and especially the most powerful ones are using their resources, including economic sanctions and military interventions, to consolidate and expand their positions, with devastating effects on people's lives.

This Charter calls on people of the world to:

1. Demand transformation of the World Trade Organisation and the global trading system so that it ceases to violate social, environmental, economic and health rights of people and begins to discriminate positively in favour of countries of the South. In order to protect public health, such transformation must include intellectual property regimes such as patents and the Trade Related aspects of Intellectual Property Rights (TRIPS) agreement.
2. Demand the cancellation of Third World debt.
3. Demand radical transformation of the World Bank and International Monetary Fund so that these institutions reflect and actively promote the rights and interests of developing countries.

4. Demand effective regulation to ensure that TNCs do not have negative effects on people's health, exploit their workforce, degrade the environment or impinge on national sovereignty.
5. Ensure that governments implement agricultural policies attuned to people's needs and not to the demands of the market, thereby guaranteeing food security and equitable access to food.
6. Demand that national governments act to protect public health rights in intellectual property laws.
7. Demand the control and taxation of speculative international capital flows.
8. Insist that all economic policies be subject to health, equity, gender and environmental impact assessments and include enforceable regulatory measures to ensure compliance.
9. Challenge growth-centred economic theories and replace them with alternatives that create humane and sustainable societies. Economic theories should recognize environmental constraints, the fundamental importance of equity and health, and the contribution of unpaid labour, especially the unrecognised work of women.

Social and Political Challenges

Comprehensive social policies have positive effects on people's lives and livelihoods.

Economic globalisation and privatisation have profoundly disrupted communities, families and cultures. Women are essential to sustaining the social fabric of societies everywhere, yet their basic needs are often ignored or denied, and their rights and persons violated.

Public institutions have been undermined and weakened. Many of their responsibilities have been transferred to the private sector, particularly corporations, or to other national and international institutions, which are rarely accountable to the people. Furthermore, the power of political parties and trade unions has been severely curtailed, while conservative and fundamentalist forces are on the rise. Participatory democracy in political organisations and civic structures should thrive. There is an urgent need to foster and ensure transparency and accountability.

This Charter calls on people of the world to:

1. Demand and support the development and implementation of comprehensive social policies with full participation of people.
2. Ensure that all women and all men have equal rights to work, livelihoods, to freedom of expression, to political participation,

to exercise religious choice, to education and to freedom from violence.

3. Pressure governments to introduce and enforce legislation to protect and promote the physical, mental and spiritual health and human rights of marginalised groups.

4. Demand that education and health are placed at the top of the political agenda. This calls for free and compulsory quality education for all children and adults, particularly girl children and women, and for quality early childhood education and care.

5. Demand that the activities of public institutions, such as child care services, food distribution systems, and housing provisions, benefit the health of individuals and communities.

6. Condemn and seek the reversal of any policies, which result in the forced displacement of people from their lands, homes or jobs.

7. Oppose fundamentalist forces that threaten the rights and liberties of individuals, particularly the lives of women, children and minorities.

8. Oppose sex tourism and the global traffic of women and children.

Environmental Challenges

Water and air pollution, rapid climate change, ozone layer depletion, nuclear energy and waste, toxic chemicals and pesticides, loss of biodiversity, deforestation and soil erosion have far-reaching effects on people's health. The root causes of this destruction include the unsustainable exploitation of natural resources, the absence of a long-term holistic vision, the spread of individualistic and profit-maximising behaviours, and over-consumption by the rich. This destruction must be confronted and reversed immediately and effectively.

This Charter calls on people of the world to:

1. Hold transnational and national corporations, public institutions and the military accountable for their destructive and hazardous activities that impact on the environment and people's health.

2. Demand that all development projects be evaluated against health and environmental criteria and that caution and restraint be applied whenever technologies or policies pose potential threats to health and the environment (the precautionary principle).

3. Demand that governments rapidly commit themselves to reductions of greenhouse gases from their own territories far stricter than those set out in the international climate change agreement, without resorting to hazardous or inappropriate technologies and practices.

4. Oppose the shifting of hazardous industries and toxic and radioactive waste to poorer countries and marginalised communities and encourage solutions that minimise waste production.

5. Reduce over-consumption and non-sustainable lifestyles - both in the North and the South. Pressure wealthy industrialised countries to reduce their consumption and pollution by 90 per cent.

6. Demand measures to ensure occupational health and safety, including worker-centred monitoring of working conditions.

7. Demand measures to prevent accidents and injuries in the workplace, the community and in homes.

8. Reject patents on life and oppose bio-piracy of traditional and indigenous knowledge and resources.

9. Develop people-centred, community-based indicators of environmental and social progress, and to press for the development and adoption of regular audits that measure environmental degradation and the health status of the population.

War, Violence, Conflict and Natural Disasters

War, violence, conflict and natural disasters devastate communities and destroy human dignity. They have a severe impact on the physical and mental health of their members, especially women and children. Increased arms procurement and an aggressive and corrupt international arms trade undermine social, political and economic stability and the allocation of resources to the social sector.

This Charter calls on people of the world to:

1. Support campaigns and movements for peace and disarmament.

2. Support campaigns against aggression, and the research, production, testing and use of weapons of mass destruction and other arms, including all types of landmines.

3. Support people's initiatives to achieve a just and lasting peace, especially in countries with experiences of civil war and genocide.

4. Condemn the use of child soldiers, and the abuse and rape, torture and killing of women and children.

5. Demand the end of occupation as one of the most destructive tools to human dignity.

6. Oppose the militarisation of humanitarian relief interventions.

7. Demand the radical transformation of the UN Security Council so that it functions democratically.

8. Demand that the United Nations and individual states end all kinds of sanctions used as an instrument of aggression which can damage the health of civilian populations.
9. Encourage independent, people-based initiatives to declare neighbourhoods, communities and cities areas of peace and zones free of weapons.
10. Support actions and campaigns for the prevention and reduction of aggressive and violent behaviour, especially in men, and the fostering of peaceful coexistence.
11. Support actions and campaigns for the prevention of natural disasters and the reduction of subsequent human suffering.

A People-Centered Health Sector

This Charter calls for the provision of universal and comprehensive primary health care, irrespective of people's ability to pay. Health services must be democratic and accountable with sufficient resources to achieve this.

This Charter calls on people of the world to:

1. Oppose international and national policies that privatise health care and turn it into a commodity.
2. Demand that governments promote, finance and provide comprehensive Primary Health Care as the most effective way of addressing health problems and organising public health services so as to ensure free and universal access.
3. Pressure governments to adopt, implement and enforce national health and drugs policies.
4. Demand that governments oppose the privatisation of public health services and ensure effective regulation of the private medical sector, including charitable and NGO medical services.
5. Demand a radical transformation of the World Health Organization (WHO) so that it responds to health challenges in a manner which benefits the poor, avoids vertical approaches, ensures intersectoral work, involves people's organisations in the World Health Assembly, and ensures independence from corporate interests.
6. Promote, support and engage in actions that encourage people's power and control in decision-making in health at all levels, including patient and consumer rights.
7. Support, recognise and promote traditional and holistic healing systems and practitioners and their integration into Primary Health Care.
8. Demand changes in the training of health personnel so that they become more problem-oriented and practice-based, understand better

the impact of global issues in their communities, and are encouraged to work with and respect the community and its diversities.

9. Demystify medical and health technologies (including medicines) and demand that they be subordinated to the health needs of the people.

10. Demand that research in health, including genetic research and the development of medicines and reproductive technologies, is carried out in a participatory, needs-based manner by accountable institutions. It should be people- and public health-oriented, respecting universal ethical principles.

11. Support people's rights to reproductive and sexual self-determination and oppose all coercive measures in population and family planning policies. This support includes the right to the full range of safe and effective methods of fertility regulation.

People's Participation for a Healthy World

Strong people's organisations and movements are fundamental to more democratic, transparent and accountable decision-making processes. It is essential that people's civil, political, economic, social and cultural rights are ensured. While governments have the primary responsibility for promoting a more equitable approach to health and human rights, a wide range of civil society groups and movements, and the media have an important role to play in ensuring people's power and control in policy development and in the monitoring of its implementation.

This Charter calls on people of the world to:

1. Build and strengthen people's organisations to create a basis for analysis and action.

2. Promote, support and engage in actions that encourage people's involvement in decision- making in public services at all levels.

3. Demand that people's organisations be represented in local, national and international fora that are relevant to health.

4. Support local initiatives towards participatory democracy through the establishment of people-centred solidarity networks across the world.

The People's Health Assembly and the Charter

The idea of a People's Health Assembly (PHA) has been discussed for more than a decade. In 1998 a number of organisations launched the PHA process and started to plan a large international Assembly meeting, held in Bangladesh at the end of 2000. A range of pre- and post-Assembly activities were initiated including regional workshops, the collection of people's health-related stories and the drafting of a *People's Charter for Health*.

The present Charter builds upon the views of citizens and people's organizations from around the world, and was first approved and opened for endorsement at the Assembly meeting in Savar, Bangladesh, in December 2000.

The Charter is an expression of our common concerns, our vision of a better and healthier world, and of our calls for radical action. It is a tool for advocacy and a rallying point around which a global health moment can gather and other networks and coalitions can be formed.

Join Us -Endorse the Charter

We call upon all individuals and organisations to join this global movement and invite you to endorse and help implement the *People's Charter for Health*
PHA Secretariat,
e-mail:gksavar@citechco.net
Web site: www.phmovement.org
Mailing address:
PHA Secretariat,
Gonoshasthaya Kendra,
Savar, Dhaka, 1344, Bangladesh.

Amendment

- After the endorsement of the PCH on December 8, 2000, it was called to the attention of the drafting group that action points number 1 and 2 under Economic challenges could be interpreted as supporting the social clause proposed by WTO, which actually serves to strengthen the WTO and its neoliberal agenda. Given that this countervails the PHA demands for change of the WTO and the global trading system, the two paragraphs were merged and amended.
- The section of War, Violence and Conflict has been amended to include natural disasters. A new action point, number 5 in this version, was added to demand the end of occupation. Furthermore, action point number 7, now number 8, was amended to read *to end all kinds of sanctions*. An additional action point number 11 was added concerning natural disasters.

Index

Note: Page number in *italics* and **bold** refers to figures and tables, respectively.

ACE. *See* Alternatives for Community and Environment
Alameda County, California
  City/County Neighborhood Initiative (CCNI), 388–392
  Framework for Health Equity
    community capacity building, 387–392
    institutional change, 385–386
    internal capacity building, 386–387
    public policy, 392–393
    working principles, 384–385
  "Latino Health Paradox," 387–388
  local policy agenda
    developing, 393–396
    implementing, 397–398
  mortality rate
    by census tract, *377*
    by neighborhood poverty level, *377*
    by race/ethnicity, *378*
  Place Matters Initiative, 410
  Public Health Department (ACPHD), 29, 376, 380, 381, 385–386, 392
    Life and Death From Unnatural Causes: Health and Social Inequity in Alameda County, 397, 398
    policy activities, 398–400
    Public Health 101 training, 29, 387
    Strategic Plan 2008–2013, 386
  public health practice, designing, 380–400
  social and health inequality in, 375–378
Allostatic load, 374
Alternatives for Community and Environment (ACE), 426
American Public Health Association, 483, 504
Association of State and Territorial Heath Officials (ASTHO), 129
ASTHO. *See* Association of State and Territorial Heath Officials

Backgrounders, 481
Baltimore City *Place Matters* team, 464–465
Barcelona Health Interview Survey, 185
BARHII. *See* Bay Area Regional Health Inequities Initiative
Barrio Adentro program, 523

Bay Area Regional Health Inequities
  Initiative (BARHII), 29, 283–294,
  380–383, *380*
  building, 285–286
  Built Environment Committee, 289
  Community Committee, 288
  Data Committee, 286–288, *287*
  future opportunities, 291–294
  history of, 284–285
  Internal Capacity Committee, 289–291,
    290
  organizing, 286
  social determinants of health ad hoc
    work group, 291
"Big Three," 478
Bill and Melinda Gates foundation,
  521, 523
Biological reductionism, 519
Black Women's Agenda, 489
Blue Cross/Blue Shield Foundation of
  Minnesota, 490
Browne, Sir Thomas, 57
Buffet, Warren, 521

CADH. *See* Connecticut Association of
  Directors of Health, Inc.
  CADH Health Equity Index (HEI),
    442–457
    application of, 449–450
      in community engagement process,
        451–454
      in LHDs, 450
      in political/governance structures,
        454–455
    constructing, 444–448
      Complementary Indicator
        framework, 445, 447–448
      Core Index, 445–447
    evaluation of, 455
    and GIS mapping, 448
    outcomes, 456–457
    testing, 448–449
California Environmental Quality Act, 337,
  341, 349
California Pan Ethnic Health Network
  (CPEHN), 490
CAM. *See* Community action model
Cancer, 168
Capitalism, 521
CBE. *See* Communities for a Better
  Environment
CBOs. *See* Community-based organizations
CBPHP. *See* Community-Based Public
  Health Practice

CBPR. *See* Community-based participatory
  research
CCNI. *See* City/County Neighborhood
  Initiative
CDC. *See* Centers for Disease Control and
  Prevention
Centers for Disease Control and Prevention
  (CDC), 490
  National Center for Environmental
    Health, 128
Chronic inflammation, 162–165
City College Foundation, 366
City/County Neighborhood Initiative
  (CCNI), 388–392
  components of, 389–391
City Health Officials, 483
City of Seattle
  Race and Social Justice Initiative, 410
Class, 11–14. *See also* Social class
  power, 12
  structure of, 11
Class/welfare regime model, *197*, 200–218.
    See also Class
  between-nation inequalities, 211–212
  decommodification effects on mortality,
    212–218, **213–214**
  within-nation inequalities, 207–211, 208,
    209–210
Clean Air Act, 7
Common good, 498
Communication misconceptions of public
  health, 505
Communities for a Better Environment
  (CBE), 426
Community(ies)
  blaming, 520
  capacity building, 387–392
  knowledge, 419–420
    and environmental health justice,
      420–423
Community action model (CAM),
    356–369, *360*
  goals of, 359–360
  implementation of, 361–362
  for tobacco divestment on college
    campuses, 362–367
    action research, 364–365
    analyzing results of, 365
    implementation of, 365–366
    maintaining/enforcing, 366–367
    skill-based training, 363–364
Community Action Toolkits, 481
Community-based organizations (CBOs),
    358, 361, 362

Community-based participatory research (CBPR). *See also* Participatory action research
    street science, 33, 350, 454, 523
Community-Based Public Health Practice (CBPHP), 134–135
Connecticut Association of Directors of Health, Inc. (CADH), 443–444
Contra Costa County
    Communities for a Better Environment in, 426
'Contradictory class location' hypothesis, 185
Coronary heart disease, 162–165
CPEHN. *See* California Pan Ethnic Health Network

DALY. *See* Disability-adjusted life years
Decommodification, 201, 206
Democracy, 20
Department of City Planning, San Francisco, 337
Disability-adjusted life years (DALY), 63–64
Discussion Guides, 481
Documentary(ies), *See also* Media, *Unnatural Causes: Is Inequality Making Us Sick?*
    for building health equity constituency, 477–492Domination and the Arts of Resistance, 505

Eastern Neighborhoods Community Health Impact Assessment (ENCHIA), 312, 313, 314
    Healthy Development Measurement Tool (HDMT), 314
Education, 374–375
    structural racism in, 151–152
Egalitarian(ism), 58, 76, 496, 522
EIA. *See* Environmental impact assessment
Elitism, 519
Empiricism, 519–520
Employment. *See also* Unemployment
    full, 202
    policies, in San Francisco, 307
    social class and, 184, 186
Empowerment, 232, 257, 297, 388, 408
ENCHIA. *See* Eastern Neighborhoods Community Health Impact Assessment
Environmental health justice
    community knowledge and, 420–423
    street science, 426–427

co-production model, 430–432
    democratic partnerships with scientific and political elites, 427–430
Environmental impact assessment (EIA), 313
    for San Francisco land use decision making, 336–350
    healthy appraisals approach for, 339
    healthy determinants of, 340–341
    use in land-use development projects, 347–348
EPA. *See* U.S. Environmental Protection Agency
Equity Gauge Alliance, 40
Ethnicity, 356, 519. *See also* Race

"Fair Health" movement, 409
Fair Housing Act of 1968, 150
Fascism, 522
Federal agencies, 128
Framing Strategy, 35
Freedom, 74

Gender, 16
    Gender inequity
        in health, 225–236
        intermediary factors, 230–234
        within organizations, removing, 234–235
        structural determinants of, 227–230
    role as social determinant of health, 227
Geographical Information System (GIS) Mapping, 448
GIS. *See* Geographical Information System Mapping
Global capitalism, 200–218
Global Health Equity Alliance, 39

Handouts, 481
Health, 73–75
    capability approach to, 74–75
    defined, 74
    medical model of, 74
    social model of, 74
Health disparities
    defined, 372
    logic diagram, *514*
Health equity, 57–68, 71–81, 276
    curriculum about, 277
    direct and indirect approaches to, 75–77
    guidelines for achieving, 549–553
    relevance for social justice, 58–68
    and social justice, 71–81
Health Equity Action Team (HEAT), 443, 450

Health Equity Impact Assessment (HEIA), 468, 469
Health equity team, 27–42
  advocacy and organizing, 38–39
  communications strategy, 34–35
    framing strategy, 35
  interagency/multidisciplinary coordination, 29–30
  leadership, 28–29
  public policy development, 35–38
  recruitment, 30
  strategic planning process, 29
  tracking and monitoring, 39–42
  training and education, 30–31
  working and collaborating with communities, 31–34
Health impact assessment (HIA), 41
  purpose of, 5
  for San Francisco land use decision making, 336–350
    informing decisions, 346–347
    predicting effects, 345–346
    stakeholder participation, 346
Health inequity(ies)
  defined, 114–116, 372
  framework for measuring, 112–122, 115
  quantification
    absolute or relative differences, 120, 120
    aggregation, 120–121
    comparison, 119, 120
    sensitivity to mean, 121–122, 121
    sensitivity to population size, 122
    subgroup considerations, 122
    unit of analysis, 118–119
    unit of time, 117–118
  as injustice indicator, 116–117
  LHDs role in eliminating, 557
  in public health practice, 3
    assumptions of, 6
    barriers to advancing, 17–19
Health Policy Institute of the Joint Center for Political and Economic Studies, 409, 493n6
Health Resources and Services Administration (HRSA)
  100 Percent Access and Zero Disparities, 128
Health Trust of Silicon Valley, 490
Healthy-migrant theory, 378
Healthy People 2010, 274, 509
Heart disease, 168
HEAT. See Health Equity Action Team
HEI, 442–457

HEIA. See Health Equity Impact Assessment
HIA. See Health Impact Assessment
Hidden transcript, 505
Homicide, 167
HRSA. See Health Resources and Services Administration
Humanitarianism, 496

Imperialism, 521
Income inequality and health, 196–220, 199. See also Class/welfare regime model
  hypothesis, 197–198
    criticisms of, 198–200
  and national wealth, 206
    between nations, 211–212
    within nations, 207–211, 208, 209–210
  in the United States, 4
Individualism, 495, 522
Ingham County, 242–269
  dialogic process in, 249–269
    action of, 260–262
    challenges of
      changing the questions, 253–254, 253
      "how for upstream?" exercise, 254–255, 255
      role-play dialogue, 254, 254
    effectiveness of, 258–260
    focus question, 249
      answering, 251–252
    health department, leadership role of, 256–258, 257
    open dialogue, 250
    summary questions, 251
    traction of, 262–263
    transformation of, 263–265
    trigger question, 249–250
    use of, 265–267
  goals for, 248
  recruitment and participation, 247
  timeline and products, 247–248
Institutionalized racism, 383. See also Racism
Interconnectedness, 495, 498–501
  cultivated, 499
  moral economy of, 499
Intersectionality, 228
Initiative to Eliminate Racial and Ethnic Disparities in Health, 512
ISAIAH/Gamaliel Interfaith Network, 489

It's on Y.O.U. (Youth with One
    Understanding), 391

Johns Hopkins School of Medicine, 523
Joint Center of Political and Economic
    Studies, 483
Joint fact-finding, 425, 432
Justice, 515

King County
    Community-Based Public Health Practice
        (CBPH), 134–135
    King County Ethnicity and Health
        Survey, 135
    social justice-oriented public health
        practice, 134–136

Labor market, structural racism in,
    152–153
Land-use development project
    environmental impact assessment of,
        347–348
    health impact assessment of
        informing decisions, 346–347
        predicting effects, 345–346
        stakeholder participation, 346
        practices for inclusive participation,
            integrating, 349–350
        rules and standards, 348–349
        tools of, 348
Language of interconnection, 495, 498–501
La Raza Centro Legal (La Raza), 308, 309
LHD. *See* Local health department
Libertarianism, 522
Living wage campaign, 42
Local health department (LHD), 21,
    129–132
    challenges to health equity, 283–284
    National Coalition for Health Equity, 25
    role in addressing health equity
        difficulties faced by, 22–24
    role in eliminating health inequality, 24–25
    role in HEI process, 450
Living wage laws, health benefits
        estimation, 324–332
    discussion, 331–332
    methods, 325–327
    results, 327–331
Louisville
    Center for Health Equity. *See* Metro
        Louisville Center for Health
        Equity
    *Health Equity through Social Justice in
        Louisville*, 274

Metro Louisville Health Department,
    272
Office of Policy Planning and Evaluation,
    274

The MacArthur Network on Socio-Economic
    Status and Health, 493n6
Marmot, Sir Michael, 60
Martin Luther King Jr. County,
    Washington, 404–416
    community partnerships, 415
    delivery of County services, 413–415
    Dellums Commission Report, 409
    Equity and Social Justice Initiative, 409
    guiding principles for promoting equity,
        411–412
    inequities in, 405–406
        formulating solutions to, 408–409
        history of inequities, correcting,
            407–408
        searching for, 406–407
    internal education and communication,
        415
    Place Matters team, 409, 466–469
    policy development and decision making,
        412–413
McKinney & Associates, 482
Media, 131. *See also* Documentary(ies)
    for building health equity constituency,
        477–492
    infrastructure, development of, 508
    planning, 506
    user network, building, 481–482
Medicalization, 512–513, 519
    racial disparities in, 171–172
Metro Louisville Center for Health Equity,
    272–282. *See also* Louisville
    challenges of, 281–282
    collaborations with agencies and
        organizations, 277–278
    collaboration with NACCHO, 281
    community organizing training, 279
    educational training project, 279
    Health Equity Grants, 278–279
    health within local government
        institutions, integrating, 276–277
    history of, 272–274
    health equity assessment, 279
    local health department, research and
        planning in, 274–276
    Office of Faith and Health, 280–281
    social marketing, 280
    West Louisville visioning process,
        279–280

The Minneapolis Foundation, A Framework
    for Social Change, 514
Morehouse School of Medicine Prevention
    Research Center, 277
Multnomah County, Oregon
    Health Equity Initiative, 410

NACCHO. See National Association
    of Country and City Health
    Officials
National Association of Counties, 483
National Association of County and City
    Health Officials (NACCHO), 25,
    130, 488, 489, 493n6
  Health Equity and Social Justice
    Strategic Direction Team,
    290, 292
  National Health Equity Work
    Group, 292
National Center for Environmental
    Health, 128
National Center for Health Statistics, 41
National Environmental Policy Act of
    1969, 336, 337, 347, 350
National Health Interview Survey (NHIS),
    90, 91
National Institute of Environmental Health
    Sciences (NIEHS), 308, 424
National Longitudinal Mortality Study
    (NLMS), 90, 91
National Minority Health Month, 273
Negro Health Week, 273
Neighborhood, 143, 513–515. See also
    Residential segregation
  environment and residential
    segregation, 103
  racial disparities in, 149, 150,
    170–171, 373–374
Neo-liberal economic globalization,
    201–218, 522
NHIS. See National Health Interview
    Survey
NIEHS. See National Institute of
    Environmental Health Sciences
Nihilism, 522
NLMS. See National Longitudinal
    Mortality Study
No Child Left Behind Act, 374

Oakland Youth Movement (OYM), 391
Occupational Safety and Health
    Administration (OSHA), 7
OECD. See Organization for Economic
    Cooperation and Development

Organizational Self Assessment Tool for
    Addressing Health Inequities, 291
Organization for Economic Cooperation
    and Development (OECD), 517
OSHA. See Occupational Safety and
    Health Administration
Ottawa Charter for Health Promotion, 296
Outreach Advisory Board, 481
OYM. See Oakland Youth Movement

PAR. See Participatory action research
Participatory action research
    (PAR). See also Community-based
    participatory research
  street science in, 423–424
Pathogenic social hierarchy, 162–165
People's Charter for Health, 559–568
  crisis of health, 560–561
  determinants of health
    economic challenges, 562–563
    environmental challenges, 564–565
    social and political challenges, 563–564
    war, violence, conflict and natural
      disasters, 565–566
  as human right, 561–562
  people-centered health sector, 566–567
  People's Health Assembly and, 567–568
  people's participation for healthy world,
    567
  principles of, 561
  vision, 559–560
People Organizing to Demand
    Environmental and Economic
    Rights (PODER), 313, 426–427
PHES. See Program on Health, Equity, and
    Sustainability
Place, 513–514
Place Matters, 458–474
  background, 458–459
  case studies
    Baltimore City team, 464–465
    King County team, 409, 466–469
    Wayne County team, 465–466
  challenges to advancing health equity,
    469–472
  health equity movement
    leveraging national/regional learning
      communities to building, 472
    partnerships role in, 472–474
  Phenomenological Social Determinants
    of Health Model, 460–464
PODER. See People Organizing to Demand
    Environmental and Economic
    Rights Policy Guides, 481

PolicyLink, 483
Political economy and academic
    institutions, 522–523
Popular epidemiology, defined, 425–426
Poverty, 373–374
    and psychiatric disorders, 181
Practice, definition, 433
Praxis Project, 483, 496n6
"Priority view," 76
Program on Health, Equity, and
    Sustainability (PHES), 304–319
    effectiveness of, 315–318
    public health practice for social justice,
        forging
        day laborers' health and safety,
            advancing, 307–309
        employment policies, health analysis
            of, 306–307
        healthy city planning, 311–315
        urban collaboration for food equity,
            309–311
Psychiatric disorders, 179–190
    class exploitation and, 186–187, 189–190
    class structure and, 183–186
    'neo-material'determinants of, 182
    poverty and, 181
    'psychosocial'determinants of, 182–183
    social inequalities in, 187–189
    social strata and, 180–181
Public awareness, strategies for building,
    504–508
Public engagement campaign, 482–490
Public health, 7–9
    misconceptions of, 505
    defined, 7, 497
    history of, 7
    as social enterprise, 130
    as social justice enterprise, 379–380,
        514–516
    in the United States, 495–501
Public Health Code of Ethics, 510, 515
Public health practice. See also Public health
    health inequities in, 3
    assumptions of, 6
    barriers to advancing, 17–19
    purpose of, 5
    research on social inequality, 86–107
        biases and limitations, 102–104
        methods, 90–92
        pathways, 104–105
        recommendations, 105–107
        results, 92–100
            disability, social inequality effects
                on, 96–100, 98–99, 100

premature mortality, social
    inequality effects on, 93–96, 94,
    95, 96–97
for social justice, forging, 296–319
    as collective responsibility, 298–299
    consensus for equity, facilitating,
        302–303
    evidence into practice, translating,
        299–300
    institutional accountability for health,
        monitoring, 301–302
    obstacles to, 303–304
    participating in social movements,
        300–301
transforming elements to, 21, 25–27
    difficulties faced by local health
        departments, 22–24
    evidence, 22
Public health practitioners, 3, 7
    consequences of health inequity for, 7
Public health surveillance data, 136–137

Quizzes, 481

Race(ism), 14–16, 356, 373–374, 519. See
        also Ethnicity
    inequality and, 15
    institutionalized, 383
    meaning of, 145
    race-consciousness, 153
    structural, 143–160
Race—The Power of an Illusion, 478
Racial and Ethnic Approaches to
        Community Health (REACH)
        program, 129
Racial Discrimination in Health Care
        Interview Project, 135–136
Racial disparities, 144
    in health, 166–175, 167
        cancer, 168
        heart disease, 168
        homicide, 167
    in medical care, 171–172
    in neighborhood residential conditions,
        170–171
    in socioeconomic status, 168–169
Racial equity, 153–155
Racial sorting, 149–150
REACH. See Racial and Ethnic
        Approaches to Community Health
        program
Realist(s)
    criticism on teaching SIH, 523–524
Research!America, 504

Residential segregation, racial disparities in, 170–171. *See also* Neighborhood
Rincon Hill Special Use District, 342–345

San Francisco Asthma Task Force, 133
San Francisco County
    Program on Health, Equity, and Sustainability. *See* Program on Health, Equity, and Sustainability, San Francisco
    a la carte system, 310–311
    Day Labor Program (DLP), 307–308
    Eastern Neighborhoods Community Health Impact Assessment, 312, 313, 314
    healthy city planning, 311–315
    La Raza Centro Legal (La Raza), 308, 309
    People Organized in Defense of Environmental and Economic Rights (PODER), 313
    Program on Health Equity and Sustainability, 25
    Department of Public Health, 304, 305–306, 309
    San Francisco Food Alliance, 309
    San Francisco Food Systems, 309, 310, 311
    San Francisco Planning Department, 312
    San Francisco Unified School District, 309, 311
San Francisco Department of Public Health (SFDPH), 132–134, 304, 305–306, 309, 337–338
    day laborers' health and safety, advancing, 307–308
    occupational and environmental health PHES statement of mission, vision and guiding principles, 305–306
San Francisco Food Alliance, 309
San Francisco Food Systems (SFFS), 309, 310, 311
San Francisco Tobacco Free Project (SFTFP), 357–359
    community action model, implementation of, 361–362
San Francisco Unified School District (SFUSD), 309, 311
Scientific Advisors, 481
Scientism, 519
Seattle-King County Healthy Homes study, 408

SEIU. *See* Service Employee International Union
Service Employee International Union (SEIU), 489
SES. *See* Socioeconomic status
Severe acute respiratory syndrome (SARS), 500–501
Sexism, 16–17
SFDPH. *See* San Francisco Department of Public Health
SFFS. *See* San Francisco Food Systems
SFTFP. *See* San Francisco Tobacco Free Project
SFUSD. *See* San Francisco Unified School District
SIH. *See* Social inequalities in health
SII. *See* Slope index of inequality
Slope index of inequality (SII), 92, 93
SNEEJ. *See* Southwest Network for Environmental and Economic Justice
Sobrante Park Time Bank (SPTB), 390
Social change, 338
Social class. *See also* Class
    exploitation in social psychiatry, 189–190
    and psychiatric disorders. See Psychiatric disorders
    relationship to productive assets, 185
    and social stratification, distinction between, 184
Social inequalities in health (SIH), 517–524
    teaching
        barriers, overcoming, **518**
        external to academia barriers, 522–523, **518**
            cultural and ideological, 522
            economic, 522–523
            political/power, 522
        internal to academia barriers, 518–521, **518**
            cultural and ideological, 519–520
            economic, 520–521
            political/power, 520
        opportunities for, 523–524
Social justice, 58–62, 555
    defined, 19–20
    health equity and, 58–68, 71–81
    message, basic elements of, 34
    practice, defined, 42–43
    public health and, 19–21
    public health practice, relationship to, 126–139
        competencies in, 137
        barriers to accepting, 138–139

federal agencies and, 128
local health departments and, 129–132
state health departments and, 128–129
tobacco epidemic as, 357
Social responsibility, 496
Social sciences, 18–19
Social Security Act, 7
Social stratification
and social class, distinction between, 184
Society(ies)
consequences of health inequity for, 6
as fair system of co-operation, 78–79
Socioecological context, of health
disparities, 513
Socioeconomic status (SES), 184–185,
356, 521
health, 12–13, 15, 17, 100–102,
324–332, **328**, **329**, **330**
racial disparities in, 168–169
"Soft money" employment contracts, 521
Solidarity, 523–524
SOMCAN. *See* South of Market
Community Action Network
South of Market Community Action
Network (SOMCAN), 314, 338
South West Organizing Project (SWOP), 427
Southwest Network for Environmental
and Economic Justice (SNEEJ),
427
SPTB. *See* Sobrante Park Time Bank
State health departments, 128–129
Status syndrome, 180–181
STEPS. *See* Steps to a Healthier United
States program
Steps to a Healthier United States (STEPS)
program, 129
Strategic Research Plan to Reduce and
Ultimately Eliminate Health
Disparities, NIH, 512–513
Street science, 33, 417–437
in community-based participatory
research, 424–425
co-production of environmental health
expertise, 430–432
as deliberative practice, 433–434
environmental health justice movement
in, 426–427
democratic partnerships with scientific
and political elites, 427–430
as environmental health practice,
434–435
as "jazz of practice," 435–436
in participatory action research,
423–424

Structural racism, 143–160. *See also*
Race(ism)
assumptions to reproducing, 158–159
community-building among social
change agents, 155–156
in education, 151–152
history of, 147–149
in labor market, 152–153
meaning of, 146–147
progress and retrenchment, 150–151
public policies and institutional practices,
156–158
sorting, 149–150
SWOP. *See* South West Organizing Project

"The Task Force Report on Black and
Minority Health" (Heckler
Report), 273
Technologies of Participation (ToP)
method, 468–469
Theory of justice as fairness, 72, 77–79,
85n46
social inequalities in health and, 79–81
Tobacco epidemic, as social justice, 357
Tobacco-Free College Campuses
Project, 366
ToP. *See* Technologies of Participation
method

Unemployment, 306, 467. *See also*
Employment
language of interconnection,
developing, 495, 498–501
Universal Declaration of Human
Rights, 226
*Unnatural Causes: Is Inequality
Making Us Sick?*, 24, 35, 288,
477–492, 510
challenges and opportunities, 490–492
public engagement strategy, 482–490
creating, 487–490
DVD distribution, 485
Partnerships, building, 484–485
press and publicity, 483
tools, 485–487
user network, building, 481–482
U.S. Bureau of the Census, 4
U.S. Department of Health and Human
Services, 296
U.S. Environmental Protection Agency
(EPA), 427
U.S. Office of Economic
Opportunity, 300
Utilitarianism, 63, 75

Violence, 500
Violence Prevention Initiative, 500

W.K. Kellogg Foundation, 25, 244, 279,
    424, 444, 458, 493n6
Washington State Governor's Interagency
    Coordinating Council on Health
    Disparities, 410
Wayne County *Place Matters* team,
    465–466
Wealth, 371–372
Weathering, 374

Welfare, 497
Welfare state
    Conservative/Corporatist/Familist,
        201–202
    Liberal, 201, 202
    Social Democratic, 201, 202
"What's Killing Our Kids," 500
WHO. *See* World Health Organization
World Health Organization
        (WHO), 296
    Commission on the Social Determinants
        of Health, 273